# Dermatology Essentials

# Dermatology Essentials

Edited by **Heidi Mueller**

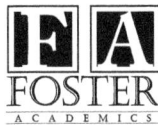

**FA**
FOSTER
ACADEMICS

New Jersey

Published by Foster Academics,
61 Van Reypen Street,
Jersey City, NJ 07306, USA
www.fosteracademics.com

**Dermatology Essentials**
Edited by Heidi Mueller

© 2016 Foster Academics

International Standard Book Number: 978-1-63242-460-0 (Hardback)

The publisher's policy is to use permanent paper from mills that operate a sustainable forestry policy. Furthermore, the publisher ensures that the text paper and cover boards used have met acceptable environmental accreditation standards.

**Trademark Notice:** Registered trademark of products or corporate names are used only for explanation and identification without intent to infringe.

Printed in the United States of America.

# Contents

**Permissions**

**List of Contributors**

# Preface

This book provides comprehensive insights into the field of dermatology. As a branch of medical science, dermatology refers to the study, diagnosis and treatment of problems related to skin, nails and hair. It also overlaps with cosmetic surgery. The different branches of this field include dermatopathology, immunodermatology, mohs surgery, teledermatology, etc. This book includes a detailed explanation of various concepts and applications of this subject. It elucidates the new techniques in a multidisciplinary approach. The topics included herein are of utmost significance and are bound to provide incredible insights to readers. It also includes contributions from experts and scientists from across the globe to help readers get a better understanding of the subject. It will serve as a valuable guide of reference for students, researchers and dermatologists alike.

This book has been the outcome of endless efforts put in by authors and researchers on various issues and topics within the field. The book is a comprehensive collection of significant researches that are addressed in a variety of chapters. It will surely enhance the knowledge of the field among readers across the globe.

It gives us an immense pleasure to thank our researchers and authors for their efforts to submit their piece of writing before the deadlines. Finally in the end, I would like to thank my family and colleagues who have been a great source of inspiration and support.

**Editor**

# Methylisothiazolinone: An Emergent Allergen in Common Pediatric Skin Care Products

**Megan J. Schlichte and Rajani Katta**

*Baylor College of Medicine, Houston, TX 77030, USA*

Correspondence should be addressed to Megan J. Schlichte; mjschlic@bcm.edu

Academic Editor: Craig G. Burkhart

Recalcitrant dermatitis, such as that of the hands, face, or genitals, may be due to allergic contact dermatitis (ACD) from ingredients in seemingly innocuous personal care products. Rising rates of allergy have been noted due to the preservative methylisothiazolinone (MI). This preservative is commonly found in skin and hair care products, especially wipes. This study evaluated the use of MI in products specifically marketed for babies and children and examined the associated marketing terms of such products. Ingredients of skin care products specifically marketed for babies and children were surveyed at two major retailers. Of 152 products surveyed, 30 products contained MI. Categories of products surveyed included facial or body wipes, antibacterial hand wipes, hair products, soaps, bubble baths, moisturizers, and sunscreens. Facial or body wipes and hair products were the categories with the greatest number of MI-containing products. MI-containing products were manufactured by a number of popular brands. Of note, products marketed as "gentle," "sensitive," "organic," or "hypoallergenic" often contained MI, thus emphasizing the importance of consumer scrutiny of product choices. These findings reinforce the importance of educating parents and providing consumer decision-making advice regarding common skin care products, in order to help prevent ACD in children.

## 1. Introduction

Could well-meaning parents who purchase personal hygiene products from their local supermarkets be exposing their children to a potentially harmful allergen? Recent reports of allergic contact dermatitis (ACD) highlight an emergent allergen—methylisothiazolinone (MI), a common preservative found in many toiletry products marketed to both children and adults [1]. Kathon CG, trade name for a 3 : 1 combination of methylchloroisothiazolinone/methylisothiazolinone (MCI/MI) produced by Dow Chemical Company, has been used as a preservative since the 1980s in the United States [2]. In response to an increasing incidence of ACD in response to MCI/MI, restrictions on concentrations of the combination preservative in cosmetics and household products were imposed, which prompted the production of more products with MI alone and in higher concentrations [3].

MI can trigger a secondary ACD in the context of skin inflammation and breakdown. In the perianal region, irritant contact dermatitis may result from a nonspecific, proinflammatory, innate immune response to the fecal enzymes of residual stool [4]. This same phenomenon may occur in the perioral region, due to the presence of salivary enzymes of residual saliva, particularly in infants. Subsequent repeated exposure to the ingredients in skin care products may eventually lead to sensitization, resulting in allergic contact dermatitis [5].

## 2. Materials and Methods

In this study, the listed ingredients of skin and hair care products targeted to pediatric populations were surveyed at two Houston grocery and supply supercenters, Target and Wal-Mart. Retailers surveyed included Houston South Central SuperTarget Store #1336 at 8500 South Main Street, 77025, and Houston Wal-Mart Supercenter Store #2066 at 2727 Dunvale Road, 77063. Products available for purchase on the day of survey may not represent full store inventory.

TABLE 1: MI or MCI/MI in facial or body wipes.

| Facial or body wipes | | | | |
|---|---|---|---|---|
| Brand | Product | MI | MCI/MI | Store |
| All-Purpose | Face, Hands, & Body | + | − | W |
| Huggies | Natural Care* | +/− | − | T, W |
| | One & Done | + | − | T, W |
| | One & Done Refreshing | + | − | T, W |
| | Simply Clean | + | − | T, W |
| | Soft Skin | + | − | T, W |
| Kleenex Cottonelle | FreshCare | + | − | W |
| | Ultra Comfort Care | + | − | W |
| Nice-Pak Products, Inc. | Baby | + | − | W |
| Pull-Ups | Big Kid | + | − | W |
| Target Brand Up & Up | Toddler | + | − | T |
| | Toddler & Family | + | − | T |
| Walmart Brand Parent's Choice | Fragrance-Free⁺ | +/− | − | W |
| Walmart Brand Parent's Choice | Fresh Scent** | +/− | − | W |

KEY

*Huggies "Natural Care" wipes sold in hard plastic dispenser indicated presence of MI. "Natural Care" wipes sold in regular, soft plastic packaging did not indicate presence of MI.

⁺Walmart Brand Parent's Choice "Fragrance-Free" wipes sold in hard plastic dispenser indicated presence of MI.

**Walmart Brand Parent's Choice "Fresh Scent" wipes indicated presence of MI in wipes contained in a package of 80 or boxes of 400 or 700, but not in box of 240 or combination of 3 packages of 80.

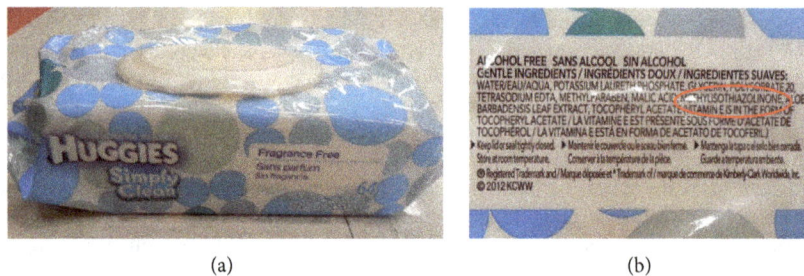

(a)                                                                 (b)

FIGURE 1: MI-containing baby wipe product, advertised to have "gentle ingredients" and found at both Target and Wal-Mart.

TABLE 2: MI or MCI/MI in antibacterial hand sanitizing wipes.

| Antibacterial hand wipes | | | | |
|---|---|---|---|---|
| Brand | Product | MI | MCI/MI | Store |
| Rockline Inc. | Pure 'n Gentle | + | − | W |
| Walmart Brand Equate | | + | + | W |

Brand names and specific products available for each of the toiletry categories were recorded, as well as the presence or absence of MI or MCI/MI and the store(s) at which the product was available.

## 3. Results

Of 152 personal care products for infants and children surveyed at both Target and Wal-Mart, 30 products contained MI. Specific products (noted with brand name) positive for the presence of MI exclusively or as part of the MCI/MI combination are reproduced in Tables 1, 2, 3, 4, 5, and 6

by category of toiletry product. Presence of MI was noted in 14 of 39 facial or body wipes, 2 of 6 antibacterial hand wipes (with 1 of the 2 products containing MI as part of the MCI/MI combination), 10 of 37 hair products (all 10 of which contained the MCI/MI combination), 1 of 17 facial or body soaps, 2 of 10 bubble bath products (both of which contained the MCI/MI combination), and 1 of 20 facial or body sunscreens. None of the 23 moisturizers surveyed, including facial and body creams and lotions, contained MI, and therefore this category is not represented in table format.

## 4. Discussion

As evidenced by this survey of pediatric products sold at typical Target or Wal-Mart stores, MI can be found in many wipes and other products applied to the skin or hair. MI-containing wipes produced by familiar brands such as Huggies (Figures 1(a) and 1(b)), Kleenex Cottonelle, and Target or Wal-Mart's own store brands, as well as MI-containing hair products produced by Suave, Target, and Wal-Mart brands,

TABLE 3: MI or MCI/MI in hair products.

| Hair products | | | | |
|---|---|---|---|---|
| Brand | Product | MI | MCI/MI | Store |
| Aussie Kids | Shampoo | + | + | T |
| Galvin & Galvin London Kids | Dubble trubble 2-in-1 shampoo & body wash | + | + | T |
| | Dubble trubble conditioner spray | + | + | T |
| MZB Accessories | 3-in-1 body wash, shampoo, and conditioner | + | + | W |
| Suave Kids | 3-in-1 shampoo, conditioner, and body wash | + | + | T, W |
| | 2-in-1 smoothers shampoo & conditioner | + | + | T, W |
| | Conditioner | + | + | T, W |
| Target Brand Up & Up | Hair detangler spray-on | + | + | T |
| Walmart Brand Equate | Detangler spray | + | + | W |
| White Rain | Kids 3-in-1 shampoo, conditioner, and body wash | + | + | W |

TABLE 4: MI or MCI/MI in facial or body soaps.

| Soap | | | | |
|---|---|---|---|---|
| Brand | Product | MI | MCI/MI | Store |
| Suave Kids | Free & gentle body wash | + | − | T |

TABLE 5: MI or MCI/MI in bubble baths.

| Bubble bath | | | | |
|---|---|---|---|---|
| Brand | Product | MI | MCI/MI | Store |
| Sanrio | Hello Kitty | + | + | W |
| Scrubbles | | + | + | W |

TABLE 6: MI or MCI/MI in facial or body sunscreens.

| Sunscreen | | | | |
|---|---|---|---|---|
| Brand | Product | MI | MCI/MI | Store |
| Neutrogena | Pure & free baby SPF 60+ | + | − | T, W |

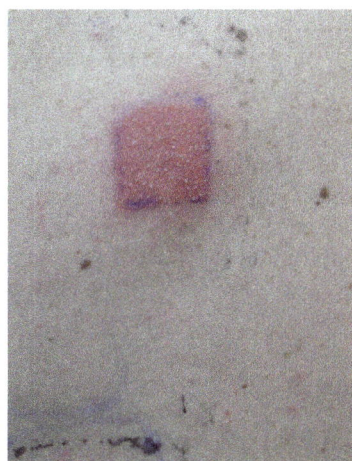

FIGURE 2: Positive reaction to MI alone by patch testing.

were all readily available for a favorable cost. In addition, this survey suggests that while many wipe producers manufacture their products with MI independent of MCI, the presence of MI in hair products was often found in combination with MCI. Also, of note, products marketed as "gentle," "sensitive," "organic," "100% natural," "dermatologist-recommended," or "hypoallergenic" often contained MI (Table 7), thus emphasizing the importance of consumer scrutiny of product choices.

If uninformed, patients with dermatologic problems may be positively predisposed towards products marketed as "hypoallergenic" or "gentle," or labeled with these other terms. However, there is no objective proof that these products pose a reduced risk for potential harm or are actually more "natural." In fact, while not being the focus of our paper, many such products did contain fragrance additives and other allergenic preservatives.

In particular, the marketing term "hypoallergenic" is intended to imply that a product is less likely to cause an allergic cutaneous reaction. However, there are no legal mandatory standards to assess the validity of a company's claim that a given product is "hypoallergenic" [6]. Historically, the US

Food and Drug Administration (FDA) mandated in 1975 that use of the claim "hypoallergenic" required objective tests to demonstrate significantly reduced rates of adverse reactions in human skin in response to "hypoallergenic" products [7]. However, this regulation was challenged and rendered null and void in the courts, leaving the term open to consumer interpretation.

While fragrances have been targeted as the most frequent causative agents in triggering ACD, they are closely followed by preservatives. Preservatives, such as MI or MCI/MI, are a necessary additive in water-based products in order to limit premature product degradation. Thus, even a fragrance-free product may disguise a potential allergic risk to consumers. Babies and children with eczema are particularly vulnerable, with compromised epidermal barrier function leaving them more susceptible to ACD in response to skin care products.

ACD of the hands or perioral or perianal regions due to MI in toiletry products can be misdiagnosed as psoriasis, eczema, or impetigo. Patch testing is the gold standard [8] for identifying MI (or other allergens) as the culprit responsible for ACD reactions (Figure 2). MI exposure and sensitization is likely to become a more common phenomenon with a cultural trend toward wipe use both in pediatric and adult

TABLE 7: Terms used in the marketing of common pediatric skin care products containing MI.

| Marketing of MI-containing pediatric products | | |
|---|---|---|
| Brand | Product | Marketing phrase(s) on product label |
| Huggies | Natural care baby wipes | "Hypoallergenic" |
| | One & done refreshing baby wipes | "Alcohol-free, gentle ingredients" |
| | Simply clean baby wipes | "Alcohol-free, gentle ingredients" |
| Nice-Pak Products | Baby wipes | "Hypoallergenic, alcohol-free" |
| Parent's Choice | Fragrance-free baby wipes | "Hypoallergenic with aloe" |
| | Fresh scent baby wipes | "Hypoallergenic with aloe" |
| Rockline Inc. | Pure 'n Gentle antibacterial hand wipes | "Hypoallergenic & alcohol-free with natural aloe & vitamin E" |
| Equate | Antibacterial hand wipes | "Hypoallergenic, with vitamin E & aloe" |
| Galvin & Galvin London Kids | Dubble trubble 2-in-1 shampoo & body wash | "Certified organic" |
| Suave | Kids body wash | "Dermatologist-tested, gentle, tear-free, dye-free" |
| Sanrio | Hello Kitty bubble bath | "Tear-free, gentle, hypoallergenic formula" |
| Neutrogena | Pure & free baby sunscreen SPF 60+ | "100% naturally sourced sunscreen ingredients, #1 dermatologist-recommended suncare" |

populations. This trend underscores the importance of raising awareness about MI as a potential allergen. Methylisothiazolinone has been deemed to be such an important emerging allergen that it was named "Contact Allergen of the Year" for 2013 by the American Contact Dermatitis Society [2].

## 5. Conclusion

In cases of recalcitrant dermatitis of the hands or perioral or perianal regions, allergic contact dermatitis to MI or other preservatives in seemingly innocuous personal care products must be considered as a possible causative factor. A thorough history of hygiene regimens and toiletry use is essential to diagnosis, as MI may trigger such reactions if found in moistened wipes, hair products, soaps, bubble baths, and sunscreens. Stopping use of the causative personal care product may provide clearance, in some cases without need for any further therapy. Parents should be educated about the potential of preservatives such as MI to cause ACD so that they can make informed consumer decisions. It is also important to inform parents that terms such as "gentle," "sensitive," "organic," or "hypoallergenic" are used for marketing purposes, and products labeled as such may still contain common allergens and result in allergic reactions.

## Conflict of Interests

The authors declare that there is no conflict of interests regarding the publication of this paper.

## Authors' Contribution

The authors had full access to all of the data in the study and take responsibility for the integrity of the data and the accuracy of the data analysis. Study concept and design were done by Rajani Katta. Analysis and interpretation of data

were done by Megan J. Schlichte. Drafting of the manuscript was done by Megan J. Schlichte. Critical revision of the manuscript for important intellectual content was done by Rajani Katta. Study supervision was done by Rajani Katta.

## References

[1] A. Scheman, S. Jacob, R. Katta et al., "Miscellaneous products: Trends and alternatives in deodorants, antiperspirants, sunblocks, shaving products, powders, and wipes: data from the American Contact Alternatives Group," *Journal of Clinical and Aesthetic Dermatology*, vol. 4, no. 10, pp. 35–39, 2011.

[2] M. P. Castanedo-Tardana and K. A. Zug, "Methylisothiazolinone," *Dermatitis*, vol. 24, no. 1, pp. 2–6, 2013.

[3] M. W. Chang and R. Nakrani, "Six children with allergic contact dermatitis to methylisothiazolinone in wet wipes (baby wipes)," *Pediatrics*, vol. 133, no. 24, pp. e434–e438, 2014.

[4] A. Bauer, J. Geier, and P. Elsner, "Allergic contact dermatitis in patients with anogenital complaints," *Journal of Reproductive Medicine for the Obstetrician and Gynecologist*, vol. 45, no. 8, pp. 649–654, 2000.

[5] A. Nosbaum, M. Vocanson, A. Rozieres, A. Hennino, and J. Nicolas, "Allergic and irritant contact dermatitis," *European Journal of Dermatology*, vol. 19, no. 4, pp. 325–332, 2009.

[6] L. A. Murphy, I. R. White, and S. C. Rastogi, "Is hypoallergenic a credible term?" *Clinical and Experimental Dermatology*, vol. 29, no. 3, pp. 325–327, 2004.

[7] V. M. Verallo-Rowell, "The validated hypoallergenic cosmetics rating system: its 30-year evolution and effect on the prevalence of cosmetic reactions," *Dermatitis*, vol. 22, no. 2, pp. 80–97, 2011.

[8] E. M. Warshaw, L. M. Furda, H. I. Maibach et al., "Anogenital dermatitis in patients referred for patch testing: retrospective analysis of cross-sectional data from the North American Contact Dermatitis Group, 1994–2004," *Archives of Dermatology*, vol. 144, no. 6, pp. 749–755, 2008.

# 2

# Retrospective Analysis of Corticosteroid Treatment in Stevens-Johnson Syndrome and/or Toxic Epidermal Necrolysis over a Period of 10 Years in Vajira Hospital, Navamindradhiraj University, Bangkok

**Wanjarus Roongpisuthipong,**[1] **Sirikarn Prompongsa,**[2] **and Theerawut Klangjareonchai**[3]

[1] *Division of Dermatology, Department of Medicine Vajira Hospital, Navamindradhiraj University, Bangkok 10300, Thailand*
[2] *Research Center, Navamindradhiraj University, Bangkok 10300, Thailand*
[3] *Department of Medicine, Faculty of Medicine, Ramathibodi Hospital, Mahidol University, Bangkok 10400, Thailand*

Correspondence should be addressed to Wanjarus Roongpisuthipong; rr_wanjarus@hotmail.com

Academic Editor: Jonathan L. Curry

*Background.* Stevens-Johnson syndrome (SJS) and/or toxic epidermal necrolysis (TEN) are uncommon and life-threatening drug reaction associated with a high morbidity and mortality. *Objective.* We studied SJS and/or TEN by conducting a retrospective analysis of 87 patients treated during a 10-year period. *Methods.* We conducted a retrospective review of the records of all patients with a diagnosis of SJS and/or TEN based on clinical features and histological confirmation of SJS and/or TEN was not available at the Department of Medicine, Vajira hospital, Bangkok, Thailand. The data were collected from two groups from 2003 to 2007 and 2008 to 2012. *Results.* A total of 87 cases of SJS and/or TEN were found, comprising 44 males and 43 females whose mean age was 46.5 years. The average length of stay was 17 days. Antibiotics, anticonvulsants, and allopurinol were the major culprit drugs in both groups. The mean SCORTEN on admission was 2.1 in first the group while 1.7 in second the group. From 2008 to 2012, thirty-nine patients (76.5%) were treated with corticosteroids while only eight patients (22.2%) were treated between 2003 and 2007. The mortality rate declined from 25% from the first group to 13.7% in the second group. Complications between first and second groups had no significant differences. *Conclusions.* Short-term corticosteroids may contribute to a reduced mortality rate in SJS and/or TEN without increasing secondary infection. Further well-designed studies are required to compare the effect of corticosteroids treatment for SJS and/or TEN.

## 1. Introduction

Steven-Johnson syndrome (SJS) and/or toxic epidermal necrolysis (TEN) are uncommon diseases with an incidence about 1.9 cases per million per year [1]. SJS and/or TEN are potentially mortal diseases, characterized by extensive blistering exanthema and epithelial sloughing, occurring with mucosal involvement (Figures 1 and 2) [2]. SJS and/or TEN are part of a spectrum, which is divided into 3 groups: SJS when the total detachment is less than 10% of the body surface area; TEN when it is over 30%; SJS-TEN overlap when it is between 10% and 30% [3]. Differential

diagnoses of SJS and/or TEN are linear IgA bullous disease, paraneoplastic pemphigus, generalized bullous fixed drug eruption, and staphylococcal scalded skin syndrome. Even though many factors have been proposed as causes of these diseases, hypersensitivity to medications reports for the most of cases. β-lactam antibiotics, sulfonamides, anticonvulsants, and allopurinol were frequent triggers of SJS and/or TEN [4]. The SCORTEN indicates a severity of illness, which is strongly correlated with the risk of death [5]. Aside from intensive supportive treatment, a normally accepted regimen for specific therapy of SJS and/or TEN is lacking. Treatment options include systemic corticosteroids,

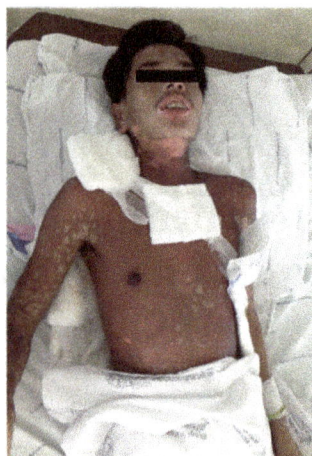

FIGURE 1: Multiple denuded areas on diffuse dusky red patches at forehead, neck, and right-sided trunk. Erosion on both upper and lower lips.

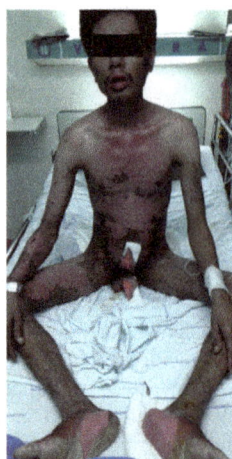

FIGURE 2: After 4 days, the patients developed progressive denuded area on previous dusky red. Patches on trunk and extremities. Erosion on both upper and lower lips, genitalia.

intravenous immunoglobulin therapy (IVIG), thalidomide, and TNF-$\alpha$ antagonist. Traditionally systemic corticosteroids were advocated until early 1990s, although no benefit has been demonstrated in case-controlled studies [6]. A retrospective single center study proposes that short-term dexamethasone therapy, given at an early stage of the disease, may contribute to a reduced mortality rate [7]. Moreover, the study from a general hospital in Singapore reports that the use of dexamethasone therapy may be a benefit [8]. The argument over systemic corticosteroid usage will still be continuously unresolved. The aim of this study was to present the etiologies, treatment, and clinical outcomes of SJS and/or TEN in Vajira Hospital, Navamindradhiraj University in Bangkok, Thailand.

## 2. Methods

A retrospective review was performed on patients admitted to Vajira Hospital, Navamindradhiraj University, with the diagnosis of SJS and/or TEN based on clinical features and histological confirmation of SJS and/or TEN was not available. The data were collected into two groups from 2003 to 2007 and 2008 to 2012 (10-year study). The ethical review board of the Faculty of Medicine Vajira Hospital, Navamindradhiraj University, approved this study.

The electronic medical database and inpatient charts were reviewed. The following data were collected: demographic information, culprit drugs, extent of mucocutaneous involvement, underlying diseases, laboratory data, treatments, complications, and mortality. Drugs that have been taken within 6 weeks before the onset of symptoms were considered as culprit drugs. If the patient had taken more than one drug, all of them were considered as culprit drugs.

## 3. Statistical Analysis

Continuous variables are reported as mean ± SD and data for categorical variables are reported as numbers and percentages. Comparisons of categorical variables among groups were performed using $\chi^2$ test or Fisher's test. Comparisons of continuous variables among groups were performed using unpaired Student's $t$-test or Mann-Whitney $U$ test. Statistical significance was set at $P < 0.05$ (two-tailed). Statistical analysis was performed with the SPSS version 18.0 (SPSS Inc., Chicago, IL, USA).

## 4. Results

Eighty-seven patients (44 males and 43 females) were admitted during this period. There were 36 cases (mean age was 42.6) since the year of 2003 until 2007 and 51 cases (mean age was 49.3) since the year of 2008 until 2012. In the first group, 36 cases were classified as SJS 26 cases (70.6%), SJS-TEN overlap 1 cases (2.8%), and TEN 9 cases (25.0%). In the second group, 51 cases were classified as SJS 36 cases (70.6%), SJS-TEN overlap 7 cases (13.7%), and TEN 8 cases (15.7%). Cardiovascular disease, diabetes mellitus, and HIV infection were not different between the first and second groups. Malignancy was 7 cases (13.7%) in the second group, while there was no case of malignancy in the first group. Mucosal involvement involved mouth more than other sites in both groups. Urethral involvement in the first group was significantly higher than the second group, while genital involvement in the second group was significantly higher than the first group. The mean of SCORTEN on the day of admission was 1.7 in the first group and 2.1 in the second group. In the second group, thirty-nine patients (76.5%) were treated with intravenous corticosteroids; the most common agent was dexamethasone. Only eight patients (22.2%) were treated with intravenous corticosteroid in the first group. The duration and dose of corticosteroid did not differ between the two groups. No patient received intravenous immunoglobulin. Table 1 shows clinical characteristics for the 87 patients.

TABLE 1: Clinical characteristics of Stevens-Johnson syndrome and/or toxic epidermal necrolysis cases from 2003 to 2012 ($n = 87$).

| | 2008–2012 ($n = 51$), $n$ (%) | 2003–2007 ($n = 36$), $n$ (%) | $P$ value |
|---|---|---|---|
| Age (years) | $49.3 \pm 19.2$ | $42.6 \pm 21.0$ | 0.104 |
| Male | 27 (52.9) | 17 (47.2) | 0.599 |
| Underlying diseases | | | |
| Cardiovascular disease | 11 (21.5) | 8 (22.2) | 0.942 |
| Diabetes mellitus | 7 (13.7) | 5 (13.8) | 0.983 |
| HIV infection | 12 (23.5) | 9 (25.0) | 0.875 |
| Malignancy* | 7 (13.7) | 0 (0) | 0.033 |
| Diagnosis | | | |
| SJS | 36 (70.6) | 26 (72.2) | 0.868 |
| SJS-TEN overlap | 7 (13.7) | 1 (2.8) | 0.082 |
| TEN | 8 (15.7) | 9 (25.0) | 0.281 |
| Mucosal involvement | | | |
| Ocular | 40 (78.4) | 32 (88.8) | 0.203 |
| Mouth | 45 (88.2) | 35 (97.2) | 0.129 |
| Genitalia* | 27 (52.9) | 11 (30.5) | 0.038 |
| Urethra* | 2 (3.9) | 7 (19.4) | 0.019 |
| Anus | 3 (5.8) | 1 (2.8) | 0.496 |
| SCORTEN | | | |
| ≤1 | 16 (31.4) | 13 (36.1) | 0.664 |
| 2 | 19 (37.3) | 19 (52.8) | 0.151 |
| 3 | 12 (23.5) | 3 (8.3) | 0.065 |
| 4 | 1 (1.9) | 1 (2.8) | 0.802 |
| ≥5 | 3 (5.8) | 0 (0) | 0.139 |
| Causes of disease | | | |
| Single drug-related | 44 (86.3) | 30 (83.3) | 0.705 |
| Multiple drug-related | 7 (13.7) | 6 (16.6) | 0.705 |
| Intravenous steroid use** | 39 (76.5) | 8 (22.2) | <0.001 |
| Dexamethasone equivalent doses (mg/day) | $13.2 \pm 6.1$ | $14.5 \pm 6.3$ | 0.914 |
| Steroid treatment duration (day) | $5.7 \pm 2.7$ | $5.4 \pm 2.5$ | 0.810 |
| Steroid treatment duration of ≥7 days | 13 (33.3) | 4 (50.0) | 0.096 |

*$P < 0.05$, **$P < 0.01$.
SJS: Stevens-Johnson syndrome.
TEN: toxic epidermal necrolysis.

TABLE 2: Percentage of intravenous steroid usage in Stevens-Johnson syndrome and/or toxic epidermal necrolysis patients stratified by SCORTEN.

| | 2008–2012 ($n = 51$) | 2003–2007 ($n = 36$) |
|---|---|---|
| SCORTEN | | |
| ≤1 | 87.5% | 15.4% |
| 2 | 63.1% | 13.0% |
| 3 | 83.3% | 33.3% |
| 4 | 100% | 0% |
| ≥5 | 66.7% | — |

TABLE 3: Comparison of incidences of culprit drugs.

| | 2008–2012 ($n = 58$), $n$ (%) | 2003–2007 ($n = 42$), $n$ (%) | $P$ value |
|---|---|---|---|
| Antibiotics | 26 (44.8) | 14 (33.3) | 0.265 |
| Penicillin | 7 (12.1) | 4 (9.5) | 0.718 |
| Cotrimoxazole | 7 (12.1) | 4 (9.5) | 0.718 |
| Cephalosporin | 5 (8.6) | 2 (4.8) | 0.473 |
| Quinolone | 3 (5.2) | 2 (4.8) | 0.949 |
| Carbapenem | 2 (3.4) | 0 (0) | 0.229 |
| Clindamycin | 1 (1.7) | 0 (0) | 0.398 |
| Tetracycline | 1 (1.7) | 0 (0) | 0.398 |
| Macrolide | 0 (0) | 2 (4.8) | 0.089 |
| Anticonvulsants | 14 (24.1) | 4 (9.5) | 0.064 |
| Phenytoin | 8 (13.8) | 3 (7.1) | 0.309 |
| Carbamazepine | 4 (6.9) | 1 (2.4) | 0.317 |
| Phenobarbital | 1 (1.7) | 0 (0) | 0.398 |
| Lamotrigine | 1 (1.7) | 0 (0) | 0.398 |
| Allopurinol | 7 (12.1) | 8 (19.1) | 0.301 |
| NSAIDs | 5 (8.6) | 4 (9.5) | 0.844 |
| Nevirapine | 3 (5.2) | 4 (9.5) | 0.377 |
| Antituberculosis[a] | 3 (5.2) | 0 (0) | 0.139 |
| Other drugs | 0 (0) | 8 (19.1) | |
| TTM | 0 (0) | 2 (4.8) | 0.089 |
| Valacyclovir | 0 (0) | 2 (4.8) | 0.089 |
| Cetirizine | 0 (0) | 1 (2.4) | 0.231 |
| Chloroquine | 0 (0) | 1 (2.4) | 0.231 |
| Cinnarizine | 0 (0) | 1 (2.4) | 0.231 |
| Silymarin | 0 (0) | 1 (2.4) | 0.231 |

[a]Antituberculosis (isoniazid, rifampicin, pyrazinamide, and ethambutol).
NSAIDs: nonsteroidal anti-inflammatory drugs.
TTM: traditional Thai medicine.

Table 2 shows percentage of intravenous steroid usage in SJS and/or TEN patients stratified by SCORTEN.

All of the patients in this study were related to drug administration. Antibiotics, anticonvulsants, and allopurinol were the major culprit drugs in both groups (Table 3). The highest culprit drugs were allopurinol (19.1%) in the first group and phenytoin (13.8%) in the second group. Penicillin and cotrimoxazole were the most frequent among antibiotics and phenytoin was the most frequent among anticonvulsants in both groups.

Many patients showed organ involvement and other complications (Table 4). Respiratory failure was the most internal organ failure in both groups. Endotracheal intubation and mechanical ventilation were needed for all of these patients. Liver and renal dysfunctions were more common in the first group than in the second group. Sepsis was more in the first group than in the second group, while skin infection and hospital-acquired pneumonia were more in the second group

TABLE 4: Organ involvement and complications in patient with Stevens-Johnson syndrome and/or toxic epidermal necrolysis cases from 2003 to 2012 ($n = 87$).

| | 2008–2012 ($n = 51$), $n$ (%) | 2003–2007 ($n = 36$), $n$ (%) | $P$ value |
|---|---|---|---|
| Internal organ involvement | | | |
| Liver failure | 3 (5.9) | 3 (8.3) | 0.657 |
| Renal failure | 6 (11.8) | 6 (16.6) | 0.514 |
| On hemodialysis | 3 (5.9) | 3 (8.3) | 0.657 |
| Respiratory failure | | | |
| On ventilator | 7 (13.7) | 6 (16.6) | 0.705 |
| Infections | | | |
| Skin infection | 9 (17.3) | 6 (16.6) | 0.905 |
| Hospital-acquired pneumonia | 7 (13.7) | 4 (11.1) | 0.718 |
| Sepsis | 7 (13.7) | 8 (22.2) | 0.301 |
| Length of stay | 19.2 ± 15.8 | 13.9 ± 9.6 | 0.287 |
| Death | 7 (13.7) | 9 (25) | 0.181 |

than in the first group. The admission duration was average 13.9 days in the first group and 19.2 days in the second group. The mortality rate declined from 25% from the first group to 13.7% in the second group.

## 5. Discussion

In our study, incidence of SJS and/or TEN was 8-9 cases per year which is similar to another report from Asia such as Thailand and Korea [9, 10]. The mean age was approximately 46 years which is as high as those reported from other countries in Asia such as Japan, Singapore, and Korea [2, 8, 10]. In contrast to earlier studies showing that females are affected with SJS and/or TEN more than males [2, 10], our series had equal numbers of males and females, which was in agreement with the study done by Tan and Tay [8]. The most common culprit drug group in this study was antibiotics (penicillin group and sulfonamide group) similar to other studies in Thailand [9, 11] and other Asian countries [2, 12]. Allopurinol showed a higher risk in this study than in previous studies [2, 9, 10]. It was the most common culprit drugs similar to EuroSCAR study [13]. The incidence of allopurinol associated with SJS or TEN increased in the EuroSCAR study because of increasing usages and dosages of this drug. This study revealed that the incidence of allopurinol associated with SJS or TEN declined from 19% in the first group to 12% in the second group. It may be hypothesized that the decreased rate is associated with physician's caution use allopurinol to accepted guidelines and adjusted dosage base on renal function. Carbapenems, a board spectrum of antibiotics, are increasingly used in clinical practice [14]. In this study, carbapenem-associated SJS or TEN was reported to be 3.4% between 2008 and 2012. In addition, Carbapenems are $\beta$-lactam; therefore, they can cross-react with penicillins or cephalosporins. There was a report of two successive episodes of cephalosporin and carbapenem associated with

TEN in the same patient; therefore, drug having chemical similarity to the initial causative compound should be strictly avoided in management of SJS or TEN [15].

Management in SJS or TEN involves sequentially rapid evaluation of the severity and prognosis of disease by using SCORTEN, prompting identification and discontinuation of all causative drugs, and initiating supportive care (such as fluid, electrolyte, wound, and nutritional management) and eventual specific treatment. Up till now, a specific treatment for SJS or TEN that has shown efficacy in controlled trials does not exist. The use of systemic corticosteroids in SJS or TEN is controversial. Although corticosteroids have pleomorphic immunomodulating effect through inhibition of various cytokines, the use of corticosteroids and prolong use of corticosteroids increase the risk of secondary infection and masking early sign of sepsis. Therefore, the use of corticosteroids is usually limited in SJS or TEN. In the present study, the use of systemic corticosteroids increased from 22% in the first group to 76% in the second group. Moreover, corticosteroid treatment duration for more than 7 days declined from 50% in the first group to 33% in the second group. In the second group, mortality and sepsis significantly declined when compared to the first group, while rate of hospital-acquired pneumonia and skin infection did not change. Additionally, the first group had lower SCORTEN than the second group but the mortality rate was higher in the first group than in the second group. In interpreting these results, short-course systemic corticosteroids such as dexamethasone in SJS or TEN reveals the benefit of decreasing the mortality rate while not increasing secondary infection such as septicemia, respiratory tract, and skin infection. In addition, two monocenter retrospective studies suggested that short-course high-dose corticosteroids (dexamethasone) might be of benefit [7, 8]. On the other hand, a retrospective case-control study conducted in France and Germany concluded that corticosteroids did not show a significant effect on mortality in comparison with supportive care only [6]. A retrospective analysis had some pitfalls; therefore, multicentre, randomized, placebo-controlled trials using standardized design are required in order to investigate further the use of corticosteroid in SJS and/or TEN. In addition, such a system might be useful for evaluation of genetic marker.

## 6. Conclusions

The most common drug-related SJS and/or TEN in Vajira hospital was allopurinol and the most common drug group was antibiotics. Short-term corticosteroids may contribute to a reduced mortality rate in SJS and/or TEN without increasing secondary infection. Further well-designed studies are required to compare the effect of corticosteroids treatment for SJS and/or TEN.

## Conflict of Interests

The authors declare that there is no conflict of interests regarding the publication of this paper.

## Acknowledgment

This work was supported by grant from Vajira Hospital, Navamindradhiraj University.

## References

[1] T. Harr and L. E. French, "Stevens-Johnson syndrome and toxic epidermal necrolysis," *Chemical Immunology and Allergy*, vol. 97, pp. 149–166, 2012.

[2] Y. Yamane, M. Aihara, and Z. Ikezawa, "Analysis of Stevens-Johnson syndrome and toxic epidermal necrolysis in Japan from 2000 to 2006," *Allergology International*, vol. 56, no. 4, pp. 419–425, 2007.

[3] S. Bastuji-Garin, B. Rzany, R. S. Stern, N. H. Shear, L. Naldi, and J.-C. Roujeau, "Clinical classification of cases of toxic epidermal necrolysis, Stevens-Johnson syndrome, and erythema multiforme," *Archives of Dermatology*, vol. 129, no. 1, pp. 92–96, 1993.

[4] T. Harr and L. E. French, "Toxic epidermal necrolysis and Stevens-Johnson syndrome," *Orphanet Journal of Rare Diseases*, vol. 5, no. 1, article 39, 2010.

[5] S. Bastuji-Garin, N. Fouchard, M. Bertocchi, J.-C. Roujeau, J. Revuz, and P. Wolkenstein, "Scorten: a severity-of-illness score for toxic epidermal necrolysis," *Journal of Investigative Dermatology*, vol. 115, no. 2, pp. 149–153, 2000.

[6] J. Schneck, J.-P. Fagot, P. Sekula, B. Sassolas, J. C. Roujeau, and M. Mockenhaupt, "Effects of treatments on the mortality of Stevens-Johnson syndrome and toxic epidermal necrolysis: a retrospective study on patients included in the prospective EuroSCAR Study," *Journal of the American Academy of Dermatology*, vol. 58, no. 1, pp. 33–40, 2008.

[7] S. H. Kardaun and M. F. Jonkman, "Dexamethasone pulse therapy for Stevens-Johnson syndrome/toxic epidermal necrolysis," *Acta Dermato-Venereologica*, vol. 87, no. 2, pp. 144–148, 2007.

[8] S.-K. Tan and Y.-K. Tay, "Profile and pattern of Stevens-Johnson syndrome and toxic epidermal necrolysis in a general hospital in Singapore: treatment outcomes," *Acta Dermato-Venereologica*, vol. 92, no. 1, pp. 62–66, 2012.

[9] V. Leenutaphong, A. Sivayathorn, P. Suthipinittharm, and P. Sunthonpalin, "Stevens-Johnson syndrome and toxic epidermal necrolysis in Thailand," *International Journal of Dermatology*, vol. 32, no. 6, pp. 428–431, 1993.

[10] H.-I. Kim, S.-W. Kim, G.-Y. Park et al., "Causes and treatment outcomes of Stevens-Johnson syndrome and toxic epidermal necrolysis in 82 adult patients," *Korean Journal of Internal Medicine*, vol. 27, no. 2, pp. 203–210, 2012.

[11] J. Thammakumpee and S. Yongsiri, "Characteristics of toxic epidermal necrolysis and stevens-johnson syndrome: a 5-year retrospective study," *Journal of the Medical Association of Thailand*, vol. 96, no. 4, pp. 399–406, 2013.

[12] M. Barvaliya, J. Sanmukhani, T. Patel, N. Paliwal, H. Shah, and C. Tripathi, "Drug-induced Stevens-Johnson syndrome (SJS), toxic epidermal necrolysis (TEN), and SJS-TEN overlap: a multicentric retrospective study," *Journal of Postgraduate Medicine*, vol. 57, no. 2, pp. 115–119, 2011.

[13] S. Halevy, P.-D. Ghislain, M. Mockenhaupt et al., "Allopurinol is the most common cause of Stevens-Johnson syndrome and toxic epidermal necrolysis in Europe and Israel," *Journal of the American Academy of Dermatology*, vol. 58, no. 1, pp. 25–32, 2008.

[14] K. M. Papp-Wallace, A. Endimiani, M. A. Taracila, and R. A. Bonomo, "Carbapenems: past, present, and future," *Antimicrobial Agents and Chemotherapy*, vol. 55, no. 11, pp. 4943–4960, 2011.

[15] P. Paquet, E. Jacob, P. Damas, and G. E. Piérard, "Recurrent fatal drug-induced toxic epidermal necrolysis (Lyell's syndrome) after putative $\beta$-lactam cross-reactivity: case report and scrutiny of antibiotic imputability," *Critical Care Medicine*, vol. 30, no. 11, pp. 2580–2583, 2002.

# 3

# Allergic Contact Dermatitis Is Associated with Significant Oxidative Stress

**S. Kaur,[1] K. Zilmer,[2] V. Leping,[3] and M. Zilmer[2]**

[1] Clinic of Dermatology, University of Tartu, 31 Raja Street, 50417 Tartu, Estonia
[2] Institute of Biomedicine and Translational Medicine, Department of Biochemistry, the Centre of Excellence for Translational Medicine, University of Tartu, 19 Ravila Street, 50411 Tartu, Estonia
[3] Institute of Computer Science, University of Tartu, 2 J. Liivi Street, 50409 Tartu, Estonia

Correspondence should be addressed to S. Kaur; sirje.kaur@kliinikum.ee

Academic Editor: Masutaka Furue

*Background.* Research has confirmed the involvement of oxidative stress (OxS) in allergic contact dermatitis whilst other inflammation-related biomarkers have been less studied. *Objective.* To evaluate systemic levels of selected inflammatory markers, OxS indices and adipokines as well as their associations in allergic contact dermatitis. *Methods.* In 40 patients, interleukin- (IL-) 6, monocyte chemoattractant protein (MCP-1), and IL-10 levels were measured in sera with the Evidence Investigator Cytokine & Growth factors High-Sensitivity Array, total peroxide concentration (TPX) and total antioxidant capacity (TAC) by means of spectrophotometry, and the plasma concentrations of adiponectin and leptin by the quantitative sandwich enzyme immunoassay technique. *Results.* TNF-$\alpha$ level ($P < 0.01$) and TPX ($P < 0.0001$) were increased whilst IL-10 ($P < 0.05$) and TAC ($P < 0.0001$) were decreased in the patients as compared to controls. Correlation and multiple linear regression analysis identified both, TPX and TAC (inversely), as possible independent markers for evaluating allergic contact dermatitis. Adiponectin level in patients was increased ($P < 0.0001$), but neither adiponectin nor leptin correlated significantly with the biomarkers of inflammation or OxS. *Conclusion.* OxS parameters, especially TPX and OSI, reflect the degree of systemic inflammation associated with allergic contact dermatitis in the best way. The relation between OxS and adiponectin level warrants further studies.

## 1. Introduction

Inflammation and oxidative stress (OxS), the latter defined as an overproduction of reactive oxygen as well as nitrogen species (ROS and RSN, resp.) with concomitant deficiency of antioxidative defenses of the body [1, 2], have been found to be inextricably connected in physiological as well as disease states [1]. In allergic contact dermatitis, elevated systemic levels of interleukin- (IL-) 6, IL-1, and tumor necrosis factor (TNF)-$\alpha$ have been found [3, 4], and ROS are proposed to participate in the initial allergen sensitization as well as in the development of pathogenic allergic responses [5].

Both, OxS and inflammatory mediators such as cytokines and C-reactive protein (CRP) have an influence on the adipokine status [6–8]. Adiponectin, a cytokine produced solely by adipose tissue, possesses antidiabetic, antiatherogenic, and potent anti-inflammatory activities [9, 10]. In accordance with its anti-inflammatory character, adiponectin levels are increased, rather than decreased, in a number of chronic inflammatory and autoimmune diseases [11]. Inverse correlations of adiponectin with markers of OxS and inflammation have been previously found [7, 9, 12]. The second most important adipokine leptin is known primarily by its ability to regulate food intake and energy expenditure [13]. Leptin has predominantly proinflammatory functions [11], promoting, for example, the activation and production of oxidative burst of inflammatory cells [13].

The current study was undertaken to concurrently examine selective biomarkers of inflammation, OxS, and inflammation-related adipokines as well as their associations in patients with acute/subacute allergic contact dermatitis involving approximately 5% of body surface.

## 2. Methods

Patients for this study were recruited from the Clinic of Dermatology of Tartu University, Estonia. The study involved 40 patients (6 male, 34 female, age 23–67 years, mean age $40.7 \pm 13.0$ years, mean BMI $25.3 \pm 5.5$ kg/m$^2$) who came to our clinic for patch testing due to acute/subacute allergic contact dermatitis, confined mostly to their hands or face (23 and 11 patients, resp.). Blood from the patients' antecubital vein was collected on the fifth day of routine patch testing after overnight fast. At the time of blood collection, 31 patients had one or more positive patch test results on their back, including 19 patients with positive patch test result to 5% nickel sulphate, nine to 0.01% methylisothiazolinone and eight patients to 1% formaldehyde. The remaining nine patients had given positive patch test results in a previous testing, and current dermatitis was associable with their contact allergy. All patients were tested with European standard series purchased from Hal Allergie GMBH, Düsseldorf, Germany, and allergens were applied on the skin with Finn Chambers on Scanpor (SmartPractice, Phoenix, USA). The patients were not treated with systemic corticosteroids at least for a month and any local corticosteroids were avoided for 24 hours before patch testing. The patients did not have active infections and concomitant chronic diseases as determined by the anamnesis, clinical assessment, and laboratory measurement of blood count, blood glucose level ($>5.5$ mmol/L), and total cholesterol ($>6.9$ mmol/L) at the time of recruitment. Collected blood samples were centrifuged at $1500 \times$g for 10 min and the serum was divided into aliquots and stored at $-70°$C for subsequent analysis.

The results obtained from the patients were compared against the data of age-matched normal weight healthy subjects from the database of the Institute of Biochemistry of Tartu University. Cytokine levels were compared with a control group (Co) consisting of 40 healthy subjects (14 male, 26 female, age $38.3 \pm 11.8$ years, range 19–58 years, mean BMI $24.8 \pm 2.7$ kg/m$^2$), OxS parameters with the data of 40 healthy individuals (25 male, 15 female, age $39.5 \pm 10.6$ years, range 20–58 years, mean BMI $23.8 \pm 3.4$ kg/m$^2$), adiponectin level with its levels in 51 healthy subjects (19 male, 32 female, age $37.1 \pm 12.00$ years, range 21–53 years, mean BMI $23.2 \pm 3.9$ kg/m$^2$), and leptin level with the data of 20 healthy women (age $34.7 \pm 11.4$ years, range 20–60 years, mean BMI $21.5 \pm 1.4$ kg/m$^2$). The study was approved by the Ethics Committee of the Faculty of Medicine of the University of Tartuand conducted after obtaining a signed consent from each participant.

*2.1. Measurement of Adiponectin, Leptin, and Cytokine Levels.* The plasma concentrations of adiponectin and leptin were analyzed by a quantitative sandwich enzyme immunoassay technique, using commercially available kits (R&D Systems, Minneapolis, MN, USA).

IL-6, monocyte chemoattractant protein (MCP-1) and IL-10 levels were measured in sera with the Evidence Investigator Cytokine & Growth factors High-Sensitivity Array (CTK HS Cat. number EV 3623 RANDOX Laboratories Ltd.,

Crumlin, United Kingdom) according to the manufacturer's protocol. Assay sensitivity varied from 0.12 pg/L to 2.12 pg/L, depending on the analyte. The reproducibility of the assay for an individual cytokine was determined using the quality controls provided with the kit.

HsCRP was analyzed by immunoturbimetry method at the Laboratory of Biochemistry of the Tartu University Hospital. The level of hsCRP 1.0 mg/L was used as a cut-off point to define a higher inflammatory status.

*2.2. Measurement of Total Peroxide Concentration.* Total peroxide concentration of samples was determined using OXY-STAT Assay Kit Cat. number BI-5007 (Biomedica Gruppe, Biomedica Medizinprodukte GmbH & Co Kg, Wien). The kit detects peroxide concentrations based on the reaction of biological peroxides with peroxidase and a subsequent color-reaction using tetramethylbenzidine (TMB) as substrate. The colored liquid is measured photometrically at 450 nm, using ELISA plate reader Photometer Sunrise (Tecan Austria GmbH, Salzburg). The concentration is stated as $H_2O_2$-equivalents ($\mu$mol/L).

*2.3. Assessment of Total Antioxidant Capacity.* The basic principle of the method is that a colourless molecule, reduced 2,2-azino-bis-3-ethylbenzothiazoline-6-sulfonicacid(ABTS), is oxidized to a characteristic blue-green ABTS, using hydrogen peroxide in acidic medium (the acetate buffer 30 mml/L pH 3,6) [14]. When the coloured ABTS is mixed with any substance, that can be oxidized, it is reduced to its original colourless ABTS form again. The ABTS is decolorized by antioxidants according to their concentrations and antioxidant capacities. This change in colour is measured as a change in absorbance at 660 nm. The reaction rate was calibrated with Trolox. The results are expressed in mmol Trolox equivalent/L. Within- and between-batch precision data obtained by TAC method were 2.5% and 2.9%, respectively.

*2.4. Oxidative Stress Index.* Percent ratio of the total peroxide concentration of plasma or other biological fluids (TPX) to the total antioxidant capacity of plasma or other biological fluids (TAC) is accepted as oxidative stress index (OSI), an indicator of the degree of oxidative stress [15]. According to this, we calculated OSI as the ratio of TPX ($\mu$mol/L) to TAC ($\mu$mol Trolox equivalent/L) $\times$ 100.

*2.5. Statistical Analysis.* Statistical analysis was performed using SAS 9.2 (SAS Institute Inc. NC, Cary, USA). All data are presented as mean $\pm$ standard deviation, and statistical significance was established as $P < 0.05$. A comparison between variables was assessed by the independent sample $t$-test. Correlations between parameters were assessed using bivariate correlation analysis (Pearson correlation coefficient) and multiple regression analysis.

## 3. Results

*3.1. Inflammatory and OxS Markers in Patients and Healthy Subjects.* As shown in Table 1, the patients had significantly increased TNF-$\alpha$ serum levels whilst the increase in MCP-1

TABLE 1: The levels of inflammatory markers and oxidative stress characteristics in the patients with acute/subacute allergic contact dermatitis covering approximately 5% of body surface as compared to healthy controls.

| | Allergic contact dermatitis ($n = 40$) | Healthy controls ($n = 40$) | $P$ |
|---|---|---|---|
| BMI kg/m$^2$ | 25.3 ± 5.5 | 24.8 ± 2.7$^*$/23.8 ± 3.4$^{**}$ | — |
| hsCRP mg/L | 1.96 ± 2.60 | <1.0 | ND |
| TNF-$\alpha$ pg/mL | 6.32 ± 7.02 | 3.33 ± 0.95 | $P < 0.01$ |
| IL-6 pg/mL | 1.34 ± 1.83 | 0.81 ± 0.30 | $P = 0.14$ |
| MCP-1 pg/mL | 245.0 ± 105.1 | 190.9 ± 53.4 | $P = 0.059$ |
| IL-10 pg/mL | 0.53 ± 0.30 | 0.68 ± 0.28 | $P < 0.05$ |
| TPX $\mu$mol/L | 719.9 ± 322.5 | 169.1 ± 58.8 | $P < 0.0001$ |
| TAC mmolTE/L | 1.32 ± 0.19 | 1.55 ± 0.23 | $P < 0.0001$ |
| OSI % | 55.9 ± 26.5 | 11.00 ± 3.7 | $P < 0.0001$ |

BMI: body mass index; hsCRP: high sensitive C-reactive protein; TNF: tumor necrosis factor; IL: interleukin; MCP: monocyte chemoattractant protein; TPX: total peroxide concentration; TAC: total antioxidant capacity; TE: Trolox equivalent; OSI: oxidative stress index.
$^*$the value for cytokine control group.
$^{**}$the value for OxS control group.
ND: not done.

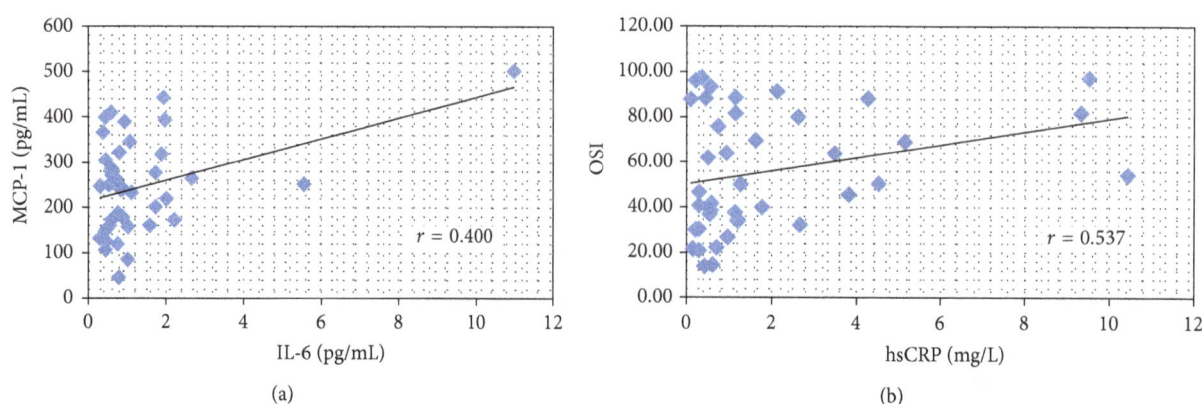

FIGURE 1: Correlations between inflammatory and oxidative stress markers in patients with acute/subacute allergic contact dermatitis approximately on 5% of body surface. MCP: monocyte chemoattractant protein; IL: interleukin; OSI: oxidative stress index; hsCRP: high sensitive C-reactive protein; TNF: tumor necrosis factor; TAC: total antioxidant capacity; TE: Trolox equivalent; TPX: total peroxide concentration.

remained below the threshold of statistical significance ($P < 0.01$ and $P = 0.059$, resp.). IL-10 levels in the patients were decreased ($P < 0.05$; Table 1). The mean concentration of hsCRP in the patients was 1.96 ± 2.60 mg/L, that is, not significantly different from the generally accepted maximum borderline value 1.0 mg/L.

The most noticeable differences between the patients and Co were established in OxS markers levels: TPX in the patients was significantly increased while TAC was decreased ($P < 0.0001$ in both) (Table 1). OSI, the percent ratio of TPX to TAC, was also significantly increased in the patients ($P < 0.0001$).

*3.2. The Relations between Markers of Inflammation and OxS.*
To confirm the possibility that inflammatory status is related to the diagnosis of allergic contact dermatitis, Pearson correlation coefficients were calculated, using combined patients' and Co data from Table 1. Significant positive correlations with the diagnosis of allergic contact dermatitis were found for TNF-$\alpha$ ($r = 0.290$, $P < 0.01$), MCP-1 ($r = 0.312$,

$P < 0.01$), TPX ($r = 0.769$, $P < 0.0001$), and OSI ($r = 0.769$, $P < 0.0001$), and negative correlations for IL-10 ($r = -0.255$, $P < 0.05$), and TAC ($r = -0.485$, $P < 0.0001$). Further multiple linear regression analysis starting with all covariates, for example, age, gender, BMI, TPX, TAC, and OSI also, revealed significant positive correlation of the diagnosis of allergic contact dermatitis with TPX ($r = 0.591$, $P < 0.0001$) and inverse correlation with TAC level ($r = -0.635$, $P = 0.006$).

We further analyzed the correlations between markers of inflammation and OxS in the group of patients and established relevant positive correlations between MCP-1 and IL-6 levels ($r = 0.400$, Figure 1(a)) as well as between hsCRP and OSI ($r = 0.537$; Figure 1(b)).

TNF-$\alpha$ level, which was most significantly increased in the patients, correlated neither with other inflammatory markers nor the indices of OxS. Both MCP-1 and IL-6 correlated positively with patients' BMI ($r = 0.380$, and $r = 0.337$, resp., Table 2). Therefore, we continued to follow the relationship between inflammatory markers and BMI,

TABLE 2: Correlations between inflammatory and oxidative stress markers and their correlations with subjects' age and BMI in patients with allergic contact dermatitis and healthy controls.

| | Patients and controls together ($n = 120$) | Patients with allergic contact dermatitis ($n = 40$) | Controls ($n = 80$) |
|---|---|---|---|
| BMI and age | $r = 0.340^{***}$ | $r = 0.303$ | $r = 0.541^{***}$ |
| BMI and IL-6 | $r = 0.327^{**}$ | $r = 0.337^{*}$ | $r = 0.206$ |
| BMI and MCP-1 | $r = 0.295^{*}$ | $r = 0.380^{*}$ | $r = -0.167$ |
| BMI and TPX | $r = 0.046$ | $r = -0.011$ | $r = 0.093$ |
| BMI and TAC | $r = -0.084$ | $r = -0.068$ | $r = -0.093$ |
| IL-6 and MCP-1 | $r = 0.391^{***}$ | $r = 0.400^{*}$ | $r = 0.013$ |
| hsCRP and OSI | ND | $r = 0.537^{***}$ | ND |
| TPX and TAC | $r = -0.380^{***}$ | $r = -0.040$ | $r = -0.087$ |

Correlations between baseline parameters were tested by Pearson rank correlation coefficient for data with a normal distribution. The $r$ and $P$ values are shown. Significant correlations are labeled as follows: $^{*}P < 0.05$, $^{**}P < 0.01$, and $^{***}P < 0.001$.
BMI: body mass index; TNF: tumor necrosis factor; IL: interleukin; MCP: monocyte chemoattractant protein; hsCPP: high sensitive C-reactive protein; TPX: total peroxide concentration; TAC: total antioxidant capacity; TE: Trolox equivalent; OSI: oxidative stress index; ND: not done.

including the analysis the patients and a corresponding Co. As shown in Table 2, subjects' BMI was positively correlated with the age ($r = 0.340$) and inflammatory markers IL-6 and MCP-1 ($r = 0.327$, and $r = 0.295$, resp., Figures 2(a) and 2(b)). At the same time, BMI was not correlated to the OxS markers in the patients and Co analyzed together (Table 2, Figures 2(c) and 2(d)). Correlation coefficients between age/TPX and age/TAC were also insignificant ($-0.059$, and $0.034$, resp.).

Other significant relations in patients and Co analyzed as whole were strong positive correlations between IL-6 and MCP-1, as well as inverse correlation between TPX and TAC (Table 2).

*3.3. Adiponectin and Leptin Levels and Their Associations with the Biomarkers of Inflammation and OxS.* Plasma concentration of adiponectin was significantly higher in the patients, compared with the mean value of 51 healthy normal weight controls with no statistically significant differences according to their age and gender ($11555 \pm 4378$ ng/mL and $6081 \pm 2422$ ng/mL, $P < 0.0001$). The levels of plasma adiponectin in the patients were inversely but nonsignificantly related to the BMI ($r = -0.225$, $P = 0.16$). We found no correlations of adiponectin level with any markers of inflammation or OxS in the patients except an inverse correlation between adiponectin and TPX ($r = -0.300$, $P = 0.06$) that, however, was only close to statistically significant relationship.

As leptin level in women exceeds the values in men two-three times [16] and our sample was predominantly female (85.0%), we calculated the mean leptin level in 34 female patients and compared it to the level in 20 female Co. The obtained values were significantly different ($13267 \pm 10435$ pg/mL, and $7318 \pm 3685$ pg/mL, resp., $P < 0.01$). On the other hand, blood leptin level positively correlates with

body weight [9, 11]. With the adjustment for BMI, which was different in our patients and Co ($25.3 \pm 5.5$ kg/m$^2$, and $21.5 \pm 1.4$ kg/m$^2$, $P = 0.0001$), the difference in leptin levels between female patients and Co became insignificant. The correlation of leptin level with BMI had only borderline significance ($r = 0.239$, $P = 0.066$) when analyzed in the patients and Co as whole ($n = 60$). There were no significant correlations between leptin levels and biomarkers of inflammation and OxS.

## 4. Discussion

The most remarkable finding of this study was that acute/subacute skin inflammation consisting of inflammatory lesions on the face or hands and positive patch test reaction site on the patients' back brought about considerable OxS.

Earlier studies have documented the rise in serum levels of several proinflammatory factors after exposure to contact allergens. The increase of TNF-$\alpha$ and, to some extent, MCP-1 levels in our patients is in concordance with the results obtained in patients with parthenium dermatitis [17] and trichloroethylene-induced hypersensitivity [18] and might be explained by the activities of activated T cells [19]. In case of inflammation, TNF-$\alpha$, which is present in healthy skin, is additionally synthesized by activated macrophages, T cells, and keratinocytes and released into circulation [19]. Furthermore, contact allergens and irritants can directly induce the expression of both TNF-$\alpha$ and MCP-1 [20]. For example, Martín et al. (2003) have demonstrated the expression of MCP-1 by basal keratinocytes and isolated dermal cells at 10 hours after antigen challenge, paralleled by dermal accumulation of mononuclear cells [21]. TNF-$\alpha$ stimulates the production of several other cyto- and chemokines, including MCP-1, by fibroblasts, endothelial cells, macrophages, and dendritic cells [21].

Though allergic contact dermatitis has been mainly associated with Th1/Th17 phenotypes, Th2-type regulatory cytokines such as IL-10 may have an important role in the downregulation of contact hypersensitivity reactions [3]. Therefore, decreased IL-10 concentrations, found in this and some previous studies [17, 22], might indicate the utilization of this cytokine in downregulation of allergic contact dermatitis.

Several inflammatory markers, including TNF-$\alpha$ and MCP-1, have been correlated with body weight [11, 23]. We found similar correlations for MCP-1 and IL-6; this demonstrates the decrease of their importance as markers of the activity of the inflammation in allergic contact dermatitis. At the same time, OxS parameters did not depend on patients' BMI.

The measurement of TPX and TAC has been currently effectively used to characterize both sides of OxS compendiously, including several conditions not related to infections or inflammation, for example, white-coat hypertension [24] and major depression [25]. In addition, the ratio of TPX to TAC (OSI) gives a single numerical value to evaluate the degree of OxS [15]. Our study of patients with restricted allergic contact dermatitis demonstrated a significant increase

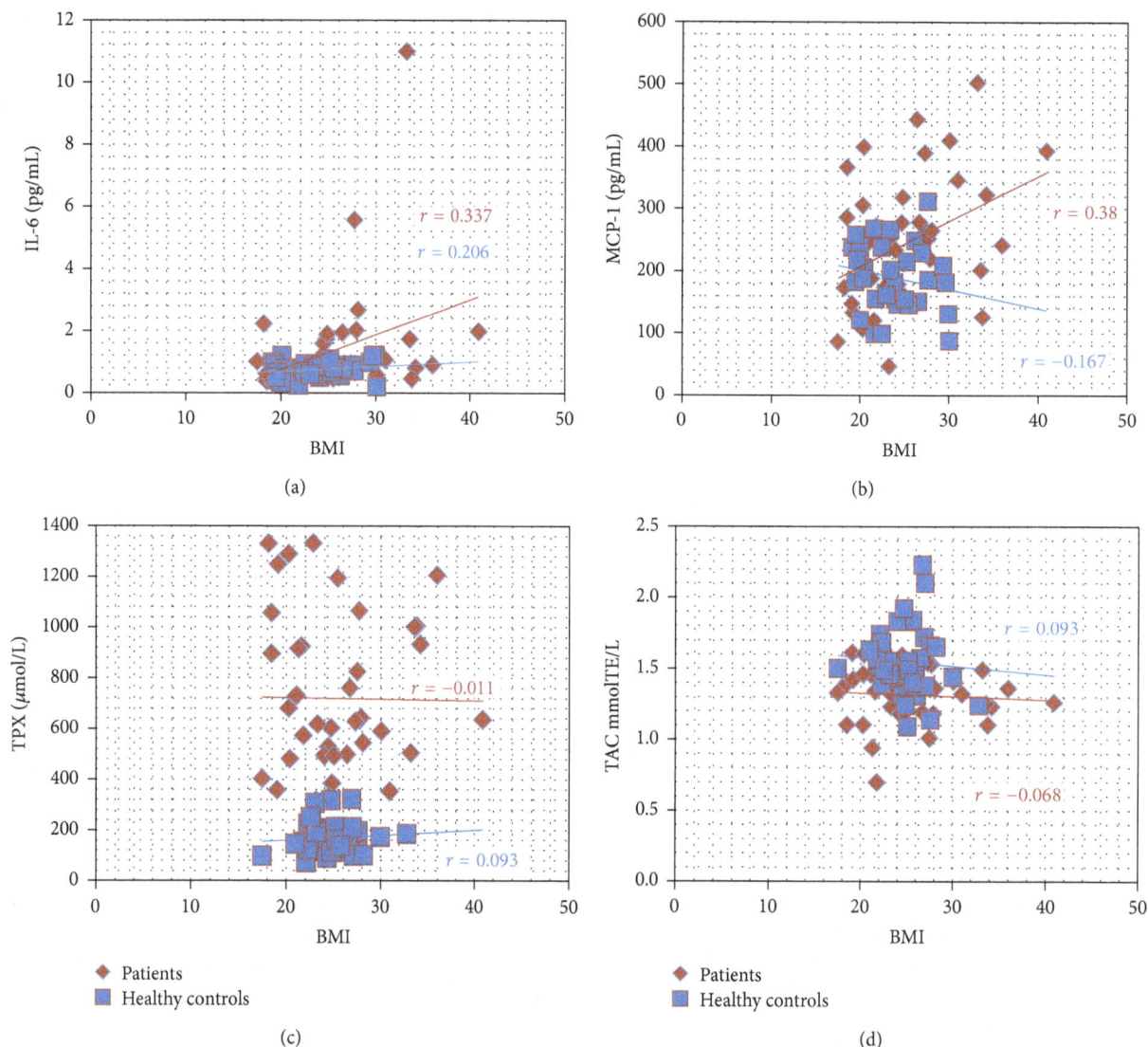

FIGURE 2: Scatterplot of correlation analysis of IL-6, MCP-1, TPX, and TAC with BMI in patients with allergic contact dermatitis and healthy controls. IL: interleukin; MCP: monocyte chemoattractant protein; TPX: total peroxide concentration; TAC: total antioxidant capacity; TE: Trolox equivalent; BMI: body mass index.

in the oxidants pool and decrease in antioxidative capacity; the latter can be explained by the consumption of radical-scavenging antioxidants due to increased free radical amounts [15]. The prevalence of OxS indices over inflammatory is in agreement with the concept that OxS may be the starter point in the pathogenesis of allergic contact dermatitis, leading to the activation of transcription factors and signaling pathways and further synthesis of inflammatory cytokines [4, 5]. Some recent studies have confirmed the ability of contact allergens to induce OxS pathway in keratinocytes [26, 27]. Our own previous study showed the decrease in antioxidants pool of the skin, evidenced by increased oxidized glutathione/reduced glutathione ratio in positive to 5% nickel sulphate patch test site [28]. The presence of contact allergen-related OxS was also confirmed by Gangemi et al. (2009) who found increased serum concentrations of nitrosylated proteins (biomarkers of OxS) in nickel-allergic female patients after oral nickel challenge [29]. Considering

all the above-mentioned facts, TPX may be the best and earliest marker of systemic changes occurring in the body after allergen challenge and before the visible inflammation. This marker could be used in the evaluation of treatment results when developing new anti-inflammatory drugs or cosmetic products.

Adiponectin and leptin, the most abundant products of the adipose tissue, have considerable effects on metabolic, inflammatory, and immune responses [16]. Well-recognized activities of adiponectin include the induction of anti-inflammatory mediators such as IL-10 and IL-1 receptor antagonist and inhibition of TNF-$\alpha$ and NF-$\kappa$B on endothelial cells [30]. The levels of adiponectin have been found to be inversely associated with marker of inflammation CRP in patients with diabetes [9] and coronary atherosclerosis [31]. However, no evidence suggests an association between plasma adiponectin and TNF-$\alpha$ in humans [32].

The relationship between adiponectin and OxS is likewise very complex. In general, low levels of adiponectin are associated with increased OxS [8], and some studies have concluded that adiponectin exerts its antiatherogenic and antidiabetic effects through the modulation of OxS [6]. In addition, higher levels of adiponectin are associated with more beneficial OxS profile in elderly population [12]. At the same time, positive as well as inverse correlations have been found between markers of OxS (isoprostanes) and adiponectin [6, 7]. An explanation for elevation of adiponectin in our allergic contact dermatitis patients may be that adiponectin represents a beneficial counter regulatory response to reduce oxidative burden similarly as it has been concluded in type 1 diabetes mellitus [8]. There was an inverse correlation between adiponectin and TPX, however, with the $P$ value below the statistical significance ($P = 0.06$). Regardless of that, these results suggest the possibility that the increase of adiponectin level may be compensatory, evoked by high TPX concentration.

Leptin that is functionally and structurally related to proinflammatory cytokines [33] polarizes T cells towards a $T_H1$ cell phenotype [11] while promoting monocyte recruitment and secretion of proinflammatory cytokines [33]. Thus, there are several mechanisms by which leptin could lead to greater inflammation. As women have markedly higher leptin concentrations as compared to men, even when adjusted for BMI [34], we investigated leptin levels only in female patients, comparing it to the value in female Co. After adjustment for BMI, we did not find differences in serum leptin levels between the patients and Co. There were no significant correlations between leptin levels and biomarkers of inflammation or OxS. Therefore, inclusion of adiponectin and leptin in severity assessment of allergic contact dermatitis may not be clinically useful.

In conclusion, the systemic effect of allergic contact dermatitis was most conspicuous in the parameters of OxS especially in TPX and OSI levels. The level of adiponectin was increased and showed a tendency to correlate inversely with TPX concentration. Therefore, as compared to inflammatory markers and adipokine levels, OxS parameters might be most helpful to assess disease activity and therapeutic response in allergic contact dermatitis.

## Conflict of Interests

The authors declare that there is no conflict of interests regarding the publication of this paper.

## Acknowledgments

The study was supported by the Estonian Science Foundation Grant no. 7549 and by targeted financing from the Ministry of Education and Science of Estonia (SF0180105s08 and SF0180043S07).

## References

[1] M. Valko, D. Leibfritz, J. Moncol, M. T. D. Cronin, M. Mazur, and J. Telser, "Free radicals and antioxidants in normal physiological functions and human disease," *International Journal of Biochemistry and Cell Biology*, vol. 39, no. 1, pp. 44–84, 2007.

[2] K. Nakai, K. Yoneda, and Y. Kubota, "Oxidative stress in allergic and irritant dermatitis: from basic research to clinical management," *Recent Patents on Inflammation & Allergy Drug Discovery*, vol. 6, no. 3, pp. 202–209, 2012.

[3] A. Cavani, O. De Pità, and G. Girolomoni, "New aspects of the molecular basis of contact allergy," *Current Opinion in Allergy and Clinical Immunology*, vol. 7, no. 5, pp. 404–408, 2007.

[4] C. Albanesi, "Keratinocytes in allergic skin diseases," *Current Opinion in Allergy and Clinical Immunology*, vol. 10, no. 5, pp. 452–456, 2010.

[5] E. Corsini, V. Galbiati, D. Nikitovic, and A. M. Tsatsakis, "Role of oxidative stress in chemical allergens induced skin cells activation," *Food and Chemical Toxicology*, vol. 61, pp. 74–81, 2013.

[6] S. Nakanishi, K. Yamane, N. Kamei, H. Nojima, M. Okubo, and N. Kohno, "A protective effect of adiponectin against oxidative stress in Japanese Americans: the association between adiponectin or leptin and urinary isoprostane," *Metabolism: Clinical and Experimental*, vol. 54, no. 2, pp. 194–199, 2005.

[7] A. Katsuki, M. Suematsu, E. C. Gabazza et al., "Increased oxidative stress is associated with decreased circulating levels of adiponectin in Japanese metabolically obese, normal-weight men with normal glucose tolerance," *Diabetes Research and Clinical Practice*, vol. 73, no. 3, pp. 310–314, 2006.

[8] S. L. Prior, T. S. Tang, G. V. Gill, S. C. Bain, and J. W. Stephens, "Adiponectin, total antioxidant status, and urine albumin excretion in the low-risk "golden Years" type 1 diabetes mellitus cohort," *Metabolism: Clinical and Experimental*, vol. 60, no. 2, pp. 173–179, 2011.

[9] G. K. Shetty, P. A. Economides, E. S. Horton, C. S. Mantzoros, and A. Veves, "Circulating adiponectin and resistin levels in relation to metabolic factors, inflammatory markers, and vascular reactivity in diabetic patients and subjects at risk for diabetes," *Diabetes Care*, vol. 27, no. 10, pp. 2450–2457, 2004.

[10] D. K. Oh, T. Ciaraldi, and R. R. Henry, "Adiponectin in health and disease," *Diabetes, Obesity and Metabolism*, vol. 9, no. 3, pp. 282–289, 2007.

[11] N. Ouchi, J. L. Parker, J. J. Lugus, and K. Walsh, "Adipokines in inflammation and metabolic disease," *Nature Reviews Immunology*, vol. 11, no. 2, pp. 85–97, 2011.

[12] S. Gustafsson, L. Lind, S. Söderberg, M. Zilmer, J. Hulthe, and E. Ingelsson, "Oxidative stress and inflammatory markers in relation to circulating levels of adiponectin," *Obesity*, vol. 21, no. 7, pp. 1467–1473, 2013.

[13] F. Lago, C. Dieguez, J. Gómez-Reino, and O. Gualillo, "The emerging role of adipokines as mediators of inflammation and immune responses," *Cytokine and Growth Factor Reviews*, vol. 18, no. 3-4, pp. 313–325, 2007.

[14] O. Erel, "A novel automated direct measurement method for total antioxidant capacity using a new generation, more stable ABTS radical cation," *Clinical Biochemistry*, vol. 37, no. 4, pp. 277–285, 2004.

[15] K. Serefhanoglu, A. Taskin, H. Turan, F. E. Timurkaynak, H. Arslan, and O. Erel, "Evaluation of oxidative status in patients with brucellosis," *Brazilian Journal of Infectious Diseases*, vol. 13, no. 4, pp. 249–251, 2009.

[16] H. Tilg and A. R. Moschen, "Adipocytokines: mediators linking adipose tissue, inflammation and immunity," *Nature Reviews Immunology*, vol. 6, no. 10, pp. 772–783, 2006.

[17] N. Akhtar, K. K. Verma, and A. Sharma, "Study of pro-and anti-inflammatory cytokine profile in the patients with parthenium dermatitis," *Contact Dermatitis*, vol. 63, no. 4, pp. 203–208, 2010.

[18] Q. Jia, D. Zang, J. Yi et al., "Cytokine expression in trichloroethylene-induced hypersensitivity dermatitis: an in vivo and in vitro study," *Toxicology Letters*, vol. 215, no. 1, pp. 31–39, 2012.

[19] A. Kerstan, E.-B. Bröcker, and A. Trautmann, "Decisive role of tumor necrosis factor-$\alpha$ for spongiosis formation in acute eczematous dermatitis," *Archives of Dermatological Research*, vol. 303, no. 9, pp. 651–658, 2011.

[20] A. Kerstan, M. Leverkus, and A. Trautmann, "Effector pathways during eczematous dermatitis: where inflammation meets cell death," *Experimental Dermatology*, vol. 18, no. 10, pp. 893–899, 2009.

[21] A. P. Martín, J. Gagliardi, C. E. Baena-Cagnani et al., "Expression of CS-1 fibronectin precedes monocyte chemoattractant protein-1 production during elicitation of allergic contact dermatitis," *Clinical and Experimental Allergy*, vol. 33, no. 8, pp. 1118–1124, 2003.

[22] S. Kaur, K. Zilmer, V. Leping, and M. Zilmer, "Comparative study of systemic inflammatory responses in psoriasis vulgaris and mild to moderate allergic contact dermatitis," *Dermatology*, vol. 225, no. 1, pp. 54–61, 2012.

[23] T. Christiansen, B. Richelsen, and J. M. Bruun, "Monocyte chemoattractant protein-1 is produced in isolated adipocytes, associated with adiposity and reduced after weight loss in morbid obese subjects," *International Journal of Obesity*, vol. 29, no. 1, pp. 146–150, 2005.

[24] A. Yildiz, M. Gür, R. Yilmaz et al., "Lymphocyte DMA damage and total antioxidant status in patients with white-coat hypertension and sustained hypertension," *Archives of the Turkish Society of Cardiology*, vol. 36, no. 4, pp. 231–238, 2008.

[25] M. Maes, I. Mihaylova, M. Kubera, M. Uytterhoeven, N. Vrydags, and E. Bosmans, "Increased plasma peroxides and serum oxidized low density lipoprotein antibodies in major depression: markers that further explain the higher incidence of neurodegeneration and coronary artery disease," *Journal of Affective Disorders*, vol. 125, no. 1–3, pp. 287–294, 2010.

[26] R. J. Vandebriel, J. L. A. Pennings, K. A. Baken et al., "Keratinocyte gene expression profiles discriminate sensitizing and irritating compounds," *Toxicological Sciences*, vol. 117, no. 1, pp. 81–89, 2010.

[27] D. H. Kim, D. Byamba, W. H. Wu, T. Kim, and M. Lee, "Different characteristics of reactive oxygen species production by human keratinocyte cell line cells in response to allergens and irritants," *Experimental Dermatology*, vol. 21, no. 2, pp. 99–103, 2012.

[28] S. Kaur, M. Zilmer, M. Eisen et al., "Nickel sulphate and epoxy resin: differences in iron status and glutathione redox ratio at the time of patch testing," *Archives of Dermatological Research*, vol. 295, no. 12, pp. 517–520, 2004.

[29] S. Gangemi, L. Ricciardi, P. L. Minciullo et al., "Serum levels of protein oxidation products in patients with nickel allergy," *Allergy and Asthma Proceedings*, vol. 30, no. 5, pp. 552–557, 2009.

[30] H. Tilg, "Adipocytokines in nonalcoholic fatty liver disease: key players regulating steatosis, inflammation and fibrosis," *Current Pharmaceutical Design*, vol. 16, no. 17, pp. 1893–1894, 2010.

[31] N. Ouchi, S. Kihara, T. Funahashi et al., "Reciprocal association of C-reactive protein with adiponectin in blood stream and adipose tissue," *Circulation*, vol. 107, no. 5, pp. 671–674, 2003.

[32] N. Ouchi and K. Walsh, "Adiponectin as an anti-inflammatory factor," *Clinica Chimica Acta*, vol. 380, no. 1-2, pp. 24–30, 2007.

[33] S. S. Martin, A. N. Qasim, D. J. Rader, and M. P. Reilly, "C-reactive protein modifies the association of plasma leptin with coronary calcium in asymptomatic overweight individuals," *Obesity*, vol. 20, no. 4, pp. 856–861, 2012.

[34] F. Lago, R. Gómez, J. J. Gómez-Reino, C. Dieguez, and O. Gualillo, "Adipokines as novel modulators of lipid metabolism," *Trends in Biochemical Sciences*, vol. 34, no. 10, pp. 500–510, 2009.

# 4

# Treatment of Nail Psoriasis: Common Concepts and New Trends

**Yasemin Oram and A. Deniz Akkaya**

*Department of Dermatology, V.K. Foundation American Hospital of Istanbul, Turkey*

Correspondence should be addressed to Yasemin Oram; dryaseminoram@mynet.com

Academic Editor: Pablo Coto-Segura

The lifetime incidence of nail involvement in psoriatic patients is estimated to be 80–90%, and the nails can be affected in 10% to 55% of psoriatic patients. Psoriasis may also solely involve the nails, without any other skin findings, in which the treatment can be more challenging. Nail psoriasis may lead to considerable impairment in quality of life due to aesthetic concerns and more importantly limitations in daily activities resulting from the associated pain, which may be overlooked by the physicians. Several topical and systemic treatment modalities, as well as radiation and light systems, have been used in the treatment of nail psoriasis. In the last decade, the introduction of biologic agents and the utilization of laser systems have brought a new insight into the treatment of nail psoriasis. This paper focuses on the recent advances, as well as the conventional methods, in treating nail psoriasis in adults and children, in reference to an extensive literature search.

## 1. Introduction

Psoriasis is a chronic skin disease that causes significant distress and morbidity. Although the skin manifestations are more characteristic, the lifetime incidence of nail involvement in psoriatic patients is estimated to be 80–90%, and the nails can be affected in 10% to 55% of psoriatic patients [1–3]. Moreover, psoriasis may involve the nails only, without any other signs of skin findings [1, 4]. Nail psoriasis has been shown to be associated with longer duration of skin lesions. There is an association between the duration of psoriasis and the severity of nail involvement [2, 3, 5]. Nail psoriasis is also associated with higher disease severity [3, 6]. However, it may also occur in 40% of patients with mild psoriasis [2]. It is slightly more common in male patients than females [3, 6]. Nail psoriasis leads to considerable impairment in quality of life due to aesthetic concerns and more importantly limitations in daily activities resulting from the associated pain [2, 7].

Nail psoriasis may show different clinical presentations according to the structure that is involved within the nail unit. Nail matrix involvement leads to irregular nail pitting (the most common finding of nail psoriasis), dystrophy, and leukonychia; nail bed involvement causes onycholysis, subungual hyperkeratosis, splinter hemorrhages, oil drop patches, and nail thickening, whereas nail fold involvement

may result in paronychia [1, 8, 9]. In cases of very severe inflammation, combined nail matrix and nail bed psoriasis may develop, forming "psoriatic crumbly nail." Psoriatic nail constitutes a risk factor for secondary mycotic infections, which can occur in up to 27% of the cases. This coexistence should be excluded by mycologic examination before treatment [10].

There is striking association between nail psoriasis and a high risk of psoriatic arthritis, a chronic inflammatory arthropathy, with a prevalence of nail involvement among patients with psoriatic arthritis as high as 70%. Nail involvement may precede arthritis or may be considered as a predictor of future psoriatic joint damage [3, 11]. Nail bed involvement prevalence has been found higher in patients with psoriatic arthritis [11]. Psoriatic arthritis mainly involves distal interphalangeal joints and is characterized by dactylitis, enthesitis, osteolysis, and periarticular new bone formation [12]. A possible explanation for this association might be the close anatomical link between the nail unit and the distal interphalangeal joint. Inflammation of the extensor tendon enthesis, which are the attachment points of ligaments, tendons, and joint capsules to bone, can extend to the nail unit and result in psoriatic nail changes [8].

The Nail Psoriasis Severity Index (NAPSI) has been developed as an objective and reproducible tool, which helps to estimate the nail involvement and therefore to standardize the treatment outcome assessments. The nail is divided into quadrants, based on the signs of involvement of the nail matrix and the nail bed, rated with 0 or 1 [13]. NAPSI scoring system has some limitations, as it does not specifically consider the severity of nail matrix or nail bed involvement. In a recent report by Mukai et al. [14], NAPSI scores were evaluated in psoriatic patients using acitretin, and it was concluded that the method was easy and rapid in measuring the improvement of the treatment; however, it did not quantify the existing lesions and might not detect small changes. In 2007, a modified NAPSI (mNAPSI) was proposed by Cassell et al. [15] in order to increase the sensitivity of NAPSI, using a qualitative gradation of severity for each parameter from 0 to 3 in each quadrant. Although it can be time consuming and impractical for the clinicians in an outpatient clinic, mNAPSI demonstrates excellent interrater reliability and validity in the assessment of psoriatic nail disease [8, 15]. Digital photography might be an easy and convenient method for monitoring the progression of the nail involvement during the treatment [8].

Although there exist several treatment options for psoriasis, there are no existing guidelines or consistent treatment algorithms for the treatment of nail psoriasis, as the amount of published evidence available is limited. Recently, a systematic review evaluating the randomized controlled trials has provided some evidence concerning the management of nail psoriasis [16]. The management of nail psoriasis has been challenging particularly when the nail involvement is the only manifestation of the disease. Low penetration of the topical medications and slow growth rate of the nails are the main factors for this difficulty. Moreover, most of the therapies require prolonged treatment and continuity, sometimes with side effects and/or disappointing results. Obviously, it may have a negative impact on patient's compliance, motivation, and quality of life [4].

## 2. General Nail Care

The Koebner, or isomorphic response, which is the formation of new psoriatic lesions at sites of physical injury to the skin, is a well-known phenomenon. Psoriatic changes of the nail unit can also be triggered by minor traumas such as manicure, biting the nails, picking or trimming the cuticle, clearing subungual debris, or wearing tight-fitting shoes. An important part of the treatment is to ensure that the patient is avoiding all the factors that may exacerbate the disease. The physical trauma should be discouraged, the hands and feet should be thoroughly wiped dry, and the nails must be kept short [8, 9].

## 3. Topical Therapy

There is limited evidence for the efficacy of topical therapies in nail psoriasis. Various topical treatment modalities have been used in nail psoriasis including corticosteroids, dithranol, fluorouracil, vitamin $D_3$ analogues, tacrolimus, cyclosporine, and tazarotene [1, 4, 7, 8] (Table 1).

The main topical treatments for nail psoriasis have traditionally comprised potent corticosteroids applied under occlusion. The clobetasol propionate at a concentration of 0.05% in cream or gel vehicle has been the most recommended topical treatment. However, they may cause atrophy, depigmentation, telangiectasia, and bone reabsorption. In 1999, Baran and Tosti [29] first described the use of 8% clobetasol propionate in nail lacquer vehicle in the treatment of 45 patients with nail psoriasis. The nail lacquer is a solution that helps to prevent the adverse effects caused by the use of intralesional corticosteroids or corticosteroids in cream or gel applied to the skin. Consequently favorable results have been observed with 8% clobetasol propionate lacquer that has effective transungual penetration and therapeutic effect both on nail bed and matrix lesions, while lacking side effects [17, 23].

Dithranol is an anthracene derivative with antiinflammatory and antiproliferative actions [8]. In a prospective study, dithranol (anthralin) ointment with a 0.4–2% concentration has been shown to be effective in 60% of 20 patients particularly in the treatment of onycholysis and subungual hyperkeratosis using daily short-contact therapy. The ointment was applied for 30 minutes daily for 5 months. Side effects included local irritation and temporary staining of the nail [31].

Fluorouracil is a pyrimidine analog, which inhibits the thymidylate synthase. Topical 5-fluorouracil (5-FU) in 1% or 5% concentrations in different vehicles has been used in nail psoriasis with unpredictable results. In a prospective study, the application of 1% fluorouracil solution twice daily for 6 months demonstrated marked improvement in nail pitting and hyperkeratosis in 85% of patients [32]. However, another small double-blinded study failed to show any benefits from topical 5-FU lotion 1%, combined with urea and propylene glycol. Besides, onycholysis was aggravated with the treatment [28]. The reported side effects such as pain, infection, nail loss, hyperpigmentation, onycholysis, and skin irritation, in the small number of studies conducted, are the reasons to limit its use.

Vitamin $D_3$ analogues of calcipotriol, calcitriol, and tacalcitol have been used in the treatment of nail psoriasis by inhibiting keratinocyte growth and differentiation and suppressing T-cell activity and cytokine production [1, 7, 21, 33]. In a double-blind study involving 58 patients with nail bed psoriasis, topical application of calcipotriol ointment twice daily was found to be as effective as twice daily application of betamethasone dipropionate in reducing subungual hyperkeratosis after 3–9 months [30]. Side effects include periungual irritation, erythema, and burning [7]. Combination therapy of topical corticosteroids with vitamin $D_3$ analogues including calcipotriol and tacalcitol has been shown to be effective, although there is no standard therapeutic regimen. The antiinflammatory effect of corticosteroids together with the antiproliferative and immunomodulatory effects of vitamin $D_3$ not only enhances the outcome of the treatment but also reduces the risk of adverse effects [8]. Rigopoulos et al. [26] demonstrated that the combined treatment with calcipotriol cream (once daily, 5 days a week) and clobetasol propionate cream (once daily, 2 days a week) for 6 months resulted in a 72% reduction at subungual hyperkeratosis. The synergistic effect of topical vitamin $D_3$, which mainly affects the nail bed,

TABLE 1: Topical therapies for treatment of nail psoriasis.

| Author | Year | n | Intervention | Comparison | Treatment protocol | Results | LoE [16] |
|---|---|---|---|---|---|---|---|
| Nakamura et al. [17] | 2012 | 15 | Clobetasol propionate at concentrations 0.05%, 1%, and 8% | Placebo (coat nail lacquer) | Twice weekly, for 4 mos | 51% improvement in treatment group (8% clobetasol more efficient) | N/A |
| Fischer-Levanchini et al. [18] | 2012 | 6 | 0.1% tazarotene ointment | — | Once daily, under occlusion, for 6 mos | 88% improvement in NAPSI scores at 6th mo | N/A |
| De Simone et al. [19] | 2012 | 21 | 0.1% tazarotene ointment | No treatment to the other hand | Once daily, to the affected nails of a randomly selected hand, for 3 mos | Statistically significant improvements in the treated hands at week 12 | N/A |
| Tzung et al. [20] | 2008 | 40 | 0.005% calcipotriol + 0.05% betamethasone dipropionate | 0.005% calcipotriol | Calcipotriol twice daily and calcipotriol + betamethasone once daily for 3 mos | Similar efficacy in both groups, significant reduction of NAPSI scores | B |
| Sánchez-Regaña et al. [21] | 2008 | 15 | 8% clobetasol in nail lacquer and tacalcitol | — | Clobetasol once daily at weekends and tacalcitol at weekdays under occlusion, for 6 mos | 78% reduction in NAPSI at 6 mos | N/A |
| Rigopoulos et al. [22] | 2007 | 46 | 0.1% tazarotene cream | 0.05% clobetasol propionate | Once daily under occlusion, for 3 mos | Similar efficacy in both groups, significant reduction of NAPSI scores | A2 |
| Regaña et al. [23] | 2005 | 10 | 8% clobetasol in nail lacquer | — | Once daily, for 3 weeks and twice weekly, for 9 mos | Reduction of all nail alterations within 1 mo | N/A |
| Cannavò et al. [24] | 2003 | 16 | 70% CsA oral solution in maize oil | Maize oil | For 3 mos | Complete resolution or substantial improvement in CsA group | A2 |
| Bianchi et al. [25] | 2003 | 25 | 0.1% tazarotene gel | — | Once daily, for 3 mos | 19/25 good clinical response | N/A |
| Rigopoulos et al. [26] | 2002 | 62 | Calcipotriol cream + clobetasol propionate | — | Calcipotriol once daily every weeknight and clobetasol once daily every weekend, for the first 6 mos and twice weekly clobetasol for the 2nd 6 mos | Reduction at subungual hyperkeratosis: 72.3% at 6 mos and 81.2% at 12 mos | N/A |
| Scher et al. [27] | 2001 | 31 | 0.1% tazarotene gel | Vehicle gel | Once daily, for 6 mos | Significant improvement of onycholysis and pitting in tazarotene group | A2/B |
| de Jong et al. [28] | 1999 | 57 | 1% 5-FU in permeation enhancer lotion (Belanyx) | Belanyx (urea and propylene glycol) | Once daily, for 3 mos | Significant improvements with both preparations | A2 |
| Baran and Tosti [29] | 1999 | 18 | 8% clobetasol nail lacquer | Placebo | Once daily in the first week, from 2nd week onwards 2-3 times weekly, for up to 9 mos | Clear improvement in 80%, complete resolution in 22% of patients in the treatment arm | B |
| Tosti et al. [30] | 1998 | 58 | Calcipotriol ointment | Betamethasone propionate + salicylic acid | Twice daily, for up to 5 months | Calcipotriol as effective as the combination of topical steroid and salicylic acid (49% versus 51% reduction of subungual hyperkeratosis in fingernails at 6 mos) | B |

TABLE 1: Continued.

| Author | Year | n | Intervention | Comparison | Treatment protocol | Results | LoE [16] |
|---|---|---|---|---|---|---|---|
| Yamamoto et al. [31] | 1998 | 20 | 0.4–2% anthralin in petrolatum | — | Once daily, for 5 mos | Effective in 12/20 patients, particularly in onycholysis and subungual hyperkeratosis | N/A |
| Fredriksson [32] | 1974 | 20 | 1% 5-FU solution | — | Twice daily, for up to 6 mos | Considerable improvement in 17/20 patients, 75% reduction of symptoms compared to baseline | N/A |

n: number of patients.
mo: month.
N/A: not applicable.
NAPSI: nail psoriasis severity index.
CsA: cyclosporine.
5-FU: 5-fluorouracil.
LoE: level of evidence (A2: randomized, double-blind, controlled trial of good quality, B: randomized controlled trial of poor quality).

togetherwith topical corticosteroid that is more effective on nail matrix, may provide safer and better treatment for nail psoriasis [20, 21, 30].

Tazarotene is a synthetic retinoid derived from vitamin A that downmodulates keratinocyte hyperproliferation, differentiation, and inflammation. Studies using tazarotene gel 0.1% have been conducted with successful results in nail psoriasis [25, 27]. Rigopoulos et al. [22] reported that tazarotene 0.1% cream was as effective as clobetasol propionate 0.05% cream in improving onycholysis, discoloration, pitting, and hyperkeratosis after 12 weeks in a double-blind study of 46 patients. In a small study, the efficacy and safety profile of tazarotene 0.1% hydrophilic ointment under occlusion was evaluated in the treatment of nail psoriasis of 6 patients. Clinically significant improvement in nail involvement, especially the subungual hyperkeratosis and onycholysis, was observed after 6 months of treatment [18]. Topical tazarotene has been generally well tolerated with mild erythema, local irritation, desquamation, and burning [25]. The combination of tazarotene with a topical corticosteroid might be helpful in decreasing the irritation caused by tazarotene while achieving an enhanced effect with two different molecules [7].

Several studies have shown that a topical calcineurin inhibitor, tacrolimus ointment, may penetrate the periungual skin and can be used to treat nail dystrophy caused by lichen planus or chronic paronychia [7, 34]. Tacrolimus in 0.1% and 0.03% ointment was found to be effective in psoriasis due to its immunosuppressive property. De Simone et al. [19] have reported good clinical results in nail psoriasis with topical tacrolimus 0.1% ointment application after 12 weeks. It seemed to be equally effective on nail bed and matrix lesions without having severe side effects.

Topical cyclosporine preparation showed to improve pitting and onycholysis in a small, placebo-controlled study. Oil-dissolved 70% solution of cyclosporine has been used in 8 patients for 12 weeks, and complete resolution or substantial improvement has been reported in all patients [24]. However, topical cyclosporine is not as effective as the systemic form in nail psoriasis, and further studies are necessary to optimize the vehicle and stability of the topical administration [35].

## 4. Intralesional Therapy

Despite a relative paucity of controlled studies, intralesional injections with corticosteroids are considered to be a standard treatment for nail psoriasis [1]. Triamcinolone acetonide is the most widely used agent in doses of 2.5–10 mg/mL at up to four injection sites (two into the proximal nail fold and two in the lateral nail fold), used bimonthly for 5-6 months. Injections to the proximal nail fold with 28- and 29-gauge needle syringes or with needle-less injectors are very effective in treating nail matrix disease such as pitting or ridging [1, 9, 36]. Up to 70–90% of psoriatic patients with both nail matrix and nail bed lesions respond to intralesional steroids, except for onycholysis, which shows a less pronounced response. Corticosteroid injections can cause considerable pain, atrophy, despigmentation, secondary infection, inclusion cysts, subungual hemorrhage, and tendon rupture [9, 36]. This treatment requires repeated injections.

Saricaoglu et al. [37] reported a case of severe psoriatic nail disease successfully treated with intralesional methotrexate at a dose of 2.5 mg of weekly injections for 6 weeks. The significant improvement in subungual hyperkeratosis and pitting was maintained after 2 years of treatment. The most important limitation of the therapy was the severe pain during injections.

## 5. Phototherapy, Radiation Therapy, and Laser Therapy

Although phototherapy with narrow-band UVB and photochemotherapy with UVA, in addition to oral psoralen (PUVA), have been successfully used in psoriasis, there is not enough evidence to support their beneficial effects in nail psoriasis. Several small studies have shown that PUVA can help psoriatic nails with variable results. The pitting and onycholysis have demonstrated poor response to PUVA treatment [38]. A recent study on the penetration of UV lights in normal human cadaveric fingernail plate showed that the nail plate completely blocks UVB light but only a minimal amount of UVA penetrates the nail [39]. This may explain the limited effect of PUVA in nail psoriasis.

Superficial radiotherapy, electron beam therapy, and Grenz rays have been infrequently used in the treatment of nail psoriasis with temporary benefits. The possibility of localized fibrosis and carcinogenesis should be considered in radiation therapy [7, 8]. Soft X-rays have been used for very thick psoriatic nails in one case, in fractionated doses of 1.5 Gy for a total of 13.5 Gy (43 kV, 25 mA, 0.6 mm aluminum filter) at 1- and 2-week intervals. The nail plates became normal after 12 months of therapy [40].

In recent years photodynamic therapy (PDT) and pulsed dye laser (PDL) have been described for the treatment of nail psoriasis regarding their proven effects on plaque type psoriasis. We have used 595 nm PDL (7 mm spot size, 1,5 ms pulse duration, 8–10 j/cm$^2$ energy) in nail psoriasis of 5 patients, once monthly for 3 months, with significant improvement, particularly of nail bed lesions [41]. Mean NAPSI scores declined from 21.2 at baseline to 3 at 1 month after 3 sessions. Treewittayapoom et al. [42] found PDL to be effective in both nail bed and matrix lesions, in a left-to-right comparison study of 20 patients, evaluating the effect of two different pulse durations (6 ms, 9 j/cm$^2$ versus 0.45 ms, 6 j/cm$^2$ both with 7 mm spot size). A significant reduction in NAPSI scores from baseline was observed in both groups after 6 months of the first treatment, while no significant difference was found between the longer and the shorter pulse duration groups. Fernández-Guarino et al. [43] evaluated the efficacy of PDT and PDL in the treatment of nail psoriasis in a left-to-right comparison study of 14 patients. Both hands were treated with 595 nm PDL (7 mm, 6 ms, 9 j/cm$^2$), following 3 hours occlusion of methyl-aminolaevulinic acid (MAL) to one hand, once a month for 6 months. After 3 hours occlusion of methyl-aminolaevulinic acid (MAL) to one hand, both hands were treated with 595 nm PDL (7 mm, 6 ms, 9 j/cm$^2$), once a month for 6 months. They showed that both treatments were equally effective in nail bed and nail matrix lesions; hence MAL did not play any role in the improvement of nail psoriasis.

## 6. Systemic Therapy

Systemic treatment can be recommended in severe localized nail psoriasis when topical or intralesional therapy has failed or in the treatment of moderate-to-severe psoriasis vulgaris accompanied with nail involvement [4, 7, 9] (Table 2).

Retinoids are vitamin A analogues that influence epidermal differentiation, proliferation, and immunomodulation. Etretinate and its active metabolite acitretin have been used in psoriasis. Tosti et al. [46] showed a 41% mean improvement in NAPSI scores after 6 months of treatment of low-dose acitretin (0.2–0.3 mg/kg/day) in nail psoriasis. Ricceri et al. [50] reported a case with severe nail psoriasis that showed marked improvement in 2 months of therapy of acitretin at a

dose of 0.5 mg/kg, combined with urea nail lacquer. Acitretin may decrease the thickness of the nail resulting in nail atrophy and fragility. Therefore patients with thickened nails and severe subungual hyperkeratosis are better candidates for acitretin treatment [8]. As retinoids are teratogenic and have been associated with significant hepatotoxicity and hypertriglyceridemia, they should be reserved for very resistant and severe nail involvement [7].

Although the efficacy of methotrexate and cyclosporine on plaque type psoriasis has been reported previously, the literature consists of few publications regarding the efficacy of the two treatment agents in the nail involvement. Syuto et al. [47] have reported that low-dose systemic cyclosporine successfully treats nail psoriasis with an improvement rate of over 90% of the patients. The initial dose was 3 mg/kg/day twice a day and was reduced to 1.5 mg/kg/day in a single administration when the improvement was observed. Oral cyclosporine (3.5–4.5 mg/kg/day) in combination with topical calcipotriol cream (50 μg/kg/day) has been shown to be more effective with a low risk of relapse in nail psoriasis when compared to the results of the patients receiving cyclosporine alone [48]. In a study by Mahrle et al. [49], 210 patients were randomly assigned for oral cyclosporine (2.5–5 mg/kg/day) or etretinate (0.5–0.75 mg/kg/day) for 10 weeks, and a significant alleviation of nail involvement was shown in both groups. At the second phase of this study, either systemic therapies were discontinued and were switched to topical dithranol or cyclosporine was tapered for 12 weeks. The tapered cyclosporine group was reported to show a significant improvement in nail involvement.

Gümüşel et al. [45] compared the efficacy and safety of methotrexate and cyclosporine in psoriatic nails of 34 patients in a randomized blinded study using NAPSI scores as an objective evaluation of the treatment outcomes. Initial methotrexate dose was 15 mg/week subcutaneously and was decreased after 3 months of treatment. The initial dose of cyclosporine was 5 mg/kg/day and was tapered to 2.5–3.5 mg/kg/day. After 6 months of treatment, they concluded that the two medications were similarly and moderately effective in nail psoriasis. Methotrexate was found to be more effective on nail matrix lesions, whereas cyclosporine was more effective in nail bed involvement.

In the retrospective study of Sánchez-Regeña et al. [44] comparing the classical and biological therapies in the treatment of nail psoriasis, all the classical and biological systemic treatments including cyclosporine, acitretin, methotrexate, and PUVA were shown to significantly reduce the severity of nail psoriasis, with the exception of narrow-band UVB (NUVB). Among the classical treatments, the improvement of nail psoriasis was more prominent in patients who had received cyclosporine. However, the percentage of change in the NAPSI score was significantly greater with biological treatments.

## 7. Biologic Treatments

In the last decade, the introduction of biological agents used for the treatment of plaque psoriasis and psoriatic arthritis has brought a safe and highly effective treatment option for

TABLE 2: Systemic therapies for treatment of nail psoriasis.

| Author | Year | n | Intervention | Comparison | Treatment protocol | Results | LoE [16] |
|---|---|---|---|---|---|---|---|
| Sánchez-Regaña et al. [44] | 2011 | 84 | Classical treatment | Biological treatment | Classical: acitretin, MTX, CsA, PUVA, NUVB, REPUVA, RENUVB Biological: infliximab, efalizumab, etanercept, adalimumab, for up to 8 mos | Significant reductions in NAPSI scores with all antipsoriatics, except for NUVB; significantly greater with CsA and biological as infliximab and adalimumab at 3 and 6 mos | N/A |
| Gümüşel et al. [45] | 2011 | 37 | MTX 15 mg/week, sc | CsA 5 mg/kg, po | MTX decreased to 10 mg/week after 3 months, for total 6 mos; CsA decreased to 2.5–3.5 mg/kg/day after 3 mos, for total 6 mos | Similar efficacy in both groups: reduction in NAPSI scores: 43% in MTX group, 37% in CsA group | A2 |
| Tosti et al. [46] | 2009 | 36 | Acitretin | — | 0.2–0.3 mg/kg/day, for 6 mos | 41% reduction in NAPSI scores | N/A |
| Syuto et al. [47] | 2007 | 16 | CsA-MEPC | — | 3 mg/kg/day and reduced to 1.5 mg/kg/day in responders | Improvement in over 90% of patients | N/A |
| Feliciani et al. [48] | 2004 | 54 | CsA | CsA + calcipotriol cream | CsA 3.5 mg/kg/day, in both groups; calcipotriol cream twice daily, for 3 mos | 79% improvement in combination group and 47% improvement in CsA alone | N/A |
| Mahrle et al. [49] | 1995 | 210 | CsA | Etretinate | Phase 1: randomly assigned for CsA (2.5–5 mg/kg/day) or etretinate (0.5–0.75 mg/kg/day) for 10 weeks Phase 2: etretinate group discontinued treatment and continued with topical dithranol; CsA group either tapered or discontinued and replaced with topical dithranol for 12 weeks | After phase 1: significant alleviation of nail involvement in both groups and after phase 2: statistically significant decrease in nail involvement for tapered cyclosporine group | B |

n: number of patients.
NAPSI: nail psoriasis severity index.
N/A: not applicable.
sc: subcutaneous.
po: peroral.
MTX: methotrexate.
CsA: cyclosporine.
MEPC: microemulsion preconcentrate.
LoE: level of evidence (A2: randomized, double-blind, controlled trial of good quality, B: randomized controlled trial of poor quality).

severe nail bed and matrix disease as well. Both antitumor necrosis-$\alpha$ (TNF-$\alpha$) and T-cell-targeted therapies have been useful for refractory severe nail psoriasis [8]. While biological therapies have been shown to be effective in nail psoriasis, infliximab appears to be the most effective option with the strongest evidence [7, 51–54] (Table 3).

Infliximab is a chimeric, human-murine IgG1 monoclonal antibody against TNF-$\alpha$, which acts by neutralizing its biological activity. It is administered intravenously, with a dose of 0.5 mg/kg at weeks 0, 2, 6 and repeated every 8 weeks. In the first study evaluating the efficacy of infliximab in nail psoriasis, 25 patients with plaque-type psoriasis or psoriatic arthritis achieved a 50% reduction in mean NAPSI scores at week 14, while at week 22, the mean NAPSI score was 0 [53]. In a 50-week RCT (randomized controlled trial)

of infliximab, 240 of 305 patients with nail psoriasis in the treatment arm started to show clearance of the nail disease as early as in week 10, with complete clearance in 44.7% of the patients at week 50. The treatment group had 26.8% and 57.2% improvements in the NAPSI scores at weeks 10 and 24, respectively, while worsening was observed in the placebo group. On the other hand, when the placebo group was switched to infliximab therapy at week 24, they achieved NAPSI scores comparable to those obtained with the original treatment group [54]. Further assessment of the results showed that the reduction of NAPSI scores was sustained, following 1 year of continuous infliximab therapy [54, 70]. A retrospective analysis of 48 patients with nail involvement confirmed the efficacy of infliximab therapy in nail psoriasis, with rapid and persistent improvements. At week 14, more

TABLE 3: Biologic therapies for treatment of nail psoriasis.

| Author | Year | n | Intervention | Comparison | Protocol | Results | LoE [16] |
|---|---|---|---|---|---|---|---|
| Fabroni et al. [55] | 2011 | 48 | Infliximab | — | 5 mg/kg, iv infusion at weeks 0, 2, 6 and every 8 weeks through week 38 | NAPSI-50 is achieved in 85% of patients at week 14, 96% at week 22, 98% at week 38; NAPSI-75 is achieved in 23% of patients at week 14, 65% at week 22, 81% at week 38; NAPSI-90 is achieved in 29% of patients at week 38 | N/A |
| Rich et al. [54] | 2008 | 305 | Infliximab | Placebo | 5 mg/kg, iv infusion at weeks 0, 2, 6 and every 8 weeks through week 46 | 26% and 57% improvements in NAPSI scores at weeks 10 and 24 and complete clearance of target nail in 45% of patients at 1 year | A2 |
| Rigopoulos et al. [56] | 2008 | 18 | Infliximab | — | 5 mg/kg iv infusion at weeks 0, 2, 6 and every 8 weeks through week 38 | Significant decrease in NAPSI scores (56 at baseline to 30 at week 14, 16 at week 22, 7 at week 30, and 3.3 at week 38) | N/A |
| Bianchi et al. [53] | 2005 | 25 | Infliximab | — | 5 mg/kg, iv, at weeks 0, 2, 6, 14, 22 | NAPSI-50 is achieved in all patients at week 14; NAPSI-75 is achieved in all patients at week 22 | N/A |
| Leonardi et al. [57] | 2011 | 36 | Adalimumab | Placebo | 80 mg, sc at week 0, 40 mg every other week starting at week 1, through week 16; patients in the placebo group were started to receive active treatment starting at week 16, through week 28 | Significantly higher improvement in NAPSI scores in the treatment arm (50% versus 8%) at week 16; once switched to adalimumab, patients in the initial placebo group improved 38% at week 28, while patients who began the study with adalimumab continued to improve to 54% | N/A |
| Van den Bosch et al. [58] | 2010 | 259 | Adalimumab | — | 40 mg, sc, at every other week through week 12 | Mean NAPSI scores are reduced by 44% at week 12 | N/A |
| Rigopoulos et al. [59] | 2010 | 21 | Adalimumab | — | 80 mg, sc at week 0, 40 mg every other week starting at week 1, through week 24 | Significant improvement in all patients after 8th injection; fingernail NAPSI decreased from 11 at baseline to 4 at week 24 in patients with just cutaneous psoriasis and from 24 to 10 in patients with psoriatic arthritis | N/A |
| Ortonne et al. [60] | 2012 | 69 | Etanercept | Etanercept | 1st group 50 mg weekly for 24 weeks and 2nd group 50 mg twice weekly for the first 12 weeks, 50 mg weekly for the other 12 weeks, sc | Both dose regimens are effective for nail psoriasis and significant improvement in NAPSI scores in both groups at week 24 | N/A |

TABLE 3: Continued.

| Author | Year | $n$ | Intervention | Comparison | Protocol | Results | LoE [16] |
|--------|------|-----|-------------|-----------|----------|---------|----------|
| Luger et al. [61] | 2009 | 564 | Etanercept | — | 25 mg twice weekly for 54 weeks or 50 mg twice weekly for 12 weeks, continued with 25 mg twice weekly in case of relapse, sc | NAPSI scores improved by 29% at week 12, by 51% at week 54, complete resolution in 30% of patients | N/A |
| Kavanaugh et al. [62] | 2009 | 287 | Golimumab | Placebo | 50 or 100 mg, sc, every 4 weeks through week 24 | Significant improvements started as early as at week 14: 25% reduction in NAPSI scores in 50 mg group, 43% reduction in 100 mg group at week 14, 33% reduction in 50 mg, and 54% reduction in 100 mg group at week 24 | B |
| Körver et al. [63] | 2006 | 8 | Alefacept | — | 15 mg weekly, im, for 12 weeks | 3 patients showed significant improvement, 3 patients unchanged, and 2 patients worsened | N/A |
| Parrish et al. [64] | 2006 | 15 | Alefacept | — | 15 mg weekly, im, for 12 weeks | 39% reduction in NAPSI scores at week 24 | N/A |
| Cassetty et al. [65] | 2005 | 6 | Alefacept | — | 15 mg weekly, im, for 12 weeks | 3 patients showed ≥30% improvement in NAPSI scores, 1 unchanged, and 2 worsened | N/A |
| Patsatsi et al. [66] | 2013 | 27 | Ustekinumab | — | 45 mg, sc, at weeks 0, 4 and every 12 weeks thereafter (90 mg if patient weight > 100 kg) | Significant improvements in NAPSI scores (43% at week 16, 86% at week 28, and 100% at week 40) | N/A |
| Vitiello et al. [67] | 2013 | 13 | Ustekinumab | — | 90 mg ($n$ = 5, patients weight > 100 kg), sc, at weeks 0, 4 and every 12 weeks thereafter or 45 mg in combination with MTX ($n$ = 6) or CsA ($n$ = 2) | 38% reduction in NAPSI scores in monotherapy group, 27% reduction in MTX combination, complete resolution in CsA combination group, at week 12 | N/A |
| Igarashi et al. [68] | 2012 | 102 | Ustekinumab | Placebo | 45 or 90 mg, sc, at weeks 0, 4 and every 12 weeks through 72 weeks, placebo group with crossover to ustekinumab at week 12 | Improvement in NAPSI scores: 57% in 45 mg group, 68% in 90 mg group at week 64 | A2 |
| Reich et al. [69] | 2011 | 317 | Briakinumab | MTX | Briakinumab 200 mg at weeks 0 and 4, 100 mg every 4 weeks through week 48, sc, MTX 5–25 mg/week for 51 weeks | NAPSI scores of the target fingernail significantly lower with the briakinumab group at weeks 24 and 52, as compared with the methotrexate group | N/A |

$n$: number of patients.
sc: subcutaneous.
iv: intravenous.
im: intramuscular.
N/A: not applicable.
NAPSI: nail psoriasis severity index.
MTX: methotrexate.
CsA: cyclosporine.
LoE: level of evidence (A2: randomized, double-blind, controlled trial of good quality, B: randomized controlled trial of poor quality).

than 50% reduction was observed in the mean NAPSI scores in 85.4% of patients. Improvement of nail psoriasis continued between weeks 14 and 38, with further reductions in NAPSI scores [55]. Similarly, in another study of 18 patients with psoriasis and psoriatic arthritis, a significant improvement was noted in most of the patients following the third infusion of infliximab, with a reduction of mean NAPSI scores from 55.8 at baseline, to 29.8 at week 14. At week 38, an almost complete resolution of psoriatic nail involvement was demonstrated [56]. Response to infliximab therapy has also been reported to be effective in patients with severe nail psoriasis refractory to other systemic therapies [71].

Adalimumab is a recombinant human IgG1 monoclonal antibody against TNF-$\alpha$. It is administered subcutaneously, at a dose of 40 mg every other week, usually preceded by an 80 mg loading dose. In a study of 21 patients treated with adalimumab for psoriasis or psoriatic arthritis, with concomitant nail disease, improvement was observed as early as at 12 weeks in both fingernails and toenails [59]. For the fingernails, there was almost a 50% reduction in mean NAPSI scores at week 12 and almost complete resolution at week 24. In another study evaluating the effectiveness of adalimumab for nail psoriasis in 259 patients with psoriatic arthritis in a 12-week study, the mean NAPSI score was reduced by 44% at week 24 [58]. In a RCT of palmoplantar psoriasis, 28 of 36 patients with nail involvement received adalimumab therapy for 16 weeks and showed a higher mean percentage of NAPSI improvement compared to placebo-treated group (50% versus 8%). At week 16, patients from the placebo group were switched to receive active treatment, and a mean improvement of 38% was reported in NAPSI at week 28 [57].

Etanercept is a soluble, human, TNF-$\alpha$ receptor fusion protein. It binds TNF-$\alpha$ with greater affinity than natural receptors, so that TNF-$\alpha$ becomes biologically inactive. Etanercept is administered subcutaneously, usually at a dose of 50 mg twice weekly for 3 months, followed by once weekly thereafter. In a prospective trial of patients with moderate to severe plaque psoriasis, 69 patients with nail psoriasis were treated with etanercept. One treatment arm received etanercept 50 mg once weekly for 24 weeks. The other treatment arm received etanercept 50 mg twice weekly for the first 12 weeks and once weekly for the following 12 weeks. There was a significant improvement in mean NAPSI scores at week 24 in both groups, with significant number of patients showing complete resolution. Both treatment regiments were found to be effective in nail psoriasis [60]. In the post hoc analysis of a RCT, in which the patients were randomized to receive either continuous (25 mg twice weekly for 54 weeks) or paused (50 mg twice weekly up to 12 weeks, followed by 25 mg twice weekly in case of relapse) etanercept therapy, 564 patients with nail involvement were evaluated. The mean NAPSI scores were improved by 28.9% at week 12 and by 51% at week 54, while complete resolution was observed in 30% of patients [61]. There are also case reports demonstrating the rapid and marked improvement of nail psoriasis with etanercept therapy [72–74].

Golimumab is a human monoclonal antibody against TNF-$\alpha$. It is administered subcutaneously. In a RCT of golimumab for psoriatic arthritis, response to nail involvement in 287 patients was assessed as a secondary outcome. Patients in the treatment arm received 50 mg or 100 mg golimumab every 4 weeks through week 24. Significant improvements in nail symptoms were observed in golimumab-treated patients as early as at week 14 in 50 mg and 100 mg group, with a reduction in NAPSI scores of 25% and 43% by week 14 and of 33% and 54% by week 24, respectively [62].

Alefacept is a recombinant human fusion protein composed of lymphocyte function-associated antigen-3 (LFA-3) and Fc portion of human IgG. It binds to CD2 receptor on T cells and thereby blocks T-cell interactions with antigen-presenting cells. In addition, it triggers the apoptosis of memory T cells and thus decreases the number of pathogenic T cells and the inflammatory response. It is administered weekly either 15 mg intramuscularly or 7.5 mg intravenously, generally for 12 weeks. There are a few studies with small number of patients in the literature, evaluating the efficacy of alefacept in nail psoriasis. In a group of 6 patients with mild nail psoriasis, after 12 weeks of intramuscular etanercept treatment, 3 demonstrated 30% or greater improvement in NAPSI scores at week 18, while 1 remained unchanged and 2 worsened [65]. Similarly in a group of 8 patients, 5 of which having moderate to severe nail psoriasis, 3 patients showed improvement, 3 remained unchanged, and 2 worsened [63]. In another study of 15 patients with severe nail psoriasis, baseline NAPSI scores were reduced by 39% at week 24, after 12 weeks of intramuscular therapy [64, 75].

Ustekinumab is a human monoclonal antibody that binds to the shared p40 subunit of the cytokines interleukin (IL)-12 and IL-23 to inhibit their biologic activity, as a consequence reduces IL-17A and IL-17F, and thus blocks the differentiation and proliferation of T helper ($T_H$)-1 and $T_H$-17 populations. It is administered subcutaneously, at a dose of 45 mg (90 mg if patient weight >100 kg), usually at weeks 0, 4 and every 12 weeks thereafter. In a case report of nail psoriasis unresponsive to etanercept, complete improvement was noted after the second injection of 45 mg subcutaneous ustekinumab at week 8 [75]. Igarashi et al. [68] randomized 158 patients with plaque psoriasis to receive ustekinumab 45 or 90 mg at weeks 0, 4 and every 12 weeks or placebo with crossover to ustekinumab at week 12. Among 102 patients with nail psoriasis, the improvements in NAPSI scores were significant at week 12 and continued to increase from week 12 to 64, with reductions of 57% at 45 mg group and 68% at 90 mg group at week 64. In a study of 27 patients with moderate-to-severe plaque psoriasis with nail involvement, excellent response to ustekinumab was demonstrated. NAPSI scores were improved by 42.5% at week 16, by 86.3% at week 28, and by 100% at week 40 [66]. Ustekinumab was also reported to be effective in a case of paradoxical psoriasis with severe scalp and nail involvement, which developed after adalimumab therapy for psoriatic arthritis [76]. In a recently published case series of 13 patients, who had been previously treated with at least four biologics with disappointing results, the patients received ustekinumab either as 90 mg monotherapy or 45 mg in combination with either methotrexate or cyclosporine. The mean percentage of reduction of the NAPSI score was 31.8% at week 12. Two patients treated in combination with cyclosporine 100 mg b.i.d. had complete resolution of their nail psoriasis at week 12 [67]. After longer term safety and efficacy are proven, ustekinumab could become an effective option for treatment of nail psoriasis.

Briakinumab, like ustekinumab, is a monoclonal antibody against p40 subunit of cytokines IL-12 and IL-23. It is administered subcutaneously. In a RCT of 317 patients with psoriasis, patients were randomized to receive either briakinumab (200 mg at weeks 0 and 4, followed by 100 mg every 4 weeks, from week 8 through 48) or methotrexate (5–25 mg per week, from week 0 through 51). Although the primary end point of the study was to assess the improvement in PASI scores, one of the secondary efficacy end points included the change in the NAPSI scores of the target fingernail, which was significantly lower with the briakinumab group at weeks 24 and 52, as compared with the methotrexate group [69].

All biologic agents currently available for the treatment of plaque psoriasis seem to be efficient in treating severe nail psoriasis, although no particular agent is approved for this purpose [7]. In an expert panel, participants strongly agreed that full nail clearance is an achievable goal using biologic therapy in psoriatic patients with nail involvement [52]. However, long-term safety data regarding use of this class of therapy is still being explored, and therefore the possible risks of treatment should be carefully weighted [52]. Most of the studies evaluating the efficacy of biologic agents in nail psoriasis are preliminary [77]. Among these only infliximab and golimumab were evaluated in RCTs, and significant improvements in nail psoriasis were achieved when compared to placebo [62, 70]. Of note, in the phase II trial of ixekizumab, an anti-IL-17 monoclonal antibody for chronic plaque psoriasis, significant improvements in NAPSI scores were reported as early as at 2 weeks with an impressive safety profile [78].

## 8. Treatment of Nail Psoriasis in Children

Despite the common onset of psoriasis in the childhood, validated clinical data on the epidemiology and the treatment of pediatric nail psoriasis is scant. In a recent multicenter study conducted in US, 39.2% of 181 children with psoriasis were found to have nail involvement [79]. Similar results were reported from Kuwait (37.81%), although in more than half of the cases the changes, pitting being the most common, were so subtle that the children were not aware of them [80]. Nail psoriasis was found to be more common in boys, probably related to koebnerization [78, 79]. There are no studies on the efficacy and safety of various treatments for nail psoriasis in children. The absence of clinical data corresponds with a lack of licensure for the pediatric use of many available treatments [81].

Data was available for the treatment of nail psoriasis from an epidemiologic study of pediatric psoriasis from Turkey. Thirteen children with nail psoriasis were treated with potent topical steroid ointments for onycholysis and nail bed hyperkeratosis; however, the results were unsatisfactory [82]. In a pilot study of 4 children to determine the efficacy of intralesional triamcinolone acetonide in the treatment of nail pitting in children, following a single dose, the degree of

pitting was reduced by a mean of 15% in the second month and 42% in the fourth month [83].

In one case report, solely of nail psoriasis in a 6-year-old girl, tazarotene 0.05% gel daily applied for 8 weeks was found to be effective, especially in nail bed hyperkeratosis [84]. A 13-year-old girl with a 3-year history of episodic pustular eruption of the right thumb and psoriasiform changes on the fingers of the right hand, with a clinical diagnosis of Acrodermatitis Continua of Hallopeau, responded well to topical application of 0.1 mg/mL indigo naturalis extract oil [85]. Indigo naturalis, a Chinese herbal remedy extracted from the leaves of indigo-bearing plants, has been demonstrated to have antipsoriatic effects. Another case report of Acrodermatitis Continua of Hallopeau, in a 2-year-old boy, revealing severe nail dystrophy of 19 nails, which was resistant to occluded clobetasol and pimecrolimus and oral acitretin and methotrexate, was reported to demonstrate an excellent response to the combined treatment of thalidomide (50 mg/day for 5 months) and broad band ultraviolet B comb (2 months) [86].

In pediatric nail psoriasis, a combination of calcipotriene (calcipotriol) and betamethasone dipropionate seems to be a rational and simple approach, as both substances have shown to be safe and efficient in children [87].

## 9. Conclusions

Since severe psoriatic nail disease can lead to functional or emotional impairment, even as a sole manifestation of psoriasis, treatment should be individualized for each patient. Topical approaches or laser treatments may be suitable for limited disease or may take part in combination therapies for more severe disease, while classical systemic agents or biologic treatments are preserved for severe cases with extensive cutaneous disease or psoriatic arthritis.

## Conflict of Interests

The authors declare that they have no conflict of interests.

## References

[1] M. M. Jiaravuthisan, D. Sasseville, R. B. Vender, F. Murphy, and C. Y. Muhn, "Psoriasis of the nail: anatomy, pathology, clinical presentation, and a review of the literature on therapy," *Journal of the American Academy of Dermatology*, vol. 57, no. 1, pp. 1–27, 2007.

[2] M. Augustin, K. Krüger, M. A. Radtke, I. Schwippl, and K. Reich, "Disease severity, quality of life and health care in plaque-type psoriasis: a multicenter cross-sectional study in Germany," *Dermatology*, vol. 216, no. 4, pp. 366–372, 2008.

[3] S. Armesto, A. Esteve, P. Coto-Segura et al., "Nail psoriasis in individuals with psoriasis vulgaris: a study of 661 patients," *Actas Dermo-Sifiliográficas*, vol. 102, no. 5, pp. 365–372, 2011.

[4] G. Wozel, "Psoriasis treatment in difficult locations: scalp, nails, and intertriginous areas," *Clinics in Dermatology*, vol. 26, no. 5, pp. 448–459, 2008.

[5] Z. Hallaji, F. Babaeijandaghi, M. Akbarzadeh et al., "A significant association exists between the severity of nail and skin

involvement in psoriasis," *Journal of the American Academy of Dermatology*, vol. 66, pp. e12–e13, 2012.

[6] M. Augustin, K. Reich, C. Blome, I. Schäfer, A. Laass, and M. A. Radtke, "Nail psoriasis in Germany: epidemiology and burden of disease," *British Journal of Dermatology*, vol. 163, no. 3, pp. 580–585, 2010.

[7] L. Dehesa and A. Tosti, "Treatment of inflammatory nail disorders," *Dermatology and Therapy*, vol. 25, pp. 525–534, 2012.

[8] E. S. Tan, W. S. Chong, and H. L. Tey, "Nail psoriasis: a review," *American Journal of Clinical Dermatology*, vol. 13, pp. 375–388, 2012.

[9] D. de Berker, "Management of psoriatic nail disease," *Seminars in Cutaneous Medicine and Surgery*, vol. 28, no. 1, pp. 39–43, 2009.

[10] A. K. Gupta, C. W. Lynde, H. C. Jain et al., "A higher prevalence of onychomycosis in psoriatics compared with non-psoriatics: a multicentre study," *British Journal of Dermatology*, vol. 136, no. 5, pp. 786–789, 1997.

[11] H. Maejima, T. Taniguchi, A. Watarai, and K. Katsuoka, "Evaluation of nail disease in psoriatic arthritis by using a modified nail psoriasis severity score index," *International Journal of Dermatology*, vol. 49, no. 8, pp. 901–906, 2010.

[12] P. J. Mease, "Measures of psoriatic arthritis: Tender and Swollen Joint Assessment, Psoriasis Area and Severity Index (PASI), Nail Psoriasis Severity Index (NAPSI), Modified Nail Psoriasis Severity Index (mNAPSI), Mander/Newcastle Enthesitis Index (MEI), Leeds Enthesitis Index (LEI), Spondyloarthritis Research Consortium of Canada (SPARCC), Maastricht Ankylosing Spondylitis Enthesis Score (MASES), Leeds Dactylitis Index (LDI), Patient Global for Psoriatic Arthritis, Dermatology Life Quality Index (DLQI), Psoriatic Arthritis Quality of Life (PsAQOL), Functional Assessment of Chronic Illness Therapy-Fatigue (FACIT-F), Psoriatic Arthritis Response Criteria (PsARC), Psoriatic Arthritis Joint Activity Index (PsAJAI), Disease Activity in Psoriatic Arthritis (DAPSA), and Composite Psoriatic Disease Activity Index (CPDAI)," *Arthritis Care & Research*, vol. 63, pp. S64–S85, 2011.

[13] P. Rich and R. K. Scher, "Nail psoriasis severity index: a useful tool for evaluation of nail psoriasis," *Journal of the American Academy of Dermatology*, vol. 49, no. 2, pp. 206–212, 2003.

[14] M. M. Mukai, I. F. Poffo, B. Werner, F. M. Brenner, and J. H. Lima Filho, "NAPSI utilization as an evaluation method of nail psoriasis in patients using acitretin," *Anais Brasileiros de Dermatologia e Sifilografia*, vol. 87, pp. 256–262, 2012.

[15] S. E. Cassell, J. D. Bieber, P. Rich et al., "The modified nail psoriasis severity index: validation of an instrument to assess psoriatic nail involvement in patients with psoriatic arthritis," *Journal of Rheumatology*, vol. 34, no. 1, pp. 123–129, 2007.

[16] A. C. de Vries, N. A. Bogaards, L. Hooft et al., "Interventions for nail psoriasis," *The Cochrane Database of Systematic Reviews*, vol. 1, Article ID CD007633, 2013.

[17] R. C. Nakamura, L. D. Abreu, B. Duque-Estrada, C. Tamler, and A. P. Leverone, "Comparison of nail lacquer clobetasol efficacy at 0.05%, 1% and 8% in nail psoriasis treatment: prospective, controlled and randomized pilot study," *Anais Brasileiros de Dermatologia e Sifilografia*, vol. 87, pp. 203–211, 2012.

[18] C. Fischer-Levancini, M. Sánchez-Regaña, F. Llambí, H. Collgros, V. Expósito-Serrano, and P. Umbert-Millet, "Nail psoriasis: treatment with tazarotene 0.1% hydrophilic ointment," *Actas Dermo-Sifiliográficas*, vol. 103, pp. 725–728, 2012.

[19] C. De Simone, A. Maiorino, F. Tassone, M. D'Agostino, and G. Caldarola, "Tacrolimus 0.1% ointment in nail psoriasis: a randomized controlled open-label study," *Journal of the European Academy of Dermatology and Venereology*, 2012.

[20] T. Y. Tzung, C. Y. Chen, C. Y. Yang, P. Y. Lo, and Y. H. Chen, "Calcipotriol used as monotherapy or combination therapy with betamethasone dipropionate in the treatment of nail psoriasis," *Acta Dermato-Venereologica*, vol. 88, no. 3, pp. 279–280, 2008.

[21] M. Sánchez Regaña, G. Márquez Balbás, and P. Umbert Millet, "Nail psoriasis: a combined treatment with 8% clobetasol nail lacquer and tacalcitol ointment," *Journal of the European Academy of Dermatology and Venereology*, vol. 22, no. 8, pp. 963–969, 2008.

[22] D. Rigopoulos, S. Gregoriou, and A. Katsambas, "Treatment of psoriatic nails with tazarotene cream 0.1% vs. clobetasol propionate 0.05% cream: a double-blind study," *Acta Dermato-Venereologica*, vol. 87, no. 2, pp. 167–168, 2007.

[23] M. S. Regaña, G. M. Ezquerra, P. U. Millet, and F. L. Mateos, "Treatment of nail psoriasis with 8% clobetasol nail lacquer: positive experience in 10 patients," *Journal of the European Academy of Dermatology and Venereology*, vol. 19, no. 5, pp. 573–577, 2005.

[24] S. P. Cannavò, F. Guarneri, M. Vaccaro, F. Borgia, and B. Guarneri, "Treatment of psoriatic nails with topical cyclosporin: a prospective, randomized placebo-controlled study," *Dermatology*, vol. 206, no. 2, pp. 153–156, 2003.

[25] L. Bianchi, R. Soda, L. Diluvio, and S. Chimenti, "Tazarotene 0-1% gel for psoriasis of the fingernails and toenails: an open, prospective study," *British Journal of Dermatology*, vol. 149, no. 1, pp. 207–209, 2003.

[26] D. Rigopoulos, D. Ioannides, N. Prastitis, and A. Katsambas, "Nail psoriasis: a combined treatment using calcipotriol cream and clobetasol propionate cream," *Acta Dermato-Venereologica*, vol. 82, no. 2, p. 140, 2002.

[27] R. K. Scher, M. Stiller, and Y. Isabel Zhu, "Tazarotene 0.1% gel in the treatment of fingernail psoriasis: a double-blind, randomized, vehicle-controlled study," *Cutis*, vol. 68, no. 5, pp. 355–358, 2001.

[28] E. M. G. J. de Jong, H. E. Menke, M. C. G. Van Praag, and P. C. M. Van De Kerkhof, "Dystrophic psoriatic fingernails treated with 1% 5-fluorouracil in a nail penetration-enhancing vehicle: a double-blind study," *Dermatology*, vol. 199, no. 4, pp. 313–318, 1999.

[29] R. Baran and A. Tosti, "Topical treatment of nail psoriasis with a new corticoid-containing nail lacquer formulation," *Journal of Dermatological Treatment*, vol. 10, no. 3, pp. 201–204, 1999.

[30] A. Tosti, B. M. Piraccini, N. Cameli et al., "Calcipotriol ointment in nail psoriasis: a controlled double-blind comparison with betamethasone dipropionate and salicylic acid," *British Journal of Dermatology*, vol. 139, no. 4, pp. 655–659, 1998.

[31] T. Yamamoto, I. Katayama, and K. Nishioka, "Topical anthralin therapy for refractory nail psoriasis," *Journal of Dermatology*, vol. 25, no. 4, pp. 231–233, 1998.

[32] T. Fredriksson, "Topically applied fluorouracil in the treatment of psoriatic nails," *Archives of Dermatology*, vol. 110, no. 5, pp. 735–736, 1974.

[33] N. Usmani and C. Wilson, "A case of nail psoriasis treated with topical calcitriol," *Clinical and Experimental Dermatology*, vol. 31, no. 5, pp. 712–713, 2006.

[34] D. Rigopoulos, S. Gregoriou, E. Belyayeva, G. Larios, G. Kontochristopoulos, and A. Katsambas, "Efficacy and safety of

tacrolimus ointment 0.1% vs. betamethasone 17-valerate 0.1% in the treatment of chronic paronychia: an unblinded randomized study," *British Journal of Dermatology*, vol. 160, no. 4, pp. 858–860, 2009.

[35] A. M. A. Prins, K. Vos, and E. J. F. Franssen, "Instability of topical ciclosporin emulsion for nail psoriasis," *Dermatology*, vol. 215, no. 4, pp. 362–363, 2007.

[36] J. J. Bleeker, "Intralesional triamcinolone acetonide using the Port O Jet and needle injections in localized dermatoses," *British Journal of Dermatology*, vol. 91, no. 1, pp. 97–101, 1974.

[37] H. Saricaoglu, A. Oz, and H. Turan, "Nail psoriasis successfully treated with intralesional methotrexate: case report," *Dermatology*, vol. 222, no. 1, pp. 5–7, 2011.

[38] J. L. Marx and R. K. Scher, "Response of psoriatic nails to oral photochemotherapy," *Archives of Dermatology*, vol. 116, no. 9, pp. 1023–1024, 1980.

[39] D. K. Stern, A. A. Creasey, J. Quijije, and M. G. Lebwohl, "UV-A and UV-B penetration of normal human cadaveric fingernail plate," *Archives of Dermatology*, vol. 147, no. 4, pp. 439–441, 2011.

[40] J. Rados, I. Dobrić, A. Pasić, J. Lipozencić, D. Ledić-Drvar, and G. Stajminger, "Normalization in the appearance of severly damaged psoriatic nails using soft x-rays. A case report," *Acta Dermatovenerologica Croatica*, vol. 15, pp. 27–32, 2007.

[41] Y. Oram, Y. Karincaòlu, E. Koyuncu, and F. Kaharaman, "Pulsed dye laser in the treatment of nail psoriasis," *Dermatologic Surgery*, vol. 36, no. 3, pp. 377–381, 2010.

[42] C. Treewittayapoom, P. Singvahanont, K. Chanprapaph, and E. Haneke, "The effect of different pulse durations in the treatment of nail psoriasis with 595-nm pulsed dye laser: a randomized, double-blind, intrapatient left-to-right study," *Journal of the American Academy of Dermatology*, vol. 66, pp. 807–812, 2012.

[43] M. Fernández-Guarino, A. Harto, M. Sánchez-Ronco, I. García-Morales, and P. Jaén, "Pulsed dye laser vs. photodynamic therapy in the treatment of refractory nail psoriasis: a comparative pilot study," *Journal of the European Academy of Dermatology and Venereology*, vol. 23, no. 8, pp. 891–895, 2009.

[44] M. Sánchez-Regaña, J. Sola-Ortigosa, M. Alsina-Gibert, M. Vidal-Fernández, and P. Umbert-Millet, "Nail psoriasis: a retrospective study on the effectiveness of systemic treatments (classical and biological therapy)," *Journal of the European Academy of Dermatology and Venereology*, vol. 25, no. 5, pp. 579–588, 2011.

[45] M. Gümüşel, M. Özdemir, I. Mevlitoğlu, and S. Bodur, "Evaluation of the efficacy of methotrexate and cyclosporine therapies on psoriatic nails: a one-blind, randomized study," *Journal of the European Academy of Dermatology and Venereology*, vol. 25, pp. 1080–1084, 2011.

[46] A. Tosti, C. Ricotti, P. Romanelli, N. Cameli, and B. M. Piraccini, "Evaluation of the efficacy of acitretin therapy for nail psoriasis," *Archives of Dermatology*, vol. 145, no. 3, pp. 269–271, 2009.

[47] T. Syuto, M. Abe, H. Ishibuchi, and O. Ishikawa, "Successful treatment of psoriatic nails with low-dose cyclosporine administration," *European Journal of Dermatology*, vol. 17, no. 3, pp. 248–249, 2007.

[48] C. Feliciani, A. Zampetti, P. Forleo et al., "Nail psoriasis: combined therapy with systemic cyclosporin and topical calcipotriol," *Journal of Cutaneous Medicine and Surgery*, vol. 8, no. 2, pp. 122–125, 2004.

[49] G. Mahrle, H. J. Schulze, L. Färber, G. Weidinger, and G. K. Steigleder, "Low-dose short-term cyclosporine versus etretinate in psoriasis: improvement of skin, nail, and joint involvement," *Journal of the American Academy of Dermatology*, vol. 32, pp. 78–88, 1995.

[50] F. Ricceri, L. Pescitelli, L. Tripo, A. Bassi, and F. Prignano, "Treatment of severe nail psoriasis with acitretin: an impressive therapeutic result," *Dermatology and Therapy*, vol. 26, pp. 77–78, 2013.

[51] S. Handa, "Newer trends in the management of psoriasis at difficult to treat locations: scalp, palmoplantar disease and nails," *Indian Journal of Dermatology, Venereology and Leprology*, vol. 76, no. 6, pp. 634–644, 2010.

[52] R. G. Langley, J. H. Saurat, and K. Reich, "Nail Psoriasis Delphi Expert Panel. Recommendations for the treatment of nail psoriasis in patients with moderate to severe psoriasis: a dermatology expert group consensus," *Journal of the European Academy of Dermatology and Venereology*, vol. 26, pp. 373–381, 2012.

[53] L. Bianchi, A. Bergamin, C. De Felice, E. Capriotti, and S. Chimenti, "Remission and time of resolution of nail psoriasis during infliximab therapy," *Journal of the American Academy of Dermatology*, vol. 52, no. 4, pp. 736–737, 2005.

[54] P. Rich, C. E. M. Griffiths, K. Reich et al., "Baseline nail disease in patients with moderate to severe psoriasis and response to treatment with infliximab during 1 year," *Journal of the American Academy of Dermatology*, vol. 58, no. 2, pp. 224–231, 2008.

[55] C. Fabroni, A. Gori, M. Troiano, F. Prignano, and T. Lotti, "Infliximab efficacy in nail psoriasis. A retrospective study in 48 patients," *Journal of the European Academy of Dermatology and Venereology*, vol. 25, no. 5, pp. 549–553, 2011.

[56] D. Rigopoulos, S. Gregoriou, A. Stratigos et al., "Evaluation of the efficacy and safety of infliximab on psoriatic nails: an unblinded, nonrandomized, open-label study," *British Journal of Dermatology*, vol. 159, no. 2, pp. 453–456, 2008.

[57] C. Leonardi, R. G. Langley, K. Papp et al., "Adalimumab for treatment of moderate to severe chronic plaque psoriasis of the hands and feet: efficacy and safety results from REACH, a randomized, placebo-controlled, double-blind trial," *Archives of Dermatology*, vol. 147, no. 4, pp. 429–436, 2011.

[58] F. Van den Bosch, B. Manger, P. Goupille et al., "Effectiveness of adalimumab in treating patients with active psoriatic arthritis and predictors of good clinical responses for arthritis, skin and nail lesions," *Annals of the Rheumatic Diseases*, vol. 69, no. 2, pp. 394–399, 2010.

[59] D. Rigopoulos, S. Gregoriou, E. Lazaridou et al., "Treatment of nail psoriasis with adalimumab: an open label unblinded study," *Journal of the European Academy of Dermatology and Venereology*, vol. 24, no. 5, pp. 530–534, 2010.

[60] J. P. Ortonne, C. Paul, E. Berardesca et al., "A 24-week randomized clinical trial investigating the efficacy and safety of two doses of etanercept in nail psoriasis," *The British Journal of Dermatology*, 2012.

[61] T. A. Luger, J. Barker, J. Lambert et al., "Sustained improvement in joint pain and nail symptoms with etanercept therapy in patients with moderate-to-severe psoriasis," *Journal of the European Academy of Dermatology and Venereology*, vol. 23, no. 8, pp. 896–904, 2009.

[62] A. Kavanaugh, I. McInnes, P. Mease et al., "Golimumab, a new human tumor necrosis factor α antibody, administered every four weeks as a subcutaneous injection in psoriatic arthritis: twenty-four-week efficacy and safety results of a randomized, placebo-controlled study," *Arthritis and Rheumatism*, vol. 60, no. 4, pp. 976–986, 2009.

[63] J. E. M. Körver, A. M. G. Langewouters, P. C. M. Van De Kerkhof, and M. C. Pasch, "Therapeutic effects of a 12-week course of alefacept on nail psoriasis," *Journal of the European*

*Academy of Dermatology and Venereology*, vol. 20, no. 10, pp. 1252–1255, 2006.

[64] C. A. Parrish, J. O. Sobera, C. M. Robbins, W. C. Cantrell, R. A. Desmond, and B. E. Elewski, "Alefacept in the treatment of psoriatic nail disease: a proof of concept study," *Journal of drugs in dermatology*, vol. 5, no. 4, pp. 339–340, 2006.

[65] C. T. Cassetty, A. F. Alexis, J. L. Shupack, and B. E. Strober, "Alefacept in the treatment of psoriatic nail disease: a small case series," *Journal of the American Academy of Dermatology*, vol. 52, no. 6, pp. 1101–1102, 2005.

[66] A. Patsatsi, A. Kyriakou, and D. Sotiriadis, "Ustekinumab in nail psoriasis: an open-label, uncontrolled, nonrandomized study," *Journal of Dermatological Treatment*, vol. 24, pp. 96–100, 2013.

[67] M. Vitiello, A. Tosti, A. Abuchar, M. Zaiac, and F. A. Kerdel, "Ustekinumab for the treatment of nail psoriasis in heavily treated psoriatic patients," *International Journal of Dermatology*, vol. 52, pp. 358–362, 2013.

[68] A. Igarashi, T. Kato, M. Kato, M. Song, and H. Nakagawa, "Efficacy and safety of ustekinumab in Japanese patients with moderate-to-severe plaque-type psoriasis: long-term results from a phase 2/3 clinical trial," *Journal of Dermatology*, vol. 39, pp. 242–252, 2012.

[69] K. Reich, R. G. Langley, K. A. Papp et al., "A 52-week trial comparing briakinumab with methotrexate in patients with psoriasis," *The New England Journal of Medicine*, vol. 365, pp. 1586–1596, 2011.

[70] K. Reich, J. P. Ortonne, U. Kerkmann et al., "Skin and nail responses after 1 year of infliximab therapy in patients with moderate-to-severe psoriasis: a retrospective analysis of the EXPRESS trial," *Dermatology*, vol. 221, no. 2, pp. 172–178, 2010.

[71] W. Hussain, I. Coulson, and C. Owen, "Severe recalcitrant nail psoriasis responding dramatically to infliximab: report of two patients," *Clinical and Experimental Dermatology*, vol. 33, no. 4, pp. 520–522, 2008.

[72] E. Rallis, E. Stavropoulou, D. Rigopoulos, and C. Verros, "Rapid response of nail psoriasis to etanercept," *Journal of Rheumatology*, vol. 35, no. 3, pp. 544–545, 2008.

[73] J. D. Coelho, F. Diamantino, S. Lestre, and A. M. Ferreira, "Treatment of severe nail psoriasis with etanercept," *Indian Journal of Dermatology, Venereology and Leprology*, vol. 77, no. 1, pp. 72–74, 2011.

[74] M. Gómez Vázquez and R. Navarra Amayuelas, "Marked improvement in nail psoriasis during treatment with etanercept," *Dermatology and Therapy*, vol. 24, pp. 498–500, 2011.

[75] M. Zaiac, "The role of biological agents in the treatment of nail psoriasis," *American Journal of Clinical Dermatology*, vol. 11, no. 1, pp. 27–29, 2010.

[76] L. Puig, C. E. Morales-Múnera, A. López-Ferrer, and C. Geli, "Ustekinumab treatment of TNF antagonist-induced paradoxical psoriasis flare in a patient with psoriatic arthritis: case report and review," *Dermatology*, vol. 225, pp. 14–17, 2012.

[77] T. Hermanns-Lê, E. Berardesca, G. E. Piérard, M. Lesuisse, and C. Piérard-Franchimont, "Challenging regional psoriasis and ustekinumab biotherapy: impact of the patterns of disease," *Journal of Biomedicine and Biotechnology*, vol. 2012, Article ID 413767, 6 pages, 2012.

[78] C. Leonardi, R. Matheson, C. Zachariae et al., "Anti-interleukin-17 monoclonal antibody ixekizumab in chronic plaque psoriasis," *The New England Journal of Medicine*, vol. 366, pp. 1190–1199, 2012.

[79] K. Mercy, M. Kwasny, K. M. Cordoro et al., "Clinical manifestations of pediatric psoriasis: results of a multicenter study in the United States," *Pediatric Dermatology*, 2013.

[80] N. Al-Mutairi, Y. Manchanda, and O. Nour-Eldin, "Nail changes in childhood psoriasis: a study from Kuwait," *Pediatric Dermatology*, vol. 24, no. 1, pp. 7–10, 2007.

[81] M. Ståhle, N. Atakan, W. H. Boehncke et al., "Juvenile psoriasis and its clinical management: a European expert group consensus," *Journal of the German Society of Dermatology*, vol. 8, no. 10, pp. 812–819, 2010.

[82] M. Seyhan, B. K. Coşkun, H. Sağlam, H. Özcan, and Y. Karincaoğlu, "Psoriasis in childhood and adolescence: evaluation of demographic and clinical features," *Pediatrics International*, vol. 48, no. 6, pp. 525–530, 2006.

[83] B. P. Khoo and Y. C. Giam, "A pilot study on the role of intralesional triamcinolone acetonide in the treatment of pitted nails in children," *Singapore Medical Journal*, vol. 41, no. 2, pp. 66–68, 2000.

[84] L. Diluvio, E. Campione, E. J. Paternò, C. Mordenti, M. E. Hachem, and S. Chimenti, "Childhood nail psoriasis: a useful treatment with tazarotene 0.05%," *Pediatric Dermatology*, vol. 24, no. 3, pp. 332–333, 2007.

[85] C. Y. Liang, T. Y. Lin, and Y. K. Lin, "Successful treatment of pediatric nail psoriasis with periodic pustular eruption using topical indigo naturalis oil extract," *Pediatric Dermatology*, vol. 30, pp. 117–119, 2013.

[86] A. E. Kiszewski, D. De Villa, I. Scheibel, and N. Ricachnevsky, "An infant with acrodermatitis continua of hallopeau: successful treatment with thalidomide and UVB therapy," *Pediatric Dermatology*, vol. 26, no. 1, pp. 105–106, 2009.

[87] B. Richert and J. André, "Nail disorders in children: diagnosis and management," *American Journal of Clinical Dermatology*, vol. 12, no. 2, pp. 101–112, 2011.

# 5

# Patch Testing in Suspected Allergic Contact Dermatitis to Cosmetics

**Pramod Kumar[1] and Rekha Paulose[2]**

[1] *Dermatology Department, KMC Hospital, Manipal University, Attavar, Mangalore 575 001, India*
[2] *Ahalia Hospital, P.O. Box 2419, Abu Dhabi, UAE*

Correspondence should be addressed to Pramod Kumar; pkderm@hotmail.com

Academic Editor: Masutaka Furue

*Background.* Increasing use of cosmetics has contributed to a rise in the incidence of allergic contact dermatitis (ACD) to cosmetics. It is estimated that 1–5.4% of the population is sensitized to a cosmetic ingredient. Patch testing helps to confirm the presence of an allergy and to identify the actual allergens which are chemical mixtures of various ingredients. *Objectives.* The aims of this study are to perform patch testing in suspected ACD to cosmetics and to identify the most common allergen and cosmetic product causing dermatitis. *Methods.* Fifty patients with suspected ACD to cosmetics were patch-tested with 38 antigens of the Indian Cosmetic Series and 12 antigens of the Indian Standard Series. *Results.* The majority (58%) of patients belonged to the 21–40 years age group. The presence of ACD to cosmetics was confirmed in 38 (76%) patients. Face creams (20%), hair dyes (14%), and soaps (12%) were the most commonly implicated. The most common allergens identified were gallate mix (40%), cetrimide (28%), and thiomersal (20%). Out of a total of 2531 patches applied, positive reactions were obtained in 3.75%. *Conclusion.* Incidence of ACD to cosmetics was greater in females. Face creams and hair dyes were the most common cosmetic products implicated. The principal allergens were gallate mix, cetrimide, and thiomersal.

## 1. Introduction

"Cosmetics" are preparations for beautifying the complexion, skin, hair, and nails. They are defined as "articles intended to be rubbed, poured, or sprayed on, introduced into, or otherwise applied to the human body or any part thereof for cleansing, beautifying, promoting attractiveness, or altering the appearance without affecting the body's structure or functions" [1].

The strong desire of individuals to improve their appearance using topical applications has resulted in the production of a variety of cosmetics throughout the world. The majority of these substances are synthetic in nature with ingredients capable of causing sensitization of the skin, thus contributing to the increased incidence of cosmetic dermatitis [2].

It is estimated that 1–5.4% of the population is sensitized to a cosmetic or cosmetic ingredient [2–4]. About 80% of reactions occur in patients aged 20–60 years and are seen more frequently in women [2, 4]. An epidemiologic survey in the UK revealed that 23% of women and 18.8% of men experience some sort of adverse reaction to a personal care product over one year [5]. Commonly used cosmetics like soaps, creams, lipsticks, foundations, sunscreens, perfumes, and eye, hair, and nail cosmetics can cause allergic contact dermatitis. The most frequently identified allergens are fragrances and preservatives [2]. Fragrance in various forms is one of the most common causes of allergies. Fragrance is used in almost all skin care products, cosmetics, and also domestic cleaning agents. This has led to a high incidence of fragrance sensitization [6].

## 2. Materials and Methods

Fifty cases with suspected allergic contact dermatitis (ACD) to cosmetics were included in the study. Cases included those with cosmetic dermatitis affecting a site of application or contact with one or more cosmetics and history of precipitation or exacerbation of the dermatitis with cosmetic use. Patients with active dermatitis were excluded from patch testing until

TABLE 1: List of antigens used (1–38 Cosmetic Series, 39–50 Standard Series).

| Number | Antigen |
|--------|---------|
| 1 | Control |
| 2 | Amercholl |
| 3 | Benzyl alcohol |
| 4 | Benzyl salicylate |
| 5 | Bronopol |
| 6 | Butylated hydroxyl anisole |
| 7 | Butylated hydroxyl toluene |
| 8 | Cetyl alcohol |
| 9 | Chloroacetamide |
| 10 | Chloroxylenol |
| 11 | Gallate mix |
| 12 | Geranium oil |
| 13 | Oxybenzone |
| 14 | Benzotriazole |
| 15 | Imidazolidinyl urea |
| 16 | Isopropyl myristate |
| 17 | Jasmine absolute |
| 18 | Lavender absolute |
| 19 | Musk mix |
| 20 | Phenyl salicylate |
| 21 | Polyxyethylenesorbitoal oleate |
| 22 | Rose oil |
| 23 | Sorbic acid |
| 24 | Sorbitan monooleate |
| 25 | Sorbitan sesquioleate |
| 26 | Stearyl alcohol |
| 27 | *tert*-Butylhydroquinone |
| 28 | Thiomersal |
| 29 | Triclosan |
| 30 | Triethanolamine |
| 31 | Vanillin |
| 32 | Cetrimide |
| 33 | Jasmine synthetic |
| 34 | Hexamine |
| 35 | Diazolidinyl urea |
| 36 | Chlorhexidine digluconate |
| 37 | Phenyl mercuric acetate |
| 38 | Cocamidopropyl betaine |
| 39 | Fragrance mix |
| 40 | Parabens |
| 41 | Propylene glycol |
| 42 | PEG-400 |
| 43 | Chlorocresol |
| 44 | Wool alcohol |
| 45 | Balsam of Peru |
| 46 | Kathon CG |
| 47 | Ethylenediamine dihydrochloride |
| 48 | Quarternium15 |
| 49 | Formaldehyde |
| 50 | 4-Phenylenediamine |

the dermatitis subsided. A detailed history regarding symptoms and cutaneous lesions was taken. Information regarding cosmetics used, duration of use, frequency of application, and precipitation or exacerbation of the dermatitis on cosmetic use was noted.

Patch testing was performed in all cases with a total of 50 allergens (Table 1), 38 allergens of the Cosmetic Series and 12 allergens of the Indian Standard Series which are common constituents of cosmetics, as per the recommendations of CODFI (Contact and Occupational Dermatoses Forum of India). The patch test kit was procured by order from Systopic Laboratories Pvt. Ltd., New Delhi. The kit consists of 42 solid allergens and 8 liquid allergens. Wherever indicated, the suspected cosmetic itself was used.

Five patch test units each consisting of ten aluminum chambers mounted on microporous tape were required per patient. The allergens were applied as 5 mm length of solid allergen from the syringes or one full drop of liquid allergen on a filter paper disc on the chamber.

After explaining the procedure in detail to the patient, informed consent was taken. The back of the patient was cleaned with spirit and five patch test units with a total of fifty antigens were applied, four on the upper back and one on the lower back. Wherever possible, a sample of the cosmetic suspected to cause the dermatitis was also included in the patch test.

The patch test units were removed after 48 hours (D2) and readings were taken one hour after removal. The patch test reactions were read according to the recommendations of the International Contact Dermatitis Research Group. The diagnosis of ACD to cosmetics was confirmed based on a positive result.

Photopatch testing and reading at D3 and D7 were not done.

## 3. Results

Age of the patients in the study group ranged from 13 to 67 years. The majority of patients were in the 21–40 years age group (58%). Among males, the majority (31.58%) belonged to the 41–50 years age group while among females the majority (38.71%) belonged to the 21–30 years age group. There were 19 males and 31 females with male : female ratio of 1 : 1.63.

The total duration of dermatitis was less than 1 year in 30 (60%) patients. The minimum duration was 1 month and the maximum duration was 20 years. The mean duration was found to be 23 months.

The most common symptom in both males and females was itching which was present in 17 (89.4%) of males and 28 (90.32%) of females. Other common symptoms were photosensitivity and burning which were present in 21 (42%) and 10 (20%) of the patients, respectively. A higher percentage of males (63.16%) gave history of photosensitivity as compared to females (29.03%). Atopy or asthma was present in 8 (16%) patients, which included 4 males and 4 females.

The face was the most common site of involvement in both males (47.37%) and females (61.29%). Face and neck (21.05%) and scalp (10.53%) were more commonly involved in males, while hands (9.68%) were more commonly involved in females.

TABLE 2: Results of patch testing with patient's own cosmetics.

| Suspected cosmetic | Patients tested | | | Positivity | | | Suspected antigens |
|---|---|---|---|---|---|---|---|
| | M | F | Total | M | F | Total | |
| Face cream | 1 | 12 | 13 | 1 | 7 | 8 | Gallate mix, cetrimide, and thiomersal |
| Hair dye | 7 | — | 7 | 5 | — | 5 | Paraphenylenediamine and gallate mix |
| Shaving cream | 5 | — | 5 | 5 | — | 5 | Gallate mix and cetrimide |
| Perfume | — | 2 | 2 | — | — | — | Thiomersal and gallate mix |
| Nail polish | — | 1 | 1 | — | 1 | 1 | Gallate mix and *tert*-butylhydroquinone |
| Foundation cream | — | 1 | 1 | — | 1 | 1 | Gallate mix and cetrimide |
| Kumkum/bindi | — | 2 | 2 | — | 1 | 1 | *Paraphenylene*diamine |

The most common lesions in both males and females were erythema and papules. The most common secondary lesions in males were hyperpigmentation (26.32%) and crusting (26.32%) and in females the most common secondary lesions were scaling (41.94%) and hyperpigmentation (29.03%). Secondary infection of the lesions was present in 7 (14%) patients.

Soap was the most common cosmetic used in both males (84.21%) and females (100%). Other cosmetics commonly used in males were hair dyes (52.63%), shaving creams (68.42%), and shampoos (31.58%). Frequently used cosmetics in females were face creams (70.97%), perfumes (41.94%), and shampoos (54.84%). Bulk of males (42.11%) had suspected allergy to hair dye, whereas face creams (45.16%) were the most commonly suspected cosmetics in females. Eighty percent of hair dye users had assumed ACD to hair dye. Incidence of ACD among users of face creams (60%), shaving creams (46.15%), and perfumes (26.32%) was also high.

Allergic contact dermatitis was confirmed in 38 cases (76%) of the study group who had positive patch test reactions, either antigens of the Cosmetic Series or the suspected cosmetic product or both. Overall, 84.21% of males and 70.97% of females had allergy to cosmetics.

In the study group, face creams (20%), hair dyes (14%), and soaps (12%) were the most common cosmetics causing allergic contact dermatitis. Shaving creams (10%), perfumes (8%), and lipsticks (4%) were the other common cosmetics identified.

On performing patch tests with the Standard Cosmetic Series in the study group, the most common antigens giving positive reactions were gallate mix (40%), cetrimide (28%), thiomersal (20%), and paraphenylenediamine (14%). On comparing positive reactions in males and females, gallate mix was the most common allergen in both groups, 47.37% and 35.48%, respectively. Other common allergens in males were cetrimide (31.58%) and paraphenylenediamine (31.58%). Cetrimide (25.81%) and thiomersal (22.58%) were the other common allergens in females.

Thirty-one patients were patch-tested with their personal cosmetics (Table 2). Twenty-two patients (71%) gave a positive reaction, thus confirming the presence of allergic contact dermatitis to cosmetics. On correlating the positive reactions to the suspected cosmetic and the positive reactions to ingredients of cosmetics, a definite causal link was established in many cases. Gallate mix was the most commonly identified allergen in face creams, paraphenylenediamine in hair dyes, gallate mix and cetrimide in shaving creams, and thiomersal in perfumes. Face creams and hair dyes gave maximum number of positive reactions in females and males, respectively.

Among the positive reactions, "1+" reactions were the most common, occurring in 67 (70.53%) patches. "2+" reactions and "3+" reactions were seen in 16 (16.84%) and 12 (12.63%) patches, respectively. Out of a total of 2531 patches applied, positive reactions were obtained in 3.75% (95/2531) patches.

## 4. Discussion

In our study of 50 patients, 19 (38%) were males and 31 (62%) were females. The male : female ratio was 1 : 1.63. Allergic contact dermatitis to cosmetics is more common in females as compared to males [2]; this was also observed in our study where females outnumbered males. In a cross-sectional retrospective study done by the North American Contact Dermatitis Group, the site and category of cosmetics differed somewhat by gender [7].

Age of the patients in the study group ranged from 13 to 67 years. In a study conducted by Adams and Maibach [8], the majority of patients with cosmetic reactions were distributed over the age group 20 to 60 years. In this study, the majority of patients (58%) belonged to the age group of 21–40 years. The majority of males (31.58%) belonged to the 41–50 years age group, whereas the majority of females (38.71%) belonged to the 21–30 years age group. The reason for this could be that the majority of males in the study had allergy to hair dyes which in most cases were first used after the age of 30 years.

Adams and Maibach [8] reported that the duration of the dermatitis prior to consulting the dermatologist was 8 days or longer in nearly all cases. In our study, the duration of dermatitis was less than one year in sixty percent of patients. Itching, which is a manifestation of allergy, was present in 45 (90%) patients of the study group. Other symptoms included photosensitivity (42%), burning (20%), pain (6%), and oozing (4%). A higher percentage of males (63.16%) gave history of photosensitivity as compared to females (29.03%). Photopatch testing was, however, not done in this study as it was out of scope of this protocol. de Groot et al. [9] reported that itching was the most frequent subjective symptom in patients with contact allergy to cosmetics.

The face is the most frequently involved site of cosmetic dermatitis [10]. In this study, face was involved in 56% of cases followed by face along with neck in 10%, face and hands in 8%, and only hands in 6%. Other sites included neck (4%) and scalp (4%). Face was the most common site affected in both males (47.37%) and females (61.29%). Face and neck (21.05%) and scalp (10.53%), the sites for hair dye allergy, were commonly involved in males, whereas hands (9.68%) were exclusively involved in females.

de Groot et al. [9] found that the most frequently reported objective symptom was erythema (61%) followed by scaling (19.3%) and pimples (14.2%). In our study, erythema (52%) was the most common objective symptom followed by papules in 40% and scaling in 34%. Other common primary lesions included plaques (20%), macules (18%), vesicles (10%), and pustules (6%). Secondary lesions commonly seen included hyperpigmentation (28%), crusting (12%), hypopigmentation (10%), and excoriation (10%).

Soap was the most common cosmetic used in both males (84.21%) and females (100%). Other commonly used cosmetics included face creams (50%), shampoos (64%), perfumes (38%), and bindi/sindoor/kumkum (32%). The prevalence of face cream usage was high in the females of the study group (70.97%), whereas hair dye usage was common in males (52.63%).

Mehta and Reddy [11] in their study on the pattern of cosmetic sensitivity in Indian patients reported that bindi, hair dye, and face creams were the most commonly suspected cosmetics in contact dermatitis due to cosmetics. In our study, face creams (30%), hair dyes (16%), and soaps (14%) were the most frequently suspected cosmetics. Males (42.11%) commonly suspected allergy to hair dye whereas females (45.16%) suspected allergy to face cream. The incidence of suspected allergic contact dermatitis was the highest among hair dye users (80%). High incidence was also seen in users of face creams (60%), shaving creams (46.15%), and perfumes (26.32%).

Several studies [10–12] have reported that skin care products (moisturizing and cleansing cream/lotion/milk) account for the majority of cases of contact allergy to cosmetics. This was confirmed in our study where face creams (20%) were the most common cosmetic causing allergic contact dermatitis. Other common cosmetics causing allergy were hair dye

(14%), soap (12%), shaving cream (10%), and perfume (8%). Hair dye, shaving cream, and perfume were the common causative agents in males, whereas face cream, soap, perfume, and lipstick were the common causative agents in females.

The most frequently identified cosmetic allergens are fragrances and preservatives [2]. In our study, gallate mix, an antioxidant, was the most common allergen. It was positive in 40% of the study group. This is probably due to the presence of propyl gallate as an antioxidant in skin creams. The other common allergens in cosmetics identified by patch testing included cetrimide (28%), thiomersal (20%), and paraphenylenediamine (14%).

In thirty-one patients, the suspected cosmetics were also included in the patch test. The cosmetics were tested "as is." Twenty-two patients (71%) gave a positive reaction to the suspected cosmetic, thus confirming the presence of cosmetic contact dermatitis. In a study conducted by Mehta and Reddy [11], patch testing with suspected cosmetics gave positive results in 50% of patients. In four cases, patients had one or more positive reactions to antigens of the cosmetic series but did not react to the suspected cosmetic product. The reason for this probably could be that the concentration of the antigen in the cosmetic was too low to elicit a positive patch test reaction.

An attempt was made to correlate the positive results of the cosmetics tested and the ingredients of cosmetics. A definite causal link was obtained in some cases such as face cream with gallate mix, shaving cream with gallate mix and cetrimide, hair dye with paraphenylenediamine, and perfume with thiomersal. Propyl gallate is an allergen in liposome containing skin creams [13]. The majority of allergy to hair dyes is caused by PPD [13].

In a study on adverse reactions to cosmetics by Dogra et al. [14], out of 2065 patches applied, positive results were obtained in 3.2% patches with standard cosmetic kit and 3.3% patches with various cosmetics. Out of a total number of 2531 patches applied in our study, positive reactions were obtained in 3.75% (95/2531) patches.

A study in Seoul found that not all antigens that are found in cosmetics are actually available in patch test kits and that these could be potential allergens which go undetected; hence, a need for regular modification of testing kits to reflect ingredients in the cosmetics is advocated [15]. In India, a study on pediatric contact dermatitis revealed that children could be sensitive to some of the cosmetic antigens and the sensitization may happen due to early age of cosmetic use [16]. Citrus being a very commonly used substance in fragrance industries should be tested for in all those who have a positive reaction to fragrance mix [17].

## 5. Conclusion

In a short communication on this study, the authors [18] highlighted the necessity for patch testing and careful use of cosmetics in India. Recent studies suggest increased incidence of cosmetic dermatitis and also of newer antigens that cause allergies [19, 20]. Patch testing is an important investigation in patients with suspected allergic contact dermatitis to cosmetics and remains a gold standard [21, 22]. In a growing economy like that of India where the market for cosmetics especially fairness creams and hair cosmetics is in high demand, the reports on cosmetic dermatitis are insignificant [23, 24]. The authors would like to make more detailed analysis and interpretation of their study to emphasize the importance of patch testing in all suspected cases and recommend use of the suspected cosmetic itself for patch testing.

## Disclosure

Part of this study has been published earlier as a short communication and cited in this paper. This is the detailed analysis and presentation of complete work.

## Conflict of Interests

The authors declare that there is no conflict of interests regarding the publication of this paper.

## References

[1] W. G. Larsen, E. M. Jackson, M. O. Barker et al., "A primer on cosmetics," *Journal of the American Academy of Dermatology*, vol. 27, pp. 469–481, 1992.

[2] S. Singh and B. S. N. Reddy, "Cosmetic dermatitis—current perspectives," *International Journal of Dermatology*, vol. 42, no. 7, pp. 533–542, 2003.

[3] M. H. Beck and S. M. Wilkinson, "Contact dermatitis," in *Rook's Textbook of Dermatology*, T. Burns, S. Breathnach, N. Cox, and C. Griffiths, Eds., pp. 20.1–20.124, Blackwell Science, Oxford, UK, 7th edition, 2004.

[4] H. I. Maibach and P. G. Engasser, "Dermatitis due to cosmetics," in *Contact Dermatitis*, A. A. Fisher, Ed., pp. 368–393, Lea & Febiger, Philadelphia, Pa, USA, 3rd edition, 1986.

[5] D. I. Orton and J. D. Wilkinson, "Cosmetic allergy: incidence, diagnosis, and management," *American Journal of Clinical Dermatology*, vol. 5, no. 5, pp. 327–337, 2004.

[6] P. L. Scheinman, "Allergic contact dermatitis to fragrance: a review," *The American Journal of Contact Dermatitis*, vol. 7, no. 2, pp. 65–76, 1996.

[7] E. M. Warshaw, H. J. Buchholz, D. V. Belsito et al., "Allergic patch test reactions associated with cosmetics: retrospective analysis of cross-sectional data from the North American Contact Dermatitis Group, 2001–2004," *Journal of the American Academy of Dermatology*, vol. 60, no. 1, pp. 23–38, 2009.

[8] R. M. Adams and H. I. Maibach, "A five-year study of cosmetic reactions," *Journal of the American Academy of Dermatology*, vol. 13, no. 6, pp. 1062–1069, 1985.

[9] A. C. de Groot, E. G. A. Beverdam, C. T. Ayong, P. J. Coenraads, and J. P. Nater, "The role of contact allergy in the spectrum of adverse effects caused by cosmetics and toiletries," *Contact Dermatitis*, vol. 19, no. 3, pp. 195–201, 1988.

[10] A. C. De Groot, "Contact allergy to cosmetics: causative ingredients," *Contact Dermatitis*, vol. 17, no. 1, pp. 26–34, 1987.

[11] S. S. Mehta and B. S. N. Reddy, "Pattern of cosmetic sensitivity in Indian patients," *Contact Dermatitis*, vol. 45, no. 5, pp. 292–293, 2001.

[12] A. C. de Groot, D. P. Bruynzeel, J. D. Bos et al., "The allergens in cosmetics," *Archives of Dermatology*, vol. 124, no. 10, pp. 1525–1529, 1988.

[13] R. L. Rietschel and J. F. Fowler, "Allergy to preservatives and vehicles in cosmetics and toiletries," in *Fisher's Contact Dermatitis*, R. L. Rietschel and J. F. Fowler, Eds., pp. 211–259, Lippincott Williams & Wilkins, Philadelphia, Pa, USA, 5th edition, 2001.

[14] A. Dogra, Y. Minocha, and S. Kaur, "Adverse reactions to cosmetics," *Indian Journal of Dermatology, Venereology and Leprology*, vol. 69, no. 2, pp. 165–167, 2003.

[15] S. H. Cheong, Y. W. Choi, K. B. Myung, and H. Y. Choi, "Comparison of marketed cosmetic products constituents with the antigens included in cosmetic-related patch test," *Annals of Dermatology*, vol. 22, no. 3, pp. 262–268, 2010.

[16] V. K. Sharma and D. P. Asati, "Pediatric contact dermatitis," *Indian Journal of Dermatology, Venereology and Leprology*, vol. 76, no. 5, pp. 514–520, 2010.

[17] A. Swerdlin, D. Rainey, and F. J. Storrs, "Fragrance mix reactions and lime allergic contact dermatitis," *Dermatitis*, vol. 21, no. 4, pp. 214–216, 2010.

[18] P. Kumar and R. Paulose, "Cosmetic dermatitis in an Indian city," *Contact Dermatitis*, vol. 55, no. 2, pp. 114–115, 2006.

[19] J. Zhao and L.-F. Li, "Contact sensitization to cosmetic series of allergens in a general population in Beijing," *Journal of Cosmetic Dermatology*, vol. 13, no. 1, pp. 68–71, 2014.

[20] M. E. Park and J. H. Zippin, "Allergic contact dermatitis to cosmetics," *Dermatologic Clinics*, vol. 32, no. 1, pp. 1–11, 2014.

[21] T. Hamilton and G. C. de Gannes, "Allergic contact dermatitis to preservatives and fragrances in cosmetics," *Skin Therapy Letter*, vol. 16, no. 4, pp. 1–4, 2011.

[22] J. I. Alani, M. D. P. Davis, and J. A. Yiannias, "Allergy to cosmetics: a literature review," *Dermatitis*, vol. 24, no. 6, pp. 283–290, 2013.

[23] A. K. Nath and D. M. Thappa, "Clinical spectrum of dermatoses caused by cosmetics in south India: high prevalence of kumkum dermatitis," *Indian Journal of Dermatology, Venereology and Leprology*, vol. 73, no. 3, pp. 195–196, 2007.

[24] N. Sarma and S. Ghosh, "Clinico-allergological pattern of allergic contact dermatitis among 70 Indian children," *Indian Journal of Dermatology, Venereology and Leprology*, vol. 76, no. 1, pp. 38–44, 2010.

# 6

# Pathogenesis of Chronic Urticaria: An Overview

**Sanjiv Jain**

*Skin Care Clinic, 108 Darya Ganj, New Delhi 110002, India*

Correspondence should be addressed to Sanjiv Jain; drsanjivjain@yahoo.com

Academic Editor: Lajos Kemeny

The pathogenesis of chronic urticaria is not well delineated and the treatment is palliative as it is not tied to the pathomechanism. The centrality of mast cells and their inappropriate activation and degranulation as the key pathophysiological event are well established. The triggering stimuli and the complexity of effector mechanisms remain speculative. Autoimmune origin of chronic urticaria, albeit controversial, is well documented. Numerical and behavioral alterations in basophils accompanied by changes in signaling molecule expression and function as well as aberrant activation of extrinsic pathway of coagulation are other alternative hypotheses. It is also probable that mast cells are involved in the pathogenesis through mechanisms that extend beyond high affinity IgE receptor stimulation. An increasing recognition of chronic urticaria as an immune mediated inflammatory disorder related to altered cytokine-chemokine network consequent to immune dysregulation resulting from disturbed innate immunity is emerging as yet another pathogenic explanation. It is likely that these different pathomechanisms are interlinked rather than independent cascades, acting either synergistically or sequentially to produce clinical expression of chronic urticaria. Insights into the complexities of pathogenesis may provide an impetus to develop safer, efficacious, and targeted immunomodulators and biological treatment for severe, refractory chronic urticaria.

## 1. Introduction

Chronic urticaria is a distressing disorder that adversely impacts the quality of life; yet its pathogenesis is not well delineated and, accordingly, the treatment is often palliative and therapeutic outcome is suboptimal. This necessitates an understanding of the pathogenesis to facilitate development of improved therapies. In the recent past rapid strides in understanding the pathomechanism of chronic urticaria have been recorded; yet, most of the evidence based, seemingly impregnable and conclusive hypotheses have been countered by alternative, equally authentic, convincing and logistic counter explanations.

The knowledge of molecular immunopathogenesis and complexities of effector mechanisms in chronic urticaria has been enhanced by immunohistologic studies performed on sequential biopsies of urticarial wheals and focused on infiltrating cell immunophenotypes and related cytokines, chemokines/chemokine receptors, and adhesion molecules [1].

The urticarial wheal is characterized by dermal edema, vasodilatation, and perivascular nonnecrotizing infiltrate comprising primarily of mononuclear cells, predominantly CD4+ lymphocytes, with variable numbers of monocytes, neutrophils, eosinophils, and basophils [2–4]. The dermal neutrophilia is strikingly evident at sixty minutes of evolution of wheal with neutrophils representing the main component of the cellular infiltrate [4]. Mast cell numbers remain unaltered and are comparable to those in uninvolved skin and healthy controls [4, 5]. The cytokine profile is characterized by an increase in interleukin-4 (IL-4), interleukin-5 (IL-5), and interferon-gamma RNA (IFN-gamma), suggestive of a mixed Th 1/Th 2 response. Chemokines are upregulated and increased expression of adhesion molecules is evident. The uninvolved skin is characterized by upregulation of soluble mediators and adhesion molecules, almost identical to lesional skin, and significantly higher T-cell numbers, while accumulation of neutrophils is an exclusivity of whealing skin [4] (Tables 1 and 2).

Chronic urticaria is initiated by inappropriate activation and degranulation of dermal mast cells. This key pathophysiological event is predominant at the very onset and the released cellular contents prime the immediate phase of inflammation, which progresses to a complex interplay of

TABLE 1: Infiltrating cells: pattern in urticarial wheal, uninvolved skin, and normal healthy control subjects [4].

| Cell type | Urticarial wheal | Uninvolved skin | Healthy control subjects |
|---|---|---|---|
| Mast cells | Normal count | Normal count | Normal count |
| Lymphocytes | Raised T-lymphocyte count | More numerous T-lymphocytes than in lesional skin | Low T-lymphocyte counts |
| Neutrophils | Major cellular infiltrate at 60 minutes of evolution of urticarial wheal | Significantly less infiltration than in lesional skin | Insignificant |
| Eosinophils | Significantly higher number | Insignificant | Insignificant |
| Basophil | Significant number, especially at 30 minutes of evolution, of urticarial wheal | Less but relevant number | Insignificant |

TABLE 2: Cytokine, chemokine, and adhesion molecule expression: urticarial wheals, uninvolved skin, and healthy control subjects [4].

| | Urticarial wheal | Uninvolved skin | Normal healthy controls |
|---|---|---|---|
| Cytokines | | | |
| Interferon gamma | High expression | Significantly low expression | Not expressed |
| Interleukin-4 | High expression | Significantly low expression | Not expressed |
| Interleukin-5 | High expression | Significantly low expression | Not expressed |
| Interleukin-8 | Moderate expression | Moderate expression | Not expressed |
| Chemokines | | | |
| C X C R 3/CC R 3 | Expression similar to control skin | High expression | Expression similar in lesional and healthy control skin |
| Adhesion molecules | | | |
| Cellular adhesion molecule | High expression | Intense expression | Significant expression |

varied proinflammatory mediators, cytokines, chemokines, chemokine receptors, and adhesion molecules that regulate vasoactivity and specific kinetics of cellular infiltration, ultimately evolving into a lymphocyte and granulocyte mediated hypersensitivity reaction, evident as urticarial wheals. The incoming inflammatory cells, in turn, release more proinflammatory mediators that serve to recruit and activate other cell types, thereby amplifying and extending the host response. The upregulation of inflammatory molecules, almost comparable expression of chemokines and adhesion molecules, and higher T-cell numbers in uninvolved skin is indicative of widespread immunologic activation, representing a low level priming of the cutaneous inflammatory and immunologic response apparatus, reconfirming the hypothesis of latent, minimal persistent inflammation in apparently uninvolved skin [4, 5]. This lowers the reactive threshold of mast cells to triggering stimuli and facilitates the maintenance of susceptibility to urticaria during clinical remission.

## 2. Autoimmunity and Chronic Urticaria

The autoimmune origin is the most accepted hypothesis advanced to explain inappropriate activation and degranulation of mast cells in urticaria. Immune tolerance is maintained by a balance between autoreactive lymphocytes and regulatory mechanisms that counteract them. An increase in number and/or function of naturally occurring autoreactive T-cells or diminished regulator mechanism manifests as autoimmunity. Regulatory T-cells (T(REG)), particularly the naturally occurring CD4(+) CD25(+) subset of T (REG),

provide a substantial component of autoimmune counterbalance. The identification of forkhead box P3 (FOX P3) as a critical determinant of CD4(+) CD25(+) T(REG) cell development and function has provided insights into the delicate balance between autoreactive and regulatory mechanisms in autoimmune disorders including chronic autoimmune urticaria. Functional assays and phenotype analysis have revealed that T(REG) isolated from patients of autoimmune disorder exhibit reduced regulatory function as opposed to those from healthy controls. It may be concluded that reduced percentage of CD4(+) CD25(+) FOX P3(+) regulator T-cells contributes to the autoimmune pathogenic process of chronic urticaria [6]. The autoimmune pathogenic mechanism has been conceptualized on the following observations that provided the initial circumstantial evidence and impetus for further clinical and laboratory investigations that reaffirmed the concept.

(i) Higher prevalence of thyroid autoantibodies in chronic urticaria [7].

(ii) A wheal-and-flare reaction on intradermal injection of autologous serum in a subpopulation of patients (positive autologous serum skin test) and reproducibility on passive transfer of serum to normal healthy control subjects [8].

(iii) Subsequent identification of IgG antibody directed to the alpha subunit of the IgE receptor, capable of inducing positive autologous serum skin test as well as histamine release from basophils [9]. The incidence of such autoantibodies is about 30 percent and an additional 5–10 percent of patients have anti-IgE antibodies rather than anti-IgE receptor antibody [10].

(iv) Positive association with HLA subtypes DRB*04 (DR4) and DQB 1*0302 (DQ8) [11].

(v) Therapeutic response to plasmapheresis [12] and intravenous immunoglobulin [13].

The evidence favouring autoimmune pathomechanism, although persuasively convincing, is incomplete. Certain issues, elucidated below, need to be addressed for unequivocal acceptance of the proposed hypothesis.

(i) The cutaneous response to intradermal injection of autologous serum may be due to the presence of nonimmunoglobulin vasoactive histamine releasing factors [14]. Moreover reactivity to autologous serum has been observed in subjects with allergic respiratory diseases and healthy controls [15]. ASST identifies subsets of patients exhibiting autoreactivity rather than establishing autoimmunity.

(ii) Animal model, mandatory to establish autoimmune status of the disorder, is yet to be developed for chronic urticaria [16].

(iii) The autoantibodies of similar specificity have been detected in sera of healthy persons and may belong to the natural repertoire. Such natural autoantibodies may become pathogenic under certain circumstances and this occurrence is dependent on the state of occupancy of the FceRI receptor by its natural ligand IgE. The urticaria results from alteration in the tissue binding of preexisting autoantibody in susceptible individuals rather than its production de novo. Thus the concept of conditional autoimmunity has evolved [17] in chronic urticaria.

(iv) It has been proposed that anti-FceRI and anti-IgE autoantibodies are not actually pathogenic but are secondary to the presence of urticaria in individuals with a predisposition to develop autoimmunity [18].

The complex pathway involved in triggering, maintaining, and controlling autoantibody formation against FceRI and/or IgE remains unexplained. The autoantibodies relevant to chronic urticaria belong to complement fixing subtypes IgG1 and IgG3 [19]. The vascular leakage of such autoantibodies by local events facilitates their binding to either FceRI or IgE, cross-linking of the receptor, and complement activation that generates C5a. C5a interacts with the receptor for complement anaphylatoxin (C5a receptor) localized on the surface of mast cell $MC_{TC}$, the subtype dominant in the skin, and participates in mast cell activation [20]. This triggers a series of intracellular events and the earliest in signal transduction involves phosphorylation of tyrosine on the beta and gamma chains of FceRI at immunoreceptor tyrosine activation motifs (ITAM). The ITAMS associate with Src-family protein tyrosine kinases (PTKs), such as Lyn and Syk, which initiate the activation of downstream effector pathways [21] and the

release of preformed granule contents such as histamine, heparin, tryptase, and tumour necrosis factor-alpha (TNF-alpha), as well as the synthesis of other proinflammatory cytokines/chemokines and eicosanoids [22]. The downregulation of signal transduction and mediator release is regulated by signal regulatory proteins (SIRP) that contain immunotyrosine inhibition motifs (ITIMS) which act by recruiting SH-2 bearing tyrosine phosphatases (SHIP 1 and 2) that dephosphorylate ITAM on beta and gamma subunits of FceRI [21].

The autoantibodies to alpha chain of FceRI and/or IgE have been detected in only 35 to 40 percent and 5 to 10 percent of patients, respectively [23]. Moreover the detection of autoantibodies in the serum does not confirm their functionality and may not be always implicated in the induction of histamine release from mast cells/basophils. It is likely that other permeabilizing factors are involved in serum mediated vascular leakage.

## 3. Nonimmunologic Agonists

Nonimmunologic agonists including substance P, endorphins, enkephalins, endogenous peptides, and somatostatin may induce regulated degranulation and liberation of proinflammatory molecules from mast cells especially when the products of activated immune system lower the cutaneous mast cell release threshold [24].

## 4. Cellular Abnormalities: Basophils

The primary abnormality in some patients of chronic urticaria might be cellular/subcellular rather than immunologically mediated autoimmune mechanism.

There is increasing evidence of altered number, structure, function, and trafficking defects in basophils. Basopenia is well documented and basophil numbers are inversely related to urticaria severity [25]. Other evidence, perhaps more convincing, is the paradoxical suppression of FceRI mediated, anti-FceRI/anti-IgE antibody induced histamine release from basophils during active disease [26]. It is still more intriguing that these basophils maintain normal response to monocyte chemotactic protein-1 (MCP-1) and bradykinin and are hyperresponsive to serum [27]. It had been reasoned that basophils in chronic autoimmune urticaria are desensitized in vivo to further FceRI induced activation. However, autoantibody mediated desensitization of IgE receptor seems unlikely as similar response of basophils has been observed in patients lacking autoimmune antibodies [27].

A more complex picture has emerged from insight into the dysregulated expression of molecules that are critical to signal propagation or its inhibition after IgE receptor activation [28]. Spleen tyrosine kinase (Syk) is a positive regulator of signaling through FceRI and its levels are a major determinant of basophil histamine release (HR) in normal basophils [29]. Src homology 2 (SH2) containing inositol phosphatases, SHIP-1 and SHIP-2, are negative regulators of signal propagation [30]. In chronic urticaria there is a shift in the paradigm of Syk dominated regulation of HR and unlike normal basophils altered levels of SHIP-1 and SHIP-2 correlate with the pattern of anti-IgE stimulated histamine release [31, 32].

In addition to these observations, based on the profile of *ex vivo* activation of basophils by optimal concentration of polyclonal anti-IgE, it has been confirmed that distinct basophil degranulation phenotypes exist in chronic urticaria and a bimodal stratification of basophils has been proposed [32]. Fifty percent of chronic urticaria subjects have significant reduction in basophil histamine release (HR) with anti-IgE stimulation. It is consequent to increased SHIP-2 levels and such subjects are designated anti-IgE nonresponders (CIU-NR). The remaining subjects have basophils that release more than 10 percent of histamine content after anti-IgE stimulation and are termed anti-IgE responders (CIU-R) and SHIP-1 levels in such basophils are reduced.

This pattern of basophil functional phenotypes (CIU-R and CIU-NR) appears to be independent of the existence and/or levels of autoantibodies [33] and remains stable in subjects with persistent disease. The salient features of basophil phenotypes in chronic urticaria are summarized in Table 3 [31–33].

The levels and/or expression of regulatory proteins is functional and normalizes during remission [33]. Such shift in basophil function is independent of the autoimmune status of urticaria and, in those with autoimmunity, is noted without a parallel decrease in antibody titres.

This profiling of signal proteins in basophils in conjunction with their stratification into distinct phenotypes has reaffirmed that abnormal basophil function may be a key factor in disease pathogenesis.

## 5. Mast Cells and Chronic Urticaria

A direct role of mast cells in CU is speculated (Table 4). The activating factors derived from inflammatory cell infiltrate surrounding dermal postcapillary venules [34] stimulate mast cells to secrete vasoactive molecules that activate endothelial cells. The expression of adhesion molecules is upregulated [35] and the increased vasopermeability promotes extravascular leakage of fluids and proteins leading to development of urticarial wheals.

In an *in vitro* study performed to evaluate permeabilizing activity of CU serum, a similar pattern of mast cell degranulation and increased endothelial monolayer permeability was observed after exposure of two distinct mast cell lines (LAD-2 and HMC-1) [36, 37] to CU serum. The CU serum evoked response remained unaltered after IgG depletion, reaffirming its nondependence on mast cell IgE receptor activation [38]. It was concluded that vasoactive molecules may be released from mast cells without degranulation [38].

It is likely that varied membrane receptors expressed on mast cells are selectively triggered by ligands such as IgG, peptides, microbial derivatives, and fragments of activated complement [39] and mast cells are stimulated by activating signals to synthesize vasoactive substances including lipid metabolites, cytokines, and chemokines [40,

41]. These newly formed permeabilizing factors include tumour necrosis factor-alpha (TNF-alpha), interleukin-6 (IL-6), vascular endothelial growth factor (VEGF), and platelet activating factor (PAF). These are secreted from mast cells independent of release of preformed mediators stored in granules such as histamine, serotonin, proteases, and proteoglycans [40, 41]. These permeabilizing factors facilitate the development of urticarial wheals. These observations provide an explanation for lack of correlation between detection of autoantibodies and degranulation of mast cells [42], quality and quantity of released vasoactive factors, increased vasopermeability, urticaria severity refractoriness of severe urticaria to standard first line management with antihistamines, and therapeutic response to immunosuppressive agents.

## 6. Chronic Urticaria: Immune Mediated Inflammatory Disorder

The concept of chronic urticaria being an immune mediated inflammatory disorder evolved from incidental observation that recommendation of targeted immunomodulator biologic therapy, directed at a particular cytokine/cell receptor, administered for some other inflammatory disorder ameliorated coexisting chronic urticaria [43]. It was indicative that inflammatory cascade in chronic urticaria may be triggered by altered chemokine-cytokine network and is attributed to immune dysregulation consequent to disturbed innate immunity in the disorder.

The investigation of early events of innate immunity through the study of dendritic cells that link innate and adaptive immune system has provided insights into the dysregulated immune response in chronic urticaria [44]. Plasmacytoid dendritic cells (pDC) express toll-like receptors (TLR) that are activated by natural and synthetic ligands triggering proinflammatory responses that play a key role in the pathogenesis of several inflammatory disorders including urticaria [45].

Accordingly, a study of early events of the immune response, through the activation of pDC by TLR sensing, was undertaken to evaluate immune dysregulation in chronic urticaria [44].

Plasmacytoid dendritic cells are unremarkably scattered amongst cellular infiltrate in the cutaneous lesion and their percentage in the peripheral blood mononuclear cells is unaltered and is similar to healthy controls. A normal degree of activation of pDC by the expression of costimulatory molecules and an increased constitutive STAT 1 phosphorylation on nonstimulated lymphocytes was observed. However, IFN-alpha secretion by pDC upon stimulation by CpGA was impaired and it was associated with altered IRF-7 and downregulation of TLR 9 expression, indicating a functional impairment of pDC, and was supportive of immune dysregulation in CU [44].

Several hypotheses have been proposed to explain the downregulation of TLR9 in pDC after CpGA stimulation. It is probable that IgE or anti-FceRI autoantibodies crosslink FceRI on immature pDC impairing immune function

TABLE 3: Basophil phenotypes: profile in chronic urticaria [31–33].

| Feature | Chronic urticarial (autoimmune/nonautoimmune) | |
| --- | --- | --- |
| | CIU-R | CIU-NR |
| (1) Anti-IgE stimulation/cross-linking: HR in active disease | >10 percent of cellular content | <10 percent of cellular content |
| (2) Regulatory proteins | Paradigm shift | Paradigm shift |
| (a) Kinase | HR not determined by kinase level | HR not determined by kinase level |
| | Normal Syk levels | Normal Syk levels |
| (b) Phosphatase | Regulates HR, reduced SHIP-1 levels | Regulates HR, increased SHIP-2 levels |
| (3) Sensitivity to anti-IgE stimulation in remission | Heightened sensitivity | Sensitivity restored to levels as in normal healthy subjects |

HR: histamine release.
CIU-R: chronic idiopathic urticaria—responders.
CIU-NR: chronic idiopathic urticaria—nonresponders.
Syk: serum tyrosine kinase.
SHIP-1: Src homology 2 (SH2) containing inositol phosphatase 1.
SHIP-2: Src homology 2 (SH2) containing inositol phosphatase 2.

TABLE 4: Mast cell mediators: relevant to chronic urticaria.

| Mediator | Effect in chronic urticaria |
| --- | --- |
| Preformed mediators | |
| Histamine | Direct potent vasoactive and smooth muscle spasmogenic effects<br>Principal mediator of vascular changes [70, 71] |
| Newly synthesised mediators | |
| Lipid mediators | |
| LTC4 | Actions similar to histamine |
| LT B4 | Potentiate vasodilatation, vascular permeability, and smooth muscle contraction |
| PGD2 | Chemotactic for neutrophils and eosinophils [72] |
| Cytokines and chemokines | |
| Tumour necrosis factor-alpha | Newly synthesised as well as preformed<br>Upregulates expression of adhesion molecules on endothelial cells<br>Promotes leukocyte rolling and adhesion<br>Chemotactic for neutrophils [73] |
| Interleukin-1 | Proinflammatory cytokine<br>Lymphocyte activator [74]<br>Activates mast cells after release from leukocyte [75] |
| Interleukin-4 | Chemotactic for neutrophils<br>Recruits eosinophils [76] |
| Interleukin-5 | Recruits eosinophils [77] |
| Interleukin-6 | Proinflammatory cytokine<br>Activates lymphocytes [78] |
| Interleukin-8/CXCL2 | Member of C X C chemokines<br>Potent neutrophil chemoattractant<br>Involved in neutrophil degranulation, respiratory burst, and adhesion to endothelial cells [79] |
| MCP-1/CCL2 | Chemoattractant for eosinophils |
| MIP-1 alpha/CCL3 | Chemoattractant for eosinophils |
| Interleukin-16 | Chemoattractant for T-lymphocytes |
| RANTES/CCL5 | Chemoattractant for eosinophils [79] |

LTC4: leukotriene C4, LTB4: leukotriene B4, PGD2: prostaglandin D2, MCP-1: monocyte chemotactic protein-1, MIP-1 alpha: monocyte inflammatory peptide-1, RANTES: regulated upon activation normal T-cell expressed and secreted.

by suppressing IFN-alpha production [46]. Alternatively, regulatory receptors including BDCA-2, ILT-7, and NKp44 downmodulate IFN production [47–49]. It is also likely that histamine released into circulation from degranulating mast cells/basophils may regulate several cell types through stimulation of histamine receptors and pDC activated by CpG respond to histamine through H2 receptors with downregulation of IFN-alpha production [50].

The dysfunctional innate immune response in CU consequent to functional impairment of pDC to TLR9 activation disturbs the cytokine production by T-cells, mainly of IL-17A and IL-10 [51]. Besides, elevated serum levels of IL-1, IL-4, IL-13, IL-18, tumour necrosis factor-alpha (TNF-alpha) [52, 53], B-cell activating factor (BAFF) [54], and factors related to inflammatory process such as neopterin [55] and C-reactive protein have been documented. These observations suggest that there is an ongoing inflammatory process, creating a proinflammatory environment in chronic urticaria that in turn is responsible for an altered pattern of secretion of chemokines.

Significantly higher serum levels of chemokines (C-C and C-X-C) including CXCL8, CXCL9, CXCL10, and CCL2 have been observed in CU and are not correlated with either the clinical parameters of the disorder or the outcome of basophil histamine release (BHR) and/or ASST assays [56]. These proinflammatory chemotactic cytokines interact with chemokine receptors on the surface of inflammatory cells to trigger chemotaxis and transendothelial migration of leukocytes to the site of inflammation.

CXCL8/IL-8 is chemotactic for neutrophils, T-lymphocytes, and monocytes [56].

CXCL9/Mig, a monokine induced by interferon- (IFN-) gamma induced protein 1 (IP-10), is a type 1 C-X-C chemokine and displays strong chemoattraction for T-helper type 1 (Th 1) lymphocytes [57, 58].

C-C ligand 2 (CCL2) (monocyte chemoattractant protein 1), prototype of C-C chemokine, is secreted mainly by monocytes, as evidenced by increased mRNA expression in CD14 + cells in CU. CCL2 activates a variety of cells including monocytes, macrophages, lymphocytes, eosinophils, and basophils and is a crucial factor for the development of Th 2 responses [59].

The upregulation of chemokines in CU contributes to the maintenance of activated status of inflammatory cell subsets. Basophils in CU display an upregulation of activation/degranulation markers, CD203c and CD63, and high responsiveness to interleukin-3 (IL-3) stimulation. It is likely that activated profile of basophils is triggered by *in vivo* priming with potent basophil activating factor such as CCL2 [60].

CCL2 induces degranulation of mast cell and has a potent basophil histamine releasing activity. Furthermore, it has been documented that an assembly of circulating chemokines CCL2, CCL5, and CXCL8 play an important role in mast cell activation and generation of histamine and serotonin [61].

It may be inferred that immunologic dysregulation consequent to disturbed innate immune response alters the cytokine-chemokine network that triggers the inflammatory status contributing to the pathogenesis of CU.

## 7. Chronic Urticaria and Coagulation System

It has been observed that autologous plasma, anticoagulated with substances other than heparin, generates positive autoreactive responses in a higher percentage of patients than autologous serum skin test (ASST) [62, 63]. As serum and plasma do not differ in their autoantibody content, this observation points to a possible role of clotting factors in wheal-and-flare reaction. It has been reasoned that plasma contains more coagulation factors and complement, while consumption of such factors in serum during formation of clot is responsible for the discrepant reactivity of autologous plasma and serum. It has thus been inferred that clotting cascade may be involved in pathogenesis of urticaria [64] and this may provide an explanation for therapeutic effects noted in some patients with drugs active on coagulation system [65, 66].

The extrinsic pathway of coagulation is activated and thrombin is generated from prothrombin by activated factor X, in the presence of activated factor V and calcium ions [64]. *In vitro* studies have confirmed that plasma of urticaria patients has significantly higher levels of prothrombin fragment $F_{1+2}$, a polypeptide of 34 kDa that is released into circulation during the activation of prothrombin to thrombin by factor X [67], and severe exacerbations of urticaria are associated with a strong activation of coagulation cascade that leads to fibrin formation and fibrinolysis as shown by elevated D-dimer plasma levels.

Thrombin is a serine protease that enhances vascular permeability, activates and degranulates mast cells, and induces generation of anaphylatoxin C5a. The activation of extrinsic pathway of coagulation is thus proposed as yet another explanation.

It is likely that different pathomechanistic pathways, namely, seroimmunologic autoimmune, inflammatory, cellular defects, coagulative, and complement system, are interlinked rather than separate independent cascades and there is extensive cross talk amongst them with mutual regulation of activation. They act synergistically or sequentially as either independent or interlinked pathomechanisms to activate mast cells with release of preformed mediators and/or secretion of newly synthesized vasoactive molecules to produce final clinical expression of urticaria [68, 69] (Figure 1).

The various mast cell mediators, preformed and newly synthesized, relevant to chronic urticaria, are summarized in Table 4.

Histamine is the principal vasoactive mediator and combined histamine-1 and -2 receptor responses are required for the full expression of histamine vasoactivity, including immediate vasodilation, alteration in vasopermeability, plasma extravasation, and dermal sensory nerve stimulation [69–71]. Its role in the pathogenesis of wheal is less certain and it is probable that nonhistamine mast cell mediators regulate cell recruitment. The leukotrienes, cytokines, and chemokines upregulate adhesion molecule expression on endothelial cells, promoting rolling and adhesion of leukocytes, followed by chemotaxis and transendothelial migration and cellular influx into whealing skin. These infiltrating cells in turn release proinflammatory cytokines and chemokines that

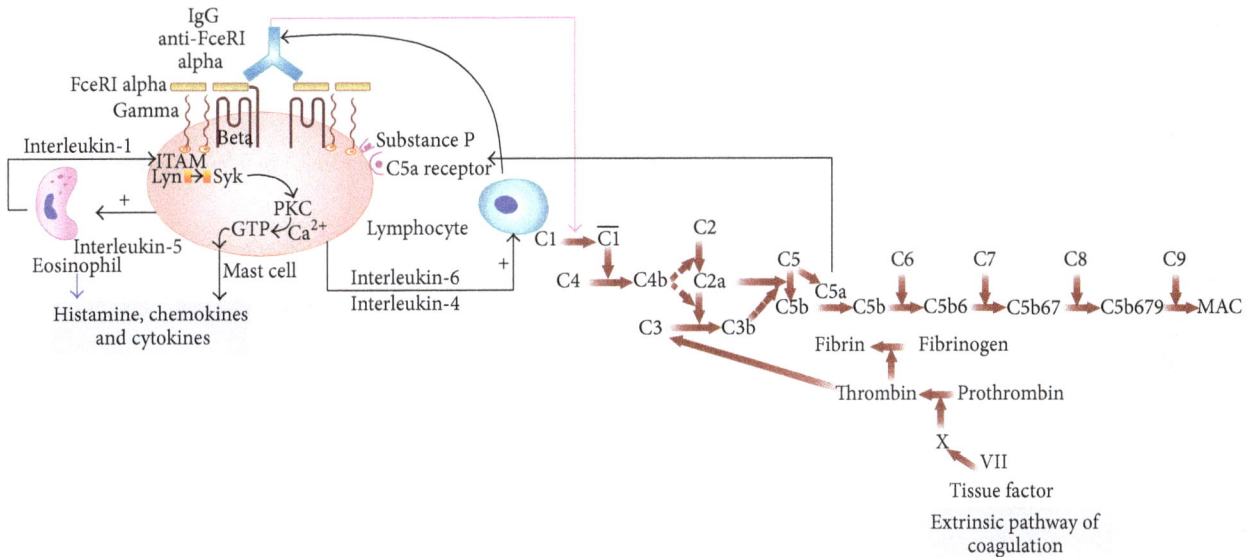

ITAM: immunotyrosine activation motif
GTP: guanosine triphosphate
Lyn, Syk: cytoplasmic tyrosine kinase

PKC: protein kinase C
MAC: membrane attack complex

FIGURE 1: Pathogenesis of chronic urticaria: molecular intercommunication between autoimmune, complement, and coagulation cascade.

serve to recruit and activate more inflammatory cells, thereby sustaining, amplifying, and extending the host response. The signals for resolution of urticaria are also not well characterized. It involves downregulation of the histamine receptor, reconstitution of integrity of the endothelial cell lining, apoptosis of the inflammatory cells, clearance of cellular debris by macrophages, and drainage of edema fluid into the vascular circulation [22].

It may be concluded that the pathogenesis of chronic urticaria is as perplexing as the disorder is intriguing and a concise pathomechanism has, as yet, not been identified that may provide a rational explanation for all cases. An incomplete understanding has hampered the search for novel, efficacious, low toxicity drugs that may be offered as alternatives in severe, unremitting urticaria, unresponsive to standard first line of management. It is, however, likely that newer insights into the complexities of pathogenesis may pave the way for evolving therapies that are more specifically tied to the pathomechanics of the disorder and provide an impetus to develop targeted immunomodulators and biological therapies that may be favorably included in therapeutic armamentarium.

## Conflict of Interests

The author declares that there is no conflict of interests regarding the publication of this paper.

## References

[1] R. A. Sabroe and M. W. Greaves, "What is urticaria ? Anatomical, physiological, and histologic consideration and classification," in *Urticaria and Angioedema*, A. P. Kaplan, Ed., pp. 1–14, Informo Health Care, New York, NY, USA, 2nd edition, 2009.

[2] J. Elias, E. Boss, and A. P. Kaplan, "Studies of the cellular infiltrate of chronic idiopathic urticaria: Prominence of T-lymphocytes, monocytes, and mast cells," *Journal of Allergy and Clinical Immunology*, vol. 78, no. 5, pp. 914–918, 1986.

[3] Y. A. Mekori, R. C. Giorno, P. Anderson, and P. F. Kohler, "Lymphocyte subpopulations in the skin of patients with chronic urticaria," *Journal of Allergy and Clinical Immunology*, vol. 72, no. 6, pp. 681–684, 1983.

[4] M. Caproni, B. Giomi, W. Volpi et al., "Chronic idiopathic urticaria: infiltrating cells and related cytokines in autologous serum-induced wheals," *Clinical Immunology*, vol. 114, no. 3, pp. 284–292, 2005.

[5] C. H. Smith, C. Kepley, L. B. Schwartz, and T. H. Lee, "Mast cell number and phenotype in chronic idiopathic urticaria," *Journal of Allergy and Clinical Immunology*, vol. 96, no. 3, pp. 360–364, 1995.

[6] X. Valencia and P. E. Lipsky, "CD4+CD25+FoxP3+ regulatory T cells in autoimmune diseases," *Nature Clinical Practice Rheumatology*, vol. 3, no. 11, pp. 619–626, 2007.

[7] A. Leznoff, R. G. Josse, J. Denburg, and J. Dolovich, "Association of chronic urticaria and angioedema with thyroid autoimmunity," *Archives of Dermatology*, vol. 119, no. 8, pp. 636–640, 1983.

[8] C. E. H. Grattan, T. B. Wallington, R. P. Warin, C. T. Kennedy, and J. W. Bradfield, "A serological mediator in chronic idiopathic urticaria—a clinical, immunological and histological evaluation," *British Journal of Dermatology*, vol. 114, no. 5, pp. 583–590, 1986.

[9] M. Hide, D. M. Francis, C. E. H. Grattan, J. Hakimi, J. P. Kochan, and M. W. Greaves, "Autoantibodies against the high-affinity IgE receptor as a cause of histamine release in chronic urticaria," *The New England Journal of Medicine*, vol. 328, no. 22, pp. 1599–1604, 1993.

[10] C. E. H. Grattan, D. M. Francis, M. Hide, and M. W. Greaves, "Detection of circulating histamine releasing autoantibodies with functional properties of anti-IgE in chronic urticaria,"

*Clinical and Experimental Allergy*, vol. 21, no. 6, pp. 695–704, 1991.

[11] B. F. O'Donnell, C. M. O'Neill, D. M. Francis et al., "Human leucocyte antigen class II associations in chronic idiopathic urticaria," *British Journal of Dermatology*, vol. 140, no. 5, pp. 853–858, 1999.

[12] C. E. H. Grattan, D. M. Francis, N. G. P. Slater, R. J. Barlow, and M. W. Greaves, "Plasmapheresis for severe, unremitting, chronic urticaria," *The Lancet*, vol. 339, no. 8801, pp. 1078–1080, 1992.

[13] B. F. O'Donnell, R. M. Barr, A. K. Black et al., "Intravenous immunoglobulin in autoimmune chronic urticaria," *British Journal of Dermatology*, vol. 138, no. 1, pp. 101–106, 1998.

[14] U. Fagiolo, F. Kricek, C. Rufb, A. Peserico, A. Amadori, and M. Cancian, "Effects of complement inactivation and IgG depletion on skin reactivity to autologous serum in chronic idiopathic urticaria," *Journal of Allergy and Clinical Immunology*, vol. 106, no. 3, pp. 567–572, 2000.

[15] E. Guttman-yassky, R. Bergman, C. Maor, M. Mamorsky, S. Pollack, and E. Shahar, "The autologous serum skin test in a cohort of chronic idiopathic urticaria patients compared to respiratory allergy patients and healthy controls," *Journal of the European Academy of Dermatology and Venereology*, vol. 21, no. 1, pp. 35–39, 2007.

[16] N. R. Rose and C. Bona, "Defining criteria for autoimmune diseases (Witebsky's postulates revisited)," *Immunology Today*, vol. 14, no. 9, pp. 426–430, 1993.

[17] M. P. Horn, J. M. Pachlopnik, M. Vogel et al., "Conditional autoimmunity mediated by human natural anti-FcεRIα autoantibodies?" *FASEB Journal*, vol. 15, no. 12, pp. 2268–2274, 2001.

[18] E. Novembre, A. Cianferoni, F. Mori et al., "Urticaria and urticaria related skin condition/disease in children," *European Annals of Allergy and Clinical Immunology*, vol. 39, no. 8, pp. 253–258, 2007.

[19] E. Fiebiger, F. Hammerschmid, G. Stingl, and D. Maurer, "Anti-FcεRIα autoantibodies in autoimmune-mediated disorders: identification of a structure-function relationship," *Journal of Clinical Investigation*, vol. 101, no. 1, pp. 243–251, 1998.

[20] Y. Kikuchi and A. P. Kaplan, "A role for C5a in augmenting IgG-dependent histamine release from basophils in chronic urticaria," *Journal of Allergy and Clinical Immunology*, vol. 109, no. 1, pp. 114–118, 2002.

[21] W. Zhao and L. B. Schwartz, "Mast cells and basophils," in *Urticaria and Angioedema*, M. W. Greaves and A. P. Kaplan, Eds., pp. 19–50, Marcel Dekker, New York, NY, USA, 2004.

[22] C. E. H. Grattan, "Autoimmune urticaria," *Immunology and Allergy Clinics of North America*, vol. 24, no. 2, pp. 163–181, 2004.

[23] A. P. Kaplan and M. Greaves, "Pathogenesis of chronic urticaria," *Clinical and Experimental Allergy*, vol. 39, no. 6, pp. 777–787, 2009.

[24] A. L. Schocket, "Chronic urticaria: pathophysiology and etiology, or the what and why," *Allergy and Asthma Proceedings*, vol. 27, no. 2, pp. 90–95, 2006.

[25] C. E. H. Grattan, G. Dawn, S. Gibbs, and D. M. Francis, "Blood basophil numbers in chronic ordinary urticaria and healthy controls: diurnal variation, influence of loratadine and prednisolone and relationship to disease activity," *Clinical & Experimental Allergy*, vol. 33, no. 3, pp. 337–341, 2003.

[26] R. A. Sabroe, D. M. Francis, R. M. Barr, A. K. Black, and M. W. Greaves, "Anti-FcεRI autoantibodies and basophil histamine releasability in chronic idiopathic urticaria," *Journal of Allergy and Clinical Immunology*, vol. 102, no. 4 I, pp. 651–658, 1998.

[27] E. Luquin, A. P. Kaplan, and M. Ferrer, "Increased responsiveness of basophils of patients with chronic urticaria to sera but hypo-responsiveness to other stimuli," *Clinical and Experimental Allergy*, vol. 35, no. 4, pp. 456–460, 2005.

[28] B. M. Vonakis and S. S. Saini, "New concepts in chronic urticaria," *Current Opinion in Immunology*, vol. 20, no. 6, pp. 709–716, 2008.

[29] D. W. MacGlashan Jr., "Relationship between spleen tyrosine kinase and phosphatidylinositol 5′ phosphatase expression and secretion from human basophils in the general population," *Journal of Allergy and Clinical Immunology*, vol. 119, no. 3, pp. 626–633, 2007.

[30] W. Leung and S. Bolland, "The inositol 5′-phosphatase SHIP-2 negatively regulates IgE-induced mast cell degranulation and cytokine production," *Journal of Immunology*, vol. 179, no. 1, pp. 95–102, 2007.

[31] B. M. Vonakis and S. S. Saini, "Syk-deficient basophils from donors with chronic idiopathic urticaria exhibit a spectrum of releasability," *Journal of Allergy and Clinical Immunology*, vol. 121, no. 1, pp. 262–264, 2008.

[32] B. M. Vonakis, K. Vasagar, S. P. Gibbons Jr. et al., "Basophil FcεRI histamine release parallels expression of Src-homology 2-containing inositol phosphatases in chronic idiopathic urticaria," *Journal of Allergy and Clinical Immunology*, vol. 119, no. 2, pp. 441–448, 2007.

[33] J. A. Eckman, R. G. Hamilton, L. M. Gober, P. M. Sterba, and S. S. Saini, "Basophil phenotypes in chronic idiopathic urticaria in relation to disease activity and autoantibodies," *Journal of Investigative Dermatology*, vol. 128, no. 8, pp. 1956–1963, 2008.

[34] A. Tedeschi, R. Asero, A. V. Marzano et al., "Plasma levels and skin-eosinophil-expression of vascular endothelial growth factor in patients with chronic urticaria," *Allergy*, vol. 64, no. 11, pp. 1616–1622, 2009.

[35] H. L. Kwang, Y. K. Ji, D. Kang, J. C. Yoo, W. Lee, and Y. R. Jai, "Increased expression of endothelial cell adhesion molecules due to mediator release from human foreskin mast cells stimulated by autoantibodies in chronic urticaria sera," *Journal of Investigative Dermatology*, vol. 118, no. 4, pp. 658–663, 2002.

[36] A. S. Kirshenbaum, C. Akin, Y. Wu et al., "Characterization of novel stem cell factor responsive human mast cell lines LAD 1 and 2 established from a patient with mast cell sarcoma/leukemia; Activation following aggregation of FcεRI or FcγRI," *Leukemia Research*, vol. 27, no. 8, pp. 677–682, 2003.

[37] G. Nilsson, T. Blom, M. Kusche-Gullberg et al., "Phenotypic characterization of the human mast-cell line HMC-1," *Scandinavian Journal of Immunology*, vol. 39, no. 5, pp. 489–498, 1994.

[38] F. Bossi, B. Frossi, O. Radillo et al., "Mast cells are critically involved in serum-mediated vascular leakage in chronic urticaria beyond high-affinity IgE receptor stimulation," *Allergy*, vol. 66, no. 12, pp. 1538–1545, 2011.

[39] B. Frossi, G. Gri, C. Tripodo, and C. Pucillo, "Exploring a regulatory role for mast cells: MCregs?" *Trends in Immunology*, vol. 31, no. 3, pp. 97–102, 2010.

[40] F. Levi-Schaffer and J. Pe'Er, "Mast cells and angiogenesis," *Clinical and Experimental Allergy*, vol. 31, no. 4, pp. 521–524, 2001.

[41] A. Hennino, F. Bérard, I. Guillot, N. Saad, A. Rozières, and J. Nicolas, "Pathophysiology of urticaria," *Clinical Reviews in Allergy and Immunology*, vol. 30, no. 1, pp. 3–11, 2006.

[42] J. A. Eckman, R. G. Hamilton, and S. S. Saini, "Independent evaluation of a commercial test for autoimmune urticaria in

normal and chronic urticaria subjects," *Journal of Investigative Dermatology*, vol. 129, no. 6, pp. 1584–1586, 2009.

[43] F. Habal and V. Huang, "Angioedema associated with Crohn's disease: response to biologics," *World Journal of Gastroenterology*, vol. 18, no. 34, pp. 4787–4790, 2012.

[44] E. Futata, M. Azor, J. Dos Santos et al., "Impaired IFN-$\alpha$ secretion by plasmacytoid dendritic cells induced by TLR9 activation in chronic idiopathic urticaria," *British Journal of Dermatology*, vol. 164, no. 6, pp. 1271–1279, 2011.

[45] G. Hartmann, J. Battiany, H. Poeck et al., "Rational design of new CpG oligonucleotides that combine B cell activation with high IFN-$\alpha$ induction in plasmacytoid dendritic cells," *European Journal of Immunology*, vol. 33, no. 6, pp. 1633–1641, 2003.

[46] J. R. Tversky, T. V. Le, A. P. Bieneman, K. L. Chichester, R. G. Hamilton, and J. T. Schroeder, "Human blood dendritic cells from allergic subjects have impaired capacity to produce interferon-$\alpha$ via toll-like receptor 9," *Clinical and Experimental Allergy*, vol. 38, no. 5, pp. 781–788, 2008.

[47] A. Dzionek, Y. Sohma, J. Nagafune et al., "BDCA-2, a novel plasmacytoid dendritic cell-specific type II C-type lectin, mediates antigen capture and is a potent inhibitor of interferon $\alpha/\beta$ induction," *Journal of Experimental Medicine*, vol. 194, no. 12, pp. 1823–1834, 2001.

[48] A. Fuchs, M. Cella, T. Kondo, and M. Colonna, "Paradoxic inhibition of human natural interferon-producing cells by the activating receptor NKp44," *Blood*, vol. 106, no. 6, pp. 2076–2082, 2005.

[49] W. Cao, D. B. Rosen, T. Ito et al., "Plasmacytoid dendritic cell-specific receptor ILT7-Fc$\varepsilon$RI$\gamma$ inhibits Toll-like receptor-induced interferon production," *Journal of Experimental Medicine*, vol. 203, no. 6, pp. 1399–1405, 2006.

[50] A. Mazzoni, C. A. Leifer, G. E. Mullen, M. N. Kennedy, D. M. Klinman, and D. M. Segal, "Cutting edge: histamine inhibits IFN-$\alpha$ release from plasmacytoid dendritic cells," *The Journal of Immunology*, vol. 170, no. 5, pp. 2269–2273, 2003.

[51] J. C. dos Santos, M. H. Azor, V. Y. Nojima et al., "Increased circulating pro-inflammatory cytokines and imbalanced regulatory T-cell cytokines production in chronic idiopathic urticaria," *International Immunopharmacology*, vol. 8, no. 10, pp. 1433–1440, 2008.

[52] M. Caproni, C. Cardinali, B. Giomi et al., "Serological detection of eotaxin, IL-4, IL-13, IFN-$\gamma$, MIP-1$\alpha$, TARC and IP-10 in chronic autoimmune urticaria and chronic idiopathic urticaria," *Journal of Dermatological Science*, vol. 36, no. 1, pp. 57–59, 2004.

[53] A. Tedeschi, M. Lorini, C. Suli, and R. Asero, "Serum interleukin-18 in patients with chronic ordinary urticaria: association with disease activity," *Clinical and Experimental Dermatology*, vol. 32, no. 5, pp. 568–570, 2007.

[54] F. Melchers, "Actions of BAFF in B-cell maturation and its effects on the development of autoimmune disease," *Annals of the Rheumatic Diseases*, vol. 62, supplement 2, pp. 1125–1127, 2013.

[55] G. Ciprandi, M. de Amici, L. Berardi et al., "Serum neopterin levels in spontaneous urticaria and atopic dermatitis," *Clinical and Experimental Dermatology*, vol. 36, no. 1, pp. 85–87, 2011.

[56] J. C. Santos, C. A. de Brito, E. A. Futata et al., "Up-regulation of chemokine C-C ligand 2 (CCL2) and C-X-C chemokine 8 (CXCL8) expression by monocytes in chronic idiopathic urticaria," *Clinical and Experimental Immunology*, vol. 167, no. 1, pp. 129–136, 2012.

[57] R. Bonecchi, G. Bianchi, P. P. Bordignon et al., "Differential expression of chemokine receptors and chemotactic responsiveness of type 1 T helper cells (Th1s) and Th2s," *Journal of Experimental Medicine*, vol. 187, no. 1, pp. 129–134, 1998.

[58] M. Rotondi, A. Rosati, A. Buonamano et al., "High pretransplant serum levels of CXCL10/IP-10 are related to increased risk of renal allograft failure," *American Journal of Transplantation*, vol. 4, no. 9, pp. 1466–1474, 2004.

[59] W. J. Karpus, N. W. Lukacs, K. J. Kennedy et al., "Differential CC chemokine-induced enhancement of T helper cell cytokine production," *The Journal of Immunology*, vol. 158, no. 9, pp. 4129–4136, 1997.

[60] F. D. Lourenço, M. H. Azor, J. C. Santos et al., "Activated status of basophils in chronic urticaria leads to interleukin-3 hyperresponsiveness and enhancement of histamine release induced by anti-IgE stimulus," *British Journal of Dermatology*, vol. 158, no. 5, pp. 979–986, 2008.

[61] M. L. Castellani, M. A. De Lutiis, E. Toniato et al., "Impact of RANTES, MCP-1 and IL-8 in mast cells," *Journal of Biological Regulators & Homeostatic Agents*, vol. 24, no. 1, pp. 1–6, 2010.

[62] R. Asero, A. Tedeschi, P. Riboldi, and M. Cugno, "Plasma of patients with chronic urticaria shows signs of thrombin generation, and its intradermal injection causes wheal-and-flare reactions much more frequently than autologous serum," *Journal of Allergy and Clinical Immunology*, vol. 117, no. 5, pp. 1113–1117, 2006.

[63] V. Safedi, M. Morahedi, A. Aghamohammed et al., "Comparison between sensitivity of autologous skin serum test and autologous plasma skin test in patients with Chronic Idiopathic Urticaria for detection of antibody against IgE or IgE receptor (Fc$\varepsilon$RI$\alpha$)," *Iranian Journal of Allergy, Asthma, and Immunology*, vol. 10, no. 2, pp. 111–117, 2011.

[64] R. Asero, A. Tedeschi, R. Coppola et al., "Activation of the tissue factor pathway of blood coagulation in patients with chronic urticaria," *Journal of Allergy and Clinical Immunology*, vol. 119, no. 3, pp. 705–710, 2007.

[65] R. Parslew, D. Pryce, J. Ashworth, and P. S. Friedmann, "Warfarin treatment of chronic idiopathic urticaria and angiooedema," *Clinical & Experimental Allergy*, vol. 30, no. 8, pp. 1161–1165, 2000.

[66] R. J. Barlow and M. W. Greaves, "Warfarin in the treatment of chronic urticaria/angio-oedema," *British Journal of Dermatology*, vol. 126, no. 4, pp. 415–416, 1992.

[67] M. Metz, A. Giménez-Arnau, E. Borzova, C. E. Grattan, M. Magerl, and M. Maurer, "Frequency and clinical implications of skin autoreactivity to serum versus plasma in patients with chronic urticaria," *Journal of Allergy and Clinical Immunology*, vol. 123, no. 3, pp. 705–706, 2009.

[68] S. S. Saini, "Chronic spontaneous urticaria: etiology and pathogenesis," *Immunology and Allergy Clinics of North America*, vol. 34, pp. 33–52, 2014.

[69] U. Amara, M. A. Flierl, D. Rittirsch et al., "Molecular intercommunication between the complement and coagulation systems," *The Journal of Immunology*, vol. 185, no. 9, pp. 5628–5636, 2010.

[70] M. Kaliner, J. H. Shelhamer, and E. A. Ottesen, "Effects of infused histamine: correlation of plasma histamine levels and symptoms," *Journal of Allergy and Clinical Immunology*, vol. 69, no. 3, pp. 283–289, 1982.

[71] W. Lorenz and A. Doenicke, "Histamine release in clinical conditions," *Mount Sinai Journal of Medicine*, vol. 45, no. 3, pp. 357–386, 1978.

[72] R. J. Flower, E. A. Harvey, and W. P. Kingston, "Inflammatory effects of prostaglandin $D_2$ in rat and human skin," *British Journal of Pharmacology*, vol. 56, no. 2, pp. 229–233, 1976.

[73] C. Grunfeld and M. A. Palladino Jr., "Tumor necrosis factor: immunologic, antitumor, metabolic, and cardiovascular activities," *Advances in Internal Medicine*, vol. 35, pp. 45–71, 1990.

[74] L. Borish, "Cytokines in allergic inflammation," in *Allergy : Principles and Practice*, E. Middleton Jr., C. E. Reed, E. F. Ellis, N. F. Adkinson, J. W. Yunginger, and W. W. Busse, Eds., vol. 1, pp. 108–119, Mosby, St. Louis, Mo, USA, 5th edition, 1998.

[75] N. Subramanian and M. A. Bray, "Interleukin 1 releases histamine from human basophils and mast cells in vitro," *The Journal of Immunology*, vol. 138, no. 1, pp. 271–275, 1987.

[76] H. Boey, R. Rosenbaum, J. Castracane, and L. Borish, "Interleukin-4 is a neutrophil activator," *Journal of Allergy and Clinical Immunology*, vol. 83, no. 5, pp. 978–984, 1989.

[77] J. M. Wang, A. Rambaldi, A. Biondi, Z. G. Chen, C. J. Sanderson, and A. Mantovani, "Recombinant human interleukin 5 is a selective eosinophil chemoattractant," *European Journal of Immunology*, vol. 19, no. 4, pp. 701–705, 1989.

[78] J. Willems, M. Joniau, S. Cinque, and J. van Damme, "Human granulocyte chemotactic peptide (IL-8) as a specific neutrophil degranulator: comparison with other monokines," *Immunology*, vol. 67, no. 4, pp. 540–542, 1989.

[79] A. D. Luster, "Mechanisms of disease: chemokines chemotactic cytokines that mediate inflammation," *The New England Journal of Medicine*, vol. 338, no. 7, pp. 436–445, 1998.

# 7

# Pyoderma Gangrenosum: A Review of Clinical Features and Outcomes of 23 Cases Requiring Inpatient Management

**Mingwei Joel Ye[1,2] and Joshua Mingsheng Ye[2]**

[1] Department of Dermatology, Western Hospital, Footscray, VIC 3011, Australia
[2] Department of Medicine, Dentistry and Health Sciences, University of Melbourne, Parkville, VIC 3010, Australia

Correspondence should be addressed to Mingwei Joel Ye; joelye_85@hotmail.com

Academic Editor: Jane M. Grant-Kels

Pyoderma gangrenosum (PG) is a rare dermatological disorder characterised by the rapid progression of a painful, necrolytic ulcer. This study retrospectively identified patients who were admitted and treated for PG during a 10-year period (2003–2013). Twenty-three patients were included in this study, 16 women and seven men. The mean age at initial admission was 62.8 years (range 30 to 89 years). Lesions were localised to lower limb in 13 patients, peristomal region in four, breast in three, and upper limb in one, and two patients had PG at multiple sites. The variants of PG noted were ulcerative (18), bullous (2), vegetative (2), and pustular (1). Associated systemic diseases were observed in 11 patients (47.8%). Systemic therapies were initiated in 21 patients while two patients received topical treatments. The mean length of hospital stay was 47 days (range 5 to 243 days) and five patients died during their admissions. Seven patients required readmissions for exacerbations of their PG. Our study showed that patients admitted for treatment of PG had high morbidity and mortality. This study also highlights the importance of early and aggressive treatment of patients admitted with PG as well as treating associated systemic diseases and wound infections.

## 1. Introduction

Pyoderma gangrenosum (PG) is a rare dermatological condition that was first described by Brocq, a French dermatologist, in 1916 [1]. It is characterized by rapidly, progressing ulceration of the skin with an ill-defined border and can occur at any age, but more frequently observed in adults than children [2]. It has a gender predilection for females [3] and commonly affects the lower extremities, in particular the pretibial area [2, 3].

The etiology of PG remains unknown but has been attributed to reactive neutrophilic dermatosis. Pathergy, a term used to describe an exaggerated skin injury occurring after trauma, can exacerbate PG [2]. Diagnosis of PG requires clinicopathologic correlation and is often a diagnosis of exclusion after common causes of skin ulceration such as infection, malignant neoplasms, and vasculitic syndromes have been ruled out. Histopathological findings of PG are not specific. Early lesions may reveal dermal neutrophilia centered on follicles, while severe skin lesions may show tissue necrosis with surrounding mononuclear cell infiltrates [2]. PG is often associated with systemic diseases such as inflammatory bowel disease (IBD), rheumatoid, and haematological conditions [4–6].

Systemic therapy such as corticosteroids and cytotoxic agents are the treatment of choice for rapidly progressing PG [7, 8]. Newer biological agents such as infliximab and adalimumab have also been found to be effective [9, 10]. Despite advances in medical therapy, the prognosis of PG remains unpredictable and, if left untreated, almost always fatal. This retrospective study was undertaken to strengthen current knowledge and experience of the outcomes of PG, as well as identifying possible factors that may exert influence over patients' outcomes.

## 2. Methods

In this study, we retrospectively analysed the characteristics of patients who were treated for PG. Twenty-three patients who were admitted and treated for PG were identified from Western Hospital Health Information Service through

TABLE 1: Demographics of 23 patients admitted with PG.

| Demographics | Number of cases (%) |
|---|---|
| Age at diagnosis (years) | |
|    30–44 | 4 |
|    45–59 | 4 |
|    60–74 | 10 |
|    75 and above | 5 |
| Mean age at diagnosis (range) | 62.8 years (30–89) |
| Sex | |
|    Male | 7 |
|    Female | 16 |
| Associated disease | 11 |
| Treatment | |
|    Topical | 2 |
|    Systemic | 21 |
| Mean length of hospital stay (range) | 47 days (5–243) |
| Outcome | |
|    Alive after 1st admission | 18 |
|    Dead at 1st admission | 5 |
|    Recurrence | 7 |

a search of medical records over a 10-year period from July 2003 to September 2013.

The medical records of these patients were reviewed and the following data were extracted: age at initial hospital admission for PG, sex, clinical variant of PG, site of ulcer, associate systemic diseases, investigation results, treatment regimes, and outcomes including length of hospital stay, deaths, and recurrence during follow-up.

## 3. Results

*3.1. Patient Demographics.* Twenty-three patients (see Table 1) were included in this study between July 2003 and September 2013. All patients were admitted for inpatient management of PG. One patient also suffered from community acquired pneumonia at the time of admission. There were 16 women and seven men (ratio of 2.3 : 1) and the mean age of onset was 62.8 years (range 30 to 89 years). The mean age of onset was 63.6 years for women and 61 years for men. The peak incidence of onset of PG was in the seventh decade ($n = 6$, 26%).

*3.2. Clinical Features.* Ulcerative PG was the most common variant and was observed in 18 patients (78.3%), vegetative PG in two (8.7%), and bullous PG in two (8.7%) and one patient suffered from pustular PG (4.3%). The lower limb was the commonest site of PG occurrence ($n = 13$, 56.5%) (see Figure 1). For the rest of the patients, lesions developed on the breasts in three patients (13%), peristomal area in four patients (17.4%), and upper limb in one patient (4.4%) and two patients had lesions in multiple sites (8.7%). Ten patients reported trauma as a precipitating cause of PG. Of these, surgery accounted for six cases.

Other associated systemic diseases were found in 11 patients (47.8%), five cases with solid tumours (three bowel and two lung cancers), two with IBD (Crohn's disease and ulcerative colitis), two with connective tissue joint diseases (CREST and ankylosing spondylitis), and two with haematological disorders (essential thrombocythemia and monoclonal gammopathy).

*3.3. Investigations.* Wound swabs and C-reactive protein (CRP) were performed on admission. Microbiological study of swabs from the ulcers revealed positive cultures in 13 patients (56.5%). *Staphylococcus aureus* was found in five, *Enterococci* in one, *Escherichia coli* in two, *Streptococci* in four, *Pseudomonas aeruginosa* in three, and *Serratia marcescens* in one. The CRP values of our patients ranged from 3 mg/L to 474 mg/L (normal reference interval, 0–10 mg/L).

In order to exclude other causes of skin ulceration and identify underlying systemic diseases, the patients also underwent a range of laboratory tests including a full blood examination, serum electrolytes, immunoelectrophoresis, antinuclear antibodies, and rheumatoid factor. Additional tests such as hepatitis serology, antineutrophilic cytoplasmic antibodies, and extractible nuclear antigen were performed in some patients according to clinical suspicion and initial investigation results. None of our patients had a positive vasculitis test. One patient had oligoclonal banding in gamma region on immunoelectrophoresis and was subsequently diagnosed with monoclonal gammopathy.

The results of skin biopsies were available for 15 patients. Neutrophil infiltration to deep dermis was seen in 12 cases, lymphocytic infiltrate in six, abscess formation in three, vasculitis in one, and leukocytoclasia in one.

*3.4. Treatment.* Systemic therapy was used in 21 patients (91.3%). Systemic therapy involved either monotherapy with prednisolone (dose of 25 mg–50 mg daily) in eight patients or combination therapy (see Figure 2) which consisted of at least prednisolone and other treatments such as tetracycline, dapsone, azathioprine, mycophenolate mofetil (MMF), and adalimumab. Potent topical steroids such as betamethasone dipropionate and mometasone furoate were used in two patients (8.7%).

Seven patients underwent surgical interventions while on immunosuppressive therapy. Five patients had minor debridement of their wounds, one patient had split skin grafts (SSG), and another had both SSG and minor debridement. None of the patients had exacerbation after these procedures.

Intravenous antibiotics were administered to 18 patients based on clinical suspicion of infected PG wound.

*3.5. Patient Outcomes*

*3.5.1. Length of Stay (LOS).* Mean length of hospital stay (LOS) till discharge or death was 47 days (range 5 to 243 days). Three patients were hospitalised for more than three months. All three suffered from concomitant wound infections during their hospital stay. Two of them grew *Staphylococcus aureus* and one grew Extended-spectrum beta-lactamase (ESBL)

TABLE 2: Characteristics of patients who died during initial admission.

| Age/sex | LOS (days) | Site | Type | Associated disease | Other comorbidities | Wound culture | CRP | Treatment | Cause of death |
|---------|-----------|------|------|-------------------|---------------------|---------------|-----|-----------|----------------|
| 85 M | 20 | Lower limb | Ulcerative | Lung and prostate cancer | Atrial fibrillation, osteoporosis | *Pseudomonas* | 65 | Prednisolone, MMF | Sepsis |
| 81 F | 15 | Lower limb | Vegetative | — | — | *Streptococcus, Enterococcus* | 88 | Prednisolone, minocycline | Sepsis |
| 72 F | 151 | Lower limb | Ulcerative | Colon cancer | Aortic valve replacement, osteoarthritis | *Staphylococcus* | 178 | Prednisolone, dapsone, MMF, and doxycycline | Sepsis |
| 72 F | 38 | Lower limb | Ulcerative | CREST | Osteoporosis, hypertension | *Staphylococcus* | 111 | Prednisolone | Multiorgan failure |
| 83 M | 29 | Lower limb | Ulcerative | Monoclonal gammopathy | Psoriasis, gout, hypertension, and osteoporosis | *Pseudomonas, Staphylococcus* | 52 | Prednisolone, azathioprine | Sepsis |

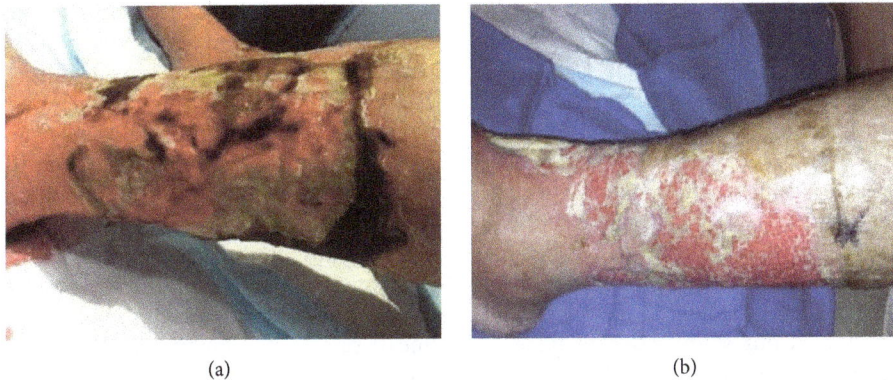

(a)                                    (b)

FIGURE 1: (a) 73-year-old female with bilateral lower limb ulcerative PG and colorectal cancer. (b) Epithelialization and granulation tissue formation after 3 months of prednisolone 30 mg/daily and mycophenolate mofetil 1 g/twice daily.

*Escherichia coli*. All three patients had abnormally high CRP levels (range 53 mg/L–178 mg/L) and one patient who also suffered from colorectal cancer died during the initial hospital admission.

*3.5.2. Death.* Five patients (21.7%) died during their initial hospital stay (see Table 2). Their mean age at time of admission was 78.8 years (range 72 to 85 years). The mean LOS till death was 50.6 days (range 15 to 151 days). All had lower limb PG. The cause of death was sepsis in four patients while one patient died of multiorgan failure secondary to hypovolemia. Four patients had ulcerative and one had vegetative PG. All patients had positive wound cultures and all had highly elevated CRP levels above 50 mg/L. Four patients had associated systemic disease. All underwent systemic therapy: three had combination therapy while two had monotherapy.

*3.5.3. Recurrence.* Seven patients had recurrence of PG requiring readmission (see Table 3). The mean number of readmissions for PG was three (range 1 to 7). Three patients died during their subsequent admissions. The mean age at diagnosis of the patients who died during subsequent

admissions was 68 years. Of those who died, two patients had concomitant gastrointestinal disorders.

## 4. Discussion

*4.1. Patient Demographics.* We retrospectively reviewed 23 patients diagnosed with PG and treated at our hospital over a 10-year period. The mean age of onset was 62.8 years which was similar to that reported in two recent studies [11, 12]. Three earlier studies reported an earlier mean age of onset with peak incidence in the fifth to sixth decade [13–15]. It is widely known that PG has a predilection for females [3] and our study has shown a similar result.

*4.2. Clinical Features.* Four variants have been described in the literature, namely, ulcerative [2], vegetative [16], bullous [6], and pustular [17]. Ulcerative PG, which is the classical variant, is the commonest form in our study as well as previous studies [11–15, 18]. It is characterised by the appearance of a painful, irregular ulcer with a violaceous border [2]. The other variants of PG are less common and usually respond well to immunosuppressive treatments [3]. In our study, the

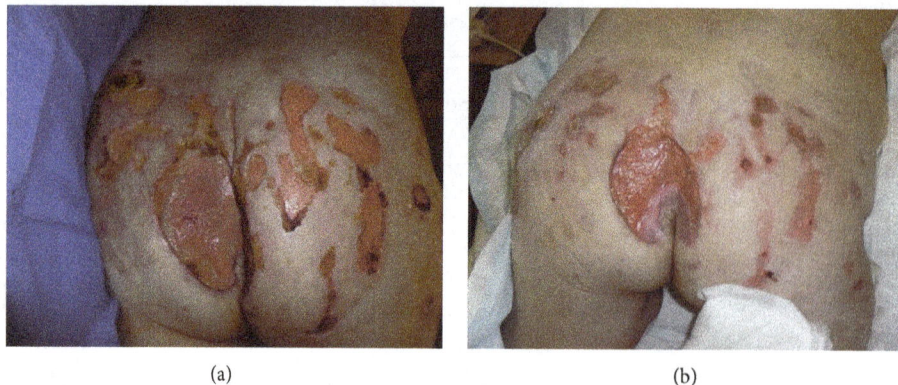

(a)                                                    (b)

FIGURE 2: (a) 51-year-old female with PG at multiple sites including sacrum. (b) Resolution of smaller lesions after 1 month of prednisolone 50 mg/daily and mycophenolate mofetil 1 g/twice daily.

lesions were more commonly localised to the lower limbs (56.5%) but this proportion was lower than other studies which reported a proportion of 70% to 80% [3, 12, 13, 15]. Pathergy was a precipitating factor in almost half the cases. One of the main causes of pathergy was surgery. It is therefore critical for clinicians to be aware and vigilant in diagnosing this complication as delayed diagnosis can potentially lead to poorer prognosis.

Many studies have reported that, in 50 to 70% of the cases, PG is associated with an underlying disease such as IBD, inflammatory arthritis, haematological disorders, and solid malignancies [11–15]. In our study, 47.8% of patients had associated systemic diseases. Most patients presented with known systemic disorders. Only one patient was newly diagnosed with an associated systemic disease during the acute admission. He was diagnosed with monoclonal gammopathy on serum protein electrophoresis. This highlights the importance of screening patients with PG for associated systemic diseases.

*4.3. Investigations.* It is not uncommon for PG to occur with wound infection. We observed that CRP alone is not specific for wound infection [6, 19, 20]. An elevated CRP can indicate either a concomitant bacterial infection or active inflammatory process associated with PG. However, an abnormally high level of CRP more than 50 mg/L, a positive wound culture, and clinical signs such as erythema and swelling indicate a wound infection which should prompt treatment with antibiotics. Immunosuppression should still be continued to prevent progression of PG [6, 19, 20] except in the presence of systemic sepsis. CRP is a valuable investigation and has been shown in previous studies to be useful in monitoring progression of PG [11].

Histology findings are nonspecific but can serve to exclude infection, malignancy, and vasculitis [2]. Neutrophilic infiltration into dermis is the histological hallmark of PG [2] and is consistent with the results of our study. Other histological findings of leukocytoclasia, abscess, and vasculitis are also seen in our patients.

*4.4. Treatment.* Systemic therapy is the mainstay of treatment for severe, progressive PG which is commonly seen in patients requiring hospital treatment for PG [7, 8]. Twenty-one patients received systemic therapy. Only two patients with mild PG received topical therapy and were discharged after a relatively short hospital stay. One patient was admitted as she was also suffering from community acquired pneumonia while the other had peristomal PG and required admission to monitor his underlying Crohn's disease.

Systemic corticosteroids have been shown to be effective in a number of studies and are therefore considered as first-line therapy [7, 8]. Combination therapy of corticosteroid and other immunosuppressive agents can be used to avoid higher doses of steroids and thus reduce the side effects associated with high doses of steroids [8]. Recently, it has been shown that antitumour necrosis factor drugs such as infliximab and adalimumab are successful in treating PG associated with IBD [9, 10]. In our study, only 1 patient received such therapy, 33-year-old female patient who was on multiple systemic immunosuppressive agents including prednisolone, MMF, azathioprine, and adalimumab. Her response to the drugs was less than satisfactory and she had six readmissions in nine months for exacerbations of lower limb PG.

Surgical intervention can worsen PG through pathergy [2, 19, 20]. Therefore, surgical intervention such as SSG should only be performed in conjunction with immunosuppression. Mild debridement of necrotic tissue may prevent bacterial infections. All our patients who underwent SSG or debridement while on immunosuppressive therapy did not have any documented evidence of postoperative exacerbation of the skin disease.

*4.5. Patient Outcomes.* A literature search revealed little information on the prognosis of patients who were admitted for treatment of PG. Our study revealed that patients had lengthy hospital admissions (mean LOS: 47 days), high death (21.7%), and recurrence rates (39%). Patients who were admitted to hospital for treatment tended to have severe and aggressive PG. There are some factors which can affect the prognosis of PG. Reichrath et al. suggested that the type

TABLE 3: Characteristics of patients who survived initial admission.

| Age/sex | Site | Type | Associated disease | Other comorbidities | Treatment | Recurrence |
|---|---|---|---|---|---|---|
| 67 M | Lower limb | Ulcerative | Ulcerative colitis | Stroke, hypertension, atrial fibrillation, and smoker | Prednisolone | Yes |
| 45 M | Upper limb | Ulcerative | — | Hypertension, hypercholesterolaemia, depression, and obstructive sleep apnoea | Prednisolone, doxycycline | Yes |
| 66 M | Peristomal | Vegetative | Crohn's disease | Ischaemic heart disease, hypertension, and peptic ulcer | Mometasone furoate ointment | Yes |
| 30 M | Multiple | Bullous | Ankylosing spondylitis | — | Prednisolone, dapsone | Yes |
| 70 F | Lower limb | Ulcerative | — | Diabetes type 2, hypertension, hypercholesterolaemia, ischaemic heart disease, congestive cardiac failure, and atrial fibrillation | Prednisolone, minocycline | Yes |
| 33 F | Lower limb | Pustular | — | Obesity | Prednisolone, azathioprine, adalimumab, and MMF | Yes |
| 53 F | Lower limb | Ulcerative | — | Obesity, osteoarthritis | Prednisolone, azathioprine | Yes |
| 71 F | Lower limb | Ulcerative | — | Diabetes type 2, hypothyroidism, and peripheral vascular disease | Prednisolone | No |
| 72 F | Lower limb | Ulcerative | — | Diabetes type 2, hypertension, and hypercholesterolaemia | Betamethasone dipropionate ointment | No |
| 51 F | Multiple | Ulcerative | — | Diabetes type 2, chronic obstructive airways disease, hypercholesterolaemia, hypertension, and peripheral vascular disease | Prednisolone, MMF, and skin grafts | No |
| 80 F | Peristomal | Ulcerative | Colon cancer | Hypertension, Guillain-Barre syndrome, diabetes type 2, and osteoarthritis | Prednisolone, minocycline | No |
| 73 F | Peristomal | Ulcerative | Lung cancer | Hypertension, hypercholesterolaemia, and osteoarthritis | Prednisolone, doxycycline | No |
| 41 F | Breast | Ulcerative | — | — | Prednisolone | No |
| 60 F | Peristomal | Ulcerative | Colon cancer | Hypertension, ischaemic heart disease, and asthma | Prednisolone | No |
| 51 M | Lower limb | Ulcerative | — | Diabetes type 2, ischaemic heart disease | Prednisolone | No |
| 37 F | Breast | Ulcerative | — | — | Prednisolone | No |
| 62 F | Breast | Ulcerative | — | Rheumatic heart disease, congestive cardiac failure, and atrial fibrillation | Prednisolone, doxycycline | No |

TABLE 3: Continued.

| Age/sex | Site | Type | Associated disease | Other comorbidities | Treatment | Recurrence |
|---------|------|------|-------------------|---------------------|-----------|------------|
| 89 F | Lower limb | Bullous | Essential thrombocytopenia | Diabetes type 2, hypertension, hypercholesterolaemia, osteoporosis, and peripheral vascular disease | Prednisolone, skin graft | No |

and severity of the associated systemic disease can affect the prognosis of PG [8]. Unresponsiveness of the associated disease to treatment resulted in a poorer prognosis. This is consistent with our findings in which 80% of the patients who died in our study had an associated systemic disease. Age is also a strong prognostic factor. The mean age of patients who died in our study was 78.8 years, 16 years older than the mean age of patients recruited for our study. In addition, the patients who died in subsequent readmissions were also old, with a mean age of 68 years at time of diagnosis of PG.

Our results also suggest a possible correlation between infected PG wounds and poorer prognosis which has never been reported in the literature. All the patients who died in our study had findings suggestive of infected lower limb PG and the cause of death was sepsis in 80% of the cases. We noted that patients with infected PG also had prolonged hospital stays. Infected PG requires urgent treatment with antibiotics and continuation of immunosuppressive medications. Reichrath et al. reported the use of topical treatments such as antiseptic or occlusive dressings in preventing wound infections [8]. However, none of these topical treatments have been used on our study patients.

Ulcerative variant of PG is more likely to be associated with poorer prognosis than other variants [3]. In our study, 80% of patients who died during initial admission had ulcerative PG. Corticosteroids remain the primary immunosuppressive treatment [7, 8]. Both monotherapy and combination therapy have similar efficacies in the treatment of aggressive PG [8]. Topical corticosteroid can be effective in treatment for small and superficial ulcers [8] and this is shown in the treatment of two of our patients with mild nonulcerative PG who received betamethasone dipropionate twice a day. Recurrence of PG requiring inpatient management was quite high (39%). Patients with lower limb PG are more likely to have recurrent PG requiring hospital admission. This highlights the importance of long term monitoring and follow-up in this group of patients.

*4.6. Limitations.* Due to the small sample size of this study, the results were not statistically analysed. PG is a rare disorder and recruiting large number of patients is extremely difficult. Other PG studies had similar number of cases to our study and all their results were not statistically significant [11–15]. Another limitation of our study is that not all our cases had wound biopsies. This raises the possibility of information bias occurring—the ulcers in patients who did not have wound biopsies may be caused by other conditions such as vasculitis

and malignancy since PG is a diagnosis of exclusion. We felt that this possibility is quite low as the diagnoses of PG in all cases were made by dermatologists and vasculitic blood tests were negative.

## 5. Conclusion

The findings of our study suggest a poor outlook for patients with PG requiring hospital admission, with long hospital stays, high death, and recurrence rates. Factors possibly associated with poorer prognosis are age, ulcerative variant of PG, presence of associated systemic disease, high CRP levels, and clinical signs of wound infections. It is hence important to treat modifiable factors such as associated systemic diseases and wound infections. The presence of abnormally high CRP levels on admission and clinical features of infection are highly suggestive of infected PG and require a combination of intravenous broad-spectrum antibiotics and immunosuppression.

## Conflict of Interests

The authors declare that there is no conflict of interests regarding the publication of this paper.

## Acknowledgment

The authors wish to thank Professor Edward Janus for his helpful discussion and critical appraisal of their paper.

## References

[1] L. Brocq, "A new contribution to the study of geometric phagedenism," *Annales de Dermatologie et de Syphiligraphie*, vol. 9, pp. 1–39, 1916.

[2] W. P. D. Su, M. D. P. Davis, R. H. Weenig, F. C. Powell, and H. O. Perry, "Pyoderma gangrenosum: clinicopathologic correlation and proposed diagnostic criteria," *International Journal of Dermatology*, vol. 43, no. 11, pp. 790–800, 2004.

[3] M. L. Bennett, J. M. Jackson, J. L. Jorizzo, A. B. Fleischer Jr., W. L. White, and J. P. Callen, "Pyoderma gangrenosum: a comparison of typical and atypical forms with an emphasis on time to remission: case review of 86 patients from 2 institutions," *Medicine*, vol. 79, no. 1, pp. 37–46, 2000.

[4] A. J. Greenstein, H. D. Janowitz, and D. B. Sachar, "The extra intestinal complications of Crohn's disease and ulcerative colitis: a study of 700 patients," *Medicine*, vol. 55, no. 5, pp. 401–412, 1976.

[5] L. P. Stolman, D. Rosenthal, R. Yaworsky, and F. Horan, "Pyoderma gangrenosum and rheumatoid arthritis," *Archives of Dermatology*, vol. 111, no. 8, pp. 1020–1023, 1975.

[6] H. O. Perry and R. K. Winkelmann, "Bullous pyoderma gangrenosum and leukemia," *Archives of Dermatology*, vol. 106, no. 6, pp. 901–905, 1972.

[7] U. Wollina, "Clinical management of pyoderma gangrenosum," *The American Journal of Clinical Dermatology*, vol. 3, no. 3, pp. 149–158, 2002.

[8] J. Reichrath, G. Bens, A. Bonowitz, and W. Tilgen, "Treatment recommendations for pyoderma gangrenosum: an evidence-based review of the literature based on more than 350 patients," *Journal of the American Academy of Dermatology*, vol. 53, no. 2, pp. 273–283, 2005.

[9] M. Regueiro, J. Valentine, S. Plevy, M. R. Fleisher, and G. R. Lichtenstein, "Infliximab for treatment of pyoderma gangrenosum associated with inflammatory bowel disease," *The American Journal of Gastroenterology*, vol. 98, no. 8, pp. 1821–1826, 2003.

[10] V. G. Hubbard, A. C. Friedmann, and P. Goldsmith, "Systemic pyoderma gangrenosum responding to infliximab and adalimumab," *British Journal of Dermatology*, vol. 152, no. 5, pp. 1059–1061, 2005.

[11] A. Saracino, R. Kelly, D. Liew, and A. Chong, "Pyoderma gangrenosum requiring inpatient management: a report of 26 cases with follow up," *Australasian Journal of Dermatology*, vol. 52, no. 3, pp. 218–221, 2011.

[12] N. Pereira, M. M. Brites, M. Gonçalo, Ó. Tellechea, and A. Figueiredo, "Pyoderma gangrenosum—a review of 24 cases observed over 10 years," *International Journal of Dermatology*, vol. 52, no. 8, pp. 938–945, 2013.

[13] D. O. Hasselmann, G. Bens, W. Tilgen, and J. Reichrath, "Pyoderma gangrenosum: clinical presentation and outcome in 18 cases and review of the literature," *Journal of the German Society of Dermatology*, vol. 5, no. 7, pp. 560–564, 2007.

[14] D. Vidal, L. Puig, M. Gilaberte, and A. Alomar, "Review of 26 cases of classical pyoderma gangrenosum: clinical and therapeutic features," *Journal of Dermatological Treatment*, vol. 15, no. 3, pp. 146–152, 2004.

[15] P. von den Driesch, "Pyoderma gangrenosum: a report of 44 cases with follow-up," *British Journal of Dermatology*, vol. 137, no. 6, pp. 1000–1005, 1997.

[16] E. Wilson-Jones and R. K. Winkelmann, "Superficial granulomatous pyoderma: a localized vegetative form of pyoderma gangrenosum," *Journal of the American Academy of Dermatology*, vol. 18, no. 3, pp. 511–521, 1988.

[17] S. O'Loughlin and H. O. Perry, "A diffuse pustular eruption associated with ulcerative colitis.," *Archives of Dermatology*, vol. 114, no. 7, pp. 1061–1064, 1978.

[18] R. B. Mlika, I. Riahi, S. Fenniche et al., "Pyoderma gangrenosum: a report of 21 cases," *International Journal of Dermatology*, vol. 41, no. 2, pp. 65–68, 2002.

[19] M. J. Ye, J. M. Ye, L. Wu, C. P. Keating, and W.-T. Choi, "A challenging diagnosis: case report of extensive pyoderma gangrenosum at multiple sites," *Clinical, Cosmetic and Investigational Dermatology*, vol. 7, pp. 105–109, 2014.

[20] M. V. Schintler, M. Grohmann, C. Donia, E. Aberer, and E. Scharnagl, "Management of an unfortunate triad after breast reconstruction: pyoderma gangrenosum, full-thickness chest wall defect and Acinetobacter Baumannii Infection," *Journal of Plastic, Reconstructive and Aesthetic Surgery*, vol. 63, no. 7, pp. e564–e567, 2010.

# 8

# Synergistic Effect of Elastic Stockings to Maintain Volume Losses after Mechanical Lymphatic Therapy

José Maria Pereira de Godoy,[1] Renata Lopes Pinto,[2]
Ana Carolina Pereira de Godoy,[2,3] and Maria de Fátima Guerreiro Godoy[2,4,5]

[1] Cardiology and Cardiovascular Surgery Department, Medicine School in São José do Rio Preto (FAMERP),
Avenida Constituição 1306, 15025-120 São José do Rio Preto, SP, Brazil
[2] Research Group Godoy Clinic, São José do Rio Preto, Brazil
[3] Medicine School of ABC, São Paulo, Brazil
[4] Medicine School in São José do Rio Preto (FAMERP), São José do Rio Preto, Brazil
[5] Post-Graduate Specialization Course on Lymphovenous Rehabilitation (FAMERP), São José do Rio Preto, Brazil

Correspondence should be addressed to José Maria Pereira de Godoy; godoyjmp@riopreto.com.br

Academic Editor: Lajos Kemeny

The objective of the current study was to assess whether Venosan elastic stockings have a synergistic effect on the maintenance of results after Mechanical Lymphatic Therapy. Eleven patients with grade II lymphedema of the legs, regardless of cause, were evaluated in the Clinica Godoy between September and November 2012. The participants' ages ranged from 53 to 83 years old with a mean of 65.1 years. Two groups were formed with Group I using Venosan elastic stockings and Group II not using any type of compression therapy. Evaluations of the lymphedematous legs were performed before and after each drainage session using bioimpedance. Patients who wore elastic stockings had a greater volume reduction than those who did not wear stockings (unpaired $t$-test: $P$ value < 0.001).

## 1. Introduction

Lymphedema is an accumulation of water, salts, electrolytes, high molecular weight proteins, and other elements in the interstitial space resulting from dynamic or mechanical changes of the lymphatic system which lead to a progressive increase in size of an extremity or body region with decreased functional and immune capacity and morphological changes [1]. Clinical staging takes into account the manifestation of the edema and the deformities observed. In grade I lymphedema, the swelling appears during the day and in grade II, the patient awakens with edema in the morning which normally worsens during the day. Grade III lymphedema is similar to grade II but more advanced and with worse deformities [2]. Severity may be mild with a volume increase of up to 20% (compared to the normal contralateral leg), medium with increases of between 20% and 40%, or severe with increases of more than 40% [1, 2].

An association of therapies is recommended to treat lymphedema with lymph drainage, compression mechanisms, and exercising constituting the cornerstone of treatment [3–6]. Management of lymphedema using drugs is also possible. The RAGodoy device, a Mechanical Lymphatic Therapy option that uses plantar flexion and extension movements, is a new addition to the armory of lymphedema treatment [7, 8]. Several studies have shown its effectiveness in reducing the volume of legs [7]. The association of therapies is a clinical option, but it is essential to assess whether combinations provide a synergistic effect.

Compression is a physical force that, when applied to the skin using elastic or nonelastic materials, exerts a pressure on the internal tissues of the body, including the microcirculation and macrocirculation structures, resulting in decreases in edema and improvements in the functioning of limbs [9, 10]. The objective of the current study was to assess whether Venosan elastic stockings have a synergistic effect on the maintenance of the results achieved by Mechanical Lymphatic Therapy.

## 2. Method

*2.1. Design.* Eleven female patients were evaluated in a randomized prospective clinical study that assessed the use of elastic stockings to maintain the results achieved by Mechanical Lymphatic Therapy performed for two hours daily to reduce the swelling of lymphedematous legs. The volume of the lymphedematous limbs was assessed using bioelectrical impedance before and after Mechanical Lymphatic Therapy and after the use of elastic stockings for maintenance between therapeutic sessions.

*2.2. Patients and Location.* Eleven female patients with grade II bilateral lymphedema of the legs from the Clinica Godoy were enrolled in this study between September and October 2012. Their ages ranged between 53 and 83 years old (mean: 65.1 years).

The inclusion criteria were grade II lymphedema, regardless of cause, as evidenced by the formation of pitting (Godet sign) but without evidence of advanced fibrosis. Patients with limited joint mobility, allergy or intolerance to elastic stockings, and infection and those without an evident Godet sign were excluded.

*2.3. Development.* All patients were submitted to Mechanical Lymphatic Therapy using the RAGodoy device for two hours per day over two weeks. Consequently they were randomly allocated to two groups by lottery: Group I (*n* = ten legs) used 20/30 Venosan elastic compression knee-length stockings between mechanical lymph drainage sessions and Group II (*n* = twelve legs) did not use any type of compression mechanism. Mechanical Lymphatic Therapy uses an electromechanical device to perform passive movements with flexion and extension of the foot [7]. The treatment sessions were daily for two weeks and differences in leg volumes were measured at the start and end of each Mechanical Lymphatic Therapy for both groups of patients.

Bioimpedance was used to calculate the volume of the limbs before and after each drainage session using the S10 InBody Body Composition Analyzer (BioSpace, Seoul, Korea).

The unpaired *t*-test was used for statistical analysis with an alpha error of 5% (*P* value < 0.05) being considered acceptable. The study was approved by the Research Ethics Committee of the Medicine School in São José do Rio Preto (FAMERP) number 58460-107-2012.

## 3. Results

Volume reductions were observed in all drainage sessions, but small gains occurred in all patients between sessions. However, a better maintenance of the volume reduction was observed in patients who wore elastic stockings than those who did not use any type of compression mechanism

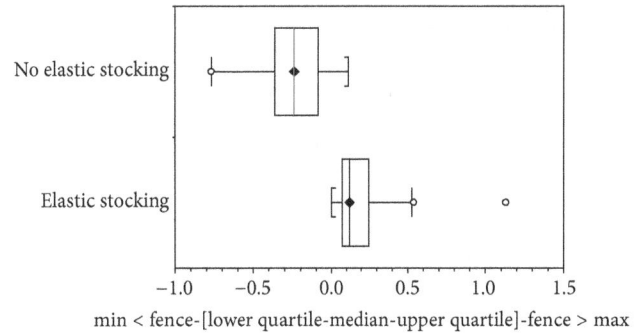

min < fence-[lower quartile-median-upper quartile]-fence > max

FIGURE 1: Box whisker plot showing leg volume changes between Mechanical Lymphatic Therapy sessions comparing patients who used elastic stockings with those without any type of compression.

(unpaired *t*-test: *P* value < 0.001). The leg volume changes between Mechanical Lymphatic Therapy sessions comparing patients who used elastic stockings with those without any type of compression can be seen in Figure 1.

## 4. Discussion

The present study demonstrates the synergetic effect of the use of elastic stockings between Mechanical Lymphatic Therapy sessions to maintain volume reductions of lymphedematous legs. An association of therapies is recommended for the treatment of lymphedema [1]; however, an evaluation of the synergistic effect of each combination is not always emphasized and there are very few publications reporting specific evaluations.

It has been observed that patients with venous insufficiency who wear elastic stockings maintain, to a great extent, the volume losses that occur at night during all the day [10]. It is common during the course of the day for an increase in volume to come about; this is normal due to the effects of gravitational pressure [10, 11]. With the use of elastic stockings, the increase in volume is within the variations of the physiological reserve.

In grade II lymphedema, the swelling persists even with rest and so the aim of treatment is to reduce the edema. An association of therapies is recommended to treat lymphedema with lymph drainage, compression mechanisms, and exercises constituting the mainstays of treatment. Nonelastic mechanisms (bandages) are recommended but require specialized professionals to apply them. Thus, elastic stockings are an option that helps to maintain the results of lymph drainage or exercises.

The limitation of elastic stockings is the fact that their effectiveness requires constant evaluation; as the volume of the limbs reduces, the elastic stockings will cease to perform their function. Hence, they must be reassessed and when necessary changed or the overlapping of stockings should be used.

Recent studies show that it is possible to reduce most lymphedema to near normality [12]. The normalization of lymphedematous legs is important as it allows patients to buy stockings that exist in the market. Even so, it is important to remember that lymphedema has no cure and an association of lymph drainage is important in the lives of these patients.

Higher compression is recommended when choosing stockings and it is necessary to carefully follow up patients to assess volume losses or gains. In the daily practice it is common to see that when stockings lose their elasticity, the leg starts to swell again.

## 5. Conclusion

Elastic stockings have a synergistic effect to maintain volume reductions achieved with lymph drainage.

## Conflict of Interests

All authors declared that they have no conflict of interests.

## References

[1] J. M. P. de Godoy, M. Andrade, W. F. Azevedo et al., "IV Latin American consensus on the treatment of lymphedema," *Journal Phlebology and Lymphology*, vol. 4, no. 1, pp. 13–16, 2011.

[2] B. Lee, M. Andrade, J. Bergan et al., "Diagnosis and treatment of primary lymphedema. Consensus document of the International Union of Phlebology (IUP)-2009," *International Angiology*, vol. 29, no. 5, pp. 454–470, 2010.

[3] H. Partsch, R. J. Damstra, and G. Mosti, "Dose finding for an optimal compression pressure to reduce chronic edema of the extremities," *International Angiology*, vol. 30, no. 6, pp. 527–533, 2011.

[4] N. Stout, H. Partsch, G. Szolnoky et al., "Chronic edema of the lower extremities: international consensus recommendations for compression therapy clinical research trials," *International Angiology*, vol. 31, no. 4, pp. 316–329, 2012.

[5] K. Kerchner, A. Fleischer, and G. Yosipovitch, "Lower extremity lymphedema. Update: pathophysiology, diagnosis, and treatment guidelines," *Journal of the American Academy of Dermatology*, vol. 59, no. 2, pp. 324–331, 2008.

[6] G. Mosti, P. Picerni, and H. Partsch, "Compression stockings with moderate pressure are able to reduce chronic leg oedema," *Phlebology*, vol. 27, no. 6, pp. 289–296, 2012.

[7] J. M. P. de Godoy and M. de Fátima Guerreiro Godoy, "Development and evaluation of a new apparatus for lymph drainage: preliminary results," *Lymphology*, vol. 37, no. 2, pp. 62–64, 2004.

[8] E. K. Symvoulakis, D. I. Anyfantakis, and C. Lionis, "Primary lower limb lymphedema: a focus on its functional, social and emotional impact," *International Journal of Medical Sciences*, vol. 7, no. 6, pp. 353–357, 2010.

[9] J. L. Cataldo, P. de Godoy, and J. de Barros, "The use of compression stockings for venous disorders in Brazil," *Phlebology*, vol. 27, no. 1, pp. 33–37, 2012.

[10] J. M. P. de Godoy, D. M. Braile, F. B. Perez, and M. de Fátima Guerreiro Godoy, "Effect of walking on pressure variations that occur at the interface between elastic stockings and the skin," *International Wound Journal*, vol. 7, no. 3, pp. 191–193, 2010.

[11] C. E. Q. Belczak, J. M. P. de Godoy, R. N. Ramos, M. A. de Oliveira, S. Q. Belczak, and R. A. Caffaro, "Is the wearing of elastic stockings for half a day as effective as wearing them for the entire day?" *British Journal of Dermatology*, vol. 162, no. 1, pp. 42–45, 2010.

[12] J. M. P. de Godoy, P. A. F. Brigidio, E. Buzato, and M. F. G. de Godoy, "Intensive outpatient treatment of elephantiasis," *International Angiology*, vol. 31, no. 5, pp. 494–499, 2012.

# 9

# Comparison the Efficacy of Fluconazole and Terbinafine in Patients with Moderate to Severe Seborrheic Dermatitis

**Narges Alizadeh,**[1] **Hamed Monadi Nori,**[1] **Javad Golchi,**[1] **Shahriar S. Eshkevari,**[1] **Ehsan Kazemnejad,**[2] **and Abbas Darjani**[1]

[1] Department of Dermatology, Razi Hospital, Guilan University of Medical Sciences, Rasht 41448, Iran
[2] Department of Preventive and Community Medicine, Guilan University of Medical Sciences, Rasht, Iran

Correspondence should be addressed to Narges Alizadeh; narges.alizadeh7@gmail.com

Academic Editor: Luigi Naldi

*Background.* Topical agents can be unpleasant due to long-term therapies in patients with moderate to severe seborrheic dermatitis. Systemic antifungal therapy is another alternative in treatment. *Aim.* This study was conducted to compare the efficacy of oral fluconazole and terbinafine in the treatment of moderate to severe seborrheic dermatitis. *Methods.* 64 patients with moderate to severe seborrheic dermatitis (SD) were enrolled in a randomized, parallel-group study. One study group took terbinafine 250 mg daily ($n = 32$) and the other one fluconazole 300 mg ($n = 32$) weekly for four weeks. Seborrheic dermatitis area severity index (SDASI) and the intensity of itching were calculated before, at the end of treatment, and two weeks after treatment. *Results.* Both drugs significantly reduced the severity of seborrheic dermatitis ($P < 0.001$). Multivariate linear regression revealed that efficacy of terbinafine is more than fluconazole ($P < 0.01$, 95% CI (0.63–4.7)). Moreover, each index of SD severity reduced 0.9 times after treatment. ($P < 0.002$, 95% CI (0.8–1.02)). The itching rate significantly diminished ($P < 0.001$); however, there was no difference between these two drugs statistically. *Conclusions.* Both systemic antifungal therapies may reduce the severity index of SD. However, terbinafine showed more reduction in the intensity of the disease. In other words, the more the primary intensity of the disease is, the more its reduction will be. This trial is resgistered with 201102205871N1.

## 1. Introduction

Seborrheic dermatitis (SD) is a common chronic inflammatory skin disorder. It is limited to specific areas of the skin such as the scalp, face, upper trunk, and flexures. It has also been found that there is a relation between overproduction of sebum and *Malassezia* yeast species, which exists naturally in the body [1].

There are different topical remedies to alleviate SD. Regarding disease progression and no response to topical therapy, patients should receive oral treatment. Alternatives are oral antifungal drugswith or without adjuvant therapies. It is the utmost to fulfill the best guideline for severe or persistent disease. Terbinafine is a good choice to decrease severity of SD. However there are alternative drugs to this choice. Recently studies have shown that the fluconazole as a broad spectrum fungistatic drug can be used in treating

seborrheic dermatitis. Despite proof of the advantages of fluconazole and terbinafine in the treatment of seborrheic dermatitis, adequate and well-controlled studies concerning the comparison of oral fluconazole and terbinafine are scarce [2–8]. The objective of this study was to compare the efficacy of two antifungal medications in treating moderate to severe seborrheic dermatitis.

## 2. Methods

*2.1. Study Population.* In this open randomized controlled parallel-group clinical study, 64 patients seeking treatment for moderate to severe seborrheic dermatitis in Department of Dermatology, Guilan University of Medical Sciences, Razi Hospital were enrolled. Four patients discontinued the study and sixty patients (28 males and 32 females) participated in this study. They were matched by age and sex in two groups.

TABLE 1: Comparison of mean SDASI in three phases study.

| Drugs | Before treatment Mean SDASI ± SD | After treatment Mean SDASI* ± SD | Two weeks after treatment Mean SDASI* ± SD |
|---|---|---|---|
| Fluconazole | 27.07 ± 11.20 | 6.64 ± 5.05[†] | 7.17 ± 3.51[†] |
| Terbinafine | 25.64 ± 8.2 | 3.81 ± 2.81[†] | 5.05 ± 3.83[†] |

SDASI: seborrheic dermatitis area severity index.

[†]$P < 0.001$ (Tukey-kramer $t$-test).

This study is launched in October 2008 to March 2011 and took three years and in order to eliminate seasonal impact, the study was conducted only in fall and winter.

Study protocol was approved by the Local Institutional Review Board of Guilan University of Medical Sciences. Before recruitment, written informed consent was obtained. Enrolled patients had no drug history of steroids, antifungal or other topical and systemic therapy for at least two weeks before entering the study (washout time).

All subjects were examined in advance by two calibrated dermatologists with the interexaminer agreement about 90% and the forms were filled out by researchers. Subjects were excluded if they had any of the followings: history of pervious diseases such as chronic renal failure and liver failure, psoriasis, documented human immunodeficiency virus infection and/or sensitivity to fluconazole and terbinafine, breast feeding, and pregnancy. Laboratory tests including CBC, BUN, Cr, AST, ALT, and ALK-Ph were requested for all patients and then the results were controlled and recorded by examiner.

*2.2. Measuring Seborrheic Dermatitis (Severity Index).* The primary endpoints of study were seborrheic dermatitis area severity index (SDASI) and itching. The scoring system used for assessment of SDASI by Baysal et al. (2004) was applied [9]. "Scalp, face, and chest are examined in the patients, graded for erythema, papule, and scale (0 = absent; 1 = mild; 2 = moderate; 3 = severe). The areas of involvement were measured on a scale of 1 to 5 (1 = less than 10%; 2 = 11–30%; 3 = 31–50%; 4 = 51–70%; 5 = more than 70%)" [9]. Severity of seborrheic dermatitis was divided into three groups based on SDASI scores (mild = 0–7.9, moderate = 8–15.9, and severe > 16).

Itching grading is quoted by Comert (0 = absent; 1 = mild; 2 = moderate; 3 = severe) [2]. The secondary endpoint of study was assessing the side effects of fluconazole and terbinafine.

*2.3. Sample Size.* We considered a one-sided test, 5% significance level with power of 90% and absolute effect size 0.75, SD = 1.2 in the terbinafine and SD = 0.65 in the fluconazole group based on the study of Scaparro et al. and Cömert et al. A sample size of 28 patients per group were determined. Regarding an anticipated dropout rate 10% during three-phase study, 64 patients are enrolled in the study [2, 7].

*2.4. Treatment.* Computerized random allocation was applied with a 1 : 1 allocation using random block size 4. The drugs were sealed in numbered, opaque envelops according to the allocation sequence. Allocation concealment was

undertaken by an independent researcher. Also, the processes of enrolling the participants and administering drugs were done by two residents of dermatology. None of them had any involvement in the trial. In one group (32 patients), fluconazole 300 mg *per week* for four weeks was applied and in another group (32 patients), terbinafine 250 mg *per day* received. Four patients discontinued study and were lost to follow-up. Patients were evaluated four weeks after initiation of treatment and two weeks after treatment and scores were noted.

Laboratory tests regarding side effects were requested for all patients at each visiting time.

*2.5. Statistical Analysis.* Data analysis is provided by SPSS software version 16. All data were statistically analyzed by means of independent $t$-test: Tukey-Kramer test, Mann-Whitney, Wilcoxon test, and repeated measure analysis of variance (ANOVA). Multivariate regression models were conducted. Statistical significance was set at $P < 0.05$.

# 3. Results

In this study, 60 patients were evaluated, 32 in the terbinafine and 28 in the fluconazole group.

On the basis of Kolmogorov-Smirnov test, the SDASI changes showed normal distribution.

Table 1 shows the comparison of SDASI in three phases of study. By Tukey-Kramer test, the SDASI changes were significant during the periods between before and after treatment as well as before treatment and two weeks after treatment in both drugs ($P < 0.001$), while there were no significant changes between after treatment and two weeks after treatment.

By repeated measure analysis, the trend of changes were followed similarly in both drugs and there was a significant downward trend ($P < 0.001$) (Figure 1).

Independent $t$-test is applied for comparison of SDASI between two drugs in each phase; there were no significant differences between two drugs (Table 2).

By using multivariate linear regression, the mean decrease of SDASI in terbinafine group was 2.7 indexes more than fluconazole ($P < 0.01$, 95% CI (0.63–4.7)). Moreover, each index of SD severity reduced 0.9 times after treatment ($P < 0.002$, 95% CI (0.8–1.02)) (Table 3).

Table 4 shows that itching was resolved by two drugs and Mann-Whitney test revealed both drugs had similar effect in each phase.

We exert Wilcoxon test to figure out the effect of drugs on itching during study and there was a significant decrease

TABLE 2: The effects of terbinafine and fluconazole on decreasing of SDASI.

| Mean decrease of SDASI | Fluconazole Mean ± SD | Terbinafine Mean ± SD | $P$ value[*] |
|---|---|---|---|
| Before and after treatment | 20.42 ± 12.34 | 21.65 ± 6.58 | 0.64 |
| After treatment and two weeks after treatment | −0.53 ± 4.5 | −1.25 ± 2.89 | 0.48 |
| Before and two weeks after treatment | 19.89 ± 10.51 | 20.4 ± 6.34 | 0.82 |

[*]Independent $t$-test.

TABLE 3: The effects of primary SDASI and drugs on decreasing of SDASI.

| | Unstandardized coefficients | | $P$ value | 95% confidence interval for $\beta$ | |
| | $B$ | Std. error | | Lower bound | Upper bound |
|---|---|---|---|---|---|
| (Constant) | −6.987 | 2.256 | 0.003 | −11.504 | −2.471 |
| Primary SDASI | 0.913 | 0.054 | 0.000 | 0.806 | 1.021 |
| Terbinafine versus fluconazole | 2.691 | 1.029 | 0.011 | 0.632 | 4.751 |

TABLE 4: Comparison of itching in three-phase study.

| | Drugs | $N$ (%) Without itching | $N$ (%) Mild itching | $N$ (%) Moderate itching | $N$ (%) Severe itching | Mean itching ± SD | $P$[*] |
|---|---|---|---|---|---|---|---|
| Before treatment | Fluconazole (28) | 0 (0%) | 15 (53.6%) | 6 (21.4%) | 7 (25%) | 1.71 ± 0.85 | 0.459 |
| | Terbinafine (32) | 4 (12.5%) | 7 (21.9%) | 11 (34.4%) | 10 (31.2%) | 1.84 ± 1.019 | |
| After treatment | Fluconazole (28) | 15 (53.6%) | 10 (35.7%) | 3 (10.7%) | 0 (0%) | 0.57 ± 0.69 | 0.220 |
| | Terbinafine (32) | 15 (46.9%) | 6 (18.8%) | 11 (34.4%) | 0 (0%) | 0. 87 ± 0.90 | |
| Two weeks after treatment | Fluconazole (28) | 16 (57.1%) | 9 (32.1%) | 3 (10.7%) | 0 (0%) | 0. 53 ± 0.69 | 0.773 |
| | Terbinafine (32) | 18 (56.2%) | 14 (43.8%) | 0 (0%) | 0 (0%) | 0. 43 ± 0.50 | |

[*]Mann-Whitney test.

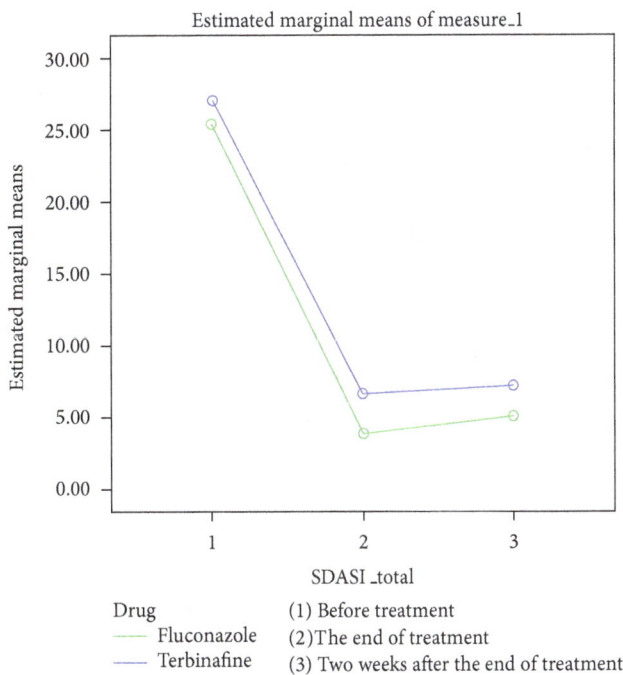

FIGURE 1: The reduction of SDASI parameters in two drugs.

Drug
— Fluconazole
— Terbinafine

(1) Before treatment
(2) The end of treatment
(3) Two weeks after the end of treatment

between before and after treatment in fluconazole ($P < 0.001$) and terbinafine group ($P < 0.001$) as well as between before treatment and two weeks after treatment in both drugs ($P < 0.001$). In comparison to fluconazole, terbinafine showed persistent effect on resolving itching after treatment ($P < 0.008$). There were no adverse drug effects. Flow diagram of this study is shown in Figure 2.

## 4. Discussion

In this study, both drugs (terbinafine and fluconazole) were effective as an independent treatment, while terbinafine reduced SDASI more than fluconazole. Also the severity of the disease or higher indexes was another determinant. It means that SD cases with higher index responded better during drug therapy and one SDASI may decrease 0.9 times in the end of treatment.

Both drugs are antifungal and fluconazole has broad spectrum antifungal activity while terbinafine is not only antifungal but also anti-inflammatory with high lipophilic properties which can be distributed into sebum. Regarding response, contribution of multiple factors rather than fungi in seborrheic dermatitis was inferred, though we eliminated seasonal impact. There are few studies regarding comparison of efficacy of systemic antifungal agents in seborrheic dermatitis. However different studies emphasize that one-month systemic therapy could delay recurrence and resolving persistent disease [5–8, 10]. It's better to point that we prescribed fluconazole with higher dose to reach the optimal minimal inhibitory concentration (MIC) [11]. It was showed that the maximum maintenance effect of drugs was for

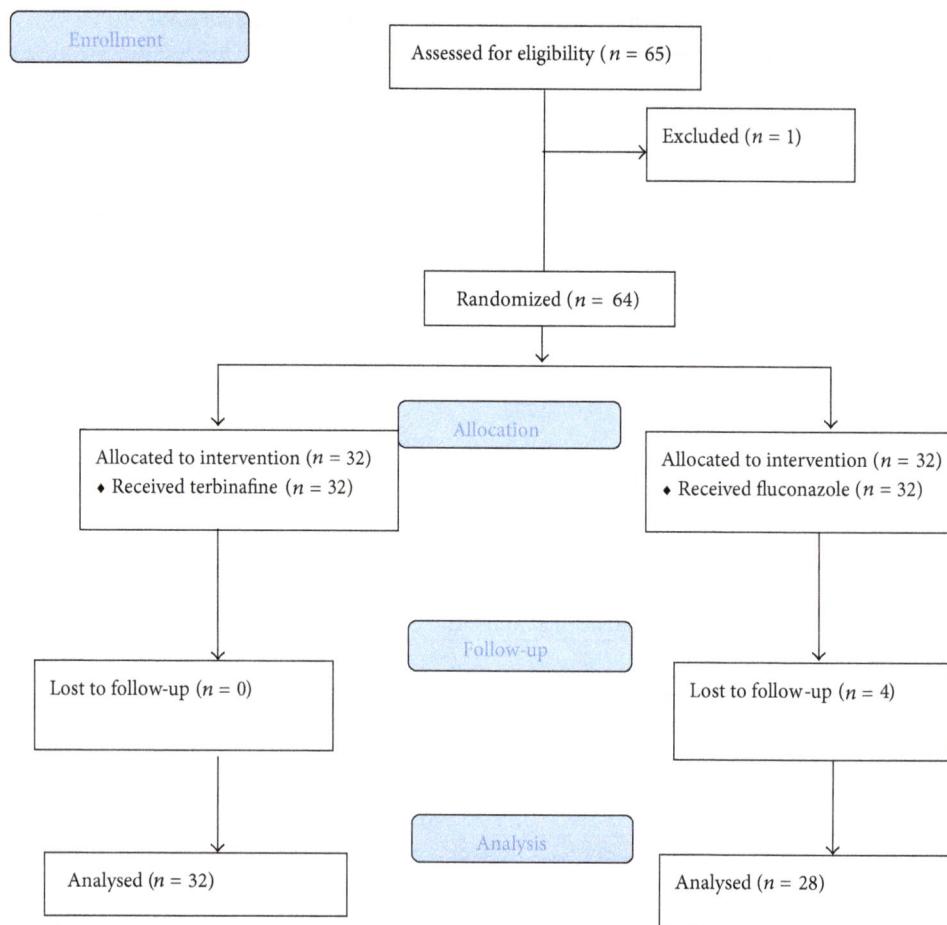

FIGURE 2: CONSORT 2010 flow diagram.

two weeks after treatment with a slightly increasing SDASI after this time, while itching was more plausible to improve without recurrence; however, terbinafine was more effective. Though findings revealed that fluconazole had advantages in decreasing severity of seborrheic dermatitis, consuming once every week is more pleasant for patients. We have to keep in mind that terbinafine and fluconazole could not resolve disease completely, but both reduce indexes.

Fortunately there were not any adverse effect during the period of study; however, some authors reported adverse reactions by therapy [2, 8].

Based on cultural factors, we considered short follow-up period as one of the limitations of this study. Also, the assessment of itching was subjective and based on patients' opinions.

Totally, although there is no definite guideline to treat moderate to severe seborrheic dermatitis, oral antifungal agents with anti-inflammatory effect may have reasonable response to disease.

## Conflict of Interests

The authors declare that there is no conflict of interests regarding the publication of this paper.

## References

[1] J. Berth-Jones, "Seborrheic dermatitis," in *Tony Burns. Rook's Text Book of Dermatology*, vol. 23, pp. 29–31, Blackwell, London, UK, 7th edition, 2010.

[2] A. Cömert, N. Bekiroglu, O. Gürbüz, and T. Ergun, "Efficacy of oral fluconazole in the treatment of seborrheic dermatitis: a placebo-controlled study," *American Journal of Clinical Dermatology*, vol. 8, no. 4, pp. 235–238, 2007.

[3] A. K. Gupta and R. Bluhm, "Seborrheic dermatitis," *Journal of the European Academy of Dermatology and Venereology*, vol. 18, no. 1, pp. 13–26, 2004.

[4] J. R. Schwartz, "Treatment of seborrheic dermatitis of the scalp," *Journal of Cosmetic Dermatology*, vol. 6, no. 1, pp. 18–22, 2007.

[5] G. Plewig and T. Jansen, "Seborrheic dermatitis," in *Fitzpatrick's Dermatology in General Medicine*, K. Wolff, Ed., pp. 219–225, McGraw-Hill, New York, NY, USA, 7th edition, 2008.

[6] L. G. Zisova, "Fluconazole and its place in the treatment of seborrheic dermatitis—new therapeutic possibilities," *Folia Medica*, vol. 48, no. 1, pp. 39–45, 2006.

[7] E. Scaparro, G. Quadri, G. Virno, C. Orifici, and M. Milani, "Evaluation of the efficacy and tolerability of oral terbinafine (Daskil®) in patients with seborrhoeic dermatitis. A multicentre, randomized, investigator-blinded, placebo-controlled trial," *British Journal of Dermatology*, vol. 144, no. 4, pp. 854–857, 2001.

[8] N. Cassano, A. Amoruso, F. Loconsole, and G. A. Vena, "Oral terbinafine for the treatment of seborrheic dermatitis in adults," *International Journal of Dermatology*, vol. 41, no. 11, pp. 821–822, 2002.

[9] V. Baysal, M. Yildirim, C. Ozcanli, and A. M. Ceyhan, "Itraconazole in the treatment of seborrheic dermatitis: a new treatment modality," *International Journal of Dermatology*, vol. 43, no. 1, pp. 63–66, 2004.

[10] G. A. Vena, G. Micali, P. Santoianni, N. Cassano, and E. Peruzzi, "Oral terbinafine in the treatment of multi-site seborrhoic dermatitis: a multicenter, double-blind placebo-controlled study," *International journal of immunopathology and pharmacology*, vol. 18, no. 4, pp. 745–753, 2005.

[11] K. C. Miranda, C. R. de Araujo, C. R. Costa, X. S. Passos, O. de Fátima Lisboa Fernandes, and M. do Rosário Rodrigues Silva, "Antifungal activities of azole agents against the Malassezia species," *International Journal of Antimicrobial Agents*, vol. 29, no. 3, pp. 281–284, 2007.

# 10

# Dermatology Residency Selection Criteria with an Emphasis on Program Characteristics: A National Program Director Survey

**Farzam Gorouhi,**[1] **Ali Alikhan,**[2] **Arash Rezaei,**[3] **and Nasim Fazel**[1]

[1] *Department of Dermatology, University of California, Davis, 3301 C Street, Sacramento, CA 95816, USA*
[2] *Department of Dermatology, Mayo Clinic, Rochester, MN, USA*
[3] *Department of Civil & Environmental Engineering, University of California, Davis, USA*

Correspondence should be addressed to Nasim Fazel; nasim.fazel@ucdmc.ucdavis.edu

Academic Editor: Iris Zalaudek

*Background.* Dermatology residency programs are relatively diverse in their resident selection process. The authors investigated the importance of 25 dermatology residency selection criteria focusing on differences in program directors' (PDs') perception based on specific program demographics. *Methods.* This cross-sectional nationwide observational survey utilized a 41-item questionnaire that was developed by literature search, brainstorming sessions, and online expert reviews. The data were analyzed utilizing the reliability test, two-step clustering, and *K*-means methods as well as other methods. The main purpose of this study was to investigate the differences in PDs' perception regarding the importance of the selection criteria based on program demographics. *Results.* Ninety-five out of 114 PDs (83.3%) responded to the survey. The top five criteria for dermatology residency selection were interview, letters of recommendation, United States Medical Licensing Examination Step I scores, medical school transcripts, and clinical rotations. The following criteria were preferentially ranked based on different program characteristics: "advanced degrees," "interest in academics," "reputation of undergraduate and medical school," "prior unsuccessful attempts to match," and "number of publications." *Conclusions.* Our survey provides up-to-date factual data on dermatology PDs' perception in this regard. Dermatology residency programs may find the reported data useful in further optimizing their residency selection process.

## 1. Introduction

The dermatology residency application process is a highly competitive and daunting endeavor. An affirmation of this is the notable finding that applicants who have successfully matched into dermatology have the second highest average USMLE Step 1 scores amongst all residency applicants [1]. Dermatology applicants usually apply to an average number of 80 out of 114 available programs and approximately 25% of candidates will attend more than 21 interviews [1].

Dermatology programs are quite variable in their demography and characteristics and the leadership style as well as the philosophy behind the leadership can be extensively different in these programs. For example, few programs have officially added a significant dedicated time to research to their residency curriculum. As a recent example, The University of Texas Medical Branch has successfully incorporated research into resident's daily activity [2]. The literature in assessing different attributes of the dermatology programs as well as its correlation with residency selection process is lacking. Considering the competitive nature of the field and the diversity of residency programs in their selection criteria, gaining a better understanding of program priorities and selection criteria would be instrumental to the respective dermatology programs and prospective applicants. We hypothesized that the programs' characteristics may contribute to the PDs' perception about selection process. Therefore, we investigated the relative importance of 25 residency selection criteria among PDs of dermatology programs in the United States. This included an assessment of PDs' perception concerning completion of a fellowship (basic science or clinical) prior to residency training. Moreover, various correlations between the PDs' perception and the characteristics of their respective programs were investigated.

## 2. Methods

### 2.1. The Development and Utilization of the Questionnaire.
This study was an online cross-sectional survey using an explicit questionnaire. A draft of the questionnaire was created by reviewing relevant published literature using PubMed and EMBASE [3, 4]. The initial draft was further developed by a brainstorming session and subsequently reviewed by five content experts, including three dermatology PDs, to generate the finalized questionnaire. The majority of the questions had a 1 to 10 analogue scale (10 = extremely important to 1 = not at all important, supplemental content 1, available online at http://dx.doi.org/10.1155/2014/692760). The survey was conducted via http://www.surveymonkey.com. The questionnaire (online appendix 1) contained a total of 41 items with 17 questions since one question included 25-item residency criteria.

The PDs from 114 accreditation council for graduate medical education ACGME-approved dermatology programs were included as eligible responders of this survey. The e-mail addresses of the PDs were obtained by a systematic search within the ACGME, American Medical Association (AMA), American Academy of Dermatology (AAD), and individual program websites. Residency coordinators and/or faculty members were contacted directly in instances where the systematic search was unsuccessful or the PD's e-mail address on record was no longer in use. A $5 Starbucks e-gift card accompanied the invitations. PDs who did not respond to the initial survey request were contacted via e-mail up to four additional times to improve compliance. Each PD had a unique uniform resource locator (URL) to access the survey.

The study protocol was approved by the IRB committee at the University of California, Davis with exemption.

### 2.2. Primary and Secondary Outcomes.
The main purpose of this study was to investigate the differences in the importance of the selection criteria according to individual program characteristics. These characteristics consisted of a total number of research grants, number of editorial board members in faculty, total number of residents and faculties, faculty to resident ratios, and the availability of postgraduate fellowships and research track positions.

The secondary outcome was to assess the general PDs' perceptions regarding the relative importance of a 25-item set of residency selection criteria. We also explored the relative importance of the following factors in residency selection: source or content of letters of recommendation (LOR), the nature of a publication/presentation, and the field of research/publication.

### 2.3. Additional Retrieval of Program Attributes.
Program attributes were extracted by searching the FRIEDA and ACGME database. They included the availability of postresidency fellowships such as pediatric dermatology, procedural dermatology, and dermatopathology.

### 2.4. Number of Residents and Faculty Members.
The total number of filled residency positions and research track positions were retrieved by searching the ACGME website. Additionally, the total number of full-time faculty was determined by inquiry of the PDs. The total number of full-time faculty members on the editorial boards in the top 20 dermatology journals (according to the ISI Web of Knowledge Journal Citation Reports) was retrieved by reviewing the journals.

### 2.5. Research Grants.
The total number and amount of National Institute of Health (NIH, 2007–2011) grants were accessed by searching the NIH RePORTER website. Dermatology foundation (DF, 2007–2011), National Rosacea Society (2006–2011), National Alopecia Areata Foundation (2006–2011), National Psoriasis Foundation (2007–2011), and Skin Cancer Foundation (2006–2011) grants were retrieved by reviewing the relevant websites or contacting the corresponding organization via e-mail.

### 2.6. Statistical Analysis.
PASW statistics 18 (SPSS Inc., Chicago, IL, USA) was utilized. Statistical significance was generally defined as a $P$ value $\leq 0.05$. Continuous variables were presented as the means $\pm$ SEM. The normality of these variables was tested by the Kolmogorov-Smirnov test. Due to the abnormal distribution of the variables with 1–10 analogue scale, the Mann-Whitney test was applied for comparisons within different selection criteria based on program characteristics. For categorical variables, the $\chi^2$ and Fisher exact tests were used when appropriate. The $K$-means method was utilized to recluster the 1–10 scoring system to a more qualitative scoring system. As shown in Figure 1, the new clusters of the 1–10 analogue scale were calculated as follows: 1-2 as "not important," 2–5 as "somewhat important," 5–8 as "fairly important," and 8–10 as "very important."

## 3. Results

Ninety-five out of 114 (83.3%) eligible dermatology PDs completed our survey. The internal consistency of the questionnaire was more than satisfactory with a Cronbach alpha of 0.861 when we assessed all 17 items of the questionnaire. Figure 1 demonstrates the graphical results of the residency selection criteria. Based on the present study, the top 5 residency selection criteria in order of importance include interview, letters of recommendation, USMLE Step I score, medical school transcripts, and rotation at the PD's institution.

When we asked about the source of an LOR, PDs considered a letter from someone they know closely (8.30 ± 0.19) of a greater importance than an LOR from a chair or PD (7.78 ± 0.24), a well-known dermatologist (7.04 ± 0.25), or a well-known expert in another field of medicine (5.58 ± 0.26). All comparisons reached statistical significance.

Peer reviewed publications (7.04 ± 0.26) were significantly preferred over oral presentations (5.97 ± 0.24), poster presentations (5.72 ± 0.23), and abstracts (5.64 ± 0.25). Although an oral presentation is likely to be more competitive, it was similarly weighted to a poster presentation in importance. When PDs were asked about the order of the authors in a publication, 44% considered a first author publication more favorably than a second-to-last author publication while 40% of PDs said that it depends on the quality of the paper.

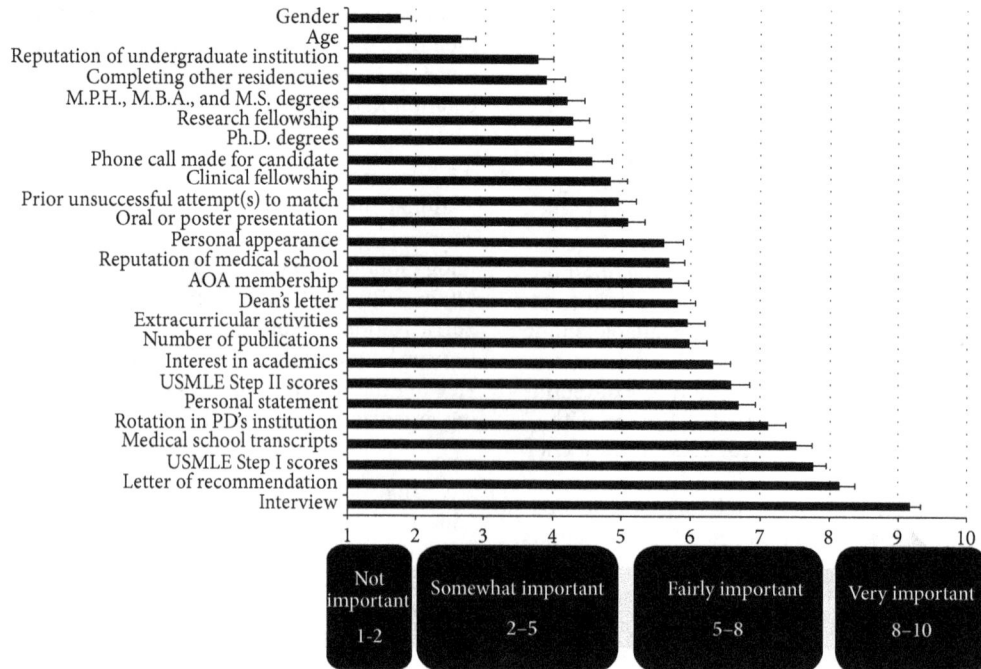

FIGURE 1: The graphical demonstration of the ranks of the 25-item residency selection criteria.

The two-step clustering method was utilized to compare program characteristics with the results of the residency selection criteria. The calculated cut points were 35 for the total number of grants, 7 for the number of non-NIH grants, 15 for the number of ACGME approved residency slots, 1.3 for the ratio of faculty to residents members, 20 for the number of full-time faculty members, 10 for the number of faculty members on a selection committee, and 6 for the number of editorial board members in the top 20 dermatology journals. The dichotomization data are presented in Figure 2.

Specifically, completion of a clinical research fellowship was deemed more favorably than a basic science research fellowship ($4.97 \pm 0.23$ versus $3.89 \pm 0.26$, resp., $P < 0.05$). However, programs with a larger number of residents and faculty members, those with a larger number of grants, and those that offered a research track position considered a basic science research fellowship comparable to a clinical fellowship (Figure 3).

Our data support two findings regarding specific areas of research. Firstly, dermatology research experience is preferable to research in other fields of medicine ($5.13 \pm 0.27$ versus $3.93 \pm 0.24$, for single or few topics in dermatology versus other fields, $P < 0.05$). Secondly, having a focus on one or a few research topics was preferred over research on a wide range of topics ($5.13 \pm 0.27$ versus $4.09 \pm 0.27$, for single or few topics versus wide range of topics in dermatology, $P < 0.05$). When we specifically asked about the importance of dermatology versus nondermatology research in the context of research fellowship training, the average importance was $4.71 \pm 0.25$, which fell into the category of "somewhat important." The reputation of the institution in which the applicant participated in research was also considered as "somewhat

important" with a mean score of $4.28 \pm 0.24$. Surprisingly, applicant research funding was not perceived as important ($2.23 \pm 0.20$).

When survey responders expressed their preference about the length of research fellowship training, 47% did not have a preference while 43% of PDs favored a duration of 1 year or less.

## 4. Discussion

To our knowledge, this is the first study to investigate the differences between dermatology PDs' perceptions of the relative importance of residency selection criteria in detail based on distinctive program characteristics. The other strength of our survey is that it achieved a response rate of 83.3%. This is substantially higher than the 2012 NRMP PD survey [5], in which the response rate for dermatology PDs was 45.3%. According to our study, "interview" and "letters of recommendation" were the only factors ranked as "very important." Many other factors were also deemed important. The 2012 NRMP dermatology PD survey results show some overlap with our study. This survey indicated that factors related to interview, interpersonal skills, evidence of professionalism and ethics, Dean's letter, grades in required clerkships, and letters of recommendation were all important factors in the selection of residency candidates [5]. Plastic surgery and orthopedic surgery, much like dermatology, are amongst the most competitive and highly sought after residencies in the US. Several of the same selection criteria overlap between dermatology, orthopedic surgery [4], and plastic surgery [3] PDs, including USMLE Step 1 score, grades, letters of recommendation, and rotation at the PD's program.

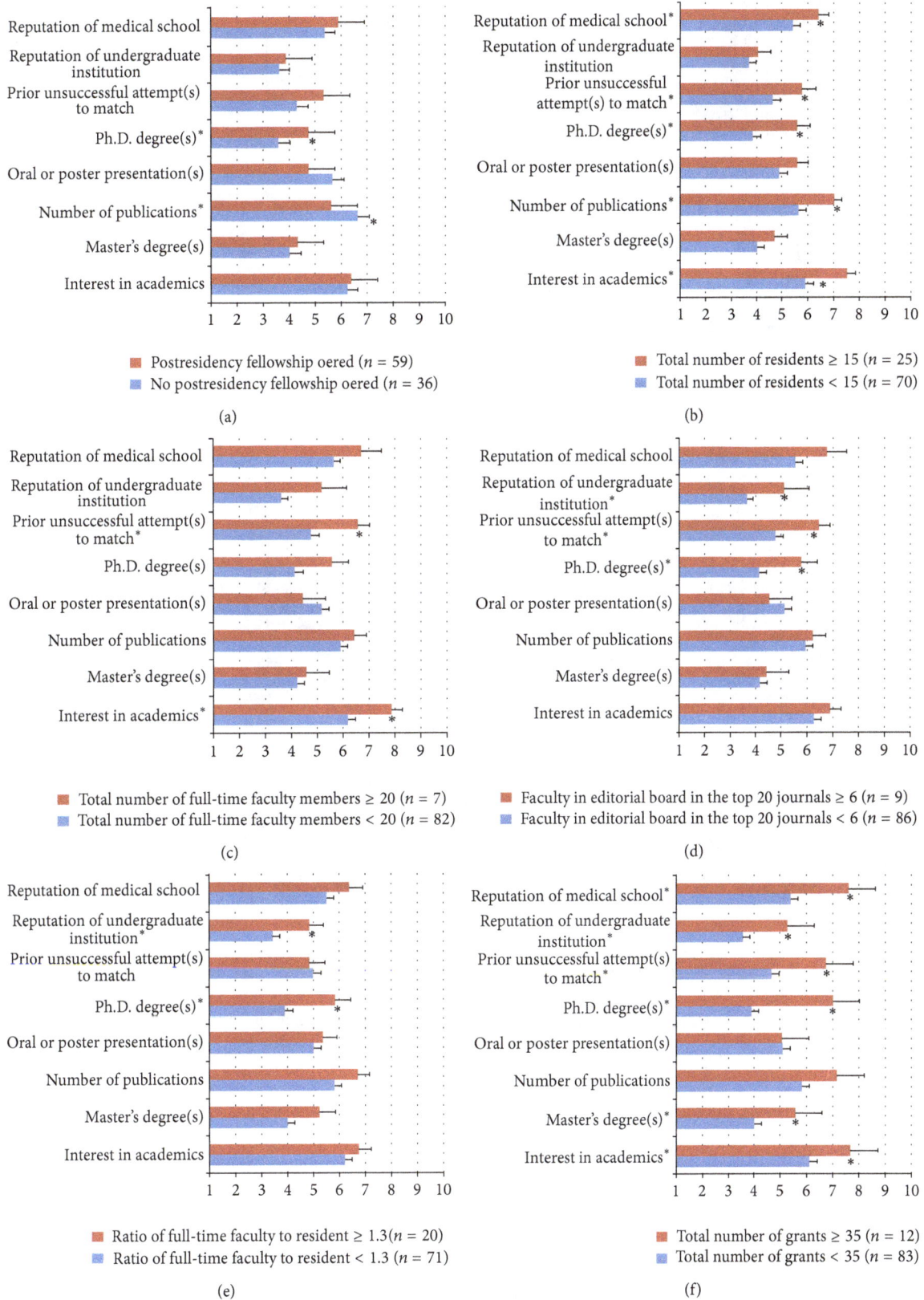

FIGURE 2: The relative importance of major academic criteria in dermatology residency selection after dichotomizing the results based on the programs that offered postresidency fellowships or not (a), the number of residents (b), the number of full-time faculty members (c), the number of faculty members on the editorial board in the top 20 dermatology journals (d), the ratio of (full-time) faculty/resident (e), and total number of grants (f). *The comparisons with asterisks are statistically significantly different from each other.

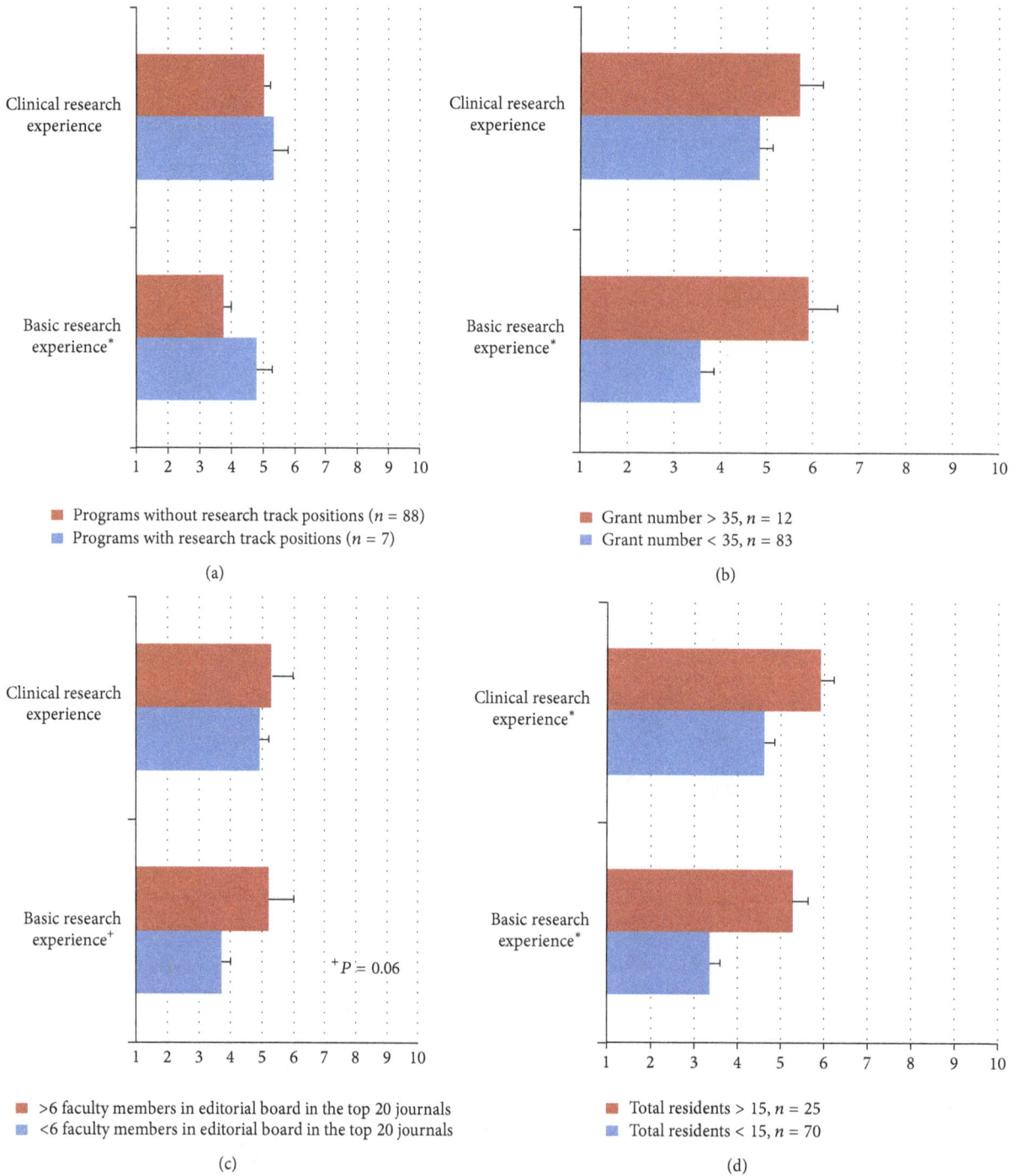

(a)

**Programs without research track positions ($n = 88$)**
**Programs with research track positions ($n = 7$)**

(b)

**Grant number > 35, $n = 12$**
**Grant number < 35, $n = 83$**

(c)

**>6 faculty members in editorial board in the top 20 journals**
**<6 faculty members in editorial board in the top 20 journals**

(d)

**Total residents > 15, $n = 25$**
**Total residents < 15, $n = 70$**

FIGURE 3: The differences in PD's attitude regarding the importance of basic and clinical research fellowship prior to beginning residency are shown. The results have been illustrated based on programs offering a research track position (a), number of grants (b), number of faculty members on the editorial board in top dermatology journals (c), and number of residents (d). *The comparisons with an asterisks reached to a statistical significance.

In our survey, interviews were the most important factor in residency candidate selection even though other factors may have been implemented before offering an interview to an applicant. This is self-explanatory because in order to receive an interview, one's application must be viewed favorably by the program and the applicant's merits are felt to be strong; hence, personal factors become more important. In general surgery programs, interview is perceived as the most important factor by PDs, chairs, and associate PDs [6]. A similar study of PDs of prosthodontic programs in dentistry also found that interviews were the most important factor when selecting candidates [7]. Furthermore, they found that the most important characteristics of the applicant considered during the interview were honesty, organization, energy, confidence, decision-making, and verbal skills. The same trend was observed in ophthalmic plastic and reconstructive surgery fellowship [8], ophthalmology [9], and otolaryngology [10]. Additionally, PDs of emergency medicine programs identified interviews as the second most important criterion [11]. Interviews, as with any other interpersonal interaction, can be biased and even potentially discriminatory as evidenced by the fact that almost all the dermatology residency applicants of one medical school were asked at least one discriminatory question during residency interviews [12]. Such biases can be minimized by using different methods like multiple mini-interviews (MMI) [13] although this method may have its own disadvantages [14, 15]. For example, pharmacy residents disagreed with the fact that MMI is more efficacious or less stressful than a traditional interview [16]. In a study, MMI method was compared to the traditional interview in a pool of interns applying to emergency medicine. Although MMI was perceived less favorably than traditional interview, MMI did correlate with emergency medicine clerkship grades as a residency selection criterion [17].

LORs were the second most important factor in residency candidate selection. These letters may have the ability to distinguish between competitive and noncompetitive applicants [18]. In terms of the source of the letter, PDs preferred letters written by dermatologists they know closely, followed by chairpersons and other PDs. Similar to our study, LORs from division chiefs were considered the most important followed by letters from clinical faculty amongst fellowship directors within the field of [16] pediatric emergency medicine [4]. Miller et al. suggested the relatively high importance of LORs written by a chair or a PD for dermatology residency applicants as compared to LORs by others [19]. Some specialties like emergency medicine [20–23] and otolaryngology [24, 25] have incorporated a standardized format for the LORs submitted by the applicants in an attempt to better assess the strengths and weaknesses of the prospective residents. This can be potentially used in dermatology.

In our study, similar to previous surveys, USMLE Step 1 scores were considered important. There has been much debate as to whether USMLE scores truly correlate with subjective clinical skill acquisition or residency performance [26–30], though there may be a moderate correlation with performance on dermatology in-training exams [31]. Interestingly, in a recent meta-analysis involving a total of 41704 participants and 80 studies, USMLE scores were among the strongest predictors of current doctor's performance [32]. USMLE Step 1 scores are often the only standardized and universally available measure of academic performance and therefore a useful screening tool within a large pool of competitive candidates. Many programs utilize USMLE Step 1 score cutoffs to initially screen applicants and cut down on the large volume of applications that come in each year for a limited number of residency positions. This is of significant importance given that many candidates are encouraged to apply to a large number of programs because of the highly competitive nature of dermatology [1].

In our study, peer reviewed publications were perceived more favorably than meeting presentations while Poirier and Pruitt noted a comparable importance placed by the PDs for publication and presentation in pediatric emergency medicine fellowship [4].

A study of plastic surgery PDs found that the most important "subjective criterion" was the candidate's performance on away/subinternship rotation [33]. Interestingly, compared to dermatology PDs, emergency medicine PDs felt that USMLE scores were less important, while rotation grades in the specialty were deemed more important [11]. Rotation at the PD's institution was ranked as the fifth most important criterion in our study, thus emphasizing the importance of dermatology rotations [34]. Away rotations may be of greater significance in the dermatology application review process as compared to other larger specialties considering that dermatology programs have a limited number of residency slots and therefore any personality conflicts may have a larger impact on the overall cohesiveness of a relatively smaller cohort of residents. The opportunity for greater interaction with the faculty and residents during the course of an away rotation can provide meaningful insight into whether or not a candidate will fit in well with the cohort of residents. Therefore, having the opportunity to get to know an applicant over the course of an away rotation rather than just the limited interaction during the course of a residency interview can be invaluable in the selection process.

Although not highly ranked on the list, "prior unsuccessful attempt to match" was perceived as a more important factor (presumably a negative factor) than an M.P.H., M.B.A., or M.S. degree, completing other residency training, and the reputation of the undergraduate institution. Stratman and Ness reported that the factors strongly associated with subsequent matching of applicants with an unsuccessful attempt included USMLE Step 3 score; LORs by academic dermatologists; completion of preliminary internships rather than transitional internship; publication record; and completion of non-ACGME approved dermatology fellowships [35].

Interesting differences were observed when program characteristics were taken into account. Advanced non-MD degrees, interest in academics, number of publications, completion of a research fellowship, reputation of undergraduate and medical school, and prior unsuccessful attempts to match were differentially ranked (Figures 2 and 3). It can be argued that the reputation of any given medical school is dependent on the degree of research conducted at the institution as is suggested by the annual *US News and World Report* rankings [36]. This finding suggests that applicants with advanced non-M.D. degrees (particularly Ph.D.) and those having completed a research fellowship would likely have a competitive edge over conventional M.D. applicants at least in some programs with more research focus. This may be partly explained by the more extensive record of scholarly achievement typically seen amongst Ph.D. candidates. A survey study of general surgery PDs demonstrated that 89.5% of respondents considered basic or clinical research "almost always" or "all the time" in the evaluation of their applicants [37].

Our data indicated that larger programs, those with more faculty members on editorial boards, those with more grant funding, and programs with postgraduate fellowships and research track positions gave greater importance to research experience and an interest in academic dermatology. These programs may have a stronger emphasis on research and more academic career opportunities.

It is possible that candidates express an interest in academics at the time of interview in order to improve their chances of matching. This is further supported by a study showing that indeed the positive predictive value of such professed interest is very low (8%) [38]. Although ranked as the eighth important factor in dermatology residency selection, it does not seem to be a reliable criterion since a prospective applicant's interests and priorities can change during the course of residency training [38, 39].

It is prudent to mention that if less important residency selection criteria indicate highly positive or negative attributes regarding any particular candidate, the effects of those relatively less important criteria may outweigh the impact of the top five. For example, a student with a *Nature* or *Science* publication will more than likely be considered a competitive candidate for a research track position or a student who has concerning comments in the Dean's letter may be less desirable independent of their credentials within the top five criteria.

A limitation to our study is that our questionnaire did not investigate the differences in the residency selection criteria for the initial screening of applicants versus subsequent selection processes. Additionally, the nature of a survey study may impose some limitations. Specifically, the results represent opinions. This makes the outcomes rather subjective.

## 5. Conclusions

Our survey provides up-to-date data on dermatology PDs' perceptions based on program characteristics and demographics. Thus, this will be useful to dermatology or other competitive similar residencies' PDs and their selection committees in comparing and potentially adjusting their selection preferences based on the aforementioned facts given the competitive nature of the specialty and the variability in program philosophies, resources, and needs.

## Disclosure

The results of this project were presented at the Dermatology Teachers Exchange Group (DTEG) session of the 70th 28 Annual American Academy of Dermatology (AAD) Meeting on March 18, 2012.

## Conflict of Interests

The authors declare that there is no conflict of interests regarding the publication of this paper.

## Authors' Contribution

Farzam Gorouhi and Arash Rezaei had access to all of the data in the study and took full responsibility of the integrity of the data and the accuracy of the data analysis. Study concept and design were made by Farzam Gorouhi, Ali Alikhan, and Nasim Fazel, acquisition of data was made by Farzam Gorouhi and Nasim Fazel, analysis and interpretation of data were made by Farzam Gorouhi and Arash Rezaei, drafting of the paper was made by Farzam Gorouhi and Ali Alikhan, critical revision of the paper was made by Farzam Gorouhi, Ali Alikhan, Arash Rezaei, and Nasim Fazel, and study supervision was made by Nasim Fazel.

## Acknowledgments

The authors would like to thank Drs. Julie Schweitzer, Alice C. Watson, Amer N. Kalaaji, Carrie Cusack, and Alka Kanaya for their valuable comments on the survey questionnaire.

## References

[1] National Resident Matching Program and Association of American Medical Colleges, *Charting Outcomes in the Match: Characteristics of Applicants Who Matched to their Preferred Specialty in the 2011 Main Residency Match*, 2011.

[2] R. F. Wagner Jr., S. S. Raimer, and B. C. Kelly, "Incorporating resident research into the dermatology residency program," *Advances in Medical Education and Practice*, vol. 2013, pp. 77–781, 2013.

[3] J. R. LaGrasso, D. A. Kennedy, J. G. Hoehn, S. Ashruf, and A. M. Przybyla, "Selection criteria for the integrated model of plastic surgery residency," *Plastic and Reconstructive Surgery*, vol. 121, no. 3, pp. 121e–125e, 2008.

[4] M. P. Poirier and C. W. Pruitt, "Factors used by pediatric emergency medicine program directors to select their fellows," *Pediatric Emergency Care*, vol. 19, no. 3, pp. 157–161, 2003.

[5] *Results of the 2012 NRMP Program Director Survey*, National Resident Matching Program, Washington, DC, USA, 2012.

[6] G. Makdisi, T. Takeuchi, J. Rodriguez, J. Rucinski, and L. Wise, "How we select our residentsa survey of selection criteria in general surgery residents," *Journal of Surgical Education*, vol. 68, no. 1, pp. 67–72, 2011.

[7] J. C.-C. Yuan, D. J. Lee, K. L. Knoernschild, S. D. Campbell, and C. Sukotjo, "Resident selection criteria for advanced education in prosthodontic programs: program directors' perspective," *Journal of Prosthodontics*, vol. 19, no. 4, pp. 307–314, 2010.

[8] D. R. Meyer and M. A. Dewan, "Fellowship selection criteria in ophthalmic plastic and reconstructive surgery," *Ophthalmic Plastic and Reconstructive Surgery*, vol. 26, no. 5, pp. 357–359, 2010.

[9] S. Nallasamy, T. Uhler, N. Nallasamy, P. J. Tapino, and N. J. Volpe, "Ophthalmology resident selection: current trends in selection criteria and improving the process," *Ophthalmology*, vol. 117, no. 5, pp. 1041–1047, 2010.

[10] L. Puscas, S. R. Sharp, B. Schwab, and W. T. Lee, "Qualities of residency applicants: comparison of otolaryngology program criteria with applicant expectations," *Archives of Otolaryngology—Head and Neck Surgery*, vol. 138, no. 1, pp. 10–14, 2012.

[11] J. T. Crane and C. M. Ferraro, "Selection criteria for emergency medicine residency applicants," *Academic Emergency Medicine*, vol. 7, no. 1, pp. 54–60, 2000.

[12] S. A. Santen, K. R. Davis, D. W. Brady, and R. R. Hemphill, "Potentially discriminatory questions during residency interviews: frequency and effects on residents' ranking of programs in the national resident matching program," *The Journal of Graduate Medical Education*, vol. 2, no. 3, pp. 336–340, 2010.

[13] A. Pau, K. Jeevaratnam, Y. S. Chen, A. A. Fall, C. Khoo, and V. D. Nadarajah, "The Multiple Mini-Interview (MMI) for student selection in health professions training—a systematic review," *Medical Teacher*, vol. 35, no. 12, pp. 1027–1041, 20132013.

[14] C. Roberts, M. Walton, I. Rothnie et al., "Factors affecting the utility of the multiple mini-interview in selecting candidates for graduate-entry medical school," *Medical Education*, vol. 42, no. 4, pp. 396–404, 2008.

[15] A. Jerant, E. Griffin, J. Rainwater et al., "Does applicant personality influence multiple mini-interview performance and medical school acceptance offers?" *Academic Medicine*, vol. 87, no. 9, pp. 1250–1259.

[16] D. R. Oyler, K. M. Smith, E. C. Elson, H. Bush, and A. M. Cook, "Incorporating multiple mini-interviews in the postgraduate year 1 pharmacy residency program selection process," *American Journal of Health-System Pharmacy*, vol. 71, no. 4, pp. 297–304, 2014.

[17] L. R. Hopson, J. C. Burkhardt, R. B. Stansfield, T. Vohra, D. Turner-Lawrence, and E. D. Losman, "The multiple mini-interview for emergency medicine resident selection," *The Journal of Emergency Medicine*, 2014.

[18] H. E. Stohl, N. A. Hueppchen, and J. L. Bienstock, "The utility of letters of recommendation in predicting resident success: can the ACGME competencies help?" *Journal of Graduate Medical Education*, vol. 3, no. 3, pp. 387–390, 2011.

[19] J. Miller, O. F. Miller III, and I. Freedberg, "Dear dermatology applicant," *Archives of Dermatology*, vol. 140, no. 7, article 884, 2004.

[20] D. V. Girzadas Jr., R. C. Harwood, N. Davis, and L. Schulze, "Gender and the council of emergency medicine residency directors standardized letter of recommendation," *Academic Emergency Medicine*, vol. 11, no. 9, pp. 988–991, 2004.

[21] S. M. Keim, J. A. Rein, C. Chisholm et al., "A standardized letter of recommendation for residency application," *Academic Emergency Medicine*, vol. 6, no. 11, pp. 1141–1146, 1999.

[22] J. N. Love, N. M. Deiorio, S. Ronan-Bentle et al., "Characterization of the Council of Emergency Medicine Residency Directors' standardized letter of recommendation in 2011-2012," *Academic Emergency Medicine*, vol. 20, no. 9, pp. 926–932, 2013.

[23] G. Tsonis, R. C. Harwood, and J. Girzadas D.V., "Standardized letter of recommendation for residency application," *Academic Emergency Medicine*, vol. 7, no. 8, article 963, 2000.

[24] A. Messner, M. Teng, E. Shimahara et al., "A case for the standardized letter of recommendation in otolaryngology residency selection," *The Laryngoscope*, vol. 124, no. 1, pp. 2–3, 2014.

[25] J. N. Perkins, C. Liang, K. McFann, M. M. Abaza, S. O. Streubel, and J. D. Prager, "Standardized letter of recommendation for otolaryngology residency selection," *The Laryngoscope*, vol. 123, no. 1, pp. 123–133, 2013.

[26] W. C. McGaghie, E. R. Cohen, and D. B. Wayne, "Are United States medical licensing exam step 1 and 2 scores valid measures for postgraduate medical residency selection decisions?" *Academic Medicine*, vol. 86, no. 1, pp. 48–52, 2011.

[27] G. F. Dillon, B. E. Clauser, and D. E. Melnick, "The role of USMLE scores in selecting residents," *Academic Medicine*, vol. 86, no. 7, p. 793, 2011.

[28] T. D. Boyse, S. K. Patterson, R. H. Cohan et al., "Does medical school performance predict radiology resident performance?" *Academic Radiology*, vol. 9, no. 4, pp. 437–445, 2002.

[29] S. M. Borowitz, F. T. Saulsbury, and W. G. Wilson, "Information collected during the residency match process does not predict clinical performance," *Archives of Pediatrics and Adolescent Medicine*, vol. 154, no. 3, pp. 256–260, 2000.

[30] H. E. Stohl, N. A. Hueppchen, and J. L. Bienstock, "Can medical school performance predict residency performance? Resident selection and predictors of successful performance in obstetrics and gynecology," *Journal of Graduate Medical Education*, vol. 2, no. 3, pp. 322–326, 2010.

[31] K. Fening, A. Vander Horst, and M. Zirwas, "Correlation of USMLE step 1 scores with performance on dermatology in-training examinations," *Journal of the American Academy of Dermatology*, vol. 64, no. 1, pp. 102–106, 2011.

[32] S. Kenny, M. McInnes, and V. Singh, "Associations between residency selection strategies and doctor performance: a meta-analysis," *Medical Education*, vol. 47, no. 8, pp. 790–800, 2013.

[33] J. E. Janis and D. A. Hatef, "Resident selection protocols in plastic surgery: A National Survey of Plastic Surgery Program Directors," *Plastic and Reconstructive Surgery*, vol. 122, no. 6, pp. 1929–1939, 2008.

[34] W. R. Heymann, "Advice to the dermatology residency applicant," *Archives of Dermatology*, vol. 136, no. 1, pp. 123–124, 2000.

[35] E. J. Stratman and R. M. Ness, "Factors associated with successful matching to dermatology residency programs by reapplicants and other applicants who previously graduated from Medical School," *Archives of Dermatology*, vol. 147, no. 2, pp. 196–202, 2011.

[36] R. Morse and S. Flanigan, "Methodology: medical school rankings," U.S. News & World Report, 2012.

[37] M. M. Melendez, X. Xu, T. R. Sexton, M. J. Shapiro, and E. P. Mohan, "The importance of basic science and clinical research as a selection criterion for general surgery residency programs," *Journal of Surgical Education*, vol. 65, no. 2, pp. 151–154, 2008.

[38] K. F. Kia, R. A. Gielczyk, and C. N. Ellis, "Academia is the life for me, I'm sure," *Archives of Dermatology*, vol. 142, no. 7, pp. 911–913, 2006.

[39] S. J. Reck, E. J. Stratman, C. Vogel, and B. N. Mukesh, "Assessment of residents' loss of interest in academic careers and identification of correctable factors," *Archives of Dermatology*, vol. 142, no. 7, pp. 855–858, 2006.

# 11

# Malignant and Noninvasive Skin Tumours in Renal Transplant Recipients

**Christopher D. Roche,[1] Joelle S. Dobson,[1] Sion K. Williams,[2] Mara Quante,[3] Joyce Popoola,[4] and Jade W. M. Chow[1,5]**

[1] St George's, University of London, Cranmer Terrace, London SW17 0RE, UK
[2] The National Hospital for Neurology, 23 Queen Square, London WC1N 3BG, UK
[3] Department of Histopathology, Royal Sussex County Hospital, Eastern Road, Brighton BN2 5BE, UK
[4] Department of Renal Medicine and Transplantation, St George's Healthcare NHS Trust, Blackshaw Road, London SW17 0QT, UK
[5] International Medical University, Jalan Jalil Perkasa 19, 57000 Kuala Lumpur, Malaysia

Correspondence should be addressed to Christopher D. Roche; croche@doctors.org.uk

Academic Editor: Jean Kanitakis

*Background.* Transplant recipients require immunosuppression to prevent graft rejection. This conveys an increased risk of malignancy, particularly skin tumours. There is a need for up-to-date data for the South of England. *Method.* Pathology records were reviewed for 709 kidney transplant recipients on immunosuppression at our hospital from 1995 to 2008. Skin tumours were recorded/analysed. *Results.* Mean age at transplant was 46 years. Mean length of follow-up was 7.2 years and total follow-up was 4926 person-years. 53 (7.5%) patients (39/458 (8.5%) males and 14/251 (5.6%) females) developed ≥1 skin malignancy. Cumulative incidences of 4.0%, 7.5%, and 12.2% were observed for those with <5, <10, and ≥10 years follow-up, respectively. The rate was 45 tumours per 1000 person-years at risk. Additionally, 21 patients (3.0%) only had noninvasive tumours. 221 malignant skin tumours were found: 50.2% were SCCs, 47.1% BCCs, and 2.7% malignant melanomas. Mean years to first tumour were 5.8. Mean number of tumours per patient was 4, with mean interval of 12 months. *Conclusions.* Despite changes in transplantation practice during the time since the last data were published in this region, these findings are similar to previous studies. This adds to the evidence allowing clinicians to inform patients in this region of their risk.

## 1. Introduction

Organ transplant recipients take immunosuppressive drugs for life to prevent graft rejection. This renders them at increased risk of many types of malignancy and they have been found to be between four [1] and fourteen [2] times more likely to develop cancer than age-matched controls. They are particularly at risk of developing nonmelanoma skin cancer (NMSC). One RCT reported that, over 20 years, 35% of their transplant patients developed NMSC alone, when for all other types of cancer the combined cumulative incidence was 19% [3]. Another study found that skin cancers accounted for 88% of cancers in the immunosuppressed patients, with the next most frequent single malignancy being lymphoma, at 1.4% [2]. Renal transplant recipients have been the most

extensively studied but the risk of malignancy applies to all patients receiving long-term immunosuppression. The cumulative dose of immunosuppression over time has been found to be the primary factor driving the tendency towards malignancy [2–10]. The other strong risk factor is UV light exposure in fair-skinned transplant patients [3, 11–15]. After 20 years of follow-up, the prevalence of NMSC for these patients has been reported to be as high as 41% in the Netherlands [14], 61% in the UK [11], and 82% in Australia [15].

In the South of England, there is a relatively low UV light burden but many patients with light, high-risk skin types. Previous regional studies have reported cumulative incidences of 5% in Oxford (1989) [16], 19% in Oxford (2004) [11], and 22% in London (1994) [17]. In the past, there was a lack of patient knowledge [18, 19], but now that more is known about the risk of sun exposure, it might be expected that patients would be better informed about the need for sun protection and clinicians would be more efficient in surveillance and detection. It is not known whether the rates have changed in this region as, in UK, there have been fewer than 10 published studies since 1987, with the most recent one in 2007 [20] and the most recent London study in 1994 [17].

With the significant advance in transplantation medicine, it is important to have up-to-date local data to inform practice. The aims of this study are to determine the risk of developing skin cancer, including noninvasive tumours, for renal transplant recipients. In addition, it will assess whether this has changed since historical published data and provide current data for the region to inform patients and clinicians.

## 2. Materials and Methods

A list of all patients receiving a renal transplant at St George's Hospital (SGH) between 1995 and 2008 was obtained and demographic data were recorded onto a spreadsheet. Where the transplant from this list was not the patient's first one, the date of their first transplant was obtained and used as the start date of their immunosuppression, with the earliest case being in 1986. The date of the most recent hospital attendance or blood test was used to mark the last date of follow-up, unless the patient had died, in which case the date of death was used.

The electronic pathology reports for each patient were reviewed at each of the three hospitals where the patients were followed up. All malignant (BCC, SCC, malignant melanoma (MM)) skin tumours developed after the dates of transplant were recorded. For completeness, noninvasive tumours (Bowen's disease (SCC in situ) and actinic keratosis) were also recorded. Keratoacanthoma behaves like SCC in immunosuppressed patients and for the purposes of this study, these were classified as well-differentiated SCC. The date of the pathology report, site of the tumour, subtype of BCC, grade of SCC, and Breslow thickness for MM were recorded.

The scope of this study was limited to skin tumours, and nonskin malignancies were not recorded or analysed. The three cohorts followed up at three sites were analysed separately and appeared similar; therefore, the combined data are analysed and those results are shown. Statistical testing was conducted with Quickcalcs (Graphpad) and XLSTAT (Addinsoft) and Fisher's exact test was used to test significance. This project was reviewed and approved by (SGH), Audit Department, and assigned a project number (DB314).

## 3. Results

Demographic data are shown in Table 1. There were 769 patients who received a kidney transplant at SGH, London, between 1995 and 2008. 20 (2.6%) transferred out of the area, 15 (2.0%) were removed from the sample for having less than 3 months follow-up time, and 25 (3.3%) were lost to follow-up. The remaining 709 patients were all followed up in South East England with 346 at SGH, 192 at St Helier Hospital, London,

TABLE 1: Patient demographic data and results at a glance. The results show the mean length of follow-up from time of transplant to time of the most recent electronic entry to the patient's record, the interval between tumours in those that developed at least two, and the mean number of tumours developed.

| Demographics and results at a glance | |
| --- | --- |
| Patients, $n$ | 709 |
| Males, $n$ (%) | 458 (65) |
| Females, $n$ (%) | 251 (35) |
| Mean length follow-up, yrs (SD) | 7.2 (3.9) |
| Total follow-up in person-years | 4926 |
| Mean age at transplant, yrs (SD) | 46 (13.0) |
| Patients with skin types I–III (white), $n$ (%) | 567 (80) |
| Patients with malignant skin tumour, $n$ (%) | 53 (7.5) |
| Mean time to 1st tumour, yrs (SD) | 5.8 (3.3) |
| Mean tumours per patient (SD) | 4 (8.5) |
| Mean tumour interval, yrs (SD) | 1 (1.4) |

and 171 at the Royal Sussex County Hospital, Brighton. On average, the medical records for these patients covered 84.3% of the maximum achievable follow-up time.

53 of 709 patients (7.5%) had at least one malignant skin tumour (Table 1). The rate of skin cancer was 45 per 1000 person-years at risk. 39 of 458 males (8.5%) and 14 of 251 females (5.6%) had at least one malignant tumour (OR 1.6, $P = 0.18$) (Figure 1). 49 (6.9%) had an NMSC. 36 (5.1%) had at least one BCC and 21 (3.0%) had an SCC, with 8 patients (11.3%) having both tumour types. 6 patients (0.8%) had an MM, with 2 (0.3%) having both MM and NMSC.

Additionally, 21 (3.0%) only developed noninvasive tumours (Bowen's disease (BD) and actinic keratosis (AK)) which may progress to invasive SCC. For those noninvasive tumours, there were 31 patients with 88 tumours. Of these, 21 never developed an SCC and these patients had a total of 23 of the noninvasive skin tumours described above.

Only one (1.9%) of the patients who developed a skin tumour following transplantation was nonwhite (Fitzpatrick skin types IV–VI) (Figure 2), compared with the ethnic mix of the local transplant population being 64% white, 14% African or Caribbean, 13% South Asian, 6% East Asian, and 3% from other ethnic groups. The rate of skin cancer for white transplant patients was 57 per 1000 person-years at risk.

Of the 247 patients with 3-month to 5-year follow-up, 10 (4.0%) developed a total of 22 malignant skin tumours (12 BCCs, 10 SCCs); of the 281 with 5–10-year follow-up, 21 (7.5%) developed a total of 49 tumours (36 BCCs, 9 SCCs, 4 MMs); of the 181 patients with over 10-year follow-up 22 (12.2%) developed 150 tumours (56 BCCs, 92 SCCs, 2 MMs). This last group included a patient who had his original transplant in 1986. After 25 years of immunosuppression, he developed 55 SCCs, 21 noninvasive tumours (BD or AK), and 2 BCCs between 1996 and 2011. Another notable patient had 8 pretransplant BCCs over 6 years and developed 22 posttransplant BCCs and none of the other tumour types over his 9 years of posttransplant follow-up.

Of the 221 malignant tumours that were found, 104 (47.1%) were BCC, 111 (50.2%) were SCC, and 6 (2.7%) were

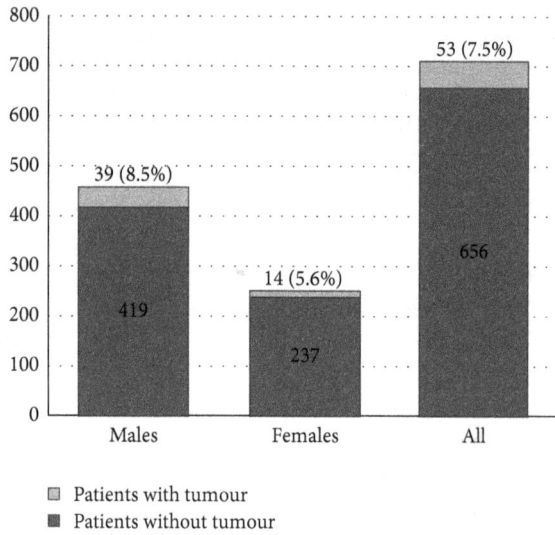

FIGURE 1: The absolute numbers and percentages of male and female kidney transplant recipients in our study population who received a renal transplant between 1995 and 2008 and had developed a malignant skin tumour at the time of data collection.

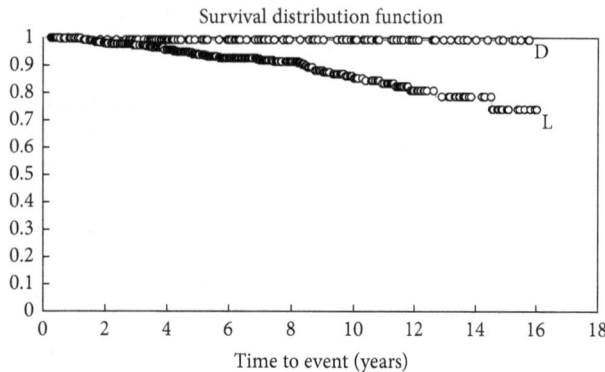

FIGURE 2: Kaplan Meier survival curve shows two groups—patients with Fitzpatrick skin types I–III (light-skinned—L) with worse times to first malignant tumour and patients with Fitzpatrick types IV–VI (dark skinned—D) where only one malignant tumour occurred.

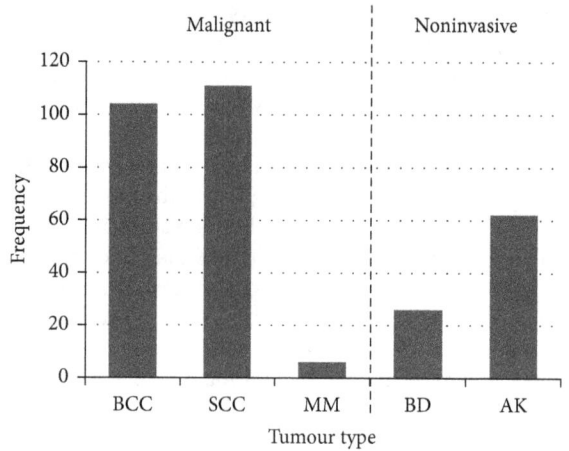

FIGURE 3: Frequency of skin tumour types among renal transplant recipients in the study population.

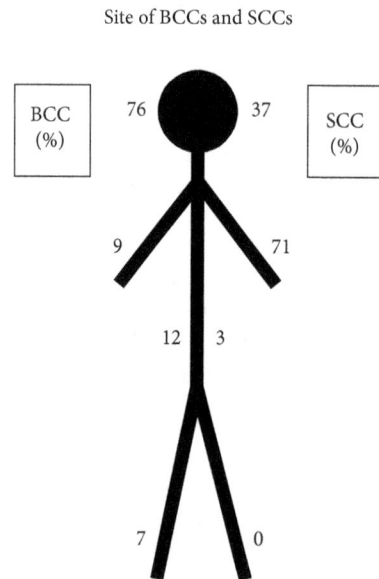

FIGURE 4: Anatomical distribution of NMSC tumours shows predominance in sun-exposed sites.

MM. In addition, there were 88 noninvasive tumours, of which 26 were BD and 62 were AK (Figure 3).

Of the BCCs, 76 were on the head and neck, 12 on the trunk, 9 on the upper limb, and 7 on the lower limb. Of the SCCs, 37 were on the head and neck, 3 on the trunk, 71 on the upper limb, and none on the lower limb (Figure 4). Of the noninvasive tumours, 33 were on the head and neck, 8 on the trunk, 38 on the upper limb, and 8 on the lower limb and in one case the location was not documented. Of the MMs, 1 was on the head and neck, 4 on the trunk, none on the upper limb, and 1 on the lower limb.

For BCC subtype, 63 (61%) were nodular; 16 (15%) were superficial type; 14 (13%) were infiltrative; 1 (1%) was basosquamous; and for 10 (10%) the subtype was not documented.

For SCC grade, 53 (48%) were well differentiated; 29 (26%) were moderately differentiated; 1 (1%) was poorly differentiated and for 28 SCCs (25%) the grade was not documented.

For the thickness of the 6 MMs, 3 were <1 mm; 1 was 1-2 mm, and 2 were 2–4 mm.

## 4. Discussion

Cumulative incidences of skin tumours following renal transplantation reported in the literature have varied according to length of follow-up of the sample and the inclusion criteria for tumours in the analysis. The 7.5% cumulative incidence of NMSC (10.5% if noninvasive tumours are added) observed in this study is comparable to those observed in other studies of similar design and follow-up period [11, 14, 16, 17].

Whilst only 4% of patients at <5 years follow-up developed a tumour, our department begins annual screening immediately after transplant as recommended by *The American Society of Transplantation* [21]. Our observed cumulative incidences of 7.5% and 12.2% for those with >5- and >10-year follow-up, respectively, contrast with 23% (>5 years) and 44% (>9 years) in sunlight-rich Australia [22]. This illustrates the importance of sun avoidance and annual screening is an opportunity to identify high-risk patients and impart education.

The BCC : SCC ratio was equalized at 1 : 1, compared to 7 : 1 in the normal population [23, 24], showing the particular risk of SCC for transplant patients. This is thought to be related to HPV which is known to be an important aetiological factor in SCC but not for BCC or MM (whereas sun exposure is an aetiological factor for all three). The precise mechanism is not clear and is the subject of some debate. There is some evidence that HPV infection, which is often transient, damages cellular DNA in a "hit and run" fashion, not by genomic integration as it does for cervical cancer [25, 26]. However, HPV genes such as E6 and E7 have been found to persist in the DNA of host SCCs, suggesting that at least some element of the pathogenesis is not entirely transient [27]. Ultimately HPV is thought to interfere with tumour suppressor genes such as p53 which would normally initiate apoptosis or repair genetic damage caused, for instance, by UV light [8, 17]. Importantly for immunosuppressed patients, they may be more susceptible to acquiring HPV infection in the first place, with 90% of transplant patients infected at a given time [28]. Furthermore, HPV types which are not known to be oncogenic (e.g., HPV 1/2) may become so in transplant patients and oncogenic strains (e.g., HPV 16/18) which are normally confined to the mucosa may manifest in the skin of transplant patients [29].

This study did not explore the role of different immunosuppressive drugs as these have been compared extensively elsewhere with no advantage between the commonly used regimes [3, 30]. The majority of our renal transplant recipients were on a calcineurin inhibitor (tacrolimus or cyclosporine) with either prednisolone or an antiproliferative agent (mycophenolate mofetil or azathioprine). There is emerging evidence to suggest that the newer m-Tor inhibitors (sirolimus/everolimus) may confer an advantage in reducing de novo malignancies in comparison to calcineurin inhibitors [4–6], though this finding applies to organ transplant recipients with a low and early SCC burden only. Longer-term evidence for the newer agents will emerge in the future, but current evidence suggests that the cumulative immunosuppressive load remains the most important risk factor [3].

Many of the limitations of this study are those inherent to the retrospective study design. In particular, it is not certain that all tumours were accounted for, as there may have been tumours which did not present to our service and therefore would not have been on the hospital records (e.g., if a patient presented to their GP and a sample was not taken). However, this scenario can be expected to be rare because of the education given to our GPs around the increased risks associated with skin malignancy in patients on immunosuppression.

Because this is a case series and the cohort is not compared to matched controls, the obtained figures are open to fluctuations depending on the nature of this cohort and baseline population rates are not accounted for. Confounding factors within the cohort such as the proportion with fair skin, age at transplant, length of follow-up, and underlying genetic susceptibilities may have influenced the results. The only randomised control trial (RCT) on this subject was recently published in Australia and found an overall NMSC cumulative incidence of 35% at 20-year median follow-up [3]. This is lower than previous retrospective studies which have been reported, even in low-sunlight areas such as Oxford where 61% was reported [10]. The cumulative incidence observed in our study approximates to the RCT's predicted incidence for low-risk patients, which was 1.9% at 5 years, 4.2% at 10 years, and 9.3% thereafter [3]. This would be expected in a region of lower sun exposure such as UK and supports the validity of our results.

Our findings being slightly lower than some previous UK studies may show the impact of patient education, as the 20-year follow-up patients in previous retrospective cohorts were transplanted before the era of increased awareness of the risk of sun exposure (e.g., the highly successful Australian "Slip! Slap! Slop!" public health campaign started in 1981) which is not the case in the RCT cohort recruited between 1983 and 1986. It also shows the importance of individual patient susceptibility, as 77% of patients in the RCT had olive or darker, less susceptible skin types (indeed the authors predict a 99% rate for fair-skinned high-risk patients). Transplant patients should be educated to understand their particular danger from sun exposure and they should avoid direct sunlight and use sun protection factor 50. Skin color is important, as highlighted by the low risk in patients in our cohort with skin types IV–VI (all but one of the malignant tumours in our cohort were seen in patients with skin types I–III). The variability in risk between different patients should be formally assessed by clinicians, with high-risk patients identified for increased surveillance.

## 5. Conclusion

This study provides recent data for London and South East England. Despite changes in transplantation practice during the time since the last data were published in this region, these findings are similar to those of previous studies. This study adds to the evidence allowing clinicians in temperate regions to inform patients of their risk of developing skin tumours after renal transplantation.

## Abbreviations

AK:      Actinic keratosis
BCC:     Basal cell carcinoma
BD:      Bowen's disease
HPV:     Human papilloma virus
MM:      Malignant melanoma
NMSC:    Nonmelanoma skin cancer
RCT:     Randomised control trial

SCC: Squamous cell carcinoma
SGH: St George's Hospital.

## Disclosure

Joyce Popoola has received sponsorship from Astellas, Novartis, and Roche (manufacturers of immunosuppressant therapy) to attend conferences and meetings and has given talks nationally and internationally relating to immunosuppressant therapy.

## Conflict of Interests

The authors declare that there is no conflict of interests regarding the publication of this paper.

## Authors' Contribution

Christopher D. Roche participated in study design, performance of the study, data analysis, and writing of the paper. Joelle S. Dobson participated in study design, performance of the study, and writing of the paper. Sion K. Williams participated in the statistical analysis and writing of the paper. Mara Quante participated in data generation and writing of the paper. Joyce Popoola participated in data generation and writing of the paper. Jade W. M. Chow participated in study design, performance of the study, data generation, data analysis, and writing of the paper.

## Acknowledgments

The authors express grateful thanks to Dr. Philip Sedgwick (Senior Lecturer in Medical Statistics, St George's, University of London, sgju511@sgul.ac.uk), for his statistical (and academic) guidance in preparation of the paper and to the Pathological Society of Great Britain and Ireland for an undergraduate bursary.

## References

[1] A. G. R. Sheil, "Cancer after transplantation," *World Journal of Surgery*, vol. 10, no. 3, pp. 389–396, 1986.

[2] F. J. Moloney, H. Comber, P. O'Lorcain, P. O'Kelly, P. J. Conlon, and G. M. Murphy, "A population-based study of skin cancer incidence and prevalence in renal transplant recipients," *British Journal of Dermatology*, vol. 154, no. 3, pp. 498–504, 2006.

[3] M. P. Gallagher, P. J. Kelly, M. Jardine et al., "Long-term cancer risk of immunosuppressive regimens after kidney transplantation," *Journal of the American Society of Nephrology*, vol. 21, no. 5, pp. 852–858, 2010.

[4] S. B. Campbell, R. Walker, S. S. Tai, Q. Jiang, and G. R. Russ, "Randomized controlled trial of sirolimus for renal transplant recipients at high risk for nonmelanoma skin cancer," *The American Journal of Transplantation*, vol. 12, no. 5, pp. 1146–1156, 2012.

[5] S. Euvrard, E. Morelon, L. Rostaing et al., "Sirolimus and secondary skin-cancer prevention in kidney transplantation," *The New England Journal of Medicine*, vol. 367, no. 4, pp. 329–339, 2012.

[6] J. M. Hoogendijk-van Den Akker, P. N. Harden, A. J. Hoitsma et al., "Two-year randomized controlled prospective trial converting treatment of stable renal transplant recipients with cutaneous invasive squamous cell carcinomas to sirolimus," *Journal of Clinical Oncology*, vol. 31, no. 10, pp. 1317–1323, 2013.

[7] J. Alberú, M. D. Pascoe, J. M. Campistol et al., "Lower malignancy rates in renal allograft recipients converted to sirolimus-based, calcineurin inhibitor-free immunotherapy: 24-month results from the CONVERT trial," *Transplantation*, vol. 92, no. 3, pp. 303–310, 2011.

[8] C. Morath, M. Mueller, H. Goldschmidt, V. Schwenger, G. Opelz, and M. Zeier, "Malignancy in renal transplantation," *Journal of the American Society of Nephrology*, vol. 15, no. 6, pp. 1582–1588, 2004.

[9] P. Jensen, S. Hansen, B. Moller et al., "Skin cancer in kidney and heart transplant recipients and different long-term immunosuppressive therapy regimens," *Journal of the American Academy of Dermatology*, vol. 40, no. 2, pp. 177–186, 1999.

[10] J. N. Bouwes Bavinck, D. R. Hardie, A. Green et al., "The risk of skin cancer in renal transplant recipients in Queensland, Australia: a follow-up study," *Transplantation*, vol. 61, no. 5, pp. 715–721, 1996.

[11] C. Bordea, F. Wojnarowska, P. R. Millard, H. Doll, K. Welsh, and P. J. Morris, "Skin cancers in renal-transplant recipients occur more frequently than previously recognized in a temperate climate," *Transplantation*, vol. 77, no. 4, pp. 574–579, 2004.

[12] I. Blohme and O. Larkö, "Premalignant and malignant skin lesions in renal transplant patients," *Transplantation*, vol. 37, no. 2, pp. 165–167, 1984.

[13] S. A. Birkeland, H. H. Storm, L. U. Lamm et al., "Cancer risk after renal transplantation in the nordic countries, 1964–1986," *International Journal of Cancer*, vol. 60, no. 2, pp. 183–189, 1995.

[14] M. M. Hartevelt, J. N. Bouwes Bavinck, A. M. Kootte m., B. J. Vermeer, and J. P. Vandenbroucke, "Incidence of skin cancer after renal transplantation in the Netherlands," *Transplantation*, vol. 49, no. 3, pp. 506–509, 1990.

[15] H. M. Ramsay, A. A. Fryer, C. M. Hawley, A. G. Smith, D. L. Nicol, and P. N. Harden, "Non-melanoma skin cancer risk in the Queensland renal transplant population," *British Journal of Dermatology*, vol. 147, no. 5, pp. 950–956, 2002.

[16] M. Liddington, A. J. Richardson, R. M. Higgins et al., "Skin cancer in renal transplant recipients," *British Journal of Surgery*, vol. 76, no. 10, pp. 1002–1005, 1989.

[17] M. T. Glover, N. Niranjan, J. T. C. Kwan, and I. M. Leigh, "Non-melanoma skin cancer in renal transplant recipients: the extent of the problem and a strategy for management," *British Journal of Plastic Surgery*, vol. 47, no. 2, pp. 80–89, 1994.

[18] P. N. Harden, S. M. Reece, A. A. Fryer, A. G. Smith, and H. M. Ramsay, "Skin cancer surveillance in renal transplant recipients: questionnaire survey of current UK practice," *British Medical Journal*, vol. 323, no. 7313, pp. 600–601, 2001.

[19] E. W. Cowen and E. M. Billingsley, "Awareness of skin cancer by kidney transplant patients," *Journal of the American Academy of Dermatology*, vol. 40, no. 5 I, pp. 697–701, 1999.

[20] H. M. Ramsay, S. M. Reece, A. A. Fryer, A. G. Smith, and P. N. Harden, "Seven-year prospective study of nonmelanoma skin cancer incidence in U.K. renal transplant recipients," *Transplantation*, vol. 84, no. 3, pp. 437–439, 2007.

[21] B. L. Kasiske, M. A. Vazquez, W. E. Harmon et al., "Recommendations for the outpatient surveillance of renal transplant recipients," *Journal of the American Society of Nephrology*, vol. 11, no. 15, pp. S1–S86, 2000.

[22] I. R. Hardie, R. W. Strong, L. C. J. Hartley, P. W. H. Woodruff, and G. J. A. Clunie, "Skin cancer in Caucasian renal allograft recipients living in a subtropical climate," *Surgery*, vol. 87, no. 2, pp. 177–183, 1980.

[23] A. Lomas, J. Leonardi-Bee, and F. Bath-Hextall, "A systematic review of worldwide incidence of nonmelanoma skin cancer," *British Journal of Dermatology*, vol. 166, no. 5, pp. 1069–1080, 2012.

[24] L. J. Christenson, T. A. Borrowman, C. M. Vachon et al., "Incidence of basal cell and squamous cell carcinomas in a population younger than 40 years," *Journal of the American Medical Association*, vol. 294, no. 6, pp. 681–690, 2005.

[25] J. Mork, A. K. Lie, E. Glattre et al., "Human papillomavirus infection as a risk factor for squamous-cell carcinoma of the head and neck," *The New England Journal of Medicine*, vol. 344, no. 15, pp. 1125–1131, 2001.

[26] S. Syrjanen, "Human papillomavirus infections and oral tumours," *Medical Microbiology and Immunology*, vol. 192, no. 3, pp. 123–128, 2003.

[27] M. L. Gillison, "Human papillomavirus and prognosis of oropharyngeal squamous cell carcinoma: implications for clinical research in head and neck cancers," *Journal of Clinical Oncology*, vol. 24, no. 36, pp. 5623–5625, 2006.

[28] D. Berg and C. C. Otley, "Skin cancer in organ transplant recipients: epidemiology, pathogenesis, and management," *Journal of the American Academy of Dermatology*, vol. 47, no. 1, pp. 1–17, 2002.

[29] B. Dreno, "Skin cancers after transplantation," *Nephrology Dialysis Transplantation*, vol. 18, no. 6, pp. 1052–1058, 2003.

[30] I. Kuijken and J. N. B. Bavinck, "Skin cancer risk associated with immunosuppressive therapy in organ transplant recipients: epidemiology and proposed mechanisms," *BioDrugs*, vol. 14, no. 5, pp. 319–329, 2000.

# 12

# Type I Interferons: Key Players in Normal Skin and Select Cutaneous Malignancies

## Aimen Ismail[1] and Nabiha Yusuf[2]

[1] *School of Medicine, University of Alabama at Birmingham, Birmingham, AL 35294, USA*
[2] *Department of Dermatology, University of Alabama at Birmingham, VH 566A, 1670 University Boulevard, Birmingham, AL 35294, USA*

Correspondence should be addressed to Nabiha Yusuf; nabiha@uab.edu

Academic Editor: Ashfaq A. Marghoob

Interferons (IFNs) are a family of naturally existing glycoproteins known for their antiviral activity and their ability to influence the behavior of normal and transformed cell types. Type I Interferons include IFN-$\alpha$ and IFN-$\beta$. Currently, IFN-$\alpha$ has numerous approved antitumor applications, including malignant melanoma, in which IFN-$\alpha$ has been shown to increase relapse free survival. Moreover, IFN-$\alpha$ has been successfully used in the intralesional treatment of cutaneous squamous cell carcinoma (SCC) and basal cell carcinoma (BCC). In spite of these promising clinical results; however, there exists a paucity of knowledge on the precise antitumor action of IFN-$\alpha/\beta$ at the cellular and molecular levels in cutaneous malignancies such as SCC, BCC, and melanoma. This review summarizes current knowledge on the extent to which Type I IFN influences proliferation, apoptosis, angiogenesis, and immune function in normal skin, cutaneous SCC, BCC, and melanoma.

## 1. Introduction

Interferons (IFNs) are a group of naturally existing glycoproteins that are secreted by cells in response to viral infections as well as synthetic and biologic inducers. Since the discovery of IFNs more than 50 years ago, *in vitro* and *in vivo* assays have demonstrated a diverse spectrum of biological activity, including antiviral, antiproliferative, and immunomodulatory properties [1]. Type I interferons include IFN-$\alpha$, IFN-$\beta$, IFN-$\varepsilon$, IFN-$\kappa$, and IFN-$\omega$. Type II interferons include IFN-$\gamma$, and type III interferons include IFN-$\lambda$ [1–3].

Type I interferons (IFN-$\alpha$, IFN-$\beta$) bind to cell surface receptors with two distinct subunits: IFN-$\alpha$ receptor 1 and IFN-$\alpha$ receptor 2. This binding triggers phosphorylation of janus kinase 1 (JAK1) and tyrosine kinase 2 (TK2), members of the Janus kinase family of receptor-associated tyrosine kinases. These kinases proceed to phosphorylate signal transducers and activators of transcriptions 1 and 2 (STAT1 and STAT2), which belong to a group of latent cytoplasmic transcription factors. The activated STAT1 and STAT2 proteins complex with p48 protein to form the IFN-stimulated

gene factor 3 (ISGF3) transcription factor. ISGF3 translocates to the nucleus, where it binds to IFN-stimulated response elements in the promoters of type I IFN-responsive genes and thereby activates transcription [4, 5].

IFN-$\gamma$ signals through the cell surface receptor IFNGR, which consists of IFNGR1 and IFNGR2 chains, impacting distinct but related pathways to those of type I IFN. IFN-$\lambda$ signals through the unique receptors IFNLR1 and IFN-10R2 [3].

Among the interferons, IFN-$\alpha$2 has been the most broadly evaluated clinically, and its three commercially available subspecies include IFN-$\alpha$2a, IFN-$\alpha$2b, and IFN-$\alpha$2c [3]. With the approval of IFN-$\alpha$2a and IFN-$\alpha$2b for the treatment of hairy cell Leukemia in 1986, IFN became the first recombinant cytokine to be licensed in the United States for the treatment of a malignancy. Since then, other approved antitumor applications for IFN-$\alpha$2a or IFN-$\alpha$2b include AIDS-related Kaposi's sarcoma, chronic myelogenous leukemia, follicular lymphoma, and malignant melanoma [6]. Currently, the only approved agents for the adjuvant treatment of resected melanoma that is at high risk of recurrence are IFN-$\alpha$2b in Europe and the United States, pegylated IFN-$\alpha$2b in the United States and Switzerland, and IFN-$\alpha$2a in Europe. High-dose IFN-$\alpha$2b (HDI) is the approved dosing regimen in the United States for American Joint Committee on Cancer (AJCC) stage IIB-III melanoma and consists of an induction phase of 20 MIU/m$^2$ intravenously (IV) 5 times/week for 4 weeks followed by a maintenance phase of 10 MIU/m$^2$ subcutaneously (SC) 3 times/week for 48 weeks [7].

The results of a metaanalysis of 18 randomized controlled trials published between 1995 and 2011 demonstrate that adjuvant IFN-$\alpha$ significantly increases both disease-free survival and, to a lesser extent, overall survival in high-risk (AJCC TNM stage II-III) cutaneous melanoma [8]. Moreover, numerous studies have demonstrated the efficacy of intralesional IFN-$\alpha$2a and IFN-$\alpha$2b for the treatment of cutaneous squamous cell carcinoma (SCC) and basal cell carcinoma (BCC) [1, 9–16]. However, there exists a dearth of knowledge on the precise antitumor action of IFN-$\alpha/\beta$ at the cellular and molecular levels in cutaneous malignancies such as SCC, BCC, and melanoma. This review serves to summarize current knowledge on the extent to which type I IFN influences proliferation, apoptosis, angiogenesis, and immune function in SCC, BCC, and melanoma. Considerably more is known regarding the mechanism of IFN action in melanoma than in SCC and BCC, and this discrepancy is reflected in the content of this review.

## 2. Effect on Normal Keratinocytes and Melanocytes

*2.1. Antiproliferative Effects.* Various studies have shown type I IFN to have an antiproliferative, prodifferentiation effect on normal keratinocytes and melanocytes. Experiments by Yaar et al. showed that cultures of human keratinocytes supplemented with 2500 units/mL of either IFN-$\alpha$ or IFN-$\beta$ demonstrated a mean growth inhibition of 70% at 7 days compared with control cultures. Moreover, IFN-$\alpha$ and -$\beta$ promoted keratinocyte terminal differentiation as demonstrated by increased cornified envelope formation and cell shedding in IFN-treated cultures compared to controls. The effects of IFN-$\alpha$ and -$\beta$ on growth and terminal differentiation were reversible upon withdrawal of IFN from the medium [17].

Similarly, Nickoloff et al. showed that incubation of cultured human keratinocytes with $19.8 \times 10^3$ units/mL IFN-$\alpha$ resulted in an approximately 30% decrease in number of attached keratinocytes at day 8 compared to control [18].

Bielenberg et al. showed that, in tissue samples of normal murine and human skin, keratinocytes in the basal layer did not express IFN-$\beta$, whereas those in the suprabasal layers did, and this expression of IFN-$\beta$ directly correlated with production of differentiation markers. The *in vitro* expression of IFN-$\beta$ by undifferentiated, growth-arrested murine keratinocytes suggested that the production of IFN-$\beta$ by terminally differentiated cells was associated with cessation of proliferation. Further, tissue samples from neither human nor transgenic mouse squamous cell carcinomas expressed significant levels of IFN-$\beta$ [19].

Krasagakis et al. demonstrated a strong growth inhibition of normal human melanocytes by IFN-$\beta$ in a dose- and time-dependant manner in 6- and 12-day assays in both RMM and CMM media (at 12 days, 10,000 IU/mL IFN-$\beta$ led to 80% growth inhibition in CMM and 77% growth inhibition in RMM compared to controls). In contrast 10,000 IU/mL of IFN-$\alpha$ showed no effect on melanocyte proliferation in RMM but did lead to a 24% growth inhibition in CMM compared to controls in 12 days. CMM is TPA- and serum-free complete melanocyte medium, and RMM is its mitogen-reduced variant [20].

*2.2. Antiangiogenesis Effects.* Mouse IFN-$\alpha/\beta$ have been shown to inhibit experimental wound healing in mice through the inhibition of proliferation of many different cell types, including endothelial, epidermal, and connective tissue cells [21].

McCarty et al. implanted gelfoam sponges in IFN-$\alpha/\beta$ receptor $-/-$ mice and IFN-$\alpha/\beta$ receptor $+/+$ mice and proceeded to induce endothelial cell migration and proliferation with 200 ng/mL of the proangiogenic factors bFGF, VEGF, and TGF-$\alpha$. Sponges that were recovered from IFN-$\alpha/\beta$ R $-/-$ mice demonstrated a significantly higher number of blood vessels than did those recovered from IFN-$\alpha/\beta$ R $+/+$ mice, indicating that IFN sensitivity of surrounding tissue was necessary for inhibition of angiogenesis around the sponges [22].

*2.3. Immunomodulatory Effects.* In experiments by Niederwieser et al., cultured human keratinocytes exposed for 72 hours to 500 units/mL IFN-$\alpha$ showed 63% class I MHC antigen expression, compared to 70% for IFN-$\gamma$ at 500 units/mL, and 51% for untreated keratinocytes. In their experiments, induction of class II MHC antigen expression was a feature of IFN-$\gamma$-, and not IFN-$\alpha$-, treated cultures [23].

Krasagakis et al. showed that 95–100% of normal cultured human melanocytes grown in melanocyte growth medium (MGM) expressed HLA class I antigens, but none of them expressed HLA-DR, a class II antigen. Treatment with 1000 IU/mL of IFN-$\alpha$ or -$\beta$ resulted in a stronger expression of HLA class I antigens, with IFN-$\beta$ having a greater effect than IFN-$\alpha$. Moreover, while IFN-$\alpha$ induced no change in HLA-DR expression by normal human melanocytes, IFN-$\beta$ induced de novo expression of HLA-DR in $\leq$20% of the cultured cells. Interestingly, IFN-$\gamma$ had the greatest effect on induction of HLA-DR, with 95% of melanocytes HLA-DR-positive at 1000 IU/mL IFN-$\gamma$ [20]. The effects of type I IFNs on keratinocytes and melanocytes have been summarized in Table 1.

## 3. Cutaneous Squamous Cell Carcinoma

*3.1. Antiproliferative Effects.* The growth inhibitory and cell cycle effects of IFNs-$\alpha,\beta$ have been evaluated in numerous human skin SCC cell lines. In SCL-1 cells, Nickoloff et al. showed that recombinant IFN-$\alpha$ at $1.98 \times 10^2$ U/mL resulted in 89% of control in cell number on day 5, compared to 78% at $2.18 \times 10^2$ U/mL of recombinant IFN-$\beta$ [24]. Naito et al.

TABLE 1: Effect of type I Interferon on normal keratinocytes and melanocytes.

| Type of effect | Description of effect | References |
|---|---|---|
| Antiproliferative | IFNs-$\alpha$, $\beta$ inhibit the growth of human keratinocytes *in vitro* and promote keratinocyte terminal differentiation. <br> IFNs-$\alpha$, $\beta$ inhibit the growth of human melanocytes *in vitro*, with IFN-$\beta$ having a greater effect than IFN-$\alpha$. | [17–20] |
| Antiangiogenesis | IFN sensitivity of surrounding tissue is necessary for inhibition of angiogenesis around gelfoam sponges implanted in mice. | [21, 22] |
| Immunomodulatory | IFN-$\alpha$ upregulates class I, but not class II, MHC antigen expression in cultured human keratinocytes. <br> IFNs-$\alpha$, $\beta$ induce increased expression of class I MHC antigens in cultured human melanocytes, with IFN-$\beta$ having a greater effect than IFN-$\alpha$. | [20, 23] |

reported that cell number of A431 human squamous cell carcinoma cells markedly decreased with IFN-$\beta$ at 5000 U/mL [25].

IFN-sensitive SRB12-p9 cells were more sensitive to the growth inhibitory effect of treatment with 100 U/mL IFN-$\alpha$ continuously for five days than were IFN-resistant SRB1-m7 cells (53.8% and 19.1% growth inhibition compared to controls, resp.). In SRB12-p9 cells, 100 U/mL IFN-$\alpha$ induced a partial G1/0 arrest (57.4% of cells in G1/0) compared to controls (48.6% of cells in G1/0), whereas this effect was not seen in SRB1-m7 cells [26].

Yaar et al. showed that growth of the human epidermal squamous cell carcinoma cell line SCC-12B.2 is inhibited to a lesser degree by IFN-$\alpha$ and IFN-$\beta$ than normal human keratinocytes *in vitro*; this result indicates that loss of sensitivity to IFN is a characteristic of malignant cells [17].

*3.2. Proapoptotic Effects.* IFN-$\alpha$ produced a greater than two-fold increase in apoptosis (4.4% apoptosed cells) compared to controls (1.9% apoptosed cells) in SRB12-p9 cells, whereas no increase in apoptosis was seen with IFN-$\alpha$ treatment in IFN-resistant SRB1-m7 cells [26].

Rodriguez-Villanueva and McDonnell reported that, beginning 48 hrs after addition of 100 IU/mL IFN-$\alpha$-2b, SRB-12 cells exhibited ultrastructural alterations associated with apoptotic cell death on transmission electron microscopy as well as DNA "laddering" on agarose gel electrophoresis. Overexpression of bcl-2 only partially blocked the direct cytotoxic effects of IFN-$\alpha$ in SRB-12. In contrast, the SRB-1 cell line showed no significant cytotoxicity to exogenous IFN-$\alpha$, even in the presence of concentrations up to $10^5$ IU/mL [27].

*3.3. Immunomodulatory Effects.* IFN-$\beta$ at doses of 50, 500, and 5000 U/mL failed to induce HLA-DR antigen expression in A431 human squamous cell carcinoma cells after a 24 hr incubation, whereas a similar treatment with IFN-$\gamma$ significantly enhanced HLA-DR expression in a dose-dependant manner. Moreover, 24 hr incubation of IFN-$\beta$ at 50 or 500 U/mL with 5 U/mL IFN-$\gamma$ was found to decrease the IFN-$\gamma$-induced expression of HLA-DR antigens and mRNA in a dose-dependant manner. It was similarly found that IFN-$\alpha$ at 500 U/mL reduced IFN-$\gamma$-induced HLA-DR expression in A431 cells [25].

*3.4. Miscellaneous Findings.* In an immunohistochemical study by Clifford et al. involving 16 surgical specimens of aggressive human skin SCCs, pairwise comparisons for STAT1$\alpha$/$\beta$, STAT2, p48, and STAT3$\alpha$/3$\beta$ revealed significantly lower staining intensity for some or all of these proteins in tumor cells compared with adjacent nonmalignant epidermal tissue. These results indicate that a decrease in IFN responsiveness may lead to tumorigenicity [4]. A follow-up immunohistochemical study by the same group revealed a significant decrease in expression of one or more ISGF-3 proteins in 19 of 25 patients with actinic keratosis compared to matched normal skin. This result indicates that a decrease in responsiveness to endogenous IFN likely represents an early event in skin carcinogenesis [5]. Since STAT2 is thought to be the only STAT specific for the IFN-$\alpha$ pathway, Clifford et al. also conducted experiments to permanently block IFN-$\alpha$ signaling in a skin cell-based system through the forced expression of double negative STAT2 protein. In experiments involving the IFN-$\alpha$ sensitive SRB12-p9 human skin SCC cell line, dnSTAT2-expressing clones treated for four days with 100 IU/mL IFN-$\alpha$ showed 15% growth inhibition compared with 47.5% for parental SRB12-p9 cells. Moreover, dnSTAT2 expression suppressed the upregulation of several IFN-$\alpha$-inducible genes identified by cDNA microarray screening. These findings led the group to conclude that the cell-growth inhibitory effect of IFN-$\alpha$ in skin cells requires an intact STAT2 protein and is therefore mediated by the ISGF-3 complex [28]. The effects of type I IFNs on squamous cell carcinoma have been summarized in Table 2.

## 4. Basal Cell Carcinoma

*4.1. Antiproliferative Effects.* One group used real-time PCR to analyze opioid growth factor receptor expression in four primary basal cell carcinoma-derived cell lines treated with imiquimod or IFN-$\alpha$ for 24 hr. IFN-$\alpha$ upregulated opioid growth factor receptor expression in 2 of the 4 cell lines, whereas imiquimod did not induce a chance in opioid growth factor receptor expression in any of the cell lines [29]. Opioid growth factor is known to act as a negative regular of cell proliferation through DNA synthesis pathways [30], so this finding may represent a novel growth-inhibitory mechanism of action for IFN-$\alpha$.

TABLE 2: Effect of type I Interferon on cutaneous squamous cell carcinoma.

| Type of effect | Description of effect | References |
|---|---|---|
| Antiproliferative | IFN-$\beta$ has greater antiproliferative effect than IFN-$\alpha$ in SCL-1 cells.<br>IFN-$\alpha$ induced a partial G1/0 arrest in SRB12-p9 cells.<br>SCC-12B.2 cell line is less sensitive than normal keratinocytes to growth inhibitory effects of IFNs-$\alpha$, $\beta$ | [17, 24–26] |
| Proapoptotic | IFN-$\alpha$ led to a twofold increase in apoptosis in SRB12-p9 cells compared to controls.<br>Upon IFN-$\alpha$ treatment, SRB-12 cells exhibited ultrastructural evidence of apoptosis on microscopy. | [26, 27] |
| Immunomodulatory | IFNs-$\alpha$, $\beta$ reduced IFN-$\gamma$-induced HLA-DR expression in A431 cells. | [25] |
| Miscellaneous | Compared to normal skin, there was decreased staining intensity for ISGF3 proteins in not only specimens of human skin SCCs but also specimens of actinic keratoses.<br>Cell growth inhibitory effect of IFN-$\alpha$ requires an intact STAT2 protein. | [4, 5, 28] |

*4.2. Proapoptotic Effects.* In a study of 15 patients with histologically proven nodular BCC, 9 of whom were treated with intralesional IFN-$\alpha$-2b, the BCC cells of untreated patients constitutively expressed CD95L, whereas the BCC cells of treated patients not only expressed CD95L but also became CD95 positive. This concomitant expression of CD95L and CD95 eventually led to cell death by suicide and fratricide, with the majority of apoptotic cells in the center, rather than the periphery, of BCC nests. The IFN-$\alpha$-induced CD95 expression in BCCs was either a direct effect of the drug or indirectly mediated through cytokines produced by the CD4$^+$ T cell predominant peritumoral lymphoid infiltrate [31].

*4.3. Immunomodulatory Effects.* IL-10 is potent immunosuppressive cytokine, and previous studies have discovered elevated levels of IL-10 mRNA in BCC and SCC compared to matched PBMCs and seborrheic keratoses, respectively. These studies have revealed that neutralization of tumor-produced IL-10 by monoclonal antibodies can restore anti-tumor T-cell recognition [32, 33]. Kim et al. found a decrease in IL-10 mRNA levels in excisional biopsy specimens from four BCCs after IFN-$\alpha$ treatment compared to pretreatment levels as well as a decrease in IL-10 mRNA levels in 2 BCC-derived cell lines and 2 SCC-derived cell lines following 24-hr IFN-$\alpha$ treatment. In these experiments, treatment of BCCs with IFN-$\alpha$ was associated with reduction in malignant cells on histologic examination [32].

Buechner treated four patients with nodular basal cell carcinomas with intralesional injections of IFN-$\alpha$-2b (1.5 million IU per injection) three times a week for two weeks. Four weeks after completion of therapy, histopathologic examination of biopsy specimens revealed resolution of BCC and a dense dermal mononuclear cell infiltrate. Immunohistochemical analysis revealed the dermal infiltrate to contain CD4$^+$ and CD8$^+$ T cells in ratios ranging from 2 : 1 to 3 : 1, CD22 cells (B cells), IL-2 receptor-expressing cells, and NK cells. CD1+ cells (Langerhans cells) were observed in the epidermis, dermoepidermal junction, and around and within dermal BCC nodules. Most of the dermal infiltrate stained for HLA-DR, although tumor cells did not; there was focal expression of HLA-DR on keratinocytes, particularly in areas of dense inflammatory infiltrate. A considerable number of

HLA-DR$^+$ dendritic cells and Langerhans cells were present at the periphery of tumor masses, in close proximity to HLA-DR$^+$-activated T cells [34].

In an analogous study by Mozzanica et al. six patients with nodular (2) or superficial (4) basal cell carcinomas were treated with intralesional injections of IFN-$\alpha$-2b (1.5 million IU per injection) three times a week for three weeks. Immunohistologic study was done before the start of IFN therapy and after two weeks of therapy. In analysis of peritumoral infiltrate, treatment with IFN-$\alpha$ led to an increased proportion of CD3$^+$ cells (53% versus 66.5%), with an increase in the CD4/CD8 ratio from 1.4 to 1.9. In analysis of intratumoral infiltrate, treatment with IFN-$\alpha$ led to an increased proportion of CD3$^+$ cells (8.0% versus 13.5%), with an increase in the CD4/CD8 ratio from 1.5 to 3.2. In both peritumoral and intratumoral infiltrates, the pre- and posttreatment changes in percentage of cells that expressed HLA-DR, CD1 (Langerhans), CD14b (monocytes/macrophages), CD56 (natural killer), CD20 (B cells), and CD15 (granulocytes) were not significant. 8 weeks after completion of therapy, 2 BCCs were cured and 4 showed clinical and histologic signs of improvement [35]. The effects of type I IFNs on basal cell carcinoma have been summarized in Table 3.

## 5. Melanoma

*5.1. Antiproliferative Effects.* Dose response curves produced by Johns et al. showed the following order of potency of inhibition for the cell lines SK-MEL-28, Hs294T, HT144, and SK-MEL-3: IFN-$\beta$ > IFN-$\alpha$-2b >IFN-$\alpha$-4a [36]. Krasagakis et al. showed that 10,000 IU/mL of IFN-$\beta$ and -$\alpha$ inhibited the proliferation of SKMel-28 melanoma cells at 5 days by 78% and 59% of the controls, respectively [20]. For the cell lines LiBr and SK-MEL-1, the order of inhibitory potency was IFN-$\beta$ > IFN-$\alpha$-2b = IFN-$\alpha$-4a. The greater antiproliferative potency of IFN-$\beta$ compared to IFN-$\alpha$-2a was also borne out in experiments using xenografts of the melanoma cell line LiBr in nude mice. In competitive binding assays in HT144, SK-MEL-28, MM418, and MM96 cell lines, the order of competition for the IFN receptor was the same as that for antiproliferative potency, IFN-$\beta$ > IFN-$\alpha$-2b > IFN-$\alpha$-4a [36].

TABLE 3: Effect of type I interferon on basal cell carcinoma.

| Type of effect | Description of effect | References |
|---|---|---|
| Antiproliferative | IFN-$\alpha$ upregulates opioid growth factor receptor expression in BCC cell lines. | [29, 30] |
| Proapoptotic | IFN-$\alpha$ leads to coexpression of CD95L and CD95 in nodular BCCs, leading to cell death by suicide and fratricide. | [31] |
| Immunomodulatory | IFN-$\alpha$ leads to decreased mRNA levels of the immunosuppressive cytokine IL-10 in BCCs. Treatment with IFN-$\alpha$ led to increased proportion of CD3[+] cells within peri- and intratumoral infiltrates of BCCs as well as an increase in the CD4/CD8 ratio in both peri- and intratumoral infiltrates. | [32–35] |

Dose-dependent inhibition of proliferation of SK-MEL-2 and SK-MEL-24 cells was seen after treatment with IFN-$\alpha$-2b or IFN-$\beta$-1a, with greater inhibition by IFN-$\beta$-1a. Treatment with IFN-$\alpha$-2b and IFN-$\beta$-1a also resulted in decreased proliferation index of human melanoma xenograft tumors as manifest by immunohistochemical staining with Ki-67; again, IFN-$\beta$-1a-treated tumors showed less staining with Ki-67 than did IFN-$\alpha$-2b-treated tumors [37]. In experiments by Garbe et al., IFN-$\alpha$ and IFN-$\beta$ both showed concentration-dependant inhibition of proliferation of three melanoma cell lines, but IFN-$\beta$ had the smallest IC$_{50}$ for all three cell lines tested. Surprisingly, IFN-$\alpha$ and IFN-$\beta$ decreased the proportion of terminally differentiated melanoma cells to 56–97% of untreated cultures [38]. Numerous other experiments have likewise demonstrated the dose-dependant antiproliferative effects of interferons as well as the greater effect of IFN-$\beta$ compared to IFN-$\alpha$, on melanoma [39–45].

As a final example, in four cell lines derived from human melanoma metastases (JKM86-4, 5, 8, and 9), IFN-$\beta$ at 50–5000 U/mL had a stronger inhibitory effect than the same concentration of IFN-$\alpha$ in all cell lines. The genes for IFN-$\alpha$ and IFN-$\beta$ are localized to chromosome 9p, and the antiproliferative effect of IFN-$\alpha$ and -$\beta$ was more pronounced in the two cell lines that expressed the highest levels of 9p per cell (4 copies and 2.8 copies in JKM86-5 and JKM86-8, resp.), indicating that cell lines with more copies of 9p are more sensitive to IFN. IFN receptor genes are located on 21q, and copies of this chromosome did not appear to influence interferon sensitivity in the four cell lines [46].

*5.2. Proapoptotic Effects.* Seventy-two-hour Annexin V apoptosis assays as well as ninety-six-hour TUNEL apoptosis assays involving three melanoma cell lines showed an increasing induction of apoptosis at higher doses of IFN-$\beta$; no increase in apoptosis occurred with IFN-$\alpha$2, even at the highest dose (1000 units/mL), in any of the three cell lines [44]. In human melanoma IGR 1 cells, the apoptosis-promoting effect of IFN-$\beta$ at 500 IU/mL was time-dependant and greater than that of IFN-$\alpha$ at all time points [39]. Kubo et al. showed that IFN-$\beta$ induced apoptosis dose-dependently in 7 melanoma cell lines as well as induced cleavage of caspase 3 in these cell lines [42]. The number of apoptotic cells in human melanoma xenograft tumors was significantly increased in IFN-$\alpha$-2b- and IFN-$\beta$-1a-treated tumors compared with untreated tumors, with IFN-$\beta$-1a having a greater apoptotic effect than IFN-$\alpha$-2b [37].

Cyt c was undetectable in the cytosolic fraction of untreated WM9 cells but increased in a time-dependant manner with IFN-$\beta$, but not IFN-$\alpha$2, treatment. This phenomenon in WM9 cells was coupled with increased activity of caspases 3, 8, and 9. Lastly, IFN-$\beta$ induced TRAIL mRNA expression in apoptosis-sensitive melanoma cell lines tested, whereas IFN-$\alpha$2 did not. Together, these findings led Chawla-Sarkar et al. to conclude that IFN-$\beta$ induces apoptosis through the production and secretion of TRAIL protein, which acts in an autocrine or paracrine manner to activate its death receptors on neighboring melanoma cells.

Regardless of their sensitivity to either cytokine alone, melanoma cell lines treated with IFN-$\beta$ for 16–24 hrs before addition of TRAIL showed apoptosis of >30% of cells. Three such cell lines demonstrated cleavage of XIAP following combination treatment, whereas resistant cell lines did not. XIAP normally inhibits caspases 3 and 9 and has been shown to be cleaved in TRAIL-treated cells. IFN-$\beta$ may sensitize cells to TRAIL through induction of XAF-1, which is a negative regulator of XIAP [47].

*5.3. Antiangiogenesis Effects.* Representative interferon-stimulated gene products were quantified in the serum of 10 patients with cutaneous metastatic melanoma after one month of daily injections with IFN-$\beta$1a at a dose of $12 \times 10^6$ IU/m$^2$ on days 1–14 and $18 \times 10^6$ IU/m$^2$ on days 15–29. The results showed significant increases in TRAIL, IL-1RA, CCL2, CCL8 (anti-angiogenic), CXCL10 (anti-angiogenic), CCL20, and CXCL8. There was a moderate decrease in the proangiogenic VEGF-A and CXCL5. In this study, IFN-$\beta$1a at a maximally tolerated dose led to tumor regression in only 1 out of 17 patients with cutaneous metastatic melanoma [48].

In a study involving 9 human melanoma cell lines, treatment of cells with 2000 U/mL IFN-$\alpha$ decreased VEGF secretion by 40–60% in VEGF-high cell lines, but not in VEGF-low cell lines [49]. Protein levels of VEGF-C and VEGFR-3 in SK-MEL-24 cells decreased in response to *in vitro* treatment with IFN-$\alpha$2b or IFN-$\beta$1a, with IFN-$\alpha$2b showing an earlier and more sustained response compared with IFN-$\beta$1a. Moreover, treatment with IFN-$\alpha$2b or IFN-$\beta$1a also decreased secretory VEGF-C levels, with a superior effect by IFN-$\alpha$2b [37]. In human melanoma IGR 1 cells, treatment with 500 IU/mL of either IFN-$\alpha$ or IFN-$\beta$ significantly and similarly led to a decrease in VEGF production compared to controls [39].

Decreased levels of VEGF-C and VEGFR-3 were also seen in human melanoma xenograft tumors following IFN-$\alpha$2b or

IFN-$\beta$1a treatment. In human melanoma xenograft tumors, microvessel density was decreased by comparable amounts in tumors treated with IFN-$\alpha$2b or IFN-$\beta$1a compared with the control. However, lymphatic vessel density was significantly decreased in xenograft tumors treated with IFN-$\alpha$2b compared with either IFN-$\beta$1a-treated tumors or controls [37].

*5.4. Immunomodulatory Effects.* Studies have suggested that the effectiveness of type I interferon against melanoma is owed largely to indirect, immunomodulatory antitumor effects. In an immunocytochemical study involving fine needle aspirates from 21 patients with systemic metastatic malignant melanoma studied before initiation of IFN-$\alpha$ treatment, 10 out of 11 patients with moderate to high numbers of infiltrating CD4$^+$ lymphocytes achieved tumor regression, while 9 out of 10 patients with low numbers of these cells had progressive disease. Similar results were found in 20 patients with regional metastatic disease. This importance of the presence of infiltrating CD4$^+$ lymphocytes for the therapeutic effect of IFN-$\alpha$ shows that one important antitumor effect of IFN-$\alpha$ is to enhance immune reactivity toward the tumor [50].

Another study measured the recruitment of CD4$^+$ cells close to tumor cells in resected metastases following treatment with IFN-$\alpha$ for 0–3 weeks in 26 IFN-treated and 10 untreated patients with regional metastatic melanoma. IFN-$\alpha$ treatment resulted in moderate to high numbers of CD4$^+$ cells infiltrating close to tumor cells in 12 out of 26 metastases compared to 1 out of 10 metastases from untreated patients [51].

Moschos et al. conducted immunohistochemical analyses on biopsy specimens from 20 patients with stage IIIB-C melanoma before and after high-dose IFN-$\alpha$-2b. Clinical responders showed a significantly greater increase in the number of tumor-infiltrating CD11c$^+$ and CD3$^+$ cells. HDI did not, however, appear to affect peritumoral infiltrates, or to alter angiogenesis, HLA expression, proliferation, or apoptosis [52].

In the first report on the testing of IFN-$\alpha$ as an adjuvant in the vaccination of cancer patients, 7 stage IV melanoma patients were injected with MART-1 and gp-100 peptides, and IFN-$\alpha$ was administered in close spatial and temporal proximity to the peptide vaccine. 3 of the 7 patients showed disease stabilization following vaccination. PBMC studies showed a significant increase in peptide- and melanoma-specific CD8$^+$ T lymphocytes in 5 patients, increase in antigen-specific effector-memory (CD45RA$^-$CCR7$^-$) cells in the 3 patients with stable disease, and increase in percentage of CD14$^+$CD16$^+$ monocytes in all 7 patients. There was enhanced antigen-presenting cell function and IP-10/CXCL10 production by postvaccination monocytes in the patients with stable disease [53].

In a study involving a cohort of 21 patients with stage II or III melanoma treated with low-dose IFN-$\alpha$ for more than 12 months, blood samples were obtained before treatment, and at 3, 6, 9, and 12 months after initiation of treatment. During this time, there was a steady decrease in the number of peripheral blood circulating total CD3$^+$ T lymphocytes as well as a decrease in the CD3$^+$CD4$^+$ and CD3$^+$CD8$^+$

lymphocyte subsets. The level of CD3-CD56$^+$ NK lymphocytes was significantly decreased by 1 year. At one year there was a significant decrease in myeloid as well as plasmacytoid dendritic cells, with a more marked depletion of the latter dendritic cell subgroup. Total blood circulating monocytes (CD14$^+$) were not significantly decreased but did show an increased fluorescence intensity of MHC class I molecules. IP-10/CXCL10 levels also increased during the treatment period [54].

Tsavaris et al. treated 14 melanoma patients with local recurrence or distant metastases with IFN-$\alpha$-2b subcutaneously 3 times per week; the dose was increased from $5 \times 10^6$ IU/day for the first week to $10 \times 10^6$ IU/day for the second week and to $15 \times 10^6$ IU/day thereafter. Two months after therapy with IFN-$\alpha$-2b, 5 patients showed partial response and 9 exhibited progressive disease. *In vitro* studies of T cell function and cytokine production showed that, during therapy with IFN-$\alpha$-2b, deficient immune responses were restored to almost normal levels in responders, whereas no significant improvement was seen in patients who had progressive disease. Specifically, responders showed a more than 25–40% increase in proliferation in autoMLR and alloMLR (MLR, mixed lymphocyte reaction), IL-2 production by T cells, IL-2 sensitivity of T cells, and IL-1 production by monocytes [55].

The effect of IFN-$\beta$ on tumor infiltration by immune cells has likewise been investigated. Excisional biopsy specimens from metastatic skin lesions that were injected with IFN-$\beta$ once weekly for four weeks showed increased tumor infiltration by TIA$^+$, CD8$^+$, and CD4$^+$ cells. Additionally, there were significant numbers of infiltrating HLA-DR$^+$ cells within the metastatic tumors that had received IFN-$\beta$ injections compared with noninjected tumors (56.3% versus 10.4%). There was no significant difference in dendritic cell infiltration with and without IFN-$\beta$ treatment [56]. After local injection of IFN-$\beta$ ($10^6$ U/injection 5 times over 5 successive days) into B16-F10 melanoma tumors in C57BL/6 mice, analysis of interstitial infiltrate showed 21–50% T cells and <5% NK cells; similarly, tumor nest infiltrate contained 5–20% T cells compared to 0% NK cells, indicating that the immune response was primarily T-cell-mediated [57].

IFN-$\alpha$ also appears to directly or indirectly modulate the expression of TNF-$\alpha$ and IL-8 in tumor cells. Melanoma metastases from 37 patients were stained for TNF-$\alpha$: 16 metastases were from untreated patients and 21 were from patients treated with IFN-$\alpha$. Significantly more metastases from IFN-$\alpha$-treated patients had a low TNF-$\alpha$ staining score compared with metastases from untreated patients. Moreover, a low TNF-$\alpha$ staining score correlated with histopathologic regression of tumors [58]. In contrast, in a study that examined serum cytokine levels in IFN-$\alpha$-treated patients, baseline levels of TNF-$\alpha$ for patients showing relapse under therapy were significantly lower than baseline levels of TNF-$\alpha$ for patients without relapse [59].

Although IFN-$\alpha$ and IFN-$\beta$ alone did not inhibit steady state IL-8 production in three metastatic melanoma variants, they did inhibit IL-1$\beta$ or TNF-$\alpha$-mediated upregulation of IL-8 mRNA, with a more potent effect by IFN-$\beta$ compared to

IFN-$\alpha$. These findings are notable since IL-8 is an autocrine growth factor for human melanoma cells and directly correlates with their metastatic potential [60].

Peripheral blood lymphocytes from three healthy donors were incubated with each of three irradiated primary melanoma cultures. 1000 U/mL IFN-$\alpha$ was added to the cocultures at days 0, 3, 6, and 9, and on day 10 the ability of PBL to lyse radiolabeled melanoma cells was measured. IFN-$\alpha$ was a potent stimulator of anti-melanoma lytic activity. When the NK cell target K562 was added to the killing assay to inhibit NK cell-mediated lysis, a considerable fraction of the IFN-$\alpha$ cytolytic activity remained, demonstrating that IFN-$\alpha$ stimulated both NK and CTL generation. To show that essentially all the lytic activity observed in the presence of K562 cells was due to a T cell receptor-mediated mechanism, they used a combination of anti-CD3 and anti-CD8 antibodies to block the activity. MHC class I, but not class II, expression was upregulated by IFN-$\alpha$ in two of the primary melanoma cultures, and this represents a possible mechanism by which IFN-$\alpha$ can stimulate CTL generation [61]. In a study assessing NK cell activity against three melanoma cell lines, IFN-$\beta$ and IFN-$\alpha$2 showed a similar, dose-dependant augmentation of NK cell-mediated cytotoxity, and this augmented NK cytotoxicity did not correlate with antiproliferative effects of the IFNs [43].

In addition to many of the studies above, numerous others have demonstrated a stimulatory effect of type I interferons on MHC classes I and II expression on melanoma and immune cells. Treatment of murine B16 melanoma cells with IFN-$\alpha$, IFN-$\alpha/\beta$ and IFN-$\gamma$ resulted in enhanced class I H2 antigen expression, with IFN-$\gamma$ having the greatest effect [62]. An increase in $\beta_2$ microglobulin cell surface expression with IFN-$\alpha$ treatment (500 units/mL for 72 hrs) was observed in Hs294T and Hs695-L melanoma cell lines [63]. In a study that involved administering escalating doses of IFN-$\alpha$ to 9 melanoma patients for three weeks, isolation of PBMCs at regular intervals revealed elevated class I MHC at mRNA, translational, and plasma membrane levels [64]. In a study of 25 patient-derived melanoma cell lines, all cell lines expressed class I MHC antigen, and all three interferons (IFNs-$\alpha$, $\beta$, $\gamma$) significantly enhanced mRNA levels, protein synthesis, and membrane expression. In the 22 cell lines displaying baseline expression of HLA class II antigen, IFN-$\gamma$ increased the levels of class II mRNA, protein synthesis, and surface expression, whereas a significant upregulation of class II transcripts and protein levels by IFN-$\alpha$ or IFN-$\beta$ was found in only two cell lines [65]. Experiments in the human melanoma cell line MeWo and its metastatic variant MeM 50-10 demonstrated increasing expression of HLA class I antigen with IFN-$\alpha$ (2000 units/mL), IFN-$\beta$ (3000 units/mL), and IFN-$\gamma$ (1000 units/mL) treatment, respectively. Induction of MHC Class II antigen was seen in MeM 50-10 cells only, and even then only with IFN-$\beta$ (3000 units/mL) or IFN-$\gamma$ (1000 units/mL), with a greater enhancement by the latter [66].

IFN-$\beta$, but not IFN-$\alpha$, was shown to increase mRNA and protein expression of melanocytic tumor-associated antigens (Melan-A/MART-1, gp100, MAGE-A1) in 15 melanoma cell lines, inducing susceptibility to lysis by cytotoxic T lymphocytes [67].

In the presence of IFN-$\alpha$ and granulocyte/macrophage colony-stimulating factor (GM-CSF), monocytes differentiate into dendritic cells termed IFN-DCs. These IFN-DCs are effective in taking up antigens, migrating to lymph nodes, producing T-helper 1 mediators, and stimulating T- and B-cell responses. IFN-DCs may therefore be promising adjuvants for cancer immunotherapy targeting melanoma [68].

*5.5. Miscellaneous Findings.* Experiments with human malignant melanoma tissues and cell lines have shown that proinflammatory cytokines, such as IL-1$\alpha/\beta$ and TNF-$\alpha$, produced by melanoma cells activate p38 kinase to promote the IFN-$\alpha/\beta$-independent pathway of IFNAR1 degradation. By linking tissue inflammation with decreased cell sensitivity to the effects of type I IFN, these findings help to explain the decreased sensitivity of melanoma to the antitumorigenic effects of endogenous as well as therapeutically administered exogenous IFN-$\alpha/\beta$ [69].

Another group found that the pSTAT1/pSTAT3 ratio in tumor cells at baseline may serve as a useful prognostic predictor in cutaneous melanoma and a predictor of therapeutic effect for IFN-$\alpha$2b. STAT1 restricts cell growth and mediates the antitumor effects of IFN-$\alpha$, while STAT3 is associated with melanoma tumor progression and host immunosuppression. Tissue samples from stage IIIB patients were obtained before and after 20 doses of HDI therapy. Higher pretreatment pSTAT1/pSTAT3 ratios in tumor cells were associated with longer overall survival, and pSTAT1/pSTAT3 ratios were augmented by HDI in melanoma cells as well as in lymphocytes. The group concluded that downregulation of STAT3 and pSTAT3 by HDI in melanoma and host immune cells is central to the immunomodulatory effect of IFN-$\alpha$ [70].

In *in vivo* prospective studies involving patients with a clinical history of resected primary melanoma who had at least four atypical nevi, systemic low dose IFN-$\alpha$ treatment for three months led to decreased detection of Stat3/Stat3 and Stat1/Stat1 homodimers and Stat1/Stat3 heterodimer in atypical nevi excised after completion of treatment compared to those resected before IFN-$\alpha$ treatment. Moreover, IFN-$\alpha$ treatment led to dephosphorylation of constitutively activated Stat3 protein in atypical nevi [71].

Simons et al. suggested a way to select patients for high-dose interferon therapy based on their peripheral blood lymphocyte (PBL) IFN signaling patterns. They measured IFN signaling responses in PBL from 14 stage IIIB-C melanoma patients taken at baseline and at day 29 of neoadjuvant HDI therapy. The induction of pSTAT1 from IFN-$\alpha$ stimulation was assessed by phosflow in PBMCs. Those patients with good clinical outcome over the 4-wk induction phase had a significant increase in STAT1 activation in peripheral blood T cells upon IFN-$\alpha$ stimulation from day 0 to day 29. Responding patients showed a lower IFN-$\alpha$-induced pSTAT1 response at day 0 compared to nonresponding patients [72].

Most clinical studies of the role of type I interferon in melanoma have focused on IFN-$\alpha$ rather than IFN-$\beta$. In Japan; however, natural IFN-$\beta$ is approved and widely used as adjuvant therapy for melanoma. In a Japanese study of 46 patients with stage II and III primary cutaneous

TABLE 4: Effect of type I interferon on melanoma.

| Type of effect | Description of effect | References |
|---|---|---|
| Antiproliferative | IFN-$\beta$ has greater antiproliferative effect than IFN-$\alpha$ in the cell lines SK-MEL-1, 2, 3, 24, and 28; LiBr; Hs294T; HT144; and JKM86-4, 5, 8, and 9. | [20, 36–46] |
| Proapoptotic | IFN-$\beta$ induced apoptosis dose-dependently in multiple cell lines, with a greater effect than IFN-$\alpha$ at all time points. In WM9 cells, IFN-$\beta$ led to increased levels of cyt c and increased activity of caspases 3, 8, and 9. IFN-$\beta$ induces TRAIL mRNA expression and XAF-1, which is a negative regulator of XIAP. | [37, 39, 42, 44, 47] |
| Anti-angiogenesis | IFN-$\beta$ increases serum levels of antiangiogenic cytokines and decreases serum levels of pro-angiogenic cytokines. IFNs-$\alpha$, $\beta$ decrease intracellular and secretory levels of VEGF in multiple cell lines, with a superior effect by IFN-$\alpha$. In human melanoma xenograft tumors, IFNs-$\alpha$, $\beta$ similarly decrease microvessel density but IFN-$\alpha$ has a superior effect over IFN-$\beta$ in decreasing lymphatic vessel density. | [37, 39, 48, 49] |
| Immunomodulatory | *IFN-$\alpha$:* tumor infiltration with CD4$^+$ cells is not only required for the therapeutic effect of IFN-$\alpha$ but is also a consequence of treatment with IFN-$\alpha$. Use of IFN-$\alpha$ as an adjuvant in the vaccination of metastatic melanoma patients has resulted in disease stabilization. Responders to IFN-$\alpha$ therapy show restoration of immune responses to almost normal levels based on *in vitro* studies of T cell function and cytokine production. Metastases from IFN-$\alpha$-treated patients show a low TNF-$\alpha$ staining score compared to those from untreated patients. IFN-$\alpha$ is a potent stimulator of antimelanoma lytic activity via natural killer cells and cytotoxic T lymphocytes. In melanoma cell lines, IFN-$\alpha$ significantly enhances class I, but not class II, MHC expression. IFN-DCs may be promising adjuvants for cancer immunotherapy targeting melanoma. *IFN-$\beta$:* treatment with IFN-$\beta$ leads to increased T cell infiltration of interstitium and tumor nests. IFN-$\beta$ has a greater effect than IFN-$\alpha$ in inhibiting the TNF-$\alpha$-mediated upregulation of IL-8, a growth factor for melanoma cells. IFN-$\beta$ augments NK cell-mediated cytotoxicity against melanoma cell lines. In melanoma cell lines, IFN-$\beta$ significantly enhances class I, but not class II, MHC expression, and augments expression of tumor-associated antigens. | [43, 50–58, 60–66, 68] |
| Miscellaneous | Proinflammatory cytokines promote degradation of IFNAR1, leading to decreased tumor responsiveness to IFN. IFN-$\alpha$ treatment leads to decreased detection of Stat3 homo- and heterodimers in atypical nevi as well as dephosphorylation of Stat3 protein in atypical nevi. Higher pretreatment pSTAT1/pSTAT3 ratios in tumor cells were associated with longer overall survival in stage IIIB patients. IFN signaling patterns in peripheral blood lymphocytes, as measured by STAT1 activation, can be used to select patients for high dose interferon therapy. IFN-$\beta$ maintenance therapy was shown to significantly increase overall and relapse-free survival in a clinical study of stage II-III melanoma patients. | [69–73] |

melanoma, 21 patients were treated with low-dose IFN-$\beta$ maintenance therapy, and 25 patients underwent observation alone. Overall survival (OS) and relapse-free survival (RFS) were significantly worse in the observation group: mean OS was 56.3 months for the observation group and 90.6 months for the IFN group, and mean RFS was 54.9 months for the observation group versus 90.3 months for the IFN group [73]. The effects of type I IFNs on melanoma have been summarized in Table 4.

## 6. Conclusion

In summary, the precise mechanism by which type I interferons exert their antitumor effects in SCC, BCC, and melanoma is the subject of ongoing study, and much remains to be elucidated. Although surgical excision remains the preferred mode of treatment for BCC and SCC, intralesional IFN-$\alpha/\beta$ is a reasonable alternative to surgery for patients with poor hemostasis, those at high risk for poor wound healing, and those in whom surgery would be deforming or destroy function (e.g., cancers of the face and fingers). Moreover, intralesional IFN can be used to shrink tumors prior to surgery or for the treatment of positive margins after surgical excision [1].

Although IFN-$\beta$ has shown more potent anti-proliferative, proapoptotic, and immunomodulatory effects than IFN-$\alpha$ in many of the above studies, further clinical trials involving larger numbers of patients are needed to establish the therapeutic profile of IFN-$\beta$ [48, 74]. Moreover, the finding that melanoma cell lines differ in their sensitivity to the same IFN may explain variations in clinical response. High-dose interferon therapy produces a clinical response and achieves relapse-free survival in only 20–33% of patients with operable high risk or metastatic melanoma [72], and therefore a better understanding of its antitumor mechanism of action would enable more selective application of this therapy to those patients who are most likely to benefit.

## Conflict of Interests

The authors have no conflict of interests to report. There was no funding provided for the production of this paper.

## References

[1] K. H. Kim, R. M. Yavel, V. L. Gross, and N. Brody, "Intralesional interferon $\alpha$-2b in the treatment of basal cell carcinoma and squamous cell carcinoma: revisited," *Dermatologic Surgery*, vol. 30, no. 1, pp. 116–120, 2004.

[2] L. M. Good, M. D. Miller, and W. A. High, "Intralesional agents in the management of cutaneous malignancy: a review," *Journal of the American Academy of Dermatology*, vol. 64, no. 2, pp. 413–422, 2011.

[3] A. A. Tarhini, H. Gogas, and J. M. Kirkwood, "IFN-$\alpha$ in the treatment of melanoma," *Journal of Immunology*, vol. 189, no. 8, pp. 3789–3793, 2012.

[4] J. L. Clifford, D. G. Menter, X. Yang et al., "Expression of protein mediators of type I interferon signaling in human squamous cell carcinoma of the skin," *Cancer Epidemiology Biomarkers and Prevention*, vol. 9, no. 9, pp. 993–997, 2000.

[5] J. L. Clifford, E. Walch, X. Yang et al., "Suppression of type I interferon signaling proteins is an early event in squamous skin carcinogenesis," *Clinical Cancer Research*, vol. 8, no. 7, pp. 2067–2072, 2002.

[6] J. Bekisz, S. Baron, C. Balinsky, A. Morrow, and K. C. Zoon, "Antiproliferative properties of type I and type II interferon," *Pharmaceuticals*, vol. 3, no. 4, pp. 994–1015, 2010.

[7] P. A. Ascierto, H. J. Gogas, J. J. Grob et al., "Adjuvant interferon alfa in malignant melanoma: an interdisciplinary and multinational expert review," *Critical Reviews in Oncology/Hematology*, vol. 85, no. 2, pp. 149–161, 2013.

[8] S. Mocellin, M. B. Lens, S. Pasquali, P. Pilati, and S. V. Chiarion, "Interferon alpha for the adjuvant treatment of cutaneous melanoma," *Cochrane Database of Systematic Reviews*, vol. 6, Article ID CD008955, 2013.

[9] S. Bostanci, P. Kocyigit, A. Alp, C. Erdem, and E. G. Gürgey, "Treatment of basal cell carcinoma located in the head and neck region with intralesional interferon $\alpha$-2a evaluation of long-term follow-up results," *Clinical Drug Investigation*, vol. 25, no. 10, pp. 661–667, 2005.

[10] B. Doğan, Y. Harmanyeri, H. Baloğlu, and I. Öztek, "Intralesional alfa-2a interferon therapy for basal cell carcinoma," *Cancer Letters*, vol. 91, no. 2, pp. 215–219, 1995.

[11] J. J. Grob, A. M. Collett, M. H. Munoz, and J. J. Bonerandi, "Treatment of large basal-cell carcinomas with intralesional interferon-alpha 2a," *Lancet*, vol. 1, no. 8590, pp. 878–879, 1988.

[12] L. Edwards, B. Berman, R. P. Rapini et al., "Treatment of cutaneous squamous cell carcinomas by intralesional interferon alfa-2b therapy," *Archives of Dermatology*, vol. 128, no. 11, pp. 1486–1489, 1992.

[13] P. A. DiLorenzo, N. Goodman, F. Lansville, and W. Markel, "Regional and intralesional treatment of invasive basal cell carcinoma with interferon alfa-n2b," *Journal of the American Academy of Dermatology*, vol. 31, no. 1, pp. 109–111, 1994.

[14] P. LeGrice, E. Baird, and L. Hodge, "Treatment of basal cell carcinoma with intralesional interferon alpha-2a," *New Zealand Medical Journal*, vol. 108, no. 1000, pp. 206–207, 1995.

[15] E. Alpsoy, E. Yilmaz, E. Başaran, and S. Yazar, "Comparison of the effects of intralesional interferon alfa-2a, 2b and the combination of 2a and 2b in the treatment of basal cell carcinoma," *Journal of Dermatology*, vol. 23, no. 6, pp. 394–396, 1996.

[16] R. R. McDonald and K. Georgouras, "Treatment of basal cell carcinoma with intralesional interferon alpha: a case report and literature review," *Australasian Journal of Dermatology*, vol. 33, no. 2, pp. 81–86, 1992.

[17] M. Yaar, R. L. Karassik, L. E. Schnipper, and B. A. Gilchrest, "Effects of alpha and beta interferons on cultured human keratinocytes," *Journal of Investigative Dermatology*, vol. 85, no. 1, pp. 70–74, 1985.

[18] B. J. Nickoloff, T. Y. Basham, T. C. Merigan, and V. B. Morhenn, "Antiproliferative effects of recombinant $\alpha$- and $\gamma$-interferons on cultured human keratinocytes," *Laboratory Investigation*, vol. 51, no. 6, pp. 697–701, 1984.

[19] D. R. Bielenberg, M. F. McCarty, C. D. Bucana et al., "Expression of interferon-$\beta$ is associated with growth arrest of murine and human epidermal cells," *Journal of Investigative Dermatology*, vol. 112, no. 5, pp. 802–809, 1999.

[20] K. Krasagakis, C. Garbe, S. Kruger, and C. E. Orfanos, "Effects of interferons on cultured human melanocytes in vitro: interferon-beta but not-alpha or -gamma inhibit proliferation and all interferons significantly modulate the cell phenotype," *Journal of Investigative Dermatology*, vol. 97, no. 2, pp. 364–372, 1991.

[21] A. J. Stout, I. Gresser, and W. D. Thompson, "Inhibition of wound healing in mice by local interferon $\alpha/\beta$ injection," *International Journal of Experimental Pathology*, vol. 74, no. 1, pp. 79–85, 1993.

[22] M. F. McCarty, D. Bielenberg, C. Donawho, C. D. Bucana, and I. J. Fidler, "Evidence for the causal role of endogenous interferon-$\alpha/\beta$ in the regulation of angiogenesis, tumorigenicity, and metastasis of cutaneous neoplasms," *Clinical and Experimental Metastasis*, vol. 19, no. 7, pp. 609–615, 2002.

[23] D. Niederwieser, J. Aubock, J. Troppmair et al., "IFN-mediated induction of MHC antigen expression on human keratinocytes and its influence on in vitro alloimmune responses," *Journal of Immunology*, vol. 140, no. 8, pp. 2556–2564, 1988.

[24] B. J. Nickoloff, T. Y. Basham, T. C. Merigan, and V. B. Morhenn, "Immunomodulatory and antiproliferative effect of recombinant alpha, beta, and gamma interferons on cultured human

malignant squamous cell lines, SCL-1 and SW-1271," *Journal of Investigative Dermatology*, vol. 84, no. 6, pp. 487–490, 1985.

[25] Y. Naito, T. Baba, H. Suzuki, and K. Uyeno, "The antagonistic effect of interferon-beta on the interferon-gamma-induced expression of HLA-DR antigen in a squamous cell carcinoma line," *Journal of Experimental Pathology*, vol. 6, no. 1-2, pp. 75–87, 1992.

[26] D. M. Shin, B. S. Glisson, F. R. Khuri et al., "Phase II and biologic study of interferon alfa, retinoic acid, and cisplatin in advanced squamous skin cancer," *Journal of Clinical Oncology*, vol. 20, no. 2, pp. 364–370, 2002.

[27] J. Rodriguez-Villaueva and T. J. McDonnell, "Induction of apoptotic cell death in non-melanoma skin cancer by interferon-$\alpha$," *International Journal of Cancer*, vol. 61, no. 1, pp. 110–114, 1995.

[28] J. L. Clifford, X. Yang, E. Walch, M. Wang, and S. M. Lippman, "Dominant negative signal transducer and activator of transcription 2 (STAT2) protein: stable expression blocks interferon alpha action in skin squamous cell carcinoma cells," *Molecular Cancer Therapeutics*, vol. 2, pp. 453–459, 2003.

[29] M. Urosevic, P. A. Oberholzer, T. Maier et al., "Imiquimod treatment induces expression of opioid growth factor receptor: a novel tumor antigen induced by interferon-$\alpha$?" *Clinical Cancer Research*, vol. 10, no. 15, pp. 4959–4970, 2004.

[30] I. S. Zagon and P. J. McLaughlin, "Opioids and the apoptotic pathway in human cancer cells," *Neuropeptides*, vol. 37, no. 2, pp. 79–88, 2003.

[31] S. A. Buechner, M. Wernli, T. Harr, S. Hahn, P. Itin, and P. Erb, "Regression of basal cell carcinoma by intralesional interferon-alpha treatment is mediated by CD95 (Apo-1/Fas)-CD95 ligand-induced suicide," *Journal of Clinical Investigation*, vol. 100, no. 11, pp. 2691–2696, 1997.

[32] J. Kim, R. L. Modlin, R. L. Moy et al., "IL-10 production in cutaneous basal and squamous cell carcinomas: a mechanism for evading the local T cell immune response," *Journal of Immunology*, vol. 155, no. 4, pp. 2240–2247, 1995.

[33] M. Yamamura, R. L. Modlin, J. D. Ohmen, and R. L. Moy, "Local expression of antiinflammatory cytokines in cancer," *Journal of Clinical Investigation*, vol. 91, no. 3, pp. 1005–1010, 1993.

[34] S. A. Buechner, "Intralesional interferon alfa-2b in the treatment of basal cell carcinoma: immunohistochemical study on cellular immune reaction leading to tumor regression," *Journal of the American Academy of Dermatology*, vol. 24, no. 5, pp. 731–734, 1991.

[35] N. Mozzanica, A. Cattaneo, V. Boneschi, L. Brambilla, E. Melotti, and A. F. Finzi, "Immunohistological evaluation of basal cell carcinoma immunoinfiltrate during intralesional treatment with alpha2-interferon," *Archives of Dermatological Research*, vol. 282, no. 5, pp. 311–317, 1990.

[36] T. G. Johns, I. R. Mackay, K. A. Callister, P. J. Hertzog, R. J. Devenish, and A. W. Linnane, "Antiproliferative potencies of interferons on melanoma cell lines and xenografts: higher efficacy of interferon $\beta$," *Journal of the National Cancer Institute*, vol. 84, no. 15, pp. 1185–1190, 1992.

[37] M. R. Roh, Z. Zheng, H. C. Jeung, S. Y. Rha, and K. Y. Chung, "Difference of interferon-alpha and interferon-beta on melanoma growth and lymph node metastasis in mice," *Melanoma Research*, vol. 23, no. 2, pp. 114–124, 2013.

[38] C. Garbe, K. Krasagakis, C. C. Zouboulis et al., "Antitumor activities of interferon alpha, beta, and gamma and their combinations on human melanoma cells in vitro: changes of proliferation, melanin synthesis, and immunophenotype," *Journal of Investigative Dermatology*, vol. 95, no. 6, pp. 231S–237S, 1990.

[39] B. Bölling, J. Fandrey, P. J. Frosch, and H. Acker, "VEGF production, cell proliferation and apoptosis of human IGR 1 melanoma cells under nIFN-$\alpha$/$\beta$ and rIFN-$\gamma$ treatment," *Experimental Dermatology*, vol. 9, no. 5, pp. 327–335, 2000.

[40] T. Horikoshi, K. Fukuzawa, N. Hanada et al., "In vitro comparative study of the antitumor effects of human interferon-$\alpha$, $\beta$ and $\gamma$ on the growth and invasive potential of human melanoma cells," *Journal of Dermatology*, vol. 22, no. 9, pp. 631–636, 1995.

[41] B. Schaber, P. Mayer, T. Schreiner, G. Rassner, and G. Fierlbeck, "Anti-proliferative activity of natural interferon-alpha, isotretinoin and their combination varies in different human melanoma cell lines," *Melanoma Research*, vol. 4, no. 5, pp. 321–326, 1994.

[42] H. Kubo, A. Ashida, K. Matsumoto, T. Kageshita, A. Yamamoto, and T. Saida, "Interferon-$\beta$ therapy for malignant melanoma: the dose is crucial for inhibition of proliferation and induction of apoptosis of melanoma cells," *Archives of Dermatological Research*, vol. 300, no. 6, pp. 297–301, 2008.

[43] C. Lossino, B. D. Wines, T. G. Johns, and I. R. Mackay, "Natural killer cell activity against cultured melanoma cells: a dye-reduction technique with studies on augmented activity by interferon subtypes," *Natural Immunity*, vol. 11, no. 4, pp. 215–224, 1992.

[44] M. Chawla-Sarkar, D. W. Leaman, and E. C. Borden, "Preferential induction of apoptosis by interferon (IFN)-$\beta$ compared with IFN-$\alpha$2: correlation with TRAIL/Apo2L induction in melanoma cell lines," *Clinical Cancer Research*, vol. 7, no. 6, pp. 1821–1831, 2001.

[45] J. H. Schiller, J. K. V. Willson, G. Bittner, W. H. Wolberg, M. J. Hawkins, and E. C. Borden, "Antiproliferative effects of interferons on human melanoma cells in the human tumor colony-forming assay," *Journal of Interferon Research*, vol. 6, no. 6, pp. 615–625, 1986.

[46] J. I. Köpf, C. Hanson, U. Delle, A. Weimarck, and U. Stierner, "Action of interferon $\alpha$ and $\beta$ on four human melanoma cell lines in vitro," *Anticancer Research*, vol. 16, no. 2, pp. 791–798, 1996.

[47] M. Chawla-Sarkar, D. W. Leaman, B. S. Jacobs, and E. C. Borden, "IFN-$\beta$ pretreatment sensitizes human melanoma cells to TRAIL/Apo2 ligand-induced apoptosis," *Journal of Immunology*, vol. 169, no. 2, pp. 847–855, 2002.

[48] E. C. Borden, B. Jacobs, E. Hollovary et al., "Gene regulatory and clinical effects of interferon $\beta$ in patients with metastatic melanoma: a phase II trial," *Journal of Interferon and Cytokine Research*, vol. 31, no. 5, pp. 433–440, 2011.

[49] E. T. Raig, N. B. Jones, K. A. Varker et al., "VEGF secretion is inhibited by interferon-alpha in several melanoma cell lines," *Journal of Interferon and Cytokine Research*, vol. 28, no. 9, pp. 553–561, 2008.

[50] A. Håkansson, B. Gustafsson, L. Krysander, and L. Håkansson, "Tumour-infiltrating lymphocytes in metastatic malignant melanoma and response to interferon alpha treatment," *The British Journal of Cancer*, vol. 74, no. 5, pp. 670–676, 1996.

[51] A. Håkansson, B. Gustafsson, L. Krysander, and L. Håkansson, "Effect of IFN-$\alpha$ on tumor-infiltrating mononuclear cells and regressive changes in metastatic malignant melanoma," *Journal of Interferon and Cytokine Research*, vol. 18, no. 1, pp. 33–39, 1998.

[52] S. J. Moschos, H. D. Edington, S. R. Land et al., "Neoadjuvant treatment of regional stage IIIB melanoma with high-dose interferon alfa-2b induces objective tumor regression in association with modulation of tumor infiltrating host cellular

immune responses," *Journal of Clinical Oncology*, vol. 24, no. 19, pp. 3164–3171, 2006.

[53] T. Di Pucchio, L. Pilla, I. Capone et al., "Immunization of stage IV melanoma patients with Melan-A/MART-1 and gplOO peptides plus IFN-$\alpha$ results in the activation of specific CD8$^+$ T cells and monocyte/dendritic cell precursors," *Cancer Research*, vol. 66, no. 9, pp. 4943–4951, 2006.

[54] A. M. Mohty, J. J. Grob, M. Mohty, M. A. Richard, D. Olive, and B. Gaugler, "Induction of IP-10/CXCL10 secretion as an immunomodulatory effect of low-dose adjuvant interferon-alpha during treatment of melanoma," *Immunobiology*, vol. 215, no. 2, pp. 113–123, 2010.

[55] N. Tsavaris, C. Baxevanis, P. Kosmidis, and M. Papamichael, "The prognostic significance of immune changes in patients with renal cancer, melanoma and colorectal cancer, treated with interferon $\alpha$2b," *Cancer Immunology Immunotherapy*, vol. 43, no. 2, pp. 94–102, 1996.

[56] T. Fujimura, R. Okuyama, T. Ohtani et al., "Perilesional treatment of metastatic melanoma with interferon-$\beta$," *Clinical and Experimental Dermatology*, vol. 34, no. 7, pp. 793–799, 2009.

[57] J. Nakayama, K. Toyofuku, A. Urabe, S. Taniguchi, and Y. Hori, "A combined therapeutic modality with hyperthermia and locally administered rIFN-$\beta$ inhibited the growth of B16 melanoma in association with the modulation of cellular infiltrates," *Journal of Dermatological Science*, vol. 6, no. 3, pp. 240–246, 1993.

[58] A. Håkansson, B. Gustafsson, L. Krysander, C. Bergenwald, B. Sander, and L. Håkansson, "Effect of interferon-$\alpha$ on the expression of tumour necrosis factor-$\alpha$ by metastatic malignant melanoma in vivo," *Melanoma Research*, vol. 7, no. 2, pp. 139–145, 1997.

[59] M. A. Hofmann, F. Kiecker, I. Kuchler, C. Kors, and U. Trefzer, "Serum TNF-a, B2M and sIL-2R levels are biological correlates of outcomes in adjuvant IFN-a2b treatment of patients with melanoma," *Journal of Cancer Research and Clinical Oncology*, vol. 137, pp. 455–462, 2011.

[60] R. K. Singh and M. L. Varney, "Regulation of interleukin 8 expression in human malignant melanoma cells," *Cancer Research*, vol. 58, no. 7, pp. 1532–1537, 1998.

[61] K. J. Palmer, M. Harries, M. E. Gore, and M. K. L. Collins, "Interferon-alpha (IFN-$\alpha$) stimulates anti-melanoma cytotoxic T lymphocyte (CTL) generation in mixed lymphocyte turnout cultures (MLTC)," *Clinical and Experimental Immunology*, vol. 119, no. 3, pp. 412–418, 2000.

[62] T. J. McMillan, J. Rao, C. A. Everett, and I. R. Hart, "Interferon-induced alterations in metastatic capacity, class-1 antigen expression and natural killer cell sensitivity of melanoma cells," *International Journal of Cancer*, vol. 40, no. 5, pp. 659–663, 1987.

[63] T. Y. Basham, M. F. Bourgeade, A. A. Creasey, and T. C. Merigan, "Interferon increases HLA synthesis in melanoma cells: interferon-resistant and -sensitive cell lines," *Proceedings of the National Academy of Sciences of the United States of America*, vol. 79, no. 10, pp. 3265–3269, 1982.

[64] P. Giacomini, R. Fraioli, A. M. Calabro, F. Di Filippo, and P. G. Natali, "Class I major histocompatibility complex enhancement by recombinant leukocyte interferon in the peripheral blood mononuclear cells and plasma of melanoma patients," *Cancer Research*, vol. 51, no. 2, pp. 652–656, 1991.

[65] P. Nistico, R. Tecce, P. Giacomini et al., "Effect of recombinant human leukocyte, fibroblast, and immune interferons on expression of class I and II major histocompatibility complex and invariant chain in early passage human melanoma cells," *Cancer Research*, vol. 50, no. 23, pp. 7422–7429, 1990.

[66] M. Maio, B. Gulwani, J. A. Langer et al., "Modulation by interferons of HLA antigen, high-molecular-weight melanoma-associated antigen, and intercellular adhesion molecule 1 expression by cultured melanoma cells with different metastatic potential," *Cancer Research*, vol. 49, no. 11, pp. 2980–2987, 1989.

[67] I. S. Dunn, T. J. Haggerty, M. Kono et al., "Enhancement of human melanoma antigen expression by IFN-$\beta$," *Journal of Immunology*, vol. 179, no. 4, pp. 2134–2142, 2007.

[68] A. Farkas and L. Kemény, "Interferon-$\alpha$ in the generation of monocyte-derived dendritic cells: recent advances and implications for dermatology," *The British Journal of Dermatology*, vol. 165, no. 2, pp. 247–254, 2011.

[69] W. C. Huangfu, J. Qian, C. Liu et al., "Inflammatory signaling compromises cell responses to interferon alpha," *Oncogene*, vol. 31, no. 2, pp. 161–172, 2012.

[70] W. Wang, H. D. Edington, U. N. M. Rao et al., "Modulation of signal transducers and activators of transcription 1 and 3 signaling in melanoma by high-dose IFN$\alpha$2b," *Clinical Cancer Research*, vol. 13, no. 5, pp. 1523–1531, 2007.

[71] J. M. Kirkwood, D. L. Farkas, A. Chakraborty et al., "Systemic interferon-$\alpha$ (IFN-$\alpha$) treatment leads to Stat3 inactivation in melanoma precursor lesions," *Molecular Medicine*, vol. 5, no. 1, pp. 11–20, 1999.

[72] D. L. Simons, G. Lee, J. M. Kirkwood, and P. P. Lee, "Interferon signaling patterns in peripheral blood lymphocytes may predict clinical outcome after high-dose interferon therapy in melanoma patients," *Journal of Translational Medicine*, vol. 9, article 52, 2011.

[73] S. Aoyagi, H. Hata, E. Homma, and H. Shimizu, "Sequential local injection of low-dose interferon-beta for maintenance therapy in stage II and III melanoma: a single-institution matched case-control study," *Oncology*, vol. 82, no. 3, pp. 139–146, 2012.

[74] J. H. Schiller, B. Storer, G. Bittner, J. K. V. Willson, and E. C. Borden, "Phase II trial of a combination of interferon-$\beta$(ser) and interferon-$\gamma$ in patients with advanced malignant melanoma," *Journal of Interferon Research*, vol. 8, no. 5, pp. 581–589, 1988.

# 13

# Comparison of Zn, Cu, and Fe Content in Hair and Serum in Alopecia Areata Patients with Normal Group

**Ladan Dastgheib,**[1] **Zohreh Mostafavi-pour,**[2] **Ahmad Adnan Abdorazagh,**[1] **Zahra Khoshdel,**[3] **Maryam Sadat Sadati,**[1] **Iman Ahrari,**[4] **Sajjad Ahrari,**[5] **and Mahsa Ghavipisheh**[6]

[1] *Molecular Dermatology Research Center, Dermatology Department, Shiraz University of Medical Sciences, Shiraz, Iran*
[2] *Maternal-Fetal Medicine Research Center, Hafez Hospital, Shiraz University of Medical Sciences, Shiraz, Iran*
[3] *Recombinant Protein Laboratory, Department of Biochemistry, Shiraz University of Medical Sciences, Shiraz, Iran*
[4] *Student Research Committee, Shiraz University of Medical Sciences, Shiraz, Iran*
[5] *Department of Biology, Shiraz University, Shiraz, Iran*
[6] *Student Research Committee, Fasa University of Medical Sciences, Fasa, Iran*

Correspondence should be addressed to Iman Ahrari; imanahrari@gmail.com and Sajjad Ahrari; sajjad_ahrari@shirazu.ac.ir

Academic Editor: Craig G. Burkhart

*Background.* Alopecia areata (AA) is an autoimmune condition, in which hair is lost from some areas of the body. Though its etiopathogenesis is not fully understood, there are claims that imbalance of trace elements may trigger the onset of AA, by distorting immune functions. In this study, we tried to investigate the relationship between AA and iron, zinc, and copper levels of serum and hair. *Materials and Methods.* Sixteen female patients with AA (14–40 years old) and 27 healthy female controls were enrolled in this study. Serum and hair level of iron, zinc, and copper were measured by flame emission spectroscopy. The resulting data was analyzed with SPSS15. *Results.* We did not detect a significant difference in the serum and hair level of iron, zinc, and copper between patients and controls. There was a significant correlation between serum and hair level of iron ($r = 0.504$, $P = 0.001$), zinc ($r = 0.684$, $P = 0.0001$), and copper ($r = 0.759$, $P = 0.0001$) in patients and controls. *Discussion and Conclusion.* According to this study, there was no statistically significant difference between trace elements among AA patients and controls. So the trace elements level in hair and serum may not be relevant to the immunologic dysfunction that exists in AA patients.

## 1. Introduction

Alopecia areata (AA) is a recurrent, nonscarring hair loss, affecting any hair-bearing area. Its incidence is 1-2%. AA is considered to be a T-cell-mediated autoimmunity occurring in genetically predisposed individuals [1]. In addition to immune function disturbance, genetic and environmental factors play a role [2]. Also, perifollicular vasculature and nerves, viruses, alterations in trace elements [3], and endocrine and thyroid abnormality [4] have been hypothesized. Complex interactions between predisposing genetic and environmental factors likely contribute to the induction of immune-mediated responses in AA [4].

Clinically, AA has many different patterns. The characteristic lesion is a flat alopetic plaque with normal skin color,

involving the scalp or any other region of the body [5]. There are claims that imbalance of trace elements may trigger the onset of AA.

Reports have been published on oral zinc sulfate therapy with encouraging results for some cases of AA [6, 7]. It has been reported that some AA patients have zinc and some other trace element deficiencies [8, 9].

Trace elements are essential cofactors for multiple enzymes and have a role in important functional activities within the hair follicle. Further, zinc accelerates hair follicle recovery and is a potent inhibitor of hair follicle regression [10]. Iron and zinc are the well-known trace elements that are associated with hair shedding [10, 11]. In spite of the fact that several studies were done on the effect of trace elements in AA, a definite result was not obtained. Therefore, in this study, we tried to investigate the relationship between AA and some trace elements in our population. At the same time, we are going to evaluate the correlation between serum and hair contents of these trace elements.

## 2. Materials and Methods

Sixteen female patients and 27 female healthy individuals were enrolled in this case control study. The patients had localized hair loss and were clinically diagnosed as AA with typical lesion. The control group was selected from healthy individuals who did not use any minerals in the last 6 months and did not have any history of hair loss. Patients with history of anemia, thalassemia, and metabolic disorders as well as patients who dyed their hair were excluded from the study. Case and control groups were matched for age. All patients were informed about the study, and their participation was voluntary.

After taking demographic data, hair analysis was made on approximately 0.5 g of hair samples obtained from the scalp of the cases and controls. The wet digestion involved the addition to the sample of 6 mL of nitric acid, which was allowed to react slowly at room temperature to prevent excessive foaming. Five milliliter of blood was obtained for determination of the level of trace elements in the serum.

After that, when warming the nitric acid digest, 1 mL of perchloric acid was added, and the digestion continued on a hot plate at about 200°C until dense white fumes of perchloric acid were evolved. At this point, the mixture was water-clear and less than 1 mL of solution remained. Each sample was transferred to a 5 mL volumetric flask and diluted to volume for copper, iron, and zinc.

Working standards for each element were prepared by dilution of 1000 micro g/mL standard solution. Dilutions were made with distilled water.

*2.1. Determination of Serum Copper with Flame Emission Method.* For determination of serum copper (Cu), the samples were diluted 1 : 4 with deionized water for flame emission spectroscopy methods. Cu standards were prepared by diluting the copper stock standard solution with deionized water. Hollow cathode lamp for Cu was used.

*2.2. Determination of Serum Zinc with Flame Emission Method.* For determination of serum zinc, the samples were diluted 1 : 5 with deionized water. Zinc standards were prepared by diluting the zinc stock standard solution with deionized water. Hollow cathode lamp for Zn was used.

*2.3. Determination of Serum Iron with Flame Emission Method.* To determine total serum iron (Fe), samples were diluted 1 : 2 with a 10% (v/v) trichloroacetic acid (TCA) solution and then centrifuged. This procedure precipitated the serum protein and removed approximately 95% of any hemoglobin iron. Hollow cathode lamp for Fe was used. Analyses were performed using a PerkinElmer model 300 atomic absorption spectrophotometer.

Data were analyzed under supervision of a statistician specialist with SPSS 15. The following statistical methods were used: Fisher's exact test, paired-sample $t$ test and two-tailed test of significance. $P$ value 0.05 and less was considered as significant. Correlation analysis was carried out using Pearson's correlation and regression analysis.

## 3. Results

Sixteen female patients and 27 female healthy individuals were enrolled in this case control study. Mean age of patients was 26.63 (±8.53) years and controls 25.07 (±5.01) years, which was not statistically significant. Only history of AA in patients and their family and occupation were different in cases and controls.

History of DM (diabetic mellitus), TY (thyroid disease), and AU (other autoimmune diseases) was not different in patients, their families, and controls. Mean duration of disease among the patients was 23.69 (±41.55) months.

The demographic data and associated disease of patients and control are illustrated in Table 1.

We did not detect a significant difference in the serum level and hair level of iron, zinc, and copper between patients and controls (Table 2).

As it is evident from Tables 3 and 4 there was no correlation found between trace element content of hair and serum when compared two by two; the $P$ values are not significant (>0.05) and Pearson correlation coefficient is very small, almost near zero. The only interesting exception was a negative relation between serum iron and zinc level evident by $P = 0.04$ (Table 4).

There was a significant correlation between serum and hair level of iron ($r = 0.524$, $P = 0.001$), zinc ($r = 0.684$, $P = 0.0001$), and copper ($r = 0.759$, $P = 0.0001$) in patients and controls.

This is also shown in Figures 1, 2, and 3 with a linear configuration.

## 4. Discussion

Our results showed that the level of zinc, iron, and copper was not significantly different in our patients compared to that of controls.

In review of the literature, there are several investigations that studied the mineral and nutritional conditions in patients with hair loss, especially AA.

Naginiene et al. [4] found a lower level of zinc in blood and urine of children with alopecia and increased levels of copper and chromium concentrations in their hair compared to healthy individuals [4]. Bruske and Salfeld [10] interpreted the statistical association of blood and serum levels of zinc, magnesium, and copper in patients with many dermatological disorders including AA. After comparing with healthy people they did not find any changes in serum levels of zinc and copper but found a significantly higher level of magnesium [10]. Kantor et al. [11] found that the mean ferritin level in patients with androgenetic alopecia and AA was statistically significantly lower than in normal individuals without hair loss [11]. The trace element concentrations of Se, Rb, Zn, Fe, Co, Cs, Mg, Ca, F, Cu, Cr, and Ag in serum and of Se, Rb, Zn, Fe, Co, and Cs in red cells of Finnish alopecia

TABLE 1: Baseline demographics and associated diseases among patients and controls.

| Parameter | | Case ($n = 16$) | Control ($n = 27$) | P value |
|---|---|---|---|---|
| Age (mean ± SD) (years) | | 26.63 ± 8.53 | 25.07 ± 5.01 | 0.515 |
| Disease duration (months) | | 23.69 ± 41.55 | | |
| Occupation | Student | 5 (31.3) | 13 (48.1) | 0.001 |
| | House wife | 9 (56.3) | 2 (7.4) | |
| | Employee | 2 (12.5) | 12 (44.4) | |
| AA | No | 9 (56.3) | 27 (100) | 0.0001 |
| | Yes | 7 (43.8) | 0 (0) | |
| DM | No | 15 (93.8) | 27 (100) | 0.372 |
| | Yes | 1 (6.3) | 0 (0) | |
| TY | No | 15 (93.8) | 26 (96.3) | 0.611 |
| | Yes | 1 (6.3) | 1 (3.7) | |
| AU | No | 16 (100) | 27 (100) | 1 |
| | Yes | 0 (0) | 0 (0) | |
| AA in family | No | 13 (81.3) | 27 (100) | 0.045 |
| | Yes | 3 (18.8) | 0 (0) | |
| DM in family | No | 12 (75) | 20 (74.1) | 0.621 |
| | Yes | 4 (25) | 7 (25.9) | |
| TY in family | No | 13 (81.3) | 26 (96.3) | 0.137 |
| | Yes | 3 (18.8) | 1 (3.7) | |
| AU in family | No | 15 (93.8) | 27 (100) | 0.327 |
| | Yes | 1 (6.3) | 0 (0) | |
| Pitting nail | No | 15 (93.8) | 27 (100) | 0.327 |
| | Yes | 1 (6.3) | 0 (0) | |

AU: other autoimmune diseases, AA: alopecia areata, DM: diabetes mellitus, TY: thyroid disease.

TABLE 2: Serum and hair level of trace elements in patients and controls.

| Parameter | Case ($n = 16$) | Control ($n = 27$) | P value* |
|---|---|---|---|
| Serum Fe ($\mu$g/dL) | 108 ± 36 | 96.01 ± 33 | 0.251 |
| Hair Fe ($\mu$g/g) | 128 ± 18 | 117.84 ± 22 | 0.121 |
| Serum Zn ($\mu$g/dL) | 134 ± 46 | 136.76 ± 41 | 0.877 |
| Hair Zn ($\mu$g/g) | 270 ± 58 | 279.35 ± 61 | 0.65 |
| Serum Cu ($\mu$g/dL) | 143 ± 38 | 128.32 ± 23 | 0.12 |
| Hair Cu ($\mu$g/g) | 52 ± 62 | 67.59 ± 59 | 0.441 |

*Two-sample $t$-test.

patients were determined in Mussalo-Rauhama study [3]. In addition, the Cu and Zn content in 24 h urine and Cu, Zn, Cd, Cr, and Se concentrations in the hair of these patients were studied. No differences in element concentrations of the samples mentioned above could be found as compared to those of the normal healthy individuals. In addition, there was no tendency of excesses or deficiencies of elements analyzed in the samples. Statistically significant difference was found between the copper content of serum in AA and alopecia universalis patients and also between the copper content of serum in AA plus alopecia totalis and alopecia universalis patients [3].

Although immunologic processes and hereditary factors are suggested to play an important role in AA, the specific etiology is unclear. Iron deficiency has been suggested to play a role, but its effect is controversial. Esfandiarpour et al. [12] found a higher mean level of serum iron and ferritin and a lower mean level of TIBC in AA patients compared

to the control subjects, but the differences did not reach significance [12]. The study of Park et al. [13] suggested that zinc supplementation could become an adjuvant therapy for AA patients with a low serum zinc level and for whom the traditional therapeutic methods have been unsuccessful [13]. Bhat et al. [14] showed in their study that copper and magnesium levels are not altered in AA, but they mentioned that the decreased level of zinc found in their study may merit further investigation of the relationship [14].

As mentioned, AA is thought to be an autoimmune disorder, in which the body attacks its own hair follicles and suppresses or stops hair growth. There is evidence that T cell lymphocytes cluster around these follicles, causing inflammation and subsequent hair loss. It is now found that nutritional deficiency of zinc and the other trace elements in human populations may distort immune function. As it has been noted, there are controversial data from different studies. The varied results of the levels of magnesium, copper,

TABLE 3: Correlation between trace elements measured in hair.

| | | Zinc (hair) | Iron (hair) | Copper (hair) |
|---|---|---|---|---|
| Zinc (hair) | Pearson correlation | 1 | .100 | .192 |
| | Sig. (2-tailed) | | .517 | .211 |
| | N | 44 | 44 | 44 |
| Iron (hair) | Pearson correlation | .100 | 1 | .177 |
| | Sig. (2-tailed) | .517 | | .251 |
| | N | 44 | 44 | 44 |
| Copper (hair) | Pearson correlation | .192 | .177 | 1 |
| | Sig. (2-tailed) | .211 | .251 | |
| | N | 44 | 44 | 44 |

TABLE 4: Correlation between serum levels of trace elements.

| | | Zinc (plasma) | Iron (plasma) | Copper (plasma) |
|---|---|---|---|---|
| Zinc (plasma) | Pearson correlation | 1 | −.319[*] | .104 |
| | Sig. (2-tailed) | | .042 | .516 |
| | N | 41 | 41 | 41 |
| Iron (plasma) | Pearson correlation | −.319[*] | 1 | .142 |
| | Sig. (2-tailed) | .042 | | .377 |
| | N | 41 | 41 | 41 |
| Copper (plasma) | Pearson correlation | .104 | .142 | 1 |
| | Sig. (2-tailed) | .516 | .377 | |
| | N | 41 | 41 | 41 |

[*] Correlation is significant at the 0.05 level (2-tailed).

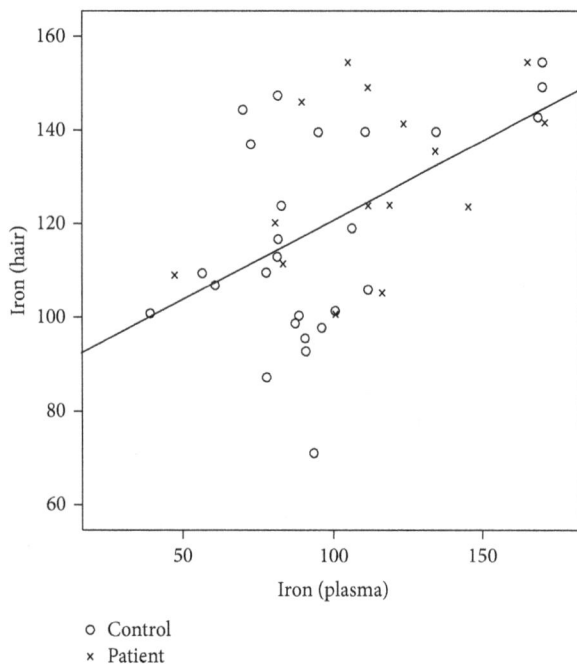

FIGURE 1: Correlation between plasma and hair iron level in patients and controls.

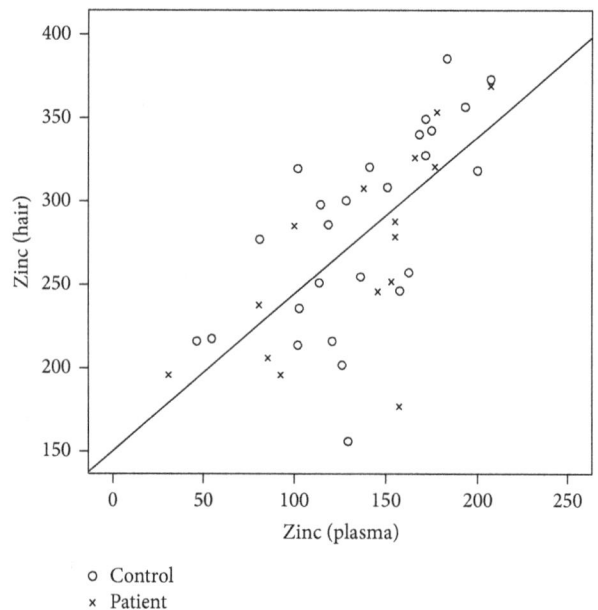

FIGURE 2: Correlation between plasma and hair zinc level in patients and controls.

and zinc in various studies can be explained on the basis of sample size, methodology, and population variations. Our study, however, suggests that low level of trace elements may

not have an important role in immunologic dysfunction in AA patients.

Although, in Bhat et al. study [14], they showed a significant difference in serum zinc levels in AA patients, it was mentioned that these results were seen in AA patients

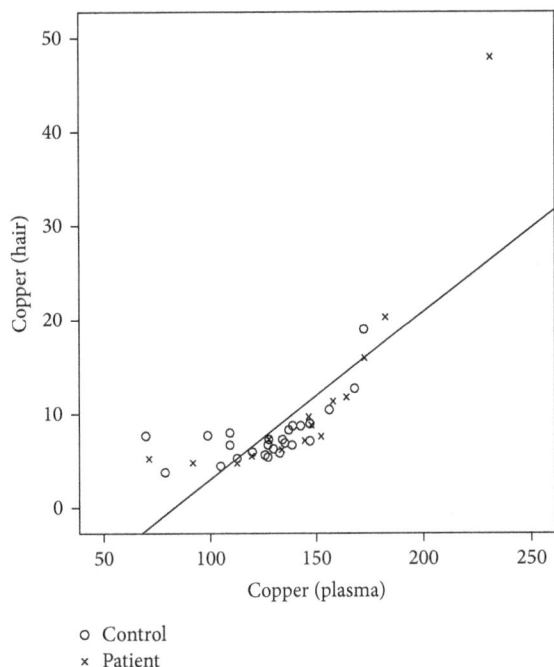

Figure 3: Correlation between plasma and hair copper level in patients and controls.

with extensive, prolonged, and resistant to treatments cases. However, most patients included in our study were mild to moderate cases. AA patients who were totalis and universalis were not enrolled in our study.

According to inconclusive data, it has been shown that the empiric therapy with mineral supplements was not very effective in the majority of AA patients. It is prudent to check the level of trace elements serum level in AA patients, and if low serum levels of trace elements are detected, it is advised to prescribe mineral supplements as an adjuvant therapy.

At the same time, we intended to evaluate the level of trace elements in the hair. The results showed a significant correlation between the level of iron and zinc in the serum and the hair. A stronger relation proved itself between the level of copper in the hair and in the serum.

Among the two groups, the results of the iron level showed a stronger relation in the normal healthy controls than in patients, while for the zinc level, results showed a strong relation in both controls and patients.

## 5. Conclusion

In conclusion, trace elements cannot be considered as a direct etiologic factor in the pathogenesis of alopecia areata and not all AA patients may benefit from receiving nutritional supplements. We rather suggest checking trace elements level in these patients and adding supplement in those with documented deficiency as an adjunct to the usual treatment.

In addition, our results showed that the measurement of hair zinc, iron, and copper level may give us an approximate estimate to its level in serum.

Our study had several limitations. First of all, we could not include male patients as 0.5–1 g sampling from male scalp would cause significant cosmetic defect. Secondly, we could not consider severe AA cases such as totalis and universalis, as they yielded no hair samples and, hence, limited the number of our patients.

## Conflict of Interests

The authors declare that there is no conflict of interests regarding the publication of this paper.

## References

[1] A. J. G. McDonagh and A. G. Messenger, "The pathogenesis of alopecia areata," *Dermatologic Clinics*, vol. 14, no. 4, pp. 661–670, 1996.

[2] A. J. G. McDonagh and A. G. Messenger, "The aetiology and pathogenesis of alopecia areata," *Journal of Dermatological Science*, vol. 7, pp. S125–S135, 1994.

[3] H. Mussalo-Rauhamaa, E. L. Lakomaa, U. Kianto, and J. Lehto, "Element concentrations in serum, erythrocytes, hair and urine of alopecia patients," *Acta Dermato-Venereologica*, vol. 66, no. 2, pp. 103–109, 1986.

[4] R. Naginiene, R. Kregzdyte, A. Abdrakhmanovas, and S. Ryselis, "Assay of trace elements, thyroid gland and blood indices in children with alopecia," *Trace Elements and Electrolytes*, vol. 21, pp. 207–210, 2004.

[5] E. A. Rivitti, "Alopecia areata: a revision and update," *Anais Brasileiros de Dermatologia*, vol. 80, no. 1, pp. 57–68, 2005.

[6] F. Wolowa and A. Stachow, "Treatment of alopecia areata with zinc sulfate," *Zeitschrift für Hautkrankheiten*, vol. 55, no. 17, pp. 1125–1134, 1980.

[7] F. Wolowa and A. Stachow, "Zinc in treatment of alopecia areata," *Przeglad Dermatologiczny*, vol. 65, no. 6, pp. 687–696, 1978.

[8] P. M. Plonka, B. Handjiski, M. Popik, D. Michalczyk, and R. Paus, "Zinc as an ambivalent but potent modulator of murine hair growth *in vivo*—preliminary observations," *Experimental Dermatology*, vol. 14, no. 11, pp. 844–853, 2005.

[9] S. Y. Lee, K. S. Nam, Y. W. Seo, J. S. Lee, and H. Chung, "Analysis of serum zinc and copper levels in alopecia areata," *Annals of Dermatology*, vol. 9, pp. 239–941, 1997.

[10] K. Bruske and K. Salfeld, "Zinc and its status in some dermatological diseases: a statistical assessment," *Zeitschrift für Hautkrankheiten*, vol. 62, pp. 125–131, 1987.

[11] J. Kantor, L. J. Kessler, D. G. Brooks, and G. Cotsarelis, "Decreased serum ferritin is associated with alopecia in women," *Journal of Investigative Dermatology*, vol. 121, no. 5, pp. 985–988, 2003.

[12] I. Esfandiarpour, S. Farajzadeh, and M. Abbaszadeh, "Evaluation of serum iron and ferritin levels in alopecia areata," *Dermatology Online Journal*, vol. 14, no. 3, article 21, 2008.

[13] H. Park, C. W. Kim, S. S. Kim, and C. W. Park, "The therapeutic effect and the changed serum zinc level after zinc supplementation in alopecia areata patients who had a low serum zinc level," *Annals of Dermatology*, vol. 21, no. 2, pp. 142–146, 2009.

[14] Y. J. Bhat, S. Manzoor, A. R. Khan, and S. Qayoom, "Trace element levels in alopecia areata," *Indian Journal of Dermatology, Venereology and Leprology*, vol. 75, pp. 29–31, 2009.

# 14

# The Preliminary Study of Effects of Tolfenamic Acid on Cell Proliferation, Cell Apoptosis, and Intracellular Collagen Deposition in Keloid Fibroblasts *In Vitro*

**Dan Yi,[1] Ji Bihl,[1] Mackenzie S. Newman,[1] Yanfang Chen,[1] and Richard Simman[1,2]**

[1] *Department of Pharmacology and Toxicology, Boonshoft School of Medicine, Wright State University, 3640 Colonel Glenn Hwy, Dayton, OH 45435, USA*

[2] *Department of Plastic and Reconstructive Surgery, Boonshoft School of Medicine, Wright State University, 3640 Colonel Glenn Hwy, Dayton, OH 45435, USA*

Correspondence should be addressed to Yanfang Chen; yanfang.chen@wright.edu and Richard Simman; plasticsimman@yahoo.com

Academic Editor: Lajos Kemény

Keloid scarring is a fibroproliferative disorder due to the accumulation of collagen type I. Tolfenamic acid (TA), a nonsteroidal anti-inflammatory drug, has been found to potentially affect the synthesis of collagen in rats. In this preliminary study, we aimed to test the effects of TA on cell proliferation, cell apoptosis, and the deposition of intracellular collagen in keloid fibroblasts. Normal fibroblasts (NFs) and keloid fibroblasts (KFs) were obtained from human dermis tissue. Within the dose range $10^{-3}$–$10^{-6}$ M and exposure times 24 h, 48 h, and 72 h, we found that $0.55 \times 10^{-3}$ M TA at 48 h exposure exhibited significantly decreased cell proliferation in both NFs and KFs. Under these experimental conditions, we demonstrated that (1) TA treatment induced a remarkable apoptotic rate in KFs compared to NFs; (2) TA treatment reduced collagen production in KFs versus NFs; (3) TA treatment decreased collagen type I expression in KFs comparing to that of NFs. In summary, our data suggest that TA decreases cell proliferation, induces cell apoptosis, and inhibits collagen accumulation in KFs.

## 1. Introduction

Keloid scarring, is a raised scar which forms by expanding beyond the boundaries of the original lesion [1]. The main histological manifestation of a keloid scar is the overgrowth of atypical fibroblasts with excessive accumulation of extracellular matrix components, especially collagen, fibronectin, elastin, and proteoglycans [1–4]. The causes of this type of scar are still unknown, but it has been pointed out that keloid scars can develop after any dermal abrasion including burns, piercing, or surgery [1–6]. Differing from normal wound healing, keloid scar formation begins with abnormal tissue growth in the dermal lesion extending beyond the borders of the original wound [7–11]. The central pathological wound healing response of keloid scarring is composed of a high density of mesenchymal cells called keloid fibroblasts (KFs) [9, 10]. Consequently, the over growth of KFs results

in overabundance of extracellular and intracellular matrix stroma, which is classified by irregularly directed and thick hyalinized spiral bundles described as keloidal collagen [5, 12]. During the formation of keloid scars, the type of collagen initially secreted by fibroblasts is granular collagen type III. Throughout the maturation of the process, collagen type I gradually replaces collagen type III and eventually comprises extracellular matrix in 99% of the wound bed [1, 5, 9–12]. Current, common treatments for keloids are often a combination of excision followed by a reconstructive surgical procedure. Glucocorticoids or 5-fluorouracil injections followed by compression therapy such as silicone sheets are frequently employed [1, 2]. Nonetheless, recurrence remains between 45% and 100% [3, 4]. Therefore, treatment of keloids continues to be a great challenge for the reconstructive surgeon.

Tolfenamic acid (TA) is a fenamic acid derivative belonging to the nonsteroidal anti-inflammatory drug (NSAID)

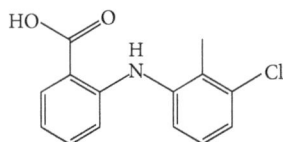

FIGURE 1: Structure of tolfenamic acid.

class that is traditionally used for rheumatic diseases [13, 14]. The predominant medical uses of this group of drugs include rheumatoid arthritis, osteoarthritis, and inflammatory arthropathies [15–18]. TA, also written as 2-([3-chloro-2-methylphenyl]-amino)-benzoic acid in IUPAC terms (Figure 1), has a low solubility in water and molecular weight of 261.7 g/mol. The exact medical applications, adverse effects, and mechanism of TA are not clear. However, previous studies have described highly specific applications of TA. Studies illustrate that TA is associated with inhibiting collagen metabolism in connective tissue in rats and has the capacity to induce cancer cell apoptosis [13, 14, 19–25]. There is an inhibition of sodium tolfenamate on the metabolism of collagen with 0.15 mol/L NaCl in rats [13]. TA reduces cell survival, growth, and angiogenesis in tumor and cancer cells, including human xenograft tumor, human pancreatic cancer, human neuroblastoma, and mouse prostate cancer by regulating the activity of transcription factor Sp1; human head and neck cancer by regulating NADAG-1; human colorectal cancer via ESE-1/EGR-1; and human oral cancer by affecting the p38 mitogen-activated protein kinase signaling pathway [14, 19–23].

## 2. Materials and Methods

*2.1. Cell Culture and Chemicals.* All skin samples were obtained under Wright State University IRB number SC4833. A sample of scar tissue (KF1) was taken from a 24-year-old African-American male with clinical and pathologic evidence of keloid scarring confirmed as previously described [10, 26]. A second keloid fibroblast cell line (KF2) was obtained from a 35-year-old African-American female was purchased from ATCC (Passage 11, ATCC, USA). One normal adult skin sample (NF) was obtained from a 29-year-old African-American female during plastic surgery [7, 8]. Skin specimens were incubated with 2 mL digestion medium containing high glucose Dulbecco's Modified Eagle's Medium (DMEM) (Gibco, Life Technologies, USA), 5 mg/mL collagenase/dispase II (RocheDiagnostics, USA), and 0.25% trypsin (Invitrogen, Life Technologies, USA) for 8 hours under 5% $CO_2$, at 37°C [7, 9, 27]. Isolated fibroblasts passages (P) 0 from keloid scar tissue and normal dermis tissue were cultured in total medium comprising of high glucose DMEM, 10% fetal bovine serum (Gibco, Life Technologies, USA), 1% pen/strep/glutamine (Invitrogen, Life Technologies, USA) in the condition of 5% $CO_2$, at 37°C. Each cell line was cultured separately. KF1 P13 to P15, KF2 P 3 to 5, and NF P3–P8 were tested in all assays. As both KF1 and KF2 were conducted in each assay, generally it will refer to KF in the following. TA was purchased from Cayman Chemical Company, USA.

*2.2. MTT.* NFs and KFs were divided into different groups for pretreatment with TA ($10^{-3}$ M, $10^{-4}$ M, $10^{-5}$ M, or $10^{-6}$ M) for different periods (24 h, 48 h, or 72 h), respectively. An MTT kit (Invitrogen, Life Technologies, USA) was used for the proliferation assay. Absorbance was detected at 535 nm in a Packard Fusion spectrophotometer [27]. Relatives of Cell proliferation rate (%) were determined with cell cultures and analyzed according to the following equation:

$$\text{Fibroblast proliferation rate (\%)} = \frac{\text{OD535 (TA treatment group)}}{\text{OD535 (Non-TA treatment group)}}. \quad (1)$$

All experiments were performed independently. Six times with keloid fibroblast cultures culture as well as normal skin dermal culture.

*2.3. Apoptosis.* NFs and KFs were divided into three groups Control ("C", only treated with medium), Vehicle ("V", medium 0.55% DMSO), and TA (550 $\mu$M TA dissolved in 0.55% DMSO with medium) for 48 h exposure separately. Annexin-binding buffer (Invitrogen, Life Technologies, USA) and propidium iodide (Invitrogen, Life Technologies, USA) working solutions were prepared at 1X. Cell apoptosis were detected by a fluorescence-activated cell sorting (FACS) Calibur Flow Cytometer (Accuri C6, Inc., USA) [20, 21]. All experiments were performed independently. Four times with keloid fibroblast cultures culture as well as normal skin dermal culture.

*2.4. Collagen Staining.* NFs and KFs were divided into three groups Control ("C", only treated with medium), Vehicle ("V", medium 0.55% DMSO), and TA (550 $\mu$M TA dissolved in 0.55% DMSO with medium) for 48 h exposure separately. Sirius red/Fast green staining kit (Chondrex, USA) was used to analyze collagen production. Absorbances at 535 nm and 600 nm were detected by a Packard Fusion spectrophotometer and analyzed by the following equation:

$$\text{Collagen (}\mu\text{g/well)} = \frac{\text{OD535} - 0.291 * \text{OD600}}{0.037}. \quad (2)$$

All experiments were performed independently. Four times with keloid fibroblast cultures culture as well as normal skin dermal culture.

*2.5. Western Blot.* NFs and KFs were divided into three groups Control ("C", only treated with medium), Vehicle ("V", medium 0.55% DMSO), and TA (550 $\mu$M TA dissolved in 0.55% DMSO with medium) for 48 h exposure separately. Proteins were extracted from each cell line and the concentrations were measured by BCA assay. Sixty micrograms of each sample were mixed with 10 $\mu$L of 5X protein sample loading buffer. The trans-blotted PVDF membrane was then blocked with blocking buffer (3% BSA; 1X TBS; and 0.05% Tween-20) for 1 h. Afterward, It was incubated with rabbit monoclonal anti-human collagen type I (dilution 1 : 2000, Thermo Fisher Scientific, USA), over two nights at 4°C.

(a)

(b)

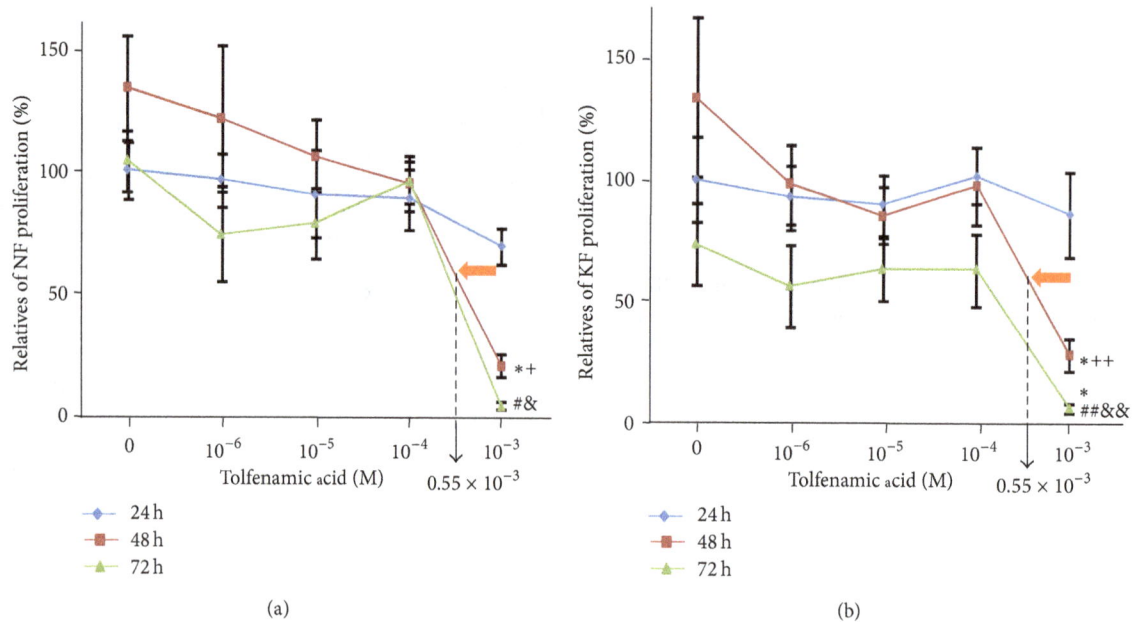

FIGURE 2: The dose- and time-responses of TA on cell proliferation in NFs and KFs. In 48 h exposure time group and 72 h exposure time group, $10^{-3}$ M TA significantly decreased cell proliferation in NFs. 0, $10^{-6}$, $10^{-5}$, $10^{-4}$, $10^{-3}$, $0.55 \times 10^{-3}$: M TA was dissolved in 1% DMSO. $^{*}P < 0.01$, $10^{-3}$ M versus 0 M; $^{+}P < 0.01$, 48 h versus 24 h; $^{\#}P < 0.01$, $10^{-3}$ M versus 0 M or $10^{-4}$ M; $^{\&}P < 0.01$, 72 h versus 24 h or 48 h; $^{**}P < 0.01$, $10^{-3}$ M versus 0 M; $^{++}P < 0.05$, 48 h versus 24 h; $^{\#\#}P < 0.05$, $10^{-3}$ M versus 0 M; $^{\&\&}P < 0.01$, 72 h versus 24 h or 48 h; $n = 6$.

Anti-rabbit HRP-conjugated secondary antibody (dilution at 1 : 20000, Sigma, USA) was then added to the membrane on a shaker for an hour at room temperature. After rinsing with TBST, the membrane was activated with chemiluminescent HRP substrate (Cell Signaling Technology, USA) for 4 min in the dark at room temperature. It was visualized and quantified using a chemiluminescent detection system (Bio-Rad, USA). Protein band intensity in each lane was scored by volume intensity and was normalized to beta-actin (dilution at 1 : 4000, Sigma, USA) [27]. All experiments were performed independently. Four times with keloid fibroblast cultures culture as well as normal skin dermal culture.

*2.6. Statistics.* Statistical analysis was performed with STA-TISTICA version 6.0 (StatSoft, Inc. USA). Data are displayed as mean ± SEM which was evaluated by one-way ANOVA between two groups in this study. $P < 0.05$ was considered statistically significant for all tests.

## 3. Results

*3.1. Dose- and Time-Response of TA on NFs and KFs Cell Proliferation.* The effect of TA on NFs and KFs proliferation was evaluated by MTT analysis and this is displayed in Figure 2. At the highest concentration of TA, cell proliferation rates appeared to decrease. As the exposure time increased, NF and KF proliferation sharply decreased at $10^{-3}$ M TA. Cell proliferation also decreased at a greater rate when TA was applied over 48 or 72 hours. Based on the results of this assay, $0.55 \times 10^{-3}$ M TA at 48 h exposure was determined to be the ideal condition for future experimentation.

*3.2. The Effect Dose and Time of TA on Inducing Cell Apoptosis in KFs.* To determine whether TA induced cell apoptosis on NFs and KFs, Annexin-V/PI labeling was administered after applying $0.55 \times 10^{-3}$ M TA dissolved in 0.55% DMSO for 48 h. Although the vehicle alone exhibited an effect on NFs, selectively significant apoptosis in TA-treated KFs compared with non-TA treatment groups of KFs and in NFs (Figure 3).

*3.3. The Effect Dose and Time of TA on Inhibiting Collagen Accumulation in KFs.* Quantitative analysis of intracellular and extracellular Sirius red fluorescent staining reflects the degree of all types of collagen produced by fibroblasts. Results indicated that collagen production was significantly reduced in KFs at the previously determined dose and time (Figure 4). Additionally, there was a considerable morphological change in KFs. Stained intensity decreased in all samples. Secreted, stained proteins and cell density were both reduced, especially in KF cultures.

*3.4. The Effect Dose and Time of TA on Reducing the Expression of Collagen Type I in KFs.* The effects of TA on collagen type I (Collagen I) protein expression were evaluated by Western blot in both cell types. Protein quantity was measured 48 hours after each treatment. Figure 5 shows a strong increased expression in KFs compared to NFs. TA significantly suppressed the expression of collagen type I in KFs compared with the other groups, while the inhibition of collagen type I expression in NFs after TA treatment was not significant. This result demonstrated that $0.55 \times 10^{-3}$ M TA for 48 h inhibits collagen I expression significantly in KFs but not, effectively in NFs.

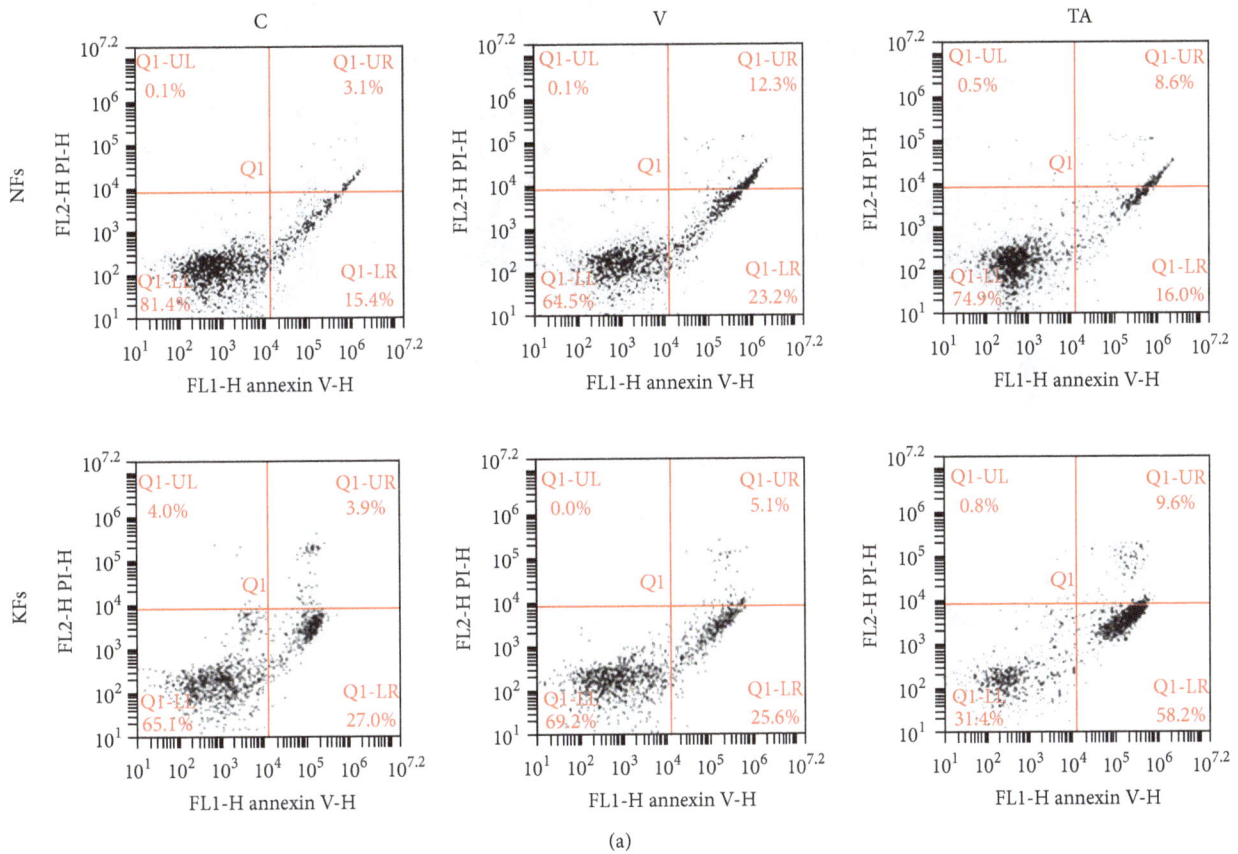

(a)

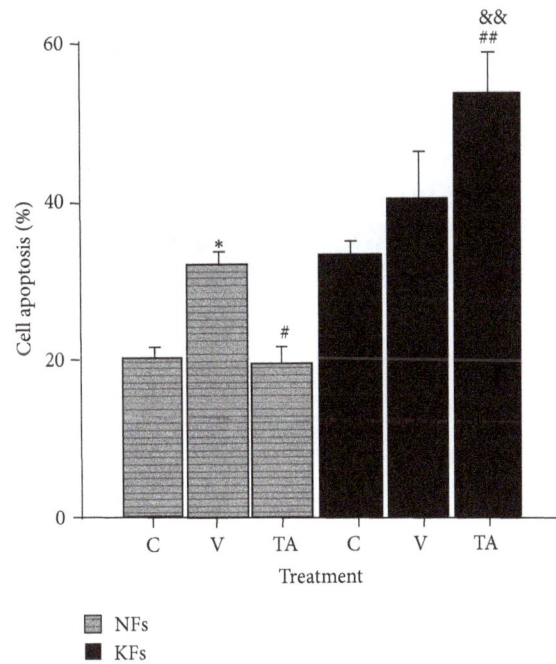

(b)

FIGURE 3: The effect of TA on cell apoptosis in NFs and KFs. DMSO induced early and late apoptosis in NFs and slightly induced early apoptosis in KFs. TA strikingly induced late apoptosis in KFs. C: control, total medium; V: vehicle, 0.55% DMSO; TA, $0.55 \times 10^{-3}$ M of TA was dissolved in 0.55% DMSO. $^{*}P < 0.01$, V versus C or TA; $^{\#}P < 0.05$, TA versus V; $^{\#\#}P < 0.05$, TA versus C; $^{\&\&}P < 0.01$, TA versus TA; $n = 6$.

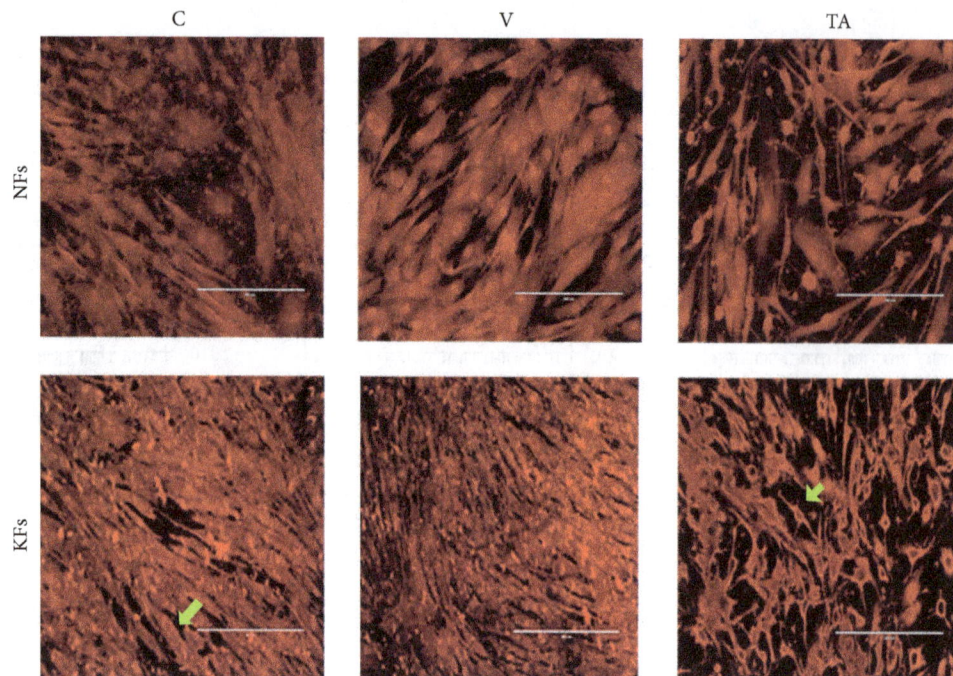

(a)

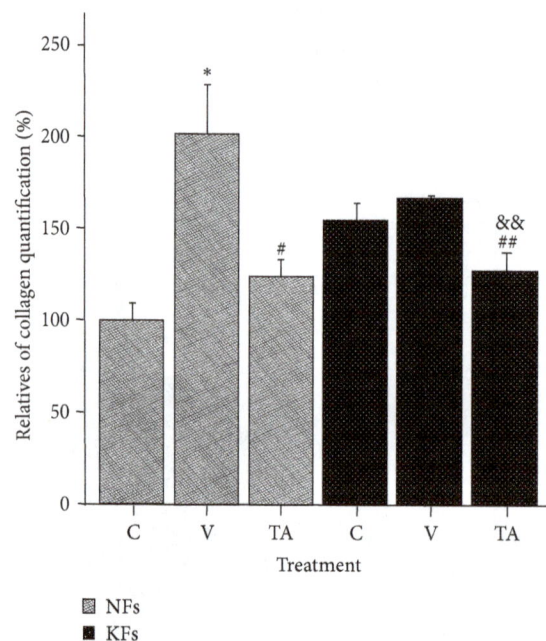

(b)

FIGURE 4: The effect of TA on collagen production in NF and KF after Sirius red staining. DMSO significantly increased collagen production in NFs. TA strikingly reduced collagen production in KFs compared with NFs. C: control, total medium; V: vehicle, 0.55% DMSO; TA, $0.55 \times 10^{-3}$ M of TA was dissolved in 0.55% DMSO. $^{*}P < 0.01$, V versus C; $^{\#}P < 0.05$, TA versus V; $^{\#\#}P < 0.05$, TA versus C; $^{\&\&}P < 0.01$, TA versus V; $n = 4$.

## 4. Discussion

Keloid scaring, a type of scars, is a fibroproliferation disease with the accumulation of collagen deposition caused by the upregulation of autocrine TGF-$\beta$ signaling during the wound healing process [5, 13, 27]. The role of TA, a fenamate and NASID, has been used recently for cancer treatments [13, 14, 19–25]. These experiments were designed to determine if the administration of TA is able to alter the proliferatory rates of keloid fibroblasts and decrease collagen production in KFs. Our preliminary study demonstrates that TA has the potential to normalize some of the characteristic

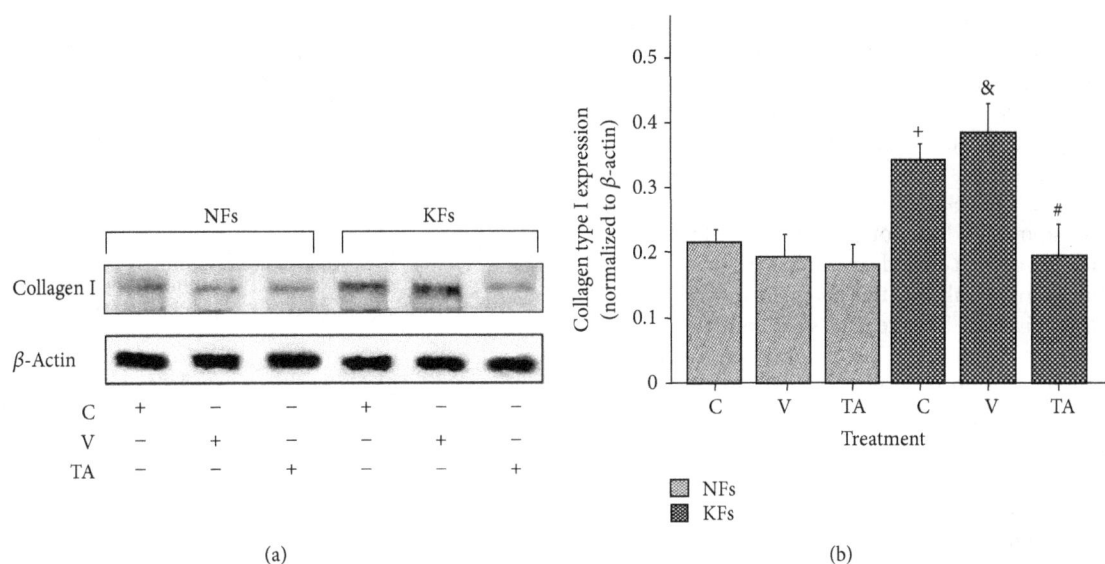

(a)                                                    (b)

FIGURE 5: The effect of TA on the expression of collagen type I in NFs and KFs. DMSO slightly increased the expression of collagen type I in KFs. TA significantly inhibited the expression of collagen type I in KFs. C: control, total medium; V: vehicle, 0.55% DMSO; TA, $0.55 \times 10^{-3}$ M of TA was dissolved in 0.55% DMSO. $^{+}P < 0.05$, C versus C; $^{\&}P < 0.05$, V versus NFs C; $^{\#}P < 0.05$, TA versus V; $n = 4$.

features of KFs such as cell apoptosis and collagen production.

Initially, we tested the effects of TA on NF and KF proliferation by applying five concentrations of TA ($10^{-3}$ M, $10^{-4}$ M, $10^{-5}$ M, and $10^{-6}$ M) for 3 different exposure times (24 h, 48 h, and 72 h) separately in order to determine the conditions at which minimal drug concentration had the greatest proportionate effect on disease fibroblasts. We found that NF and KF proliferation rates were decreased with the $10^{-3}$ M TA after 48 h exposure. This indicated that the diversity of NF and KF proliferation were significantly reduced by certain higher amount of TA. Linear extrapolation of cell proliferation assay, data at 48 h revealed that the effective concentration of TA which can result in half reduction of NF proliferation was 550 $\mu$M. This concentration of TA at 48 h exposure did not show a significant reduction in KFs proliferation, but other effects were still expected to be present. At 72 hours, there was a large reduction in proliferation of KF cultures versus NFs. This may be due to a long-phase response to TA toxicity in KF or a side effect of changing culture media every three days. To further qualify the effects of this TA does and time exposure treatment, we conducted cell apoptosis assays with $0.55 \times 10^{-3}$ M TA and with 48 h time exposure. A group exposed to 0.55% DMSO in medium was added to control for vehicle effects. Though 0.55% DMSO induced a proportional apoptotic rate in NFs and KFs, cell apoptosis in KFs after TA treatment induced a selectively significant apoptotic rate compared to NFs. This indicated that cell apoptosis was significantly influenced by TA. According to the typical histological changes in KFs [1–4], reducing collagen production is a primary pharmacological target to treat keloid scarring. In our study, we tested the effects of TA on decreasing the accumulation of collagen and furthermore tried to verify a relationship between cell apoptosis and

collagen deposition. Based on our data, a high inhibition rate of collagen production was detected in KFs after $0.55 \times 10^{-3}$ M TA with 48 h exposure time compared with NFs. Although the effect of 0.55% DMSO increased collagen production in NFs, the production caused by 0.55% DMSO did not show specific significance in KFs. Concurrently, after TA treatment, cell number also decreased. Therefore, TA reduced collagen production in KFs with high efficiency. The Sirius red collagen quantification assay targets the helical collagen repeat bundles and is therefore nonspecific for specific types of collagens. The majority of collagen produced by KFs is collagen type I, and our results were specific for collagen type I after TA treatment [1, 2, 12, 26–28]. Our study confirms that collagen I is overexpressed in KFs versus NFs. Treatment with TA *in vitro* significantly decreased collagen expression in KFs over NFs.

In the cell apoptosis and collagen expression experiments, DMSO vehicle alone did have some effects compared to control group. The underlying mechanism for this is not apparent from our study. In cell apoptosis assays, compared with the treatment group, the vehicle group had more significant effect in NFs while the effect in KFs is not significant. This may be further considered for clinical studies. In collagen expression assays, DMSO did not significantly induce collagen expression in NFs. In KFs, it significantly increased the expression of collagen but this effect can be reversed by TA. In summary, DMSO did not influence the performance of TA on cell apoptosis and collagen expression in KFs. The present study is limited by the number of samples. Nonetheless, statistically significant effects were seen from TA treatment in KF cells. A potential mechanism for the activity of TA in keloid is its capacity to induce degradation of the Sp2 transcription factor. Sp1 has a role in the canonical TGF-$\beta$ transduction pathway. Because TGF-$\beta$ is widely regarded as the central progenitor of fibrotic scars and has a large capacity for autocrine signaling, the degradation of Sp1 may serve as a putative pharmacological target in keloids. Future studies may include the use of TGF-$\beta$ receptor blockers and measuring intracellular phosphorylated SMAD family members. Other studies may include work to refine the dosage with respect to solubility without a vehicle. Although a genetic mouse model does not yet exist for keloids, there are still valid models of keloid and hypertrophic scarring that may function to validate the mechanism and activity of TA in this disease. Despite the shortcomings of this preliminary study, TA has clear potential to selectively treat keloid fibroblasts over normal dermal fibroblasts. Numerous other small-molecule treatments have been tested in keloids, but TA and fenamates on the whole, have not been explored.

Generally speaking, our current novel data demonstrated that tolfenamic acid induced cell apoptosis and inhibited collagen production in keloid fibroblasts. TA could be the new therapeutic application for treating keloid scars. With the development of the advanced technologies, hundreds and thousands of treatments on keloid scar have been reported. However, this is the first time where TA was successfully used *in vitro* to induce cell apoptosis and reduce collagen accumulation in KFs. Furthermore, TA is an available commercial formulation chemical. Thereby, TA is recommended for clinical trials to confirm our findings.

## Conflict of Interests

The authors declare that there is no conflict of interests regarding the publication of this paper.

## References

[1] C. Chipev, R. Simman, G. Hatch, A. E. Katz, D. M. Siegel, and M. Simon, "Myofibroblast phenotype and apoptosis in keloid and palmar fibroblasts in vitro," *Cell Death and Differentiation*, vol. 7, no. 2, pp. 166–176, 2000.

[2] R. Simman, H. Alani, and F. Williams, "Effect of mitomycin C on keloid fibroblasts: an in vitro study," *Annals of Plastic Surgery*, vol. 50, no. 1, pp. 71–76, 2003.

[3] C. H. Ricketts, L. Martin, D. T. Faria, G. M. Saed, and D. P. Fivenson, "Cytokine mRNA changes during the treatment of hypertrophic scars with silicone and nonsilicone gel dressings," *Dermatologic Surgery*, vol. 22, no. 11, pp. 955–959, 1996.

[4] J. Meenakshi, V. Jayaraman, K. M. Ramakrishnan, and M. Babu, "Ultrastructural differentiation of abnormal scars," *Annals of Burns and Fire Disasters*, vol. 18, pp. 83–88, 2005.

[5] H. Wang and S. Luo, "Establishment of an animal model for human keloid scars using tissue engineering method," *Journal of Burn Care and Research*, vol. 34, no. 4, pp. 439–446, 2013.

[6] A. Asilian, A. Darougheh, and F. Shariati, "New combination of triamcinolone, 5-fluorouracil, and pulsed-dye laser for treatment of keloid and hypertrophic scars," *Dermatologic Surgery*, vol. 32, no. 7, pp. 907–915, 2006.

[7] C.-C. E. Lan, I.-H. Liu, A.-H. Fang, C.-H. Wen, and C.-S. Wu, "Hyperglycaemic conditions decrease cultured keratinocyte mobility: implications for impaired wound healing in patients with diabetes," *The British Journal of Dermatology*, vol. 159, no. 5, pp. 1103–1115, 2008.

[8] T. T. Phan, I. J. Lim, O. Aalami et al., "Smad3 signalling plays an important role in keloid pathogenesis via epithelial-mesenchymal interactions," *Journal of Pathology*, vol. 207, no. 2, pp. 232–242, 2005.

[9] Y. Yagi, E. Muroga, M. Naitoh et al., "An ex vivo model employing keloid-derived cell-seeded collagen sponges for therapy development," *Journal of Investigative Dermatology*, vol. 133, no. 2, pp. 386–393, 2013.

[10] F. Syed, D. Sherris, R. Paus, S. Varmeh, P. P. Pandolfi, and A. Bayat, "Keloid disease can be inhibited by antagonizing excessive mTOR signaling with a novel dual TORC1/2 inhibitor," *The American Journal of Pathology*, vol. 181, no. 5, pp. 1642–1658, 2012.

[11] F. Syed and A. Bayat, "Notch signaling pathway in keloid disease: enhanced fibroblast activity in a Jagged-1 peptide-dependent manner in lesional vs. extralesional fibroblasts," *Wound Repair and Regeneration*, vol. 20, no. 5, pp. 688–706, 2012.

[12] W. J. Lee, I.-K. Choi, J. H. Lee et al., "Relaxin-expressing adenovirus decreases collagen synthesis and up-regulates matrix metalloproteinase expression in keloid fibroblasts: in vitro experiments," *Plastic and Reconstructive Surgery*, vol. 130, no. 3, pp. 407e–417e, 2012.

[13] J. Krajickova, V. Pesakova, M. Adam, and K. E. Senius, "Effect of tolfenamic acid on the metabolism of the main connective tissue components in rats," *Arzneimittel-Forschung*, vol. 37, no. 2, pp. 177–180, 1987.

[14] J.-H. Kim, J.-Y. Jung, J.-H. Shim et al., "Apoptotic effect of tolfenamic acid in KB human oral cancer cells: possible involvement of the p38 MAPK pathway," *Journal of Clinical Biochemistry and Nutrition*, vol. 47, no. 1, pp. 74–80, 2010.

[15] P. D. Gotzsche, "Meta-analysis of grip strength: most common, but superfluous variable in comparative NSAID trials," *Danish Medical Bulletin*, vol. 36, no. 5, pp. 493–495, 1989.

[16] P. C. Gotzsche, "Review of dose-response studies of NSAIDs in rheumatoid arthritis," *Danish Medical Bulletin*, vol. 36, no. 4, pp. 395–399, 1989.

[17] P. C. Gotzsche, "Methodology and overt and hidden bias in reports of 196 double-blind trials of nonsteroidal antiinflammatory drugs in rheumatoid arthritis," *Controlled Clinical Trials*, vol. 10, no. 1, pp. 31–56, 1989.

[18] S. Rossi, W. Ou, D. Tang et al., "Gastrointestinal stromal tumours overexpress fatty acid synthase," *Journal of Pathology*, vol. 209, no. 3, pp. 369–375, 2006.

[19] E.-S. Choi, J.-H. Shim, J.-Y. Jung et al., "Apoptotic effect of tolfenamic acid in androgen receptor-independent prostate cancer cell and xenograft tumor through specificity protein 1," *Cancer Science*, vol. 102, no. 4, pp. 742–748, 2011.

[20] S. U. Kang, Y. S. Shin, H. S. Hwang, S. J. Baek, S.-H. Lee, and C.-H. Kim, "Tolfenamic acid induces apoptosis and growth inhibition in head and neck cancer: involvement of NAG-1 expression," *PLoS ONE*, vol. 7, no. 4, Article ID e34988, 2012.

[21] D. Eslin, U. T. Sankpal, C. Lee et al., "Tolfenamic acid inhibits neuroblastoma cell proliferation and induces apoptosis: a novel therapeutic agent for neuroblastoma," *Molecular Carcinogenesis*, vol. 52, no. 5, pp. 377–386, 2013.

[22] M. Abdelrahim, C. H. Baker, J. L. Abbruzzese, and S. Safe, "Tolfenamic acid and pancreatic cancer growth, angiogenesis, and Sp protein degradation," *Journal of the National Cancer Institute*, vol. 98, no. 12, pp. 855–868, 2006.

[23] S.-H. Lee, H. B. Jae, K. C. Chang et al., "ESE-1/EGR-1 pathway plays a role in tolfenamic acid-induced apoptosis in colorectal

cancer cells," *Molecular Cancer Therapeutics*, vol. 7, no. 12, pp. 3739–3750, 2008.

[24] M. Abdelrahim, C. H. Baker, J. L. Abbruzzese et al., "Regulation of vascular endothelial growth factor receptor-1 expression by specificity proteins 1, 3, and 4 in pancreatic cancer cells," *Cancer Research*, vol. 67, no. 7, pp. 3286–3294, 2007.

[25] U. T. Sankpal, M. Abdelrahim, S. F. Connelly et al., "Small molecule tolfenamic acid inhibits PC-3 cell proliferation and invasion in vitro, and tumor growth in orthotopic mouse model for prostate cancer," *Prostate*, vol. 72, no. 15, pp. 1648–1658, 2012.

[26] D.-L. Fan, W.-J. Zhao, Y.-X. Wang, S.-Y. Han, and S. Guo, "Oxymatrine inhibits collagen synthesis in keloid fibroblasts via inhibition of transforming growth factor-$\beta$1/Smad signaling pathway," *International Journal of Dermatology*, vol. 51, no. 4, pp. 463–472, 2012.

[27] C. K. Lim, A. S. Halim, N. S. Yaacob, I. Zainol, and K. Noorsal, "Keloid pathogenesis via Drosophila similar to mothers against decapentaplegic (SMAD) signaling in a primary epithelial-mesenchymal in vitro model treated with biomedical-grade chitosan porous skin regenerating template," *Journal of Bioscience and Bioengineering*, vol. 115, no. 4, pp. 453–458, 2013.

[28] C.-S. Wu, P.-H. Wu, A.-H. Fang, and C.-C. E. Lan, "FK506 inhibits the enhancing effects of transforming growth factor (TGF)-$\beta$1 on collagen expression and TGF-$\beta$/Smad signalling in keloid fibroblasts: implication for new therapeutic approach," *The British Journal of Dermatology*, vol. 167, no. 3, pp. 532–541, 2012.

# 15

# The Prevalence and Pattern of Superficial Fungal Infections among School Children in Ile-Ife, South-Western Nigeria

**Olaide Olutoyin Oke,[1] Olaniyi Onayemi,[2] Olayinka Abimbola Olasode,[2] Akinlolu Gabriel Omisore,[3] and Olumayowa Abimbola Oninla[2]**

[1]*Dermatology Unit, Department of Internal Medicine, Federal Medical Centre, Abeokuta 110222, Nigeria*
[2]*Department of Dermatology & Venereology, Obafemi Awolowo University, Ile-Ife, Nigeria*
[3]*Department of Community Medicine, Osun State University, Osogbo, Nigeria*

Correspondence should be addressed to Olaide Olutoyin Oke; laidekolawole@yahoo.com

Academic Editor: Masutaka Furue

Fungal infections of the skin and nails are common global problems with attendant morbidity among affected individuals. Children are mostly affected due to predisposing factors such as overcrowding and low socioeconomic factors. The aim of this study was to determine the prevalence and the clinical patterns of superficial fungal infections among primary school children in Ile-Ife. A multistage sampling was conducted to select eight hundred pupils from ten primary schools in Ile-Ife. Data on epidemiological characteristics and clinical history was collected using a semistructured questionnaire and skin scrapings were done. The prevalence of superficial fungal infections among the 800 respondents was 35.0%. Male pupils constituted 51.0% of respondents while the females were 49.0%. The mean age for all the respondents was 9.42 ± 2.00. Tinea capitis was the commonest infection with a prevalence of 26.9% and tinea unguium, tinea corporis, and tinea faciei had a prevalence of 0.8%, 0.6%, and 0.5%, respectively. Tinea manuum had the least prevalence of 0.1%. Pityriasis versicolor had a prevalence of 4.4%. *Microsporum audouinii* was the leading organism isolated. The study shows that the prevalence of superficial fungal infection (SFI) among primary school children in Ile-Ife is high with tinea capitis as the commonest SFI.

## 1. Introduction

Fungal infections of the skin and nails have been found in the last few decades to affect 20–25% of the world's population, making them one of the most frequent forms of infection [1]. They represent a major public health problem in school-age children especially in low- and middle-income countries (LMICs) like Nigeria where possible predisposing factors to acquiring the infection such as hygiene, overcrowding, and low socioeconomic factors remain present [2]. Prevalence of superficial fungal infection (SFI) in Nigeria as reported ranges from 3.4% to 55% [3–6].

The superficial fungal infections include those caused by dermatophytes (such as tinea capitis, tinea faciei, tinea corporis, tinea unguium, tinea manuum, and tinea pedis) and nondermatophytes such as pityriasis versicolor, cutaneous candidiasis, tinea nigra, black piedra, and white piedra [2].

Tinea capitis is the commonest superficial fungal infection among primary school children [1]. In developing countries including Africa, *Microsporum audouinii* and *Trichophyton soudanense* are most frequently isolated aetiological agents whereas this has been displaced by *Microsporum canis* and *Trichophyton tonsurans* in most European countries [3]. The most common and most widely distributed aetiological agent is *Trichophyton rubrum*, which causes different types of infection in different parts of the world [1].

Many studies have been done on SFI in Nigeria; however, most of them are limited and are not recent; therefore, a more recent and comprehensive study is needed to assess the impact of this problem. The quality of life has been shown to be impaired in children with tinea capitis [5]. It has also been documented that prevalence and aetiological agents vary from time to time with geographic zone, age, humidity, and sex [3]; thus it becomes imperative not only to know the prevalence of SFI but also to ascertain the pattern of SFI, not only in terms of sociodemographic characteristics but also in terms of the specific causative organisms. Thus, this study was designed to determine the current prevalence and pattern of SFI in an urban area of Nigeria, and thus can provide additional information on the trends of SFI in Nigeria. Findings from this study will provide up-to-date information on SFI for evidence-based action aimed at reducing the morbidity of the infection.

## 2. Subjects, Materials, and Methods

This cross sectional study was conducted between January and March 2011 in Ile-Ife, Osun State, South-Western Nigeria. Ile-Ife is an ancient city that is believed to be the source of the Yoruba people.

A multistage sampling technique was used that involved selection along local governments, schools (both public and private), classes, and proportionate pupils from selected class strata.

A total of 800 school children were recruited from 10 schools—6 publicly funded and 4 privately owned primary schools in Ile-Ife, Nigeria. Calculated minimum sample size using prevalence from a previous study [5] was 255 but this was increased to 800. The purpose and benefits of the study were explained to the pupils, their parents/guardians, teachers, and head-teachers. Only pupils whose parents/guardians gave informed consent were eventually included in the study.

Ethical clearance was obtained from the Ethical Committee, Obafemi Awolowo University Teaching Hospitals Complex, Ile-Ife, Osun State, Nigeria.

Quantitative data was collected from pupils in selected schools using an interviewer administered questionnaire. The semistructured precoded questionnaire had sections focusing on the sociodemographic details of the respondents, possible predisposing factors for developing superficial fungal infections, and socioeconomic status of parents. Physical examination was conducted in a well-lit room and the pupils were examined thoroughly from head to toe with minimal clothing for the presence of any superficial fungal infection. The fungal infections were then classified.

Diagnosis was made clinically, and appropriate skin scrapings or nail clippings were taken to confirm diagnosis. Pupils who had superficial fungal infections were treated appropriately by the authors.

*2.1. Sample Collection and Processing.* Areas of the skin suspected to have fungal infections were scraped using disposable scalpel blades after first cleaning with alcohol. The scrapings were collected on a sterile brown paper and transported to the laboratory within 2 hours for microscopic and culture analysis. The scrapings were handled separately ensuring that no individual scrapings mixed. Nail clippings were also done as required. For direct microscopy, each specimen was placed on a slide and a drop of 10% potassium hydroxide added before covering with a cover slip. This was then heated gently (for about five minutes) to soften it and it was then examined for the presence of hyphae and/or arthroconidia under low (X10) and high (X40) power objective.

Diagnosis of dermatophytes in hair pieces was made by the visualisation of arthroconidia arranged along the length of the hair in chains or masses around the hair (ectothrix infection) or in the hair substance (endothrix infection). The scrapings and the pieces of hair were plated out separately on Sabouraud's dextrose agar. Cycloheximide was employed because saprophytic fungi and yeasts normally present as contaminants will be inhibited by it. Chloramphenicol and streptomycin were the antibiotics used to inhibit bacterial contaminants. Culture plates were incubated at $27°C$ for 4 weeks and then examined for the presence of dermatophytes. Macro- and micromorphological studies of cultured colonies were done for the presence of dermatophytes.

*2.2. Data Analysis.* The data obtained were entered and analysed using Statistical Package for Social Sciences version 16.0 (SPSS, IBM Corporation, Armonk, NY, USA). Some of the variables were regrouped and/or recoded before the data analysis was done. Continuous data were expressed as means $\pm$ standard deviation (SD) and categorical data as percentages. Differences between categorical variables were analyzed using chi-square test. The level of statistical significance for all the tests was a $P$ value $<0.05$.

## 3. Results

*3.1. General Characteristics/Prevalence.* A total of 800 pupils were recruited for the study. The mean age for all the respondents was $9.42 \pm 2.00$. Males made up 51% (408 pupils) of the respondents while the females were 49% (392 pupils).

Out of the 800 pupils, 280 pupils were found to have superficial fungal infection (SFI) giving a prevalence of 35%. Highest prevalence was found among the age group 9–12 years. Males were more affected than the females as it occurred in 40.6% and 29.1% of them, respectively, and this difference was statistically significant. Similarly, more respondents from the Hausa ethnic group had SFI compared to other tribes (Table 1).

*3.2. Clinical Types of SFI Seen.* In terms of clinical types, tinea capitis was the commonest accounting for 26.9% of the prevalence. Tinea unguium, tinea corporis, and tinea faciei had a prevalence of 0.8%, 0.6%, and 0.5%, respectively. Tinea manuum had the least prevalence of 0.1%. Pityriasis versicolor, a nondermatophytosis was seen with a prevalence of 4.4%. In some pupils, more than one type of superficial fungal infection was seen. Tinea capitis with pityriasis versicolor was seen in 12 cases (1.5%); tinea capitis with tinea unguium and tinea capitis with tinea faciei were seen in 0.1% of total prevalence, respectively. There was no case of tinea pedis or any form of candidiasis seen in the course of the study (Table 2) (see Figures 1, 2, 3, 4, 5, 6, 7, and 8).

*3.3. Clinical Pattern of SFI Seen.* Two hundred and nine pupils (95%) with tinea capitis, either singly or in combination had noninflammatory form with the grey patch type accounting for 46.3%. This was followed by the black dot type and then seborrheic dermatitis-like tinea capitis that constituted 27.1% and 17.9%, respectively. As regards

TABLE 1: Relationship between the sociodemographic characteristics and the presence of superficial fungal infections.

| | Presence of superficial fungal infections Yes $n = 280$ (%) | Fungal Infections No $n = 520$ (%) | Total $n = 800$ | $\chi^2$ | df | P value |
|---|---|---|---|---|---|---|
| Age in years | | | | | | |
| 5–8 | 94 (31.97) | 199 (67.9) | 293 | | | |
| 9–12 | 164 (37.61) | 274 (62.6) | 438 | 2.936 | 2 | 0.230 |
| 13–16 | 22 (31.43) | 47 (68.1) | 69 | | | |
| Sex | | | | | | |
| Male | 166 (40.7) | 242 (59.3) | 408 | 12.293 | 1 | 0.001 |
| Female | 114 (29.1) | 278 (70.9) | 392 | | | |
| Class | | | | | | |
| Pry 1–3 | 140 (34.3) | 268 (65.7) | 408 | 0.026 | 1 | 0.678 |
| Pry 4–6 | 140 (35.7) | 252 (64.3) | 392 | | | |
| Religion | | | | | | |
| Christianity | 214 (34.6) | 404 (65.4) | 618 | | | |
| Islam | 66 (36.5) | 115 (63.5) | 181 | 0.662 | 2 | 0.586 |
| Traditional | 0 (0) | 1 (1.0) | 1 | | | |
| Ethnicity | | | | | | |
| Yoruba | 265 (35.7) | 477 | 742 | | | |
| Hausa | 7 (50.0) | 7 | 14 | 11.097 | 3 | 0.011 |
| Igbo | 2 (8.3) | 22 | 24 | | | |
| Others | 6 (30.0) | 14 | 20 | | | |

TABLE 2: Prevalence and Clinical types of superficial fungal infections among primary school children in Ile-Ife.

| Type | Frequency | % Prevalence among all children examined ($n = 800$) | % Prevalence among those with infections ($n = 280$) |
|---|---|---|---|
| Tinea capitis alone | 215 | 26.9 | 76.8 |
| Pityriasis versicolor | 35 | 4.4 | 12.5 |
| Pityriasis versicolor and tinea capitis | 12 | 1.5 | 4.3 |
| Tinea unguium | 6 | 0.8 | 2.1 |
| Tinea corporis | 5 | 0.6 | 1.8 |
| Tinea faciei | 4 | 0.5 | 1.4 |
| Tinea manuum | 1 | 0.1 | 0.4 |
| Tinea capitis and tinea faciei | 1 | 0.1 | 0.4 |
| Tinea capitis and tinea unguium | 1 | 0.1 | 0.4 |
| Total | **280** | **35** | **100.0** |

the inflammatory form, the pustular type was the most common (6.5%) of all types of tinea capitis seen, while 2.2% of the pupils were found to have kerion. There was no case of favus seen among all the pupils that were examined. The back was the commonest site (60%) of tinea corporis, while the face was the commonest site (95.7%) for pityriasis versicolor. Tinea unguium involving the fingernails was seen in 85.7% of cases while involvement of the toenails occurred in the remaining 14.3% (Table 3).

3.4. Characteristics of Aetiological Agents Isolated. The distribution of the species isolated from the pupils with clinically suspected superficial fungal infections (according to age, gender, and clinical types) is as shown in Tables 4(a) and 4(b).

Of the 800 pupils recruited for the study, 280 pupils were found to have lesions with clinical suspicion of superficial

fungal infection. 35 of the pupils did not give consent to have their skin or nail scraped. Of the 245 pupils that had skin scrapings or nail clippings done for suspected superficial fungal infection, 157 (64.1%) samples were mycologically proven and 88 (35.9%) were culture negative.

Dermatophytes constituted 72.7% of the samples (first five species in Table 4) while nondermatophyte molds were 27.3%. Concerning the dermatophytes, the 3 genera, Microsporum, Trichophyton, and Epidermophyton, were represented with 5 different species that included Microsporum audouinii as the leading organism isolated (28%). This was followed by Trichophyton rubrum (21.7%). Epidermophyton floccosum was the least isolated (5.1%). Other isolates in the study were Trichophyton mentagrophytes and Trichophyton schoenleinii. The nondermatophyte molds identified were Penicillium (12%), Aspergillus fumigatus (8.4%), and Aspergillus niger (6.4%).

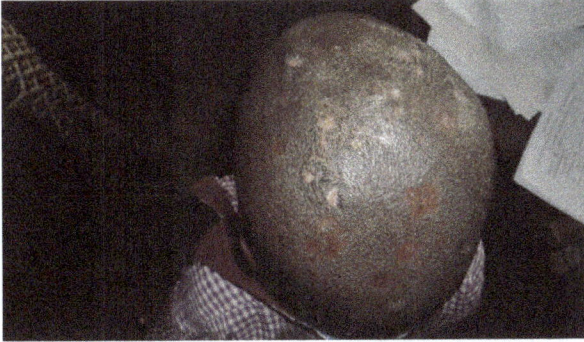

FIGURE 1: Tinea capitis with scarring alopecia.

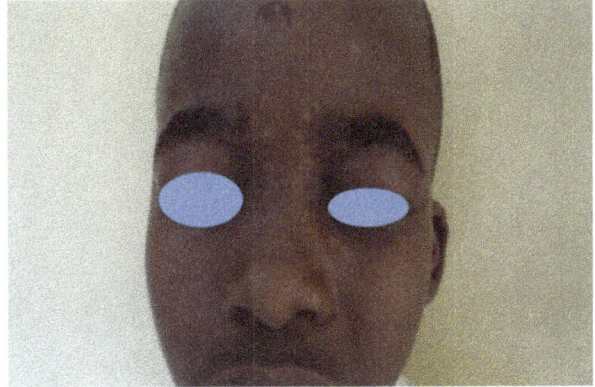

FIGURE 2: Tinea capitis.

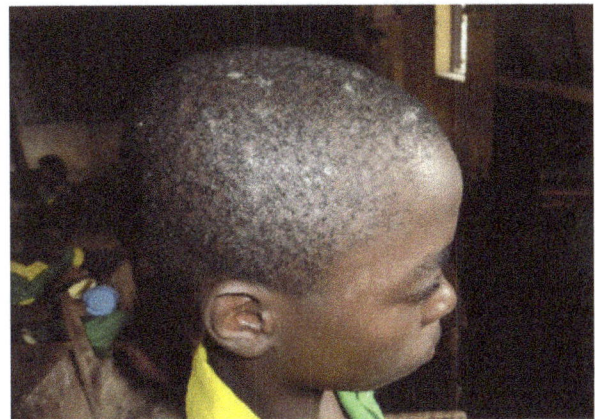

FIGURE 3: Pityriasis versicolor on the face.

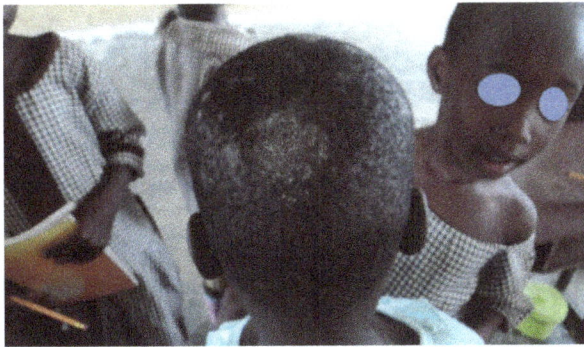

FIGURE 4: Tinea capitis and pityriasis versicolor.

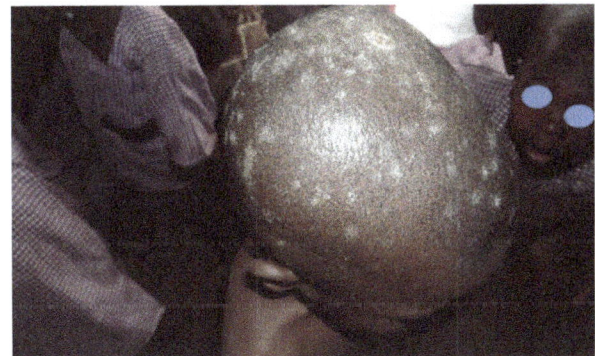

FIGURE 5: Tinea capitis.

About half of the isolates of the dermatophytes were from pupils aged 4–6 years and 7–11 years (49% and 49.7%, resp.). Only 1.3% were from the age group 12–16 years.

The frequency distribution of the positive cases among the males and females was statistically significant with positive isolates being more among males than females (Table 4).

## 4. Discussion

*4.1. Prevalence of Superficial Fungal Infection.* Superficial fungal infections are common and remain an important public health problem among children worldwide and particularly in Nigeria [5–7]. This is evident in this study where prevalence of superficial fungal infection was 35%. This prevalence is comparably slightly higher than the 21% observed in a study in Ebonyi State, South-Eastern Nigeria [4]. Similar studies in Iraq and Egypt had a low prevalence of 2.7% and 7.4%, respectively [8]. It has been suggested that differences in the prevalence of superficial fungal infection in different regions may be due to variation in climatic and environmental conditions of the areas being studied [5, 9].

Tinea capitis, a dermatophytosis, was the predominant superficial fungal infection and this corroborates other studies that showed that tinea capitis is the commonest superficial fungal infection among children [6, 9–11]. Reasons that can explain the predominance of tinea capitis among children of primary school age include use of local barbers, poor personal hygiene, short hair that promotes transmission from one scalp to the other, and increased frequent contacts with playmates at school and younger siblings at home [12, 13].

The noninflammatory form of tinea capitis was the commoner tinea capitis lesion and out of this the grey patch type was the most common. This is comparable to other studies [11, 14, 15]. Kerion has been observed to occur more in males compared to females and this was also observed in this study [5]. Tinea capitis was also found in association with tinea faciei, tinea unguium, and pityriasis versicolor in some

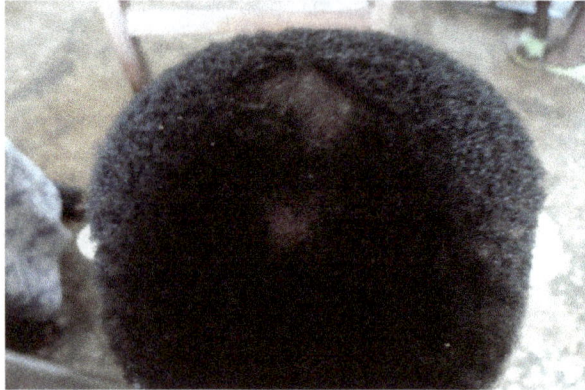

FIGURE 6: Tinea capitis with alopecia.

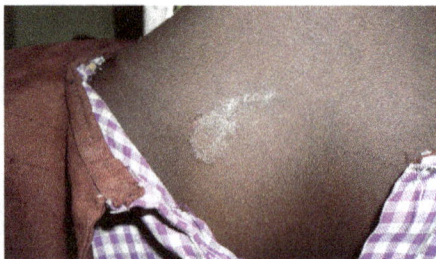

FIGURE 8: Tinea faciei.

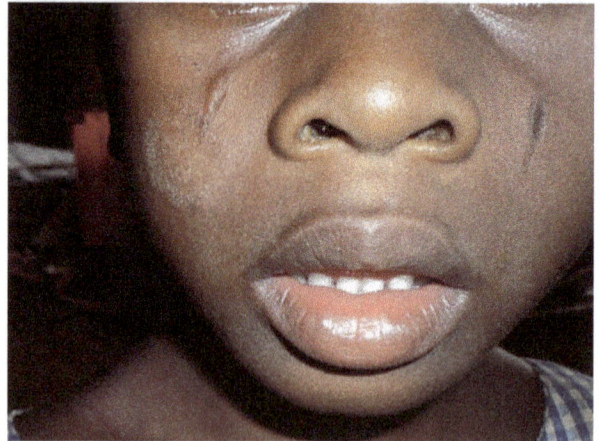

FIGURE 7: Tinea corporis.

TABLE 3: Clinical Patterns of SFI seen.

| Tinea capitis | Number (%) |
| --- | --- |
| Noninflammatory types | |
| Grey patch type | 106 (46.3) |
| Black dot type | 62 (27.1) |
| Seborrheic dermatitis-like | 41 (17.9 |
| Inflammatory types | |
| Pustular | 15 (6.5) |
| Kerion | 5 (2.2) |
| Favus | 0 (0) |
| Tinea corporis site | |
| Abdomen | 1 (20) |
| Back | 3 (60) |
| Limbs | 1 (20) |
| Tinea unguium site | |
| Right middle finger | 3 (42.8) |
| Right fourth finger | 2 (28.6) |
| Left fourth and fifth fingers | 1 (14.3) |
| Left great toe | 1 (14.3) |
| Pityriasis versicolor site | |
| Face | 45 (95.7) |
| Chest | 2 (4.3) |

pupils. This is possible as the dermatophytes can spread from the scalp to other regions through autoinoculation.

Pityriasis versicolor which was the next common type of superficial fungal infection is a nondermatophytosis. Its prevalence of 4.4% is similar to that found in Ibadan, South-Western Nigeria, and in Abakaliki, South-Eastern Nigeria, where the prevalence was 4.6% and 4.7%, respectively [10, 11], and in Taiwan where they also recorded a prevalence of 4.4%, but comparatively higher than what was obtained in Bamako, Mali (1.6%) [11]. Other dermatophytoses such as tinea unguium, tinea corporis, tinea faciei, and tinea manuum all had a prevalence that was <1%. This is corroborated by previous studies that show these infections to be uncommon in the age group being studied as they are not usually exposed to the predisposing factors such as involvement in gardening which predispose them to tinea manuum [16, 17].

There was no case of tinea pedis or candidiasis found in this study. This is probably due to the age group that is being studied. Tinea pedis has been found more with older age group as documented by Moon et al. [18]. It is also believed that the older age groups are likely to wear their shoes more constantly and this with the hot and humid environment promoting moisture will favour susceptibility to the infection [12].

### 4.2. Sociodemographic Characteristics and the Presence of Superficial Fungal Infections.
This study showed that superficial fungal infection was commoner in males (40.7%) than females, in a ratio of 1.4 : 1. Males usually keep short hair and

visit the barbers' shop more, have more frequent contacts with playmates, play with sand more, and are less concerned about hygiene and personal grooming than the females [12]. Also females usually weave their hair and visit the barbers less [12]. This male predominance was also observed in previous studies done both within and outside Nigeria [1, 9, 19].

Superficial fungal infection has a higher prevalence amongst children less than twelve years of age. This is comparable to what Nweze obtained in North-Eastern Nigeria and in other studies [3, 20]. Tinea capitis in particular was higher in children less than seven years of age. Presence of superficial fungal infection in younger age group observed in this study supports the suggestion that infection is related to the poor hygiene at the younger age and absence of saturated fatty acids that provide a natural protective mechanism against fungal

TABLE 4: (a) Distribution of dermatophytic isolates according to age and gender grouping of primary pupils in Ile-Ife ($n = 157$). (b) Distribution of dermatophytic isolates according to clinical types.

(a)

| Species | Total (%) | Isolates according to age group | | | Isolates according to gender | |
|---|---|---|---|---|---|---|
| | | 4–6 yrs | 7–11 yrs | 12–16 yrs | Male (%) | Female (%) |
| *Microsporum audouinii* | 44 (28.0) | 13 (30.0) | 31 (70.0) | 0 (0.0) | 32 (72.3) | 12 (27.7) |
| *Trichophyton rubrum* | 34 (21.7) | 19 (55.9) | 14 (41.2) | 1 (2.9) | 20 (58.8) | 14 (41.2) |
| *Trichophyton mentagrophytes* | 18 (11.5) | 14 (77.8) | 4 (22.2) | 0 (0.0) | 12 (66.7) | 6 (33.3) |
| *Trichophyton schoenleinii* | 10 (6.4) | 8 (80.0) | 2 (20.0) | 0 (0.0) | 7 (70.0) | 3 (30.0) |
| *Epidermophyton floccosum* | 8 (5.1) | 2 (25.0) | 6 (75.0) | 0 (0.0) | 4 (50.0) | 4 (50.0) |
| *Aspergillus fumigatus* | 14 (8.9) | 8 (57.1) | 6 (42.9) | 0 (0.0) | 11 (78.6) | 3 (21.4) |
| *Aspergillus niger* | 10 (6.4) | 5 (50.0) | 5 (50.0) | 0 (0.0) | 6 (60.0) | 4 (40.0) |
| *Penicillium* | 19 (12.0) | 8 (42.1) | 10 (52.6) | 1 (5.3) | 17 (89.5) | 2 (10.5) |
| Total number (%) | **157 (100.0)** | **77 (49.0)** | **78 (49.7)** | **2 (1.3)** | **109 (69.4)** | **48 (30.6)** |

*yrs—years.

(b)

| Clinical type | Isolate according to clinical type $n = 157$ | | | | | | | |
|---|---|---|---|---|---|---|---|---|
| | *Microsporum audouinii* (%) | *Trichophyton rubrum* (%) | *Trichophyton mentagrophytes* (%) | *Trichophyton schoenleinii* (%) | *Epidermophyton floccosum* (%) | *Aspergillus fumigatus* (%) | *Aspergillus niger* (%) | *Penicillium* (%) |
| Tinea capitis | 44 (100.0) | 25 (73.5) | 17 (94.4) | 10 (100.0) | — | 14 (100.0) | 10 (100.0) | 18 (94.7) |
| Tinea faciei | — | 2 (5.9) | 1 (5.6) | — | 2 (25.0) | — | — | |
| Tinea corporis | — | 4 (11.8) | — | — | 1 (12.5) | — | — | 1 (5.3) |
| Tinea manuum | — | 1 (2.9) | — | — | — | — | — | |
| Tinea unguium | — | 2 (5.9) | — | — | 5 (62.5) | — | — | |
| Total | **44** | **34** | **18** | **10** | **8** | **14** | **10** | **19** |

infections [21]. Furthermore, Ayanbimpe et al. attributed the highest rate of infection amongst them to the fact that they are the group active at playgrounds and will thus have closer contact with sources of pathogens [19].

*4.3. Characteristics of Aetiological Agents Identified.* The dermatophyte species isolated in this study belonged to the three genera *Trichophyton, Microsporum,* and *Epidermophyton* of which five species, mostly anthropophilic, were identified. *Microsporum audouinii* was the commonest specie followed by *Trichophyton rubrum.* Others included *T. mentagrophytes, T. schoenleinii,* and *Epidermophyton floccosum.* The nondermatophyte mould identified were *Aspergillus fumigatus, Aspergillus niger,* and *Penicillium.* Most of the species were more predominant in the males. Studies have established variability in the species of dermatophytes isolated from one geographical region to the other and also per time [19]. In Nigeria, Nweze documented that the spectrum of pathogens and their clinical presentations in West Africa are different from those seen in other continents [22]. This finding was corroborated in this study.

*Microsporum audouinii* was the commonest dermatophyte species isolated (28%) and this is similar to findings done by

Soyinka decades ago and also by Ajao and Akintunde both in Ile-Ife (the study site) on superficial fungal infections and tinea capitis, respectively, and by Enweani et al. at Ekpoma located in a different geopolitical zone from Ile-Ife [6, 12, 23]. In other parts of the country, it seems *Microsporum audouinii* has ceased to be the dominant aetiological agent where *Trichophyton soudanese, Trichophyton mentagrophytes,* and other species predominate [17, 19, 24]. *Microsporum audouinii* is mainly a human pathogen but occasionally it infects animals and has been observed to resolve as pupils approach puberty [5, 6, 12]; thus, in this study, it was only found among the age group 4–11 years.

*Trichophyton* species (*rubrum, mentagrophytes,* and *schoenleinii*) were isolated from 39.6% pupils with *Trichophyton rubrum* being the dominant species in 21.7% and these were the fungi most recovered among pupils with tinea unguium, tinea corporis, and tinea faciei. This is similar to findings obtained elsewhere [17, 25].

*Epidermophyton floccosum* was the least isolated (5.1%) and this is not unusual as it is usually isolated more in tinea pedis and there was no case of this fungal infection in the study [12].

Presence of nondermatophyte molds such as *Aspergillus* and *Penicillium* is becoming increasingly common and one of the factors attributed is the ubiquitous nature of their spores in our environment that makes it to be carried transiently on healthy skin [25, 26].

## 5. Conclusion

The prevalence of superficial fungal infection among primary school children in Ile-Ife, South-Western Nigeria, remains high. Tinea capitis was the most common fungal infection and the noninflammatory clinical type was most prevalent among them. *Microsporum audouinii* was the commonest organism isolated.

Regular health education about fungal infections that highlights their morbidities and modes of spread, should be given to school children, their parents and teachers, in order to truly reduce the prevalence and burden of superficial fungal infections in low and middle income countries (LMICs) such as Nigeria. Establishment of school-based dermatological services for primary school pupils will also be of immense help.

## Conflict of Interests

The authors declare that there is no conflict of interests regarding the publication of this paper.

## References

[1] B. Havlickova, V. A. Czaika, and M. Friedrich, "Epidemiological trends in skin mycoses worldwide," *Mycoses*, vol. 51, supplement 4, pp. 2–15, 2008.

[2] S. Verma and M. P. Heffernan, "Superficial fungal infections," in *Fitzpatrick's Dermatology in General Medicine*, pp. 1807–1831, McGraw Hill Professional, 7th edition, 2008.

[3] E. I. Nweze and J. I. Okafor, "Prevalence of dermatophytic fungal infections in children: a recent study in Anambra State, Nigeria," *Mycopathologia*, vol. 160, no. 3, pp. 239–243, 2005.

[4] J. C. Anosike, I. R. Keke, J. C. Uwaezuoke et al., "Prevalence and distribution of ringworm infection in primary school children in parts of Eastern, Nigeria," *Journal of Applied Sciences and Environmental Management*, vol. 9, no. 3, pp. 21–25, 2005.

[5] A. O. Akinboro, O. A. Olasode, O. Onayemi, and D. A. Mejiuni, "The impacts of *Tinea capitis* on quality of life: a community based cross sectional study among Nigerian children," *Clinical Medicine Insights: Dermatology*, vol. 6, pp. 9–17, 2013.

[6] A. O. Ajao and C. Akintunde, "Studies on the prevalence of tinea capitis infection in Ile-Ife, Nigeria," *Mycopathologia*, vol. 89, no. 1, pp. 43–48, 1985.

[7] M. R. Vander Straten, M. A. Hossain, and M. A. Ghannoum, "Cutaneous infections dermatophytosis, onychomycosis, and tinea versicolor," *Infectious Disease Clinics of North America*, vol. 17, no. 1, pp. 87–112, 2003.

[8] H. I. Fathi and A. G. M. Al-Samarai, "Prevalence of tinea capitis among schoolchildren in Iraq," *Eastern Mediterranean Health Journal*, vol. 6, no. 1, pp. 128–137, 2000.

[9] C. I. C. Ogbonna, R. O. Robinson, and J. M. Abubakar, "The distribution of ringworm infections among primary school children in Jos, Plateau State of Nigeria," *Mycopathologia*, vol. 89, no. 2, pp. 101–106, 1985.

[10] A. O. Ogunbiyi, E. Owoaje, and A. Ndahi, "Prevalence of skin disorders in school children in Ibadan, Nigeria," *Pediatric Dermatology*, vol. 22, no. 1, pp. 6–10, 2005.

[11] C. J. Uneke, B. A. Ngwu, and O. Egemba, "Tinea capitis and pityriasis versicolor infections among school children in the south-eastern nigeria: the public health implications," *The Internet Journal of Dermatology*, vol. 4, no. 2, 2006.

[12] F. Soyinka, "Epidemiologic study of dermatophyte infections in Nigeria (clinical survey and laboratory investigations)," *Mycopathologia*, vol. 63, no. 2, pp. 99–103, 1978.

[13] Y.-H. Wu, H.-Y. Su, and Y.-J. Hsieh, "Survey of infectious skin diseases and skin infestations among primary school students of Taitung County, eastern Taiwan," *Journal of the Formosan Medical Association*, vol. 99, no. 2, pp. 128–134, 2000.

[14] A. O. Akinboro, O. A. Olasode, and O. Onayemi, "The pattern, risk factors and clinic-aetiological correlate of Tinea capitis among the children in a tropical community setting of Osogbo, South-Western Nigeria," *Afro-Egyptian Journal of Infectious and Endemic Diseases*, vol. 1, no. 2, pp. 53–64, 2011.

[15] E. N. Nnoruka, I. Obiagboso, and C. Maduechesi, "Hair loss in children in South-East Nigeria: common and uncommon cases," *International Journal of Dermatology*, vol. 46, no. 1, pp. 18–22, 2007.

[16] H. Degreef, "Clinical forms of dermatophytosis," *Mycopathologia*, vol. 166, no. 5-6, pp. 257–265, 2008.

[17] C. A. Oyeka and I. I. Eze, "Fungal skin infections among prison inmates in Abakaliki, Nigeria," *Mycoses*, vol. 51, no. 1, pp. 50–54, 2008.

[18] H. Moon, J. Moon, J. Lee, S. Kim, Y. Won, and S. Lee, "Epidemiologic study of superficial fungal infections in outpatients of dermatologic Clinic and Healthy individuals," *Chonnam Medical Journal*, vol. 37, no. 4, pp. 409–413, 2001.

[19] G. M. Ayanbimpe, H. Taghir, A. Diya, and S. Wapwera, "Tinea capitis among primary school children in some parts of central Nigeria," *Mycoses*, vol. 51, no. 4, pp. 336–340, 2008.

[20] A. A. Omar, "Ringworm of the scalp in primary-school children in Alexandria: infection and carriage," *Eastern Mediterranean Health Journal*, vol. 6, no. 5-6, pp. 961–967, 2000.

[21] F. Fisher and N. B. Cook, *Fundamentals of Diagnostic Mycology*, WB Saunders Company, Philadelphia, Pa, USA, 7th edition, 1998.

[22] E. I. Nweze, "Dermatophytosis in Western Africa: a review," *Pakistan Journal of Biological Sciences*, vol. 13, no. 13, pp. 649–656, 2010.

[23] I. B. Enweani, C. C. Ozan, D. E. Agbonlahor, and R. N. Ndip, "Dermatophytosis in schoolchildren in Ekpoma, Nigeria," *Mycoses*, vol. 39, no. 7-8, pp. 303–305, 1996.

[24] T. Mbata and C. Nwajagu, "Dermatophytes and other fungi associated with hair-scalp of nursery and primary school children in Awka, Nigeria," *The Internet Journal of Microbiology*, vol. 3, no. 2, 2007.

[25] S. A. Adefemi, L. O. Odeigah, and K. M. Alabi, "Prevalence of dermatophytosis among primary school children in Oke-oyi community of Kwara state," *Nigerian Journal of Clinical Practice*, vol. 14, no. 1, pp. 23–28, 2011.

[26] A. Chepchirchir, C. Bii, and J. O. Ndinya-Achola, "Dermatophyte infections in primary school children in Kibera slums of Nairobi," *East African Medical Journal*, vol. 86, no. 2, pp. 59–68, 2009.

# 16

# Metabolic Changes and Serum Ghrelin Level in Patients with Psoriasis

**Haydar Ucak,[1] Betul Demir,[2] Demet Cicek,[2] Ilker Erden,[3] Suleyman Aydin,[4] Selma Bakar Dertlioglu,[2] and Mustafa Arica[1]**

[1]*Department of Dermatology, Faculty of Medicine, Dicle University, 21070 Diyarbakir, Turkey*
[2]*Department of Dermatology, Faculty of Medicine, Firat University, Elazig, Turkey*
[3]*Department of Dermatology, Elazig Training and Research Hospital, Elazig, Turkey*
[4]*Department of Biochemistry, Faculty of Medicine, Firat University, Elazig, Turkey*

Correspondence should be addressed to Haydar Ucak; ucak23@mynet.com

Academic Editor: Kiyofumi Yamanishi

*Background.* Serum ghrelin levels may be related to metabolic and clinical changes in patients with psoriasis. *Objective.* This study was performed to determine the possible effects of serum ghrelin in patients with psoriasis. *Methods.* The study population consisted of 25 patients with plaque psoriasis. The patients were questioned with regard to age, gender, age of onset, duration of disease, height, weight, and body mass index (BMI). In addition, fasting blood sugar, triglyceride, cholesterol levels, insulin, and ghrelin levels were measured. *Results.* The mean serum ghrelin level was $45.41 \pm 22.41$ in the psoriasis group and $29.92 \pm 14.65$ in the healthy control group. Serum ghrelin level was significantly higher in the psoriasis group compared with the controls ($P = 0.01$). The mean ghrelin level in patients with a lower PASI score was significantly higher than in those with a higher PASI score ($P = 0.02$). *Conclusion.* The present study was performed to determine the effects of ghrelin in psoriasis patients. We found a negative correlation between severity of psoriasis and ghrelin level. Larger and especially experimental studies focusing on correlation of immune system-ghrelin levels and severity of psoriasis may be valuable to clarify the etiopathogenesis of the disease.

## 1. Introduction

Psoriasis is a chronic inflammatory disease that affects approximately 1–3% of the general population [1]. In addition, psoriasis is characterized by local and systemic increases in levels of proinflammatory cytokines, such as interleukin-6 (IL-6) and tumor necrosis factor-alpha (TNF-$\alpha$) [2]. Proinflammatory cytokines in chronic inflammation lead to atherogenesis and peripheral insulin resistance, which in turn cause hypertension and type II diabetes mellitus (DM) [3, 4]. In addition, recent studies have indicated a relationship between psoriasis and metabolic syndrome [5, 6].

Ghrelin is a 28-amino acid peptide hormone secreted mainly by the mucosa of the stomach [7]. Ghrelin, thought to be a stimulator of growth hormone (GH) secretion [7] and food intake [8], also shows potent inhibitory effects on proinflammatory mediators via its effect on T cells and monocytes [9].

Previous studies have focused on the relationship between metabolic syndrome and psoriasis. The present study was performed to determine the effects of ghrelin on metabolic changes and the correlation between ghrelin level and disease severity in patients with psoriasis.

## 2. Patients and Methods

The study population consisted of 25 patients with chronic plaque psoriasis patients (11 males and 14 females) all of whom had been referred to the Department of Dermatology of Elazig Education and Research Hospital and Department of Dermatology of Firat University Hospital. Twenty-five healthy control subjects were also enrolled in the present study. All psoriasis patients had symptoms for at least 6 months and had not received any systemic or local antipsoriatic treatment for the last 4 weeks.

## 2.1. Exclusion Criteria

(1) Patients with pustular psoriasis, erythroderma, and psoriatic arthritis,

(2) Systemic diseases (diabetes and hypertension),

(3) Age < 18 years,

(4) Pregnancy,

(5) Acute or chronic infection,

(6) Acute or chronic neurological disorders,

(7) Polycystic ovary syndrome or amenorrhea,

(8) Hyperthyroidism or hypothyroidism.

*2.2. Study Plan.* The patients enrolled in the present study were questioned regarding age, gender, age of onset, duration of disease, history of smoking and alcohol use, height, weight, body mass index (BMI), and waist circumference. In addition, fasting blood sugar, triglyceride, low-density lipoprotein (LDL), very-low-density lipoprotein (VLDL), high-density lipoprotein (HDL), total cholesterol, HbA1c, insulin, C-peptide levels, thyroid stimulating hormone (TSH), T3, T4, and ghrelin levels were measured. Ghrelin levels may be affected by many metabolic factors, so patients and controls had similar BMI to decrease the different metabolic factors in patients with psoriasis.

The extent and severity of lesions were determined using the psoriasis area severity index (PASI) scoring system [10], body surface area (BSA) [11], and quality of life (QOL) was evaluated by calculating the Dermatology Life Quality Index score, which was tested previously for validity and reliability in Turkish by Öztürkcan et al. [12].

BMI was calculated as weight/height ($kg/m^2$) and metabolic syndrome was diagnosed in the presence of central obesity in addition to two or more criteria of the international Diabetes Foundation: waist circumference ≥94 cm in males or ≥80 cm in females; hypertriglyceridemia ≥150 mg/dL; HDL <40 mg/dL in males or <50 mg/dL in females; blood pressure ≥130/85 mmHg; fasting blood glucose ≥ 100 mg/dL [13]. In addition, insulin resistance was calculated according to the homeostasis model assessment of insulin resistance (HOMA-IR) formula: (0 min glucose mg/dL × 0 min insulin $\mu$U/mL)/405. Cases with a HOMA-IR index of >3.2 were diagnosed as having insulin resistance [14].

The control group comprised age-, sex-, and BMI-matched individuals who did not have any systemic or neurological diseases and did not use drugs or alcohol.

*2.3. Collection and Storage of Biological Samples.* As ghrelin is a peptide hormone and can be broken down by proteases, aprotinin (500 Kallikrein units per mL) was added to plain biochemistry tubes before collection of blood samples from the participants to prevent proteolysis. Blood samples were collected at 09.00–10.00 in the morning after an overnight fast to avoid any effects associated with circadian rhythm. Samples (5 mL) were collected from each participant after fasting and centrifuged at 3000 ×g for 5 min. The sera obtained were

TABLE 1: Demographical and clinical findings of groups.

| | *Psoriasis vulgaris* | Control | *P* |
|---|---|---|---|
| *n* | 25 | 25 | |
| Gender (F/M) | 14/11 | 14/11 | *P* > 0.05 |
| Age* (year) | 32.24 ± 7.54 | 31.40 ± 6.77 | *P* > 0.05 |
| BMI* ($kg/m^2$) | 24.96 ± 2.53 | 23.80 ± 1.50 | *P* > 0.05 |
| BMI score* | 2.48 ± 0.65 | 2.28 ± 0.45 | *P* > 0.05 |
| Waist circumference* (cm) | 86.84 ± 10.22 | 83.72 ± 8.48 | *P* > 0.05 |

*(Mean ± SD).

transferred to Eppendorf tubes and frozen at −80°C until the day of analysis.

Serum ghrelin levels were studied using a Human ghrelin kit (Cat. No. A05106; SPI-Bio, Montigny le Bretonneux, France) by the enzyme-linked immunosorbent assay (ELISA) method according to the manufacturer's instructions. According to the kit's supplier, the intra- and interassay coefficients of variation (CV) for this kit are <7% and <8.1%, respectively.

*2.4. Statistical Analysis.* SPSS version 12.0 (SPSS, Chicago, IL) was used for statistical analyses. The data obtained in the study are expressed as the means ± SD. The independent samples *t*-test and Mann-Whitney *U* test were used to compare groups. In all analyses, *P* < 0.05 was taken to indicate statistical significance.

## 3. Results

The study population consisted of 25 patients with psoriasis who presented at the Dermatology Polyclinics of Elazig Training and Research Hospital and Firat University Medical School Hospital. Twenty-five healthy volunteers were also included in the control group. The mean ages of the participants were 32.24 ± 7.54 years for the patients with psoriasis and 31.40 ± 6.77 years for the control subjects. The female-to-male ratio (F/M) was 14/11 in all groups. There were no significant differences between the groups in terms of mean age or gender (*P* > 0.05). Similarly, there was no significant difference in BMI between the psoriasis and control groups (*P* > 0.05). The demographic characteristics and clinical findings of the two groups are presented in Table 1.

The mean disease duration in psoriasis patients was 11.84±7.79 years. In addition, nail involvement was observed in 5 patients (20.0%), genital involvement in 3 patients (12.0%), and scalp involvement in 20 patients (80.0%). Disease involvement score, PASI scores, and DLQI scores are presented in Table 2.

The relationships between involvement/severity of psoriasis and QOL were examined, and higher PASI score was shown to be associated with poorer QOL—the QOL scores were 6.00 ± 3.42, 6.37 ± 2.61, and 7.50 ± 4.78 in patients with low, moderate, and high PASI scores, respectively. However,

TABLE 2: Body involvement percentage and PASI and DLQI values of patients with psoriasis.

| | Patients with psoriasis | $n$ (%) |
|---|---|---|
| PASI* | 5.59 ± 4.38 | |
| PASI score* | 1.96 ± 0.84 | |
| PASI score dissociation | Mild | 9 (36.0) |
| | Moderate | 8 (32.0) |
| | Severe | 8 (32.0) |
| Body involvement percentage* | 18.72 ± 16.49 | |
| DLQI* | 6.60 ± 3.60 | |
| DLQI score* | 1.72 ± 0.73 | |
| DLQI score dissociation | No efficacy | 1 (4.0) |
| | Low efficacy | 8 (32.0) |
| | Moderate efficacy | 13 (52.0) |
| | Major efficacy | 3 (12.0) |
| | Colossal efficacy | 0 (0) |

*(Mean ± SD).

TABLE 3: Laboratory findings of patient and control groups.

| Parameter | Psoriasis vulgaris | Control | $P$ |
|---|---|---|---|
| Glucose* (mg/dL) | 85.80 ± 11.88 | 84.96 ± 10.94 | $P > 0.05$ |
| Triglycerides* (mg/dL) | 129.52 ± 71.80 | 125.08 ± 90.56 | $P > 0.05$ |
| LDL-cholesterol* (mg/dL) | 112.75 ± 33.77 | 103.02 ± 34.88 | $P > 0.05$ |
| HDL-cholesterol* (mg/dL) | 44.48 ± 13.47 | 47.48 ± 13.26 | $P > 0.05$ |
| Total cholesterol* (mg/dL) | 182.64 ± 37.29 | 179.92 ± 26.87 | $P > 0.05$ |
| Insulin* ($\mu$IU/mL) | 4.79 ± 3.46 | 8.56 ± 4.33 | **$P = 0.002$** |
| C-peptide* (ng/mL) | 1.95 ± 0.73 | 1.88 ± 0.66 | $P > 0.05$ |
| HOMA-IR values* | 0.99 ± 0.70 | 1.80 ± 0.97 | **$P = 0.001$** |
| Ghrelin* (pg/mL) | 45.41 ± 22.41 | 29.92 ± 14.65 | **$P = 0.01$** |

*(Mean ± SD).

the differences among these groups were not statistically significant ($P > 0.05$).

The mean serum ghrelin level was 45.41 ± 22.41 in the psoriasis group and 29.92 ± 14.65 in the healthy control group, and this difference was significant ($P = 0.01$) (Table 3, Figure 1).

Mean serum insulin level and HOMA-IR index in the psoriasis group (4.79 ± 3.46 and 0.99 ± 0.70, resp.) were significantly lower than those in the healthy controls (8.56 ± 4.33 and 1.80 ± 0.97, resp.) ($P = 0.002$ and $P = 0.001$, resp.) (Table 3, Figure 1). Insulin resistance was observed in two patients in the psoriasis group (8.0%) and four subjects in the control group (16.0%). As the number of patients with insulin resistance was low, it was not possible to statistically

compare the ghrelin levels of the subjects with and without insulin resistance. In addition, insulin level showed positive correlations with both C-peptide and HOMA-IR levels ($r = 0.64$, $P < 0.001$; $r = 0.98$, $P < 0.001$, resp.).

Metabolic syndrome was found in 10 (40.0%) psoriasis patients and 9 (36.0%) controls. The mean serum ghrelin level was higher in psoriasis patients with than in those without metabolic syndrome but the difference was not significant (54.21 ± 23.02 and 39.55 ± 20.69, resp.; $P > 0.05$). In addition, mean age and BSA in psoriasis patients with metabolic syndrome (36.20 ± 8.65, 27.62 ± 19.98, resp.) were significantly higher than those in patients without metabolic syndrome (29.60 ± 5.55, 12.78 ± 10.74, resp.) ($P = 0.02$, $P = 0.02$, resp.). In our study 10 psoriasis patients had MetS. 3 patients (30%) had mild psoriasis, 4 patients (40%) has moderate psoriasis, and 3 patients (30%) had severe psoriasis. MetS ratio in patients who had low PASI score was not higher than the other groups.

There were no significant differences in PASI, DLQI, or disease duration between the psoriasis patients with and without metabolic syndrome (all $P > 0.05$). The mean serum ghrelin levels were not significantly different between female and male patients (48.04 ± 23.99 and 42.07 ± 20.85, resp.; $P > 0.05$).

The relation between severity of psoriasis and ghrelin level was examined, and the results indicated that higher PASI score was associated with lower ghrelin level. The ghrelin levels were 62.66 ± 25.00, 37.89 ± 11.35, and 33.53 ± 16.43 in patients with low, moderate, and high PASI scores, respectively. The mean ghrelin level in patients with a lower PASI score was significantly higher than in those with a higher PASI score ($P = 0.02$) (Figure 2).

There was a positive correlation between BMI and DLQI ($r = 0.46$, $P < 0.05$). Therefore, higher BMI negatively affects QOL in patients with psoriasis. Interestingly, there was a negative correlation between PASI and serum ghrelin level ($r = 0.49$, $P < 0.05$).

## 4. Discussion

Metabolic syndrome affects approximately 15–25% of the general population [15, 16]. In addition, recent studies suggested that psoriasis patients may have an increased prevalence of metabolic syndrome. The reported prevalence of metabolic syndrome among patients with psoriasis ranges from 14% to 40% [17]. In the present study, metabolic syndrome was seen in 40% of psoriasis patients, which is consistent with the incidences reported in the literature.

The mechanism underlying the etiology of metabolic syndrome in patients with psoriasis is not fully understood. Some studies have suggested that psoriasis predisposes patients to the development of obesity or hypertension related to stress and reduced physical activity [18]. Therefore, insulin resistance and abdominal obesity are considered to play important roles in the pathogenesis of metabolic syndrome [19, 20]. In addition, Sommer et al. [21] found significant associations between psoriasis and type II DM, hypertension, hyperlipidemia, and coronary artery disease in a study of

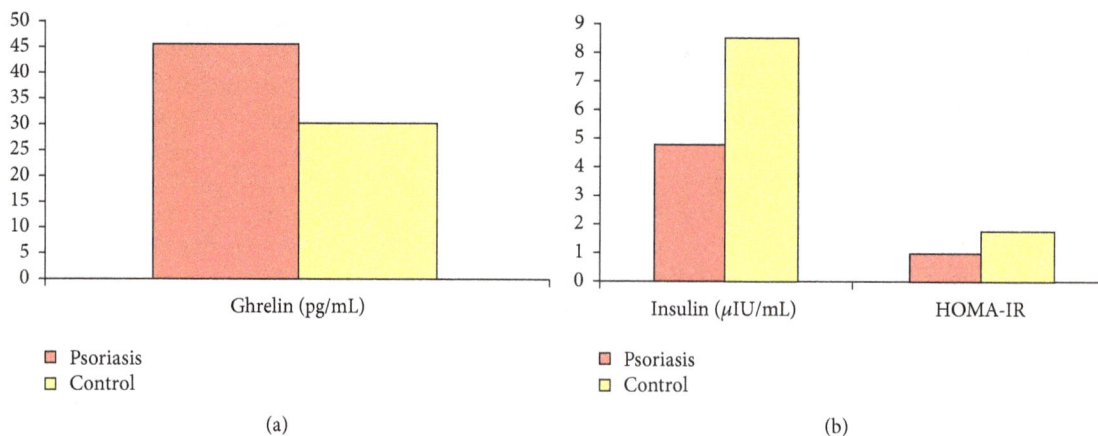

FIGURE 1: Serum ghrelin, insulin, and HOMA-IR levels.

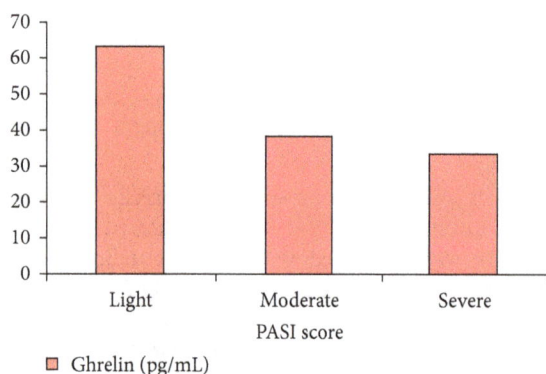

FIGURE 2: Serum ghrelin levels according to PASI score.

581 patients. In the present study, we found no differences between psoriasis patients and controls with regard to fasting blood glucose, triglyceride, cholesterol, HDL, LDL, or VLDL levels. In addition, Naldi et al. [22] reported an association between BMI and psoriasis, and found a higher risk of psoriasis in the obese population. However, we found no differences in BMI or waist circumference among groups in the present study. These discrepancies between the present and previous studies may have been related to the similarity in BMI between patients and controls in our study.

There is controversy in the literature about the relationship between metabolic syndrome and severity of psoriasis. Sommer et al. [21] reported a positive correlation between metabolic syndrome and severity of the disease, while Gisondi et al. [23] reported no such correlation. We did not find a positive correlation between PASI and metabolic syndrome in the present study, but BSA was positively correlated with metabolic syndrome in our subjects.

A few studies have indicated relationships between elevated levels of inflammatory mediators, such as IL-6, TNF-$\alpha$, and C-reactive protein levels, and metabolic syndrome [24]. In addition, psoriasis is a chronic inflammatory skin disorder characterized by a variety of immunological and inflammatory changes. Therefore, the link between psoriasis and metabolic syndrome may be related to the effects of chronic inflammatory changes and the secretion of proinflammatory cytokines [25].

Ghrelin is produced predominantly by the stomach, but is also expressed in other tissues, such as the hypothalamus, pituitary gland, intestine, pancreas, kidney, placenta, testes, ovary, and lymphocytes [26]. There has been only one previous study regarding ghrelin levels in patients with psoriasis. Özdemir et al. [27] reported that the ghrelin level was higher in psoriasis patients than in controls, but the difference was not statistically significant. In the present study, ghrelin levels were significantly higher in psoriasis patients compared to controls. In addition, the levels of insulin and HOMA-IR were significantly lower in patients than in controls. These observations may be related to possible effects of ghrelin on insulin homeostasis. In addition, we found higher levels of ghrelin in psoriasis patients with than without metabolic syndrome, although the difference was not significant. This finding may have been related to the presence of many factors that affect ghrelin levels in psoriasis and metabolic syndrome.

Özdemir et al. [27] reported a negative correlation between ghrelin level and the severity of psoriasis. Interestingly, we also found a negative correlation between ghrelin level and PASI score. Some studies indicated that ghrelin has potent inhibitory effects on the mRNA and protein expression levels of proinflammatory cytokines, such as IL-6 and TNF-$\alpha$ [28], which are important in the pathogenesis of psoriasis. In addition, Xia et al. [29] reported that ghrelin inhibits proliferation of anti-CD3-activated murine T cells and nonspecifically inhibits both Th1 (IL-1 and INF-$\gamma$) and Th2 (IL-4 and IL-10) cytokines. Arican et al. [30] reported positive correlations between the severity of psoriasis and serum TNF-$\alpha$, IL-6, and IL-8 levels. This correlation may have been responsible for the negative correlation between PASI score and ghrelin levels observed in the present study.

This study had some limitations, such as the small number of patients. In addition, serum levels of ghrelin may be affected by various endogenous and exogenous factors, such as diet and decreased physical activity, which could not be compared in our study. Moreover, we could not study immunological parameters associated with metabolic syndrome and psoriasis that may have been affected by ghrelin.

## 5. Conclusions

The pathogenesis of psoriasis and presence of metabolic syndrome in psoriasis are not fully understood. Recent studies discussed the relations between serum ghrelin levels and both metabolic syndrome and psoriasis. The present study was performed to determine the effects of ghrelin in psoriasis patients. We found a negative correlation between severity of psoriasis and ghrelin level. In addition, we found correlations between ghrelin levels and some metabolic changes. Larger and especially experimental studies focusing on the correlations between the immune system, ghrelin levels, and severity of psoriasis may be valuable to clarify the etiopathogenesis of the disease and to improve treatment alternatives in patients with psoriasis.

## Disclosure

The English in this document has been checked by at least two professional editors, both native speakers of English. For a certificate, please see, http://www.textcheck.com/certificate/XNwBiR.

## Conflict of Interests

Authors have no financial interest with regard to the paper.

## References

[1] J. M. Gelfand, R. Weinstein, S. B. Porter, A. L. Neimann, J. A. Berlin, and D. J. Margolis, "Prevalence and treatment of psoriasis in the United Kingdom: a population-based study," *Archives of Dermatology*, vol. 141, no. 12, pp. 1537–1541, 2005.

[2] M. P. Schon and W. H. Boehncke, "Psoriasis," *The New England Journal of Medicine*, vol. 352, pp. 1899–1912, 2005.

[3] T. Henseler and E. Christophers, "Disease concomitance in psoriasis," *Journal of the American Academy of Dermatology*, vol. 32, no. 6, pp. 982–986, 1995.

[4] D. M. Sommer, S. Jenisch, M. Suchan, E. Christophers, and M. Weichenthal, "Increased prevalence of the metabolic syndrome in patients with moderate to severe psoriasis," *Archives of Dermatological Research*, vol. 298, no. 7, pp. 321–328, 2006.

[5] I. Zindanci, O. Albayrak, M. Kavala et al., "Prevalence of metabolic syndrome in patients with psoriasis," *The Scientific World Journal*, vol. 2012, Article ID 312463, 5 pages, 2012.

[6] A. Gerkowicz, A. Pietrzak, J. C. Szepietowski, S. Radej, and G. Chodorowska, "Biochemical markers of psoriasis as a metabolic disease," *Folia Histochemica et Cytobiologica*, vol. 50, no. 2, pp. 155–170, 2012.

[7] M. Kojima, H. Hosoda, Y. Date, M. Nakazato, H. Matsuo, and K. Kangawa, "Ghrelin is a growth-hormone-releasing acylated peptide from stomach," *Nature*, vol. 402, no. 6762, pp. 656–660, 1999.

[8] M. Nakazato, N. Murakami, Y. Date et al., "A role for ghrelin in the central regulation of feeding," *Nature*, vol. 409, no. 6817, pp. 194–198, 2001.

[9] V. D. Dixit, E. M. Schaffer, R. S. Pyle et al., "Ghrelin inhibits leptin- and activation-induced proinflammatory cytokine expression by human monocytes and T cells," *The Journal of Clinical Investigation*, vol. 114, no. 1, pp. 57–66, 2004.

[10] T. Fredriksson and U. Pettersson, "Severe psoriasis—oral therapy with a new retinoid," *Dermatologica*, vol. 157, no. 4, pp. 238–244, 1978.

[11] T. Henseler and K. Schmitt-Rau, "A comparison between BSA, PASI, PLASI and SAPASI as measures of disease severity and improvement by therapy in patients with psoriasis," *International Journal of Dermatology*, vol. 47, no. 10, pp. 1019–1023, 2008.

[12] S. Öztürkcan, A. T. Ermertcan, E. Eser, and M. Turhan Şahin, "Cross validation of the Turkish version of dermatology life quality index," *International Journal of Dermatology*, vol. 45, no. 11, pp. 1300–1307, 2006.

[13] P. I. Sidiropoulos, S. A. Karvounaris, and D. T. Boumpas, "Metabolic syndrome in rheumatic diseases: epidemiology, pathophysiology, and clinical implications," *Arthritis Research and Therapy*, vol. 10, article 207, 2008.

[14] N. Kondo, M. Nomura, Y. Nakaya, S. Ito, and T. Ohguro, "Association of inflammatory marker and highly sensitive C-reactive protein with aerobic exercise capacity, maximum oxygen uptake and insulin resistance in healthy middle-aged volunteers," *Circulation Journal*, vol. 69, no. 4, pp. 452–457, 2005.

[15] E. S. Ford, W. H. Giles, and W. H. Dietz, "Prevalence of the metabolic syndrome among US adults: findings from the Third National Health and Nutrition Examination Survey," *The Journal of the American Medical Association*, vol. 287, no. 3, pp. 356–359, 2002.

[16] G. Hu, Q. Qiao, J. Tuomilehto, B. Balkau, K. Borch-Johnsen, and K. Pyorala, "Prevalence of the metabolic syndrome and its relation to all-cause and cardiovascular mortality in nondiabetic European men and women," *Archives of Internal Medicine*, vol. 164, no. 10, pp. 1066–1076, 2004.

[17] A. W. Armstrong, C. T. Harskamp, and E. J. Armstrong, "Psoriasis and metabolic syndrome: a systematic review and meta-analysis of observational studies," *Journal of the American Academy of Dermatology*, vol. 68, no. 4, pp. 654–662, 2013.

[18] A. L. Neimann, D. B. Shin, X. Wang, D. J. Margolis, A. B. Troxel, and J. M. Gelfand, "Prevalence of cardiovascular risk factors in patients with psoriasis," *Journal of the American Academy of Dermatology*, vol. 55, no. 5, pp. 829–835, 2006.

[19] R. H. Eckel, S. M. Grundy, and P. Z. Zimmet, "The metabolic syndrome," *The Lancet*, vol. 365, no. 9468, pp. 1415–1428, 2005.

[20] The IDF consensus worldwide definition of the metabolic syndrome, 2011, http://www.idf.org/webdata/docs/MetSyndrome_FINAL.pdf.

[21] D. M. Sommer, S. Jenisch, M. Suchan, E. Christophers, and M. Weichenthal, "Increased prevalence of the metabolic syndrome in patients with moderate to severe psoriasis," *Archives of Dermatological Research*, vol. 298, no. 7, pp. 321–328, 2006.

[22] L. Naldi, L. Chatenoud, D. Linder et al., "Cigarette smoking, body mass index, and stressful life events as risk factors for psoriasis: results from an Italian case-control study," *Journal of Investigative Dermatology*, vol. 125, no. 1, pp. 61–67, 2005.

[23] P. Gisondi, G. Tessari, A. Conti et al., "Prevalence of metabolic syndrome in patients with psoriasis: a hospital-based case-control study," *British Journal of Dermatology*, vol. 157, no. 1, pp. 68–73, 2007.

[24] J. S. Yudkin, C. D. A. Stehouwer, J. J. Emeis, and S. W. Coppack, "C-reactive protein in healthy subjects: associations

with obesity, insulin resistance, and endothelial dysfunction: a potential role for cytokines originating from adipose tissue?" *Arteriosclerosis, Thrombosis, and Vascular Biology*, vol. 19, no. 4, pp. 972–978, 1999.

[25] H. Nakajima, K. Nakajima, M. Tarutani, and S. Sano, "The role of pigment epithelium-derived factor as an adipokine in psoriasis," *Archives of Dermatological Research*, vol. 304, no. 1, pp. 81–84, 2012.

[26] S. Ghelardoni, V. Carnicelli, S. Frascarelli, S. Ronca-Testoni, and R. Zucchi, "Ghrelin tissue distribution: comparison between gene and protein expression," *Journal of Endocrinological Investigation*, vol. 29, no. 2, pp. 115–121, 2006.

[27] M. Özdemir, M. Yüksel, H. Gökbel, N. Okudan, and I. Mevlitoğlu, "Serum leptin, adiponectin, resistin and ghrelin levels in psoriatic patients treated with cyclosporin," *Journal of Dermatology*, vol. 39, no. 5, pp. 443–448, 2012.

[28] V. D. Dixit, E. M. Schaffer, R. S. Pyle et al., "Ghrelin inhibits leptin- and activation-induced proinflammatory cytokine expression by human monocytes and T cells," *The Journal of Clinical Investigation*, vol. 114, no. 1, pp. 57–66, 2004.

[29] Q. Xia, W. Pang, H. Pan, Y. Zheng, J.-S. Kang, and S.-G. Zhu, "Effects of ghrelin on the proliferation and secretion of splenic T lymphocytes in mice," *Regulatory Peptides*, vol. 122, no. 3, pp. 173–178, 2004.

[30] O. Arican, M. Aral, S. Sasmaz, and P. Ciragil, "Serum levels of TNF-$\alpha$, IFN-$\gamma$, IL-6, IL-8, IL-12, IL-17, and IL-18 in patients with active psoriasis and correlation with disease severity," *Mediators of Inflammation*, vol. 2005, no. 5, pp. 273–279, 2005.

# 17

# Narrow-Band Ultraviolet B versus Oral Minocycline in Treatment of Unstable Vitiligo: A Prospective Comparative Trial

**Amir Hossein Siadat,[1] Naser Zeinali,[1] Fariba Iraji,[1] Bahareh Abtahi-Naeini,[2] Mohammad Ali Nilforoushzadeh,[3] Kioumars Jamshidi,[1] and Parastoo Khosravani[1]**

[1] *Department of Dermatology, Skin Diseases and Leishmaniasis Research Center, Isfahan University of Medical Sciences, Isfahan, Iran*
[2] *Department of Dermatology, Skin Diseases and Leishmaniasis Research Center, Students' Research Committee, Isfahan University of Medical Sciences, Isfahan, Iran*
[3] *Skin and Stem Cell Research Center, Tehran University of Medical Sciences, Tehran, Iran*

Correspondence should be addressed to Naser Zeinali; pr.zeinali@yahoo.com

Academic Editor: Desmond Tobin

*Background.* We have compared NB-UVB and oral minocycline in stabilizing vitiligo for the first time. *Subjects and Methods.* 42 patients were divided equally into two groups: the NB-UVB and minocycline groups. Phototherapy was administered twice a week on nonconsecutive days. In the minocycline group, patients were advised to take minocycline 100 mg once daily. The treatment period was 3 months. Vitiligo disease activity (VIDA) score was noted every 4 weeks for 12 months. Digital photographs were taken at baseline and monthly intervals. *Results.* Before the therapy, disease activity was present in 100% of the patients, which was reduced to 23.8% and 66.1% by the end of therapy in the NB-UVB and minocycline groups retrospectively ($P < 0.05$). 16 of the 21 (76/1%) patients with unstable disease in the NB-UVB group achieved stability, whereas this was the case for only 7 of the 21 (33.3%) in the minocycline group ($P < 0.001$). The diameter changes were statistically significant at the end of treatment in the NB-UVB group compared to the minocycline group ($P = 0.031$). Side effects in both groups were mild. *Conclusion.* NB-UVB was statistically more advantageous than oral minocycline in unstable vitiligo in terms of efficacy and the resulting stability.

## 1. Introduction

Vitiligo is an acquired cutaneous disorder of pigmentation, manifested by the selective destruction of melanocytes in the skin, with a 1% to 2% incidence worldwide, without predilection for sex or race [1, 2]. There are some major hypotheses for the pathogenesis of vitiligo; the convergence theory is one. This theory states that stress, accumulation of toxic compounds, infection, autoimmunity, mutations, altered cellular environment, and impaired melanocyte migration and proliferation can all contribute in varying proportions to the etiopathogenesis of the disease [3]. High $H_2O_2$ level has been suggested to be responsible for the disappearance of melanocytes in vitiligo. Minocycline, an antibiotic possessing antioxidant activity, is capable of attenuating oxidative stress-induced neurotoxicity [2]. Song et al. showed that $H_2O_2$ decreases cell viability in a concentration-dependent manner

which is attenuated by minocycline [2]. They suggest that minocycline may be used to prevent melanocyte loss in the early stage of vitiligo [2]. Since a causative treatment is not available, current treatment modalities are directed towards stopping the progression of vitiligo and achieving repigmentation in order to repair the morphology and functional deficiencies of the depigmented skin areas [4, 5]. The concept of stability in vitiligo is multifaceted, and no consensus has yet been reached on defining the criteria for this so far. An objective criterion, the vitiligo disease activity score (VIDA), was suggested by Njoo et al. in 1999 to follow the course of lesions. It is a 6-point scale on which the activity of the disease is evaluated by appearance of new vitiligo lesions or enlargement of preexisting lesions gauged during a period ranging from <6 weeks to 1 year [6] (Table 1).

Recently, minocycline has been proposed as an alternative therapy for unstable vitiligo [7]. But minocycline should

Table 1: Vitiligo disease activity score (VIDA): 6-point score for activity evaluation of unstable vitiligo [6].

| Disease activity | VIDA score |
|---|---|
| Active in past 6 weeks | +4 |
| Active in past 3 months | +3 |
| Active in past 6 months | +2 |
| Active in past 1 year | +1 |
| Stable for at least 1 year | 0 |
| Stable for at least 1 year and spontaneous repigmentation | −1 |

be used with caution. Some of side effects of minocycline include light-headedness and vertigo, lack of concentration, gastrointestinal disturbance, increase of intracranial pressure, and unwanted skin and mucosal hyperpigmentation which should be considered before administration [2, 7]. To the best of our knowledge, this is the first instance of clinical evidence that compares the effectiveness of oral minocycline and NB-UVB in the treatment of unstable vitiligo.

## 2. Patients and Methods

A randomized clinical trial was done on patients with clinically diagnosed vitiligo vulgaris. The study included 42 consecutive patients of unstable vitiligo attending the clinic of Al-Zahra Hospital, a referral clinic of dermatology in Isfahan, Iran. The unstable vitiligo was defined as score 1–4 in vitiligo disease activity (VIDA) score [8].

Also the stability was defined as score 0, −1 in VIDA score. The patients were randomly, using a table of random numbers, allocated to one of two groups (NB-UVB or minocycline); 21 patients were thus allocated to each group. Reasons for exclusion were age ≤ 8 years or ≥50 years; pregnancy or intention to become pregnant; breastfeeding; other severe systemic diseases, for example, cardiovascular, renal, and hepatic failure; segmental vitiligo; acral vitiligo, taking any other vitiligo treatment within the previous 3 months; history of having taken any medication that could interact with minocycline (e.g., isotretinoin, oral contraceptive pills, etc.) within the previous 3 months; history of photomediated disorders such as systemic lupus erythematous and xeroderma pigmentosum (XP) and known hypersensitivity to the study medication. All patients provided written consent of informed participation beforehand.

### 2.1. Group A: The NB-UVB Group.

All patients were treated with NB-UVB as monotherapy (V care UV therapy unit, Surya 440 ANB comprising Phillips Holland lamps with emission spectrum 311 nm, irradiance 1800–2000 $\mu W/cm^2$, calibrated twice yearly). Phototherapy was given twice a week on nonconsecutive days. Initial phototesting was not done. An initial dose of 0.25–0.75 J/cm$^2$ was administered to all patients in the group. Standard photoprotection protocol for NB-UVB was observed. The optimal constant dose was achieved when minimal erythema appeared in the lesions. Otherwise, dose increment was carried out at the rate of

20% amount of the previous week. The phototherapy was continued until 100% repigmentation was achieved, or the treatment period was complete, whichever occurred earlier.

### 2.2. Group B: The Oral Minocycline Group.

Patients were advised to take minocycline hydrochloride (MINOCIN) 100 mg once daily until 100% repigmentation was achieved or the 3-month treatment period was complete, whichever occurred earlier. During the study period, no other therapy was prescribed.

### 2.3. Procedures.

In response to the treatment, using VIDA score, a 6-point score for activity evaluation of unstable vitiligo (Table 1) [8] was evaluated by observing the appearance of new lesions or any increase in the size of existing ones; repigmentation of existing lesions was also noted.

The treatment period was 3 months. During the study, the point of time at which stability was achieved was noted. Stability refers to no new and no increase in size of existing lesions for at least 3 months. On each visit, repigmentation was assessed and graded in the topographical area as follows. The patients were assessed every week 4 for 12 months by a blinded dermatologist. Baseline VIDA score was calculated, and disease activity was noted on each visit as follows.

### 2.4. Statistical Analysis.

Statistical evaluation was done using SPSS for Windows version 16.0 (SPSS Inc., II, USA). Data were shown as frequency (percentage) or mean ± standard deviation (SD). The results of the study were analyzed by using "$t$-test," $\chi^2$-test of proportions.

## 3. Results

A total of 42 patients (24 females and 18 males) (range 15–44) in NB-UBV group (27.6 ± 9.4 years) and in minocycline group (25.4 ± 10.3 years, $P > 0.05$) were included in this study during a one-year period. All patients completed the study. The basic patient data and clinical characteristics of each group are summarized in Table 2.

All patients had stopped any method of therapy at least 3 months before entering the study, the NB-UVB group (21 patients), and the oral minocycline group (21 patients). Comparison of the demographic and disease parameters in the two groups showed no statistically significant difference in any of the variables ($P > 0.05$). 16 of the 21 (76/1%) patients with unstable disease in the NB-UVB group achieved stability (VIDA score 0, −1), whereas this was only 7 of the 21 (33.3%) patients in the minocycline group ($P < 0.001$) (Table 3).

In our study disease stabilization is more frequent in the NB-UVB group compared with the minocycline group ($P = 0.019$). There were patches of unstable vitiligo in all patients in both groups before the initiation of the study ($P > 0.05$). VIDA 3 or 4 (new lesions 3 months before) was seen in 11 of the 21 (52.3%) and 9 of the 21 (42.8%) patients in the NB-UVB and oral minocycline groups, respectively ($P > 0.05$). At the end of the therapy, activity was present in 5 (23.9%) and 13 patients (66.1%) in the NB-UVB and oral minocycline groups, respectively ($P = 0.019$). The difference

TABLE 2: Demographics and disease parameters of the 42 patients.

|  | NB-UVB | Minocycline |
|---|---|---|
| Number of patients | 21 | 21 |
| Age in years (mean ± SD) | 27.6 ± 9.4 | 25.4 ± 10.3 |
| Sex (male/female) | 8/13 | 10/11 |
| Duration of disease before commencing therapy in years (mean ± SD) | 15.13 ± 6.30 | 9.76 ± 3.84 |
| Positive family history ($n$) | 2 | 4 |
| Skin type |  |  |
| Type 3 (%) | 16 (76.19%) | 18 (85.71%) |
| Type 4 (%) | 5 (23.81%) | 3 (14.29%) |
| Mean body surface involved (mean ± SD) | 30.5 ± 10.5 | 35.5 ± 11.5 |
| Anatomical |  |  |
| Head and neck | 9 | 12 |
| Trunk | 13 | 7 |
| Upper limb (proximal) | 6 | 4 |
| Upper limb (distal) | 8 | 6 |
| Lower limb (proximal) | 5 | 6 |
| Lower limb (distal) | 4 | 3 |

TABLE 3: Stability achieved by using NB-UVB and minocycline in each group.

| VIDA score | Beginning of therapy NB-UVB group | End of therapy NB-UVB group | Beginning of therapy Minocycline group | End of therapy Minocycline group |
|---|---|---|---|---|
| +4 | 6 | 0 | 4 | 2 |
| +3 | 5 | 0 | 5 | 5 |
| +2 | 4 | 3 | 6 | 4 |
| +1 | 6 | 2 | 6 | 3 |
| 0 | 0 | 10 | 0 | 3 |
| −1 | 0 | 6 | 0 | 4 |

in the percentage of patients showing activity at the start and end of therapy was statistically significant in both groups ($P = 0.027$). Of the five patients in the NB-UVB group with activity at the end of the study, three were initially unstable, whereas the remaining two were stable. The total mean size of the lesions in the NB-UVB group and the minocycline group changed from 25.68 cm$^2$ to 14.20 cm$^2$ and from 25.12 cm$^2$ to 20.82 cm$^2$, respectively. The difference in diameter changes was statistically significant at the end of treatment in the NB-UVB group compared to the minocycline group ($P = 0.031$). NB-UVB was generally well tolerated and adverse reactions were erythema and pruritus. Side effects were reported by 3 (14.2%) of the minocycline users. These included oral mucosal pigmentation, gastrointestinal complaint, and headache. All of these side effects were mild or moderately severe and no patient left the study due to side effects.

## 4. Discussion

In our study it was shown that, regarding NB-UVB versus oral minocycline in terms of stability, the former was more statistically advantageous with respect to the stability achieved in unstable vitiligo when assessed by the VIDA score. Most

studies on the clinical aspects of stability in vitiligo have not been able to establish cut-off values that could be helpful in classifying the disease as active or stable in a patient. In this study, we use an objective measure: the VIDA score.

In the previous study by Parsad and Kanwar it has been suggested that oral minocycline was a new effective drug in the treatment of unstable vitiligo. They evaluated the efficacy of minocycline 100 mg once daily in 32 patients. They showed an arrest in the progression of disease in 29/32 patients and only three patients showed development of new lesions and/or enlargement of existing lesions. Ten patients showed arrest of depigmentation after 4 weeks of treatment. Seven patients showed moderate to marked repigmentation [7].

Recently Singh et al. performed a randomized controlled study to evaluate the effectiveness of dexamethasone oral minipulse (OMP) therapy versus oral minocycline in patients with active vitiligo vulgaris. They observed that, of the 25 patients in minocycline group, only 6 (24%) patients developed new lesions during 24 weeks of follow-up period, whereas in OMP group only 3 (12%) patients showed activity of disease [9]. These results in minocycline group were comparable to those observed in previous study by Parsad and Kanwar.

Our result shows that although the minocycline can have a role as a treatment for unstable vitiligo NB-UVB was more statistically advantageous.

NB-UVB therapy has emerged as one of the most effective treatment options in vitiligo over the last decade. A number of clinical studies have been conducted all over the world and all of these studies have documented a positive effect of narrow-band UVB therapy in vitiligo [6, 10, 11].

How narrow-band UVB therapy helps in vitiligo is not known with certainty but it has been postulated that NB-UVB acts in two different steps in vitiligo treatment. The first step is the stabilization of the depigmenting process and the second is the stimulation of residual follicular melanocytes [12, 13]. The stabilization of the depigmenting process is explained by the immunomodulatory effect of NB-UVB on the local and systemic immune responses [13, 14].

The limitations of the study include lack of blinding due to the nature of phototherapy, small sample size, and short treatment period. In summary, although the previous study of Parsad and Kanwar regarding treatment of unstable vitiligo by oral minocycline makes sense, the comparison of oral minocycline and NB-UVB in our study showed that the effect of oral minocycline is only attributable to the sunscreen effect and not quantitatively significant.

## 5. Conclusion

The results of our study reiterate the fact that minocycline is an effective and safe drug to control the activity of vitiligo but NB-UVB is more effective in reaching the activity of vitiligo comparable to oral minocycline. To the best of our knowledge, our study is the first to compare the efficacy and tolerability of oral minocycline with narrow-band ultraviolet B (NB-UVB) corticosteroids. In future studies, a comparison between minocycline and other modalities in the treatment of both stable and unstable vitiligo should be used to better compare treatment outcomes. In addition clarifying the exact mechanism of minocycline action in cellular biology is an issue that helps us design more accurate models of study.

## Conflict of Interests

The authors declare that there is no conflict of interests regarding the publication of this paper.

## References

[1] S. Moretti, L. Amato, S. Bellandi, and P. Fabbri, "Focus on vitiligo: a generalized skin disorder," *European Journal of Inflammation*, vol. 4, no. 1, pp. 21–30, 2006.

[2] X. Song, A. Xu, W. Pan et al., "Minocycline protects melanocytes against $H_2O_2$-induced cell death via JNK and p38 MAPK pathways," *International Journal of Molecular Medicine*, vol. 22, no. 1, pp. 9–16, 2008.

[3] I. C. le Poole, P. K. das, R. M. J. G. J. van den Wijngaard, J. D. Bos, and W. Westerhof, "Review of the etiopathomechanism of vitiligo: a convergence theory," *Experimental Dermatology*, vol. 2, no. 4, pp. 145–153, 1993.

[4] M. D. Njoo, P. I. Spuls, J. D. Bos, W. Westerhof, and P. M. M. Bossuyt, "Nonsurgical repigmentation therapies in vitiligo: meta-analysis of the literature," *Archives of Dermatology*, vol. 134, no. 12, pp. 1532–1540, 1998.

[5] R. M. Bacigalupi, A. Postolova, and R. S. Davis, "Evidence-based, non-surgical treatments for vitiligo: a review," *The American Journal of Clinical Dermatology*, vol. 13, no. 4, pp. 217–237, 2012.

[6] A. Bhatnagar, A. J. Kanwar, D. Parsad, and D. De, "Psoralen and ultraviolet A and narrow-band ultraviolet B in inducing stability in vitiligo, assessed by vitiligo disease activity score: an open prospective comparative study," *Journal of the European Academy of Dermatology and Venereology*, vol. 21, no. 10, pp. 1381–1385, 2007.

[7] D. Parsad and A. Kanwar, "Oral minocycline in the treatment of vitiligo: a preliminary study," *Dermatologic Therapy*, vol. 23, no. 3, pp. 305–307, 2010.

[8] M. D. Njoo, P. K. Das, J. D. Bos, and W. Westerhof, "Association of the Kobner phenomenon with disease activity and therapeutic responsiveness in vitiligo vulgaris," *Archives of Dermatology*, vol. 135, no. 4, pp. 407–413, 1999.

[9] A. Singh, A. J. Kanwar, D. Parsad, and R. Mahajan, "Randomized controlled study to evaluate the effectiveness of dexamethasone oral minipulse therapy versus oral minocycline in patients with active vitiligo vulgaris," *Indian Journal of Dermatology, Venereology and Leprology*, vol. 80, no. 1, pp. 29–35, 2014.

[10] A. C. Borderé, J. Lambert, and N. van Geel, "Current and emerging therapy for the management of vitiligo," *Clinical, Cosmetic and Investigational Dermatology*, vol. 2, pp. 15–25, 2009.

[11] S. Bansal, B. Sahoo, and V. Garg, "Psoralen-narrowband UVB phototherapy in treatment of vitiligo in comparison to narrowband UVB phototherapy," *Photodermatol Photoimmunol Photomed*, vol. 29, no. 6, pp. 311–317, 2013.

[12] I. Hamzavi, H. Jain, D. McLean, J. Shapiro, H. Zeng, and H. Lui, "Parametric modeling of narrowband UV-B phototherapy for vitiligo, using a novel quantitative tool: the vitiligo area scoring index," *Archives of Dermatology*, vol. 140, no. 6, pp. 677–683, 2004.

[13] J. Cui, L. Y. Shen, and G. C. Wang, "Role of hair follicles in the repigmentation of vitiligo," *Journal of Investigative Dermatology*, vol. 97, no. 3, pp. 410–416, 1991.

[14] T. B. Fitzpatrick, "Mechanisms of phototherapy of vitiligo," *Archives of Dermatology*, vol. 133, no. 12, pp. 1591–1592, 1997.

# 18

# Newer Hemostatic Agents Used in the Practice of Dermatologic Surgery

## Jill Henley[1] and Jerry D. Brewer[2]

[1] College of Osteopathic Medicine Glendale, Midwestern University, 13989 N59th Avenue, Glendale, AZ 85308, USA
[2] Division of Dermatologic Surgery, Department of Dermatology Mayo Clinic, Mayo Clinic College of Medicine Rochester, 200 First Street SW, Rochester, MN 55905, USA

Correspondence should be addressed to Jerry D. Brewer; brewer.jerry@mayo.edu

Academic Editor: Giuseppe Argenziano

Minor postoperative bleeding is the most common complication of cutaneous surgery. Because of the commonality of this complication, hemostasis is an important concept to address when considering dermatologic procedures. Patients that have a bleeding diathesis, an inherited/acquired coagulopathy, or who are on anticoagulant/antiplatelet medications pose a greater risk for bleeding complications during the postoperative period. Knowledge of these conditions preoperatively is of the utmost importance, allowing for proper preparation and prevention. Also, it is important to be aware of the various hemostatic modalities available, including electrocoagulation, which is among the most effective and widely used techniques. Prompt recognition of hematoma formation and knowledge of postoperative wound care can prevent further complications such as wound dehiscence, infection, or skin-graft necrosis, minimizing poor outcomes.

## 1. Introduction

Dermatologists are estimated to perform over 3.9 million procedures each year [1]. Although the risks and complications of dermatologic surgery are generally very low, even the most talented surgeon can experience complications related to hemostasis during both the intraoperative and postoperative periods. Minor bleeding complications are the most frequently encountered complications of cutaneous surgery, which can predispose the patient to hematoma formation, increased risk of infection, skin graft necrosis, and wound dehiscence. This chapter will highlight proper hemostasis technique to prevent complications.

## 2. Overview of Hemostasis

By understanding the mechanism behind the physiologic clotting system, it is easier to understand how the different hemostatic agents work in the body. The body's primary response to injury is reflex vasoconstriction of the blood vessels in the surrounding tissues, followed by formation of the platelet plug and activation of the fibrinolytic clotting cascade. There are two separate pathways of the fibrinolytic clotting system, that lead to the final common pathway and formation of the insoluble fibrin clot. Function of the body's hemostatic system can be monitored by various laboratory tests. These tests can be helpful to assess the degree of anticoagulation in patients on antiplatelet and anticoagulant medications or who have inherited coagulopathies before proceeding with dermatologic procedures (see Table 1).

## 3. Preoperative Evaluation

One of the most important steps that the dermatologist can take to prevent bleeding complications is to gain a thorough preoperative history of the patient before performing any kind of dermatologic procedure. This allows the physician to gain a better understanding of the patient's overall health and should include a detailed history of the patient's comorbidities, prior surgeries including complications, current medications, social history, and family history, which can help reveal any potential bleeding diatheses.

TABLE 1: Overview of hemostasis.

| Stages of hemostasis | Physiology | Monitoring |
|---|---|---|
| Primary hemostasis | | |
| Formation of the platelet plug | Platelets first adhere to the exposed collagen and von Willebrand's factor on the subendothelium. Then, circulating stimuli activate the platelets, causing shape changes in the platelets [2]. Upon activation, platelet receptors get transferred to the surface, allowing for platelet aggregation. Platelets then release granules that stimulate further platelet aggregation and vasoconstriction [2, 3]. | BT, PFA-100 analysis |
| Secondary hemostasis | | |
| Intrinsic pathway | Plasma proteins get activated in contact with negatively charged surfaces, leading to activation of factor XII and other clotting factors, ultimately leading to the final common pathway and formation of the fibrin clot [4]. | aPTT |
| Extrinsic pathway | Damaged endothelium exposes tissue factor, activating the extrinsic pathway, leading to thrombin production, and activation of other clotting factors, ultimately leading to the final common pathway and formation of the fibrin clot [2, 4]. | PT |
| Final common pathway | Both pathways lead to activation of factor X, which converts prothrombin into thrombin. Thrombin leads to formation of the insoluble fibrin clot, by converting fibrinogen into fibrin [5]. The clot is then stabilized by factor XIII [6]. | |

Abbreviations: ADP: adenosine diphosphate, aPTT: activated partial thromboplastin time, BT: bleeding time, PFA-100 analysis: platelet function analysis, PT: prothrombin time, and $TX_{A_2}$: thromboxane $A_2$.

Specifically, questions regarding comorbid illnesses that can lead to coagulopathies, such as chronic renal and liver disease, hematologic disorders, and malignancies, should be asked, in addition to prior diagnoses of inherited bleeding disorders such as von Willebrand's disease and hemophilia [7]. Many mild forms of bleeding disorders go undiagnosed until later in life and should be investigated by thorough questioning of bleeding complications in prior minor surgical procedures (dental/oral surgery), prolonged episodes of epistaxis, menorrhagia, bruising, history of prior blood transfusions, and any family history of bleeding disorders. On physical exam, it is important to look for any indications of hemostatic abnormalities such as increased bruising or petechiae. For more details on how to manage a patient with a bleeding disorder, please see the section titled, "Approach to the Patient with a Bleeding Disorder." It is also important to investigate the patient's cardiac history including the presence of a pacemaker or implantable cardiac defibrillator (estimated that 4% of Mohs patients are estimated to have one), because the use of certain electrosurgical agents used for hemostatic purposes may be prohibited in these patients [8]. Also, alcohol is a natural anticoagulant, and obtaining information regarding consumption could be beneficial as part of the preoperative evaluation.

## 4. Pharmacologic Agents and Their Effects on Anticoagulation

Many patients that are going to have dermatologic surgery are on anticoagulant and antiplatelet medications. One question many healthcare providers face prior to cutaneous surgery is whether to continue anticoagulation medications prior to surgery. The discrepancy lies between keeping the patient on their current medication regimen, potentially increasing the patient's risk for bleeding complications during the perioperative period, or discontinuing their medication, which has now been proven to increase the patient's risk of life-threatening thromboembolic events during the postoperative period. For a list of some of the most widely used anticoagulant and antiplatelet medications today, including pharmacodynamics of the different medications, and various recommendations regarding usage during the perioperative period see Table 2.

Due to several clinical studies conducted in the past ten years, the general consensus between dermatologic surgeons has been to continue patients on their anticoagulant medications preoperatively, because the benefit of these medications significantly outweighs the risk of bleeding complications during or after procedure [1, 9, 12–18]. The overall risk of hemorrhagic complications in cutaneous surgeries, such as continuous bleeding or hematoma formation in a patient who is not on anticoagulant medications, is very low (1.4%) [18].

In a 2005 nationwide survey of Mohs surgeons, 66% were found to continue Warfarin during the perioperative period [19]. Some studies have shown that there is an increase in minor bleeding complications for patients taking Warfarin chronically, which includes: minor bleeding defined as bleeding less than 24 hours postoperatively, hematoma formation, bleeding that is controlled in the office setting, and bleeding controlled with manual compression [1, 20]. For patients taking Warfarin, checking the international normalized ratio (INR) within 48 hours to one week prior to the surgery can give the surgeon a better idea of the current magnitude of anticoagulation. It is generally recommended that the INR level be within the therapeutic range of 2–3.5 preoperatively [21]. There is a suggestion that the higher the INR level (especially >3.5), the higher the risk for hemorrhagic complications [15]. Because minor bleeding can

TABLE 2: Anticoagulant and antiplatelet medications [9–11].

| Drug | Pharmacodynamics | Indications and monitoring | Discontinuation | Reversal |
|---|---|---|---|---|
| Warfarin | Coumarin inhibits the enzyme epoxide reductase, inhibiting the $\gamma$-carboxylation of Vitamin K-dependent clotting factors: II, VII, IX, X, Protein C, and S [11]. | Indications: acute/chronic venous thromboembolism, pulmonary embolism, atrial fibrillation, prosthetic heart valves. Monitoring: PT and INR. When combined with aspirin, heparin, herbal supplements, or other acquired coagulopathies, can lead to potentiated increase in PT/INR in the patient. Generally recommend a PT/INR level 1 week prior to surgery (2–3.5 range recommended). | Discontinuation not recommended for dermatologic surgery. If patient is at high risk for bleeding during the procedure, consider delaying the surgery until better hemostatic control is obtained. | Reversal generally not needed. If an emergent situation arises, fresh frozen plasma, prothrombin complex concentrates, or recombinant Factor VIIa can be used. Parenteral Vitamin K administration can also be used, but takes longer for effects to be seen. |
| Unfractionated Heparin | Binds to antithrombin III which leads to inactivation of thrombin and Factor Xa. | Indications: DVT, pulmonary embolism, acute arterial occlusion, as a bridge in conjunction with Warfarin until Warfarin levels become therapeutic. Monitoring: aPTT. Check aPTT level 1 week prior to surgery as well as a CBC to check for platelet levels. | Discontinuation not recommended for dermatologic surgery. | Reversal generally not needed. If an emergent situation, 1 mg of protamine sulfate for every 100 units of heparin in vivo can be given. |
| Dabigatran | Direct thrombin inhibitor. | Indications: Atrial fibrillation. Monitoring: Not recommended. | Discontinuation not recommended for dermatologic surgery. | No reversal agent. Control bleeding site, give supportive care. |
| Aspirin | Irreversibly inhibits the cyclooxygenase enzymes, which decreases the levels of $TX_{A_2}$, decreasing platelet aggregation. | Indications: MI, TIA/stroke prevention, CAD, fever, pain, inflammatory diseases (RA), cardiac stent placement. Monitoring: Not recommended, but platelet inhibition can be monitored by bleeding time or PFA-100. | Prophylactic aspirin with no prior history of myocardial infarction or cerebral vascular events should be discontinued 10–14 days prior to procedure due to irreversible effect on platelets and started 1 week postoperatively. ASA used for therapeutic purposes or prophylactically in high risk individuals should be continued. | Reversal generally not needed. |
| Ticlopidine and Clopidogrel | Thienopyridines that irreversibly inhibit adenosine-diphosphate receptors, decreasing platelet aggregation [12]. | Indications: Drug eluding stent, TIA/stroke, MI, PVD. Monitoring: Not recommended. Can be monitored by bleeding time or PFA-100. | Discontinuation not recommended, although Clopidogrel has been shown to lead to greater bleeding complications than other antiplatelet agents [12]. | Reversal generally not needed. |
| Cilostazol | Vasodilator that inhibits cellular phosphodiesterase, decreasing platelet aggregation. | Indications: Commonly used in treatment of peripheral arterial disease for intermittent claudication. Monitoring: Not recommended. | No recommendations have been made regarding discontinuation. | Reversal generally not needed. |
| Dipyridamole | Vasodilator that inhibits cGMP phosphodiesterase and cellular uptake of adenosine. | Indications: Mostly used in combination with other drugs such as aspirin (Aggrenox) or warfarin after cardiac valve replacement. Monitoring: Not recommended. | No recommendations have been made regarding discontinuation. | Reversal generally not needed. |
| NSAIDs (Ibuprofen, diclofenac) | Reversibly inhibit cyclooxygenase, inhibiting $TX_{A_2}$, decreasing platelet aggregation. | Indications: Pain, inflammatory conditions (RA), fever, dysmenorrhea, HA. Monitoring: Not recommended. | Recommended to be discontinued 3–5 days preoperatively, with resumption 1 week post-operatively. | Reversal generally not needed. |

Abbreviations: aPTT: activated partial thromboplastin time, ASA: aspirin, CAD: coronary artery disease, DVT: deep venous thrombosis, INR: international normalized ratio, MI: myocardial infarction, PVD: peripheral vascular disease, PFA-100: platelet function analyzer, PT: prothrombin time, RA: rheumatoid arthritis, TIA: transient ischemic attack, and $TX_{A_2}$: Thromboxane $A_2$.

be psychologically disturbing, an elevated INR level above the therapeutic range can be an indication for postponing the procedure depending on the urgency of the surgery.

In comparison to Warfarin, the 2005 survey of Mohs surgeons found that a majority of surgeons (87%) discontinue prophylactic (not medically necessary) aspirin use 7–10 days prior to surgery, with a majority (77%) continuing medically necessary aspirin [19]. There is a consensus that the benefits of continuing medically necessary aspirin outweigh the risk of discontinuation. Patients taking another antiplatelet agent, Clopidogrel, have been found to be at increased risk of bleeding complications during cutaneous surgery. In a recent study conducted at Mayo Clinic, patients were found to be twenty eight times more likely to have a severe complication (defined as bleeding for <1 hour, bleeding not stopped with pressure, acute hematoma formation, flap or graft necrosis, or wound dehiscence >2 mm) with Clopidogrel use during surgery [13]. Patients were also found to be eight times more likely to experience a severe complication when taking Clopidogrel in combination with aspirin than aspirin monotherapy [13]. Although anatomical site has been speculated as a possible risk factor for postoperative bleeding complications, it appears that flaps and grafts are the biggest associated risk [13]. There have been reports in the literature of patients on anticoagulation medications who unfortunately developed either a thromboembolic stroke or acute myocardial infraction after stopping their anticoagulation medications to undergo cutaneous surgery [17]. Thus it is the current consensus of dermatologic surgeons in the United States, and the opinion of the authors, no matter what the increased risk of a postoperative bleeding complication might be whether influenced by anatomic site or anticoagulation, that these anticoagulation medications should not be stopped prior to cutaneous surgery regardless of the anatomic site or anticipated complicated nature of the cutaneous surgery. Although bleeding risk has been found to be significantly increased in these patients, continuation of the medication during surgery is still recommended due to the increased risk of life-threatening thromboembolic events that can accompany the discontinuation of these medications.

Many patients are not just on one type of anticoagulation or antiplatelet agent but a combination. Certain combinations of anticoagulation medications, especially with Clopidogrel, have been shown to have a more profound effect on bleeding complications. Distinctly, the combination of Warfarin and Clopidogrel is 40 times more likely to lead to increased perioperative and postoperative bleeding complications, including hematoma formation in comparison to other anticoagulant agents [1]. Patients with recent drug eluding stent placement are advised to remain on dual antiplatelet therapy with Clopidogrel and aspirin for six months to one year and are highly advised to continue both of these medications in the perioperative period due to high risk of stent restenosis [22, 23].

Although most studies support continuation of anticoagulant medications perioperatively, a 2005 survey of 271 Mohs surgeons found that 37% still discontinued medically necessary aspirin and 44% still discontinued Warfarin [19]. Discontinuation of these medications can lead to life-threatening

thromboembolic events such as deep venous thromboses, pulmonary embolism, myocardial infarctions, cerebrovascular accidents, cardiac stent thrombosis, or clotted prosthetic heart valves [17, 23]. Alam and Goldberg presented two cases that led to pulmonary embolus and a clotted prosthetic heart valve within 36 hours after operative cutaneous surgery due to the patients' antiplatelet and anticoagulant medications being discontinued [17]. It appears that prophylactic aspirin use can be discontinued 7–10 days prior to the procedure without significant risk of thrombotic events.

## 5. Alternative Medicine and Herbal Supplements

According to the 2007 National Health Interview Survey, 4 out of 10 adults in the United States were found to have used some form of complementary alternative medicine during the past year. It has been shown that up to 70% of people do not tell their physicians that they are taking a herbal supplement [24]. Many popular alternative supplements contain a dietary ingredient, such as garlic, *ginkgo biloba*, feverfew, ginseng, and ginger [25]. Although it has become increasingly common for patients to be using alternative therapies such as those mentioned above, they are unlikely to volunteer this information to their physician [26]. Along with western pharmacotherapy, alternative therapies can have dose-related antiplatelet side effects especially in combination with other anticoagulant/antiplatelet pharmacologic agents (see Table 3).

## 6. Approach to the Patient with a Bleeding Disorder

Whether discovered upon taking a thorough preoperative history or a previously diagnosed condition, knowledge of an inherited or acquired bleeding disorder is of great importance before proceeding with dermatologic surgery. This section discusses how to approach patients with acquired disorders of coagulation due to chronic illnesses such as uremia secondary to chronic renal failure, severe liver cirrhosis, and the most commonly encountered hereditary bleeding disorders such as von Willebrand's disease and hemophilia A/B.

The rates of chronic illnesses such as chronic renal failure are on the rise in the United States, with an increase in population longevity and chronic debilitating illnesses such as hypertension and type II diabetes mellitus. Uremia secondary to chronic renal failure causes a qualitative platelet defect that can lead to a bleeding diathesis and can be monitored by checking a bleeding time or PFA-100. Knowledge of this condition can help prevent bleeding complications, and by working in conjunction with the patient's nephrologist, the platelet defects can often be improved with hemodialysis or desmopressin prior to the procedure [31]. Desmopressin improves platelet defects, providing improvement of the bleeding time for up to 24 hours [32]. Severe liver cirrhosis can also cause a coagulopathy, leading to increased risk for bleeding complications. Liver damage decreases production of the clotting factors decreasing the body's ability to form

TABLE 3: Dietary supplements and anticoagulant properties.

| Type of supplement | Mechanism of action | Comments |
|---|---|---|
| Garlic | Allicin, adenosine, and paraffinic sulfide in garlic inhibit platelet aggregation, increasing bleeding time [26, 27]. | Should be used in caution in conjunction with other anticoagulants such as Coumadin and heparin [27]. |
| Ginkgo-biloba | Inhibits platelet activating factor [26]. Platelet aggregation thought to be inhibited by terpene ginkgolide B [24, 28]. | Discontinue 36 hours before surgery [27]. One energy drink contains more than recommended dosage [28]. Caution should be used when combining with Cilostazil [28]. Some studies have shown no increase in bleeding when compared to a placebo [29]. |
| Ginseng | Inhibits platelet aggregation by altering inhibiting thromboxane function [24, 27]. | Large ingredient in energy drinks. |
| Ginger | Gingerol in ginger inhibits platelet function by inhibiting platelet activation also decreases synthesis of thromboxane [24, 27]. | Has not shown to interact with NSAIDs or warfarin. More studies need to be performed on the extent of ginger's anticoagulant properties. |
| Vitamin E | Decreased platelet adhesion and aggregation [24]. | Anticoagulant properties are dosedependent. Because it is a fat soluble vitamin, large doses can be stored in the body causing toxicity as well as increased propensity to bleed [27]. |
| Omega-3-fish oil | Decreased platelet adhesion and aggregation [24]. | Has not been shown to increase bleeding complications in spinal surgery [30]. In conjunction with other anticoagulant medications, may lead to increased effect [27]. |

a fibrin clot, and many patients will exhibit concurrent portal hypertension causing splenic sequestration of platelets and thrombocytopenia. The patient's risk for bleeding can be monitored preoperatively by the PT, aPTT, platelet count, and bleeding time. The patient's gastroenterologist should be consulted prior to the operation, and administration of recombinant tissue factor VIIa, fresh frozen plasma, or prothrombin complex concentrates may need to be given pre/postoperatively to help manage bleeding [33].

Although relatively rare in general, von Willebrand's disease is the most common inherited bleeding disorder affecting up to 1% of the population [34]. With the proper management of these conditions both pre- and postoperatively in collaboration with the patient's hematologist, the patient's risk for bleeding complications decreases substantially. The severity of the inherited defect (amount of clotting factor absent) corresponds to the amount of preoperative preparation needed. For minor surgeries, such as dermatologic surgery, it is generally recommended that coagulation factor levels approach 40–50% of normal serum levels before proceeding with the operation, with continued factor replacement 5–7 days postoperatively [34].

Although von Willebrand's disease comprises up to 1% of the population, significant bleeding has been shown to occur in only 10% of the affected patients [34]. Desmopressin is commonly given to patients with this disease preoperatively to help increase release of vWF from the endothelial cells [34]. Severely affected patients also exhibit decreased Factor VIII levels (20%) and can be given Factor VIII concentrates pre/postoperatively [34]. Hemophilia A is more common than hemophilia B, and this is due to a decrease or absence of Factor VIII (Hemophilia B has decreased Factor IX) and is most often discovered in childhood due to greater risk for developing deeper hemorrhages such as: hemarthroses, CNS bleeds, hematomas, or hematuria [31]. In conjunction

with the patient's hematologist, factor VIII and IX concentrates can be given to the patient preoperatively and should be continued for up to 5–7 days postoperatively [34]. Hematoma formation is the most common complication for hemophiliacs, even with factor replacement, so patients should be monitored closely during the postoperative period (see Table 4).

The importance of the preoperative history and physical exam cannot be underestimated. If there is any suspicion by the surgeon that a bleeding diathesis is present, the patient should undergo further laboratory testing to assess coagulation status.

## 7. Introduction to Hemostatic Agents

There are many different hemostatic modalities that can be implemented during surgical procedures. The specific types of modalities used depend upon the surgeon's preference, the efficacy and ease of use of the products, expense, and the bleeding risks of the particular patient at hand. The next few sections explore the various hemostatic techniques used today to provide optimal outcomes for the patient.

## 8. Anesthetic Techniques Promoting Hemostasis

The anesthetic agent chosen for the operation can provide hemostatic benefits to the patient when applicable. Anesthetic agents can lead to vasodilation of blood vessels increasing blood loss. Thus, the addition of a vasoconstrictive agent such as epinephrine or norepinephrine can improve intraoperative hemostasis. Not only do vasoconstrictive agents decrease bleeding, but they also increase the duration of action of the anesthetics, leading to decreased anesthetics

TABLE 4: Acquired and inherited coagulopathies and management.

| | Mechanism | Monitoring | Treatment |
|---|---|---|---|
| Acquired coagulopathies | | | |
| Uremia (chronic renal failure) | Qualitative defect in platelets with a normal platelet count. | BT or PFA-100 | DDAVP; per patients nephrologist, hemodialysis, or peritoneal dialysis [31, 32]. |
| Liver cirrhosis | Decreased production of the clotting factors; coincident splenomegaly can lead to sequestration of platelets and thrombocytopenia. | PT, aPTT, BT, and platelet count | Vitamin K, FFP, recombinant Factor VIIa, Cryoprecipitate, Platelet transfusions, Prothrombin complex concentrates, and Desmopressin [33]. |
| Inherited coagulopathies | | | |
| Von-Willebrand's disease | Decreased production of von-Willebrand's factor and factor VIII. | BT, aPTT | DDAVP, factor VIII concentrates, Cryoprecipitate [34]. |
| Hemophilia A | Decreased Factor VIII. | aPTT | Factor VIII concentrates, DDAVP [34]. |
| Hemophilia B | Decreased factor IX. | aPTT | Factor IX concentrates [34]. |

Abbreviations: aPTT: activated partial thromboplastin time, BT: bleeding time, DDAVP: desmopressin, FFP: fresh frozen plasma, PFA-100: platelet function analyzer, and PT: prothrombin time.

required and prolonged anesthetic effect after procedure. Premixed concentrations of epinephrine in 1 : 100,000 or 1 : 200,000 are generally considered safe and effective [10]. Caution should be taken in pregnant and breastfeeding patients because epinephrine is considered Category C and can be secreted in breast milk [10]. Epinephrine infused anesthetic agents should also be used cautiously in patients who have vascular compromise or who take beta blockers. In patients on beta blockers, epinephrine leads to unopposed alpha$_1$-receptor stimulation which can lead to life-threatening increases in blood pressure [11]. Epinephrine is absolutely contraindicated in patients with severe cardiovascular disease, severe hypertension, pheochromocytoma, or severe hyperthyroidism [10]. In the past, it was generally recommended that epinephrine be avoided in procedures involving the nose, ear lobes, fingers, toes, or genitals, including the penis, but recent studies have shown that certain concentrations of anesthetic with epinephrine (0.5% lidocaine with 1 : 200,000 epinephrine for example) show no evidence of ischemia or necrosis when injected into the digits [35]. Caution, however, should be used when operating on these special sites in patients with peripheral vascular disease and compromised circulation.

Another anesthetic technique that provides excellent hemostasis is tumescent anesthesia. This technique is often used in liposuction surgery or in areas of the body associated with increased risk for bleeding. The technique is accomplished by injecting extremely dilute concentrations of lidocaine (0.1%) and epinephrine (1 : 1,000,000) subcutaneously into the tissues providing anesthesia to the superficial and deeper tissues while vasoconstricting the surrounding blood vessels [10, 36]. Dr. Jeffrey Klein, the innovator of the tumescent anesthesia technique, created the original formula, adding 1,000 mg of lidocaine and 1 amp of 1 : 1,000 epinephrine to one liter of normal saline, creating the concentration of 0.1% lidocaine with 1 : 1,000,000 epinephrine [10]. The large amount of fluid injected leads to swelling and induration of the tissues, placing pressure on the surrounding

nerves and vascular structures, providing anesthetic and hemostatic effects on the tissue [36, 38]. For full hemostatic effect, the surgeon should wait 20–30 minutes after tumescent anesthesia is started before beginning with the procedure; however most of the time, the anesthetic effect of tumescence anesthesia is almost instantaneous, especially when it involves the superficial layers of the skin [10]. This technique provides prolonged anesthesia to the patient post-procedurally for up to 48 hours [37].

## 9. Electrosurgery

Electrosurgery is by far the most common hemostatic technique used in cutaneous surgery due to its accessibility, multifunctionality, ease of use, low expense, and effectiveness. There are different types of electrosurgical units depending on the surgeon's desired use of the product. The electrosurgical unit can be monoterminal or biterminal depending on the number of electrodes. The biterminal electrosurgical unit works by producing a high frequency, low voltage electrical current that is transmitted from an electrosurgical generator through an active electrode to the patient's tissues, and then back to the generator through a return electrode [10, 39]. The electrical current can be transmitted through the active electrode to the skin through one tissue contact point (monopolar) or through two tissue contact points (bipolar). An example of bipolar electrocoagulation would be the use of tissue forceps. Some studies suggest that the use of bipolar electrocoagulation produces less surrounding tissue damage, due to the ability of the forceps to grasp the specific hemorrhagic vessel providing hemostasis to a localized area [40]. The waveforms that are transmitted to the tissues can be categorized as damped or undamped. Damped waveforms provide the best hemostasis by generating heat to the tissues, leading to sealing of blood vessels; however these techniques can be more destructive [8].

The most common types of electrosurgery used by dermatologic surgeons are electrodesiccation, electrosection, electrocoagulation, and electrocautery [8]. A unit such as the Bovie, capable of conducting electrosection and electrocoagulation, provides the physician the ability to cut through the tissues and simultaneously provide hemostasis in a biterminal fashion. The unit produces high amplitude, low voltage currents that can be damped or undamped depending on the desire to cut or provide coagulation. Electrocoagulation produces damped waveforms providing excellent hemostasis, while electrosection produces mainly undamped waveforms that slice through tissue layers [8]. Because these methods generate an electrical current, they can alter implantable cardioverter defibrillators and pacemakers, potentially producing premature firing of the devices, generating arrhythmias, or causing asystole. A method called electrocautery can be used in this select group of patients, because it works by generating heat from a high resistance wire instead of producing electricity [8]. Less heat can be generated in areas of increased blood flow; therefore, electrocautery is generally only used for hemostasis of small cutaneous vessels. Pooling of blood in areas of increased blood flow not only hinders the visualization of the specific bleeding vessels to be cauterized but also decreases the effectiveness of the cauterization by decreasing the conduction of electrical current to the tissues. This problem can be prevented by dabbing the site with gauze or a cotton tipped applicator followed by quick cauterization.

Electrosurgery can produce thermal damage to the surrounding healthy tissues during the procedure [41]. Excess charring of the tissues can lead to decreased wound healing and slower recovery of the tissues postoperatively. This side-effect can be prevented by using the lowest power setting for the shortest amount of time during electrocoagulation or by touching a hemostat with the tip of a monopolar unit to produce pin-point coagulation (see Figure 1). Another potentially worrisome complication of electrosurgery is the risk of fire and electrical shock. This can be prevented by ensuring that the surgical area is not prepped with ethanol based products and through the use of insulated disposable tips on the electrosurgical device [10]. 35% aluminum chloride, a popular topical hemostatic agent used for shave biopsies, should not be used in conjunction with electrosurgery as well, because of the risk of fire. Also, the active electrode transmitting the electrical current to the tissue has an insulated shaft and base preventing electrical shock to the patient and surgeon [39]. It is important to keep in mind when removing lesions caused by human papillomavirus and other viral pathogens in the skin or when operating on patients who are suffering from a concomitant viral illness such as HIV or hepatitis, that these infections have the potential to be transmitted through the smoke plume [42]. Because of this, proper protection is warranted such as protective eye wear, masks, and gloves along with a smoke evacuator, and it is generally recommended that the smoke evacuator be held within 2 cm of the area being cauterized [42].

## 10. Physical Hemostatic Techniques

Among the cheapest and most accessible of all the hemostatic modalities is that of manual compression. This is by far one

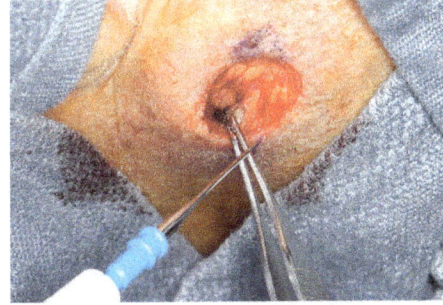

FIGURE 1: Minimizing the amount of surrounding tissue damage by using a monopolar electrocoagulation device applied to tissue forceps.

of the most basic techniques and has been used throughout history to stop bleeding and enhance coagulation. Downward pressure should be applied firmly to the affected area for 15–20 minutes depending on the extent of bleeding to tamponade the vessel(s). If the bleeding is severe, applying pressure to the supplying artery further upstream in addition to the wound area can help decrease blood flow to the affected area. This pressure applied allows time for platelets to adhere and initiation of the clotting cascade, as well as time to gather additional hemostatic agents to aid in the process. Sterile gauze pads and cotton tipped applicators can facilitate the process by soaking up the excess blood allowing better visualization of the surgical field and by providing counter pressure to aid in hemostasis. Cotton tipped applicators, (applicators with 8-inch handles and oversized cotton tips), are often used in nasal procedures, providing counterforce to the surgical field when entered in the nares for providing stabilization and hemostasis to the tissues [43]. Surgical instruments, chalazion clamp, can also provide hemostasis by manually compressing tissue during surgery [44, 45].

Tourniquets have also been used to decrease blood flow to the procedural area. An example is a digital tourniquet made out of a single finger of a surgical glove. A small hole is pierced at the end of the finger of the glove, and the glove is rolled down the patient's digit, causing exsanguination. This digital tourniquet is then rolled tightly to the base of the metacarpophalangeal joint and stabilized with a hemostat that clamps and tightens the tourniquet [46] (see Figure 2).

Another physical method providing hemostasis for smaller wounds with minimal tension is through the use of acrylates. Octyl-2-cyanoacrylate (Dermabond) is a liquid that acts by polymerization to create a barrier, reaching its full strength in 2.5 minutes [47, 48]. This adhesive is approved for skin closure and is especially beneficial in children and patients with cognitive deficits who may not tolerate suturing or the removal of nonabsorbant sutures. Studies have shown other benefits with acrylates, including lower rates of bacterial contamination [47]. An animal study conducted in 2001 also showed earlier re-epithelization as well as decreased irritation with the use of Dermabond [49]. Another study showed that compared to using an adhesive bandage, acrylates provided significant hemostasis and pain relief. Band-Aid Liquid Bandage, an acrylate available over

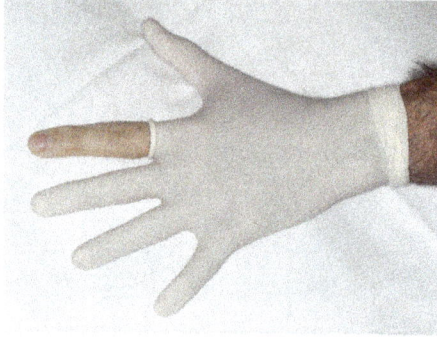

FIGURE 2: A surgical glove acting as a digital tourniquet.

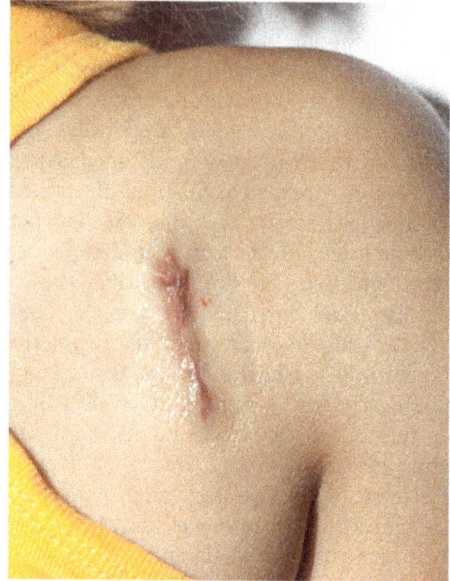

FIGURE 3: Dermabond liquid adhesive providing hemostasis to a child's laceration when applied topically.

the counter, is a less expensive, more accessible option [48] (see Figure 3).

## 11. Suturing Techniques

When performing punch biopsies and excisions of cutaneous lesions, preliminary sutures can be placed to decrease the hemorrhagic propensity of the procedure. One example is placing horizontal mattress sutures under the desired area prior to performing a punch biopsy. This can be very effective in areas that have an increased tendency to bleed such as the scalp [50].

Another suturing technique that can be particularly useful for larger defects and removal of non-melanoma skin cancers is the purse-string technique [51]. This suture applies tension to the wound edge and compresses vessels in the reticular and papillary dermis decreasing bleeding complications [51].

When bleeding from larger vessels (>2 mm) and cannot be controlled with manual compression or electrocoagulation, the vessels can be ligated or clamped with a hemostat. A figure-of-eight is most commonly placed around the vessel to tamponade the bleeding.

## 12. Caustic Hemostatic Agents

This category of topical hemostatic agents is used with less frequency in dermatologic procedures today due to the corrosive effects that the agents have on the surrounding tissues. Caustic agents cause hemostasis by precipitating proteins in the tissues, causing occlusion of smaller vessels [48, 52]. One of the oldest topical hemostatic agents known as "Moh's paste" was created by Frederic Mohs in 1941 [53]. Zinc chloride is the main component of the paste, and it can be applied with a tongue depressor, cotton tipped applicator, or incorporated into gauze (product sold as Z-squares) [48]. Studies have shown that Moh's paste has been successful in providing hemostasis to friable tissues such as breast carcinomas that are metastatic to the skin [53].

Another topical agent that is still used in dermatologic and gynecologic procedures, but with decreased frequency, is Monsel's solution, which is composed of 20% ferric subsulfate [48]. Monsel's solution has an acidic pH which is thought to contribute to its hemostatic properties eliciting protein precipitation in vessels and oxidization [51]. Monsel's solution is effective after punch or shave biopsies but is used less frequently due to its tattooing effect on the skin. Upon application, iron particles deposit into the dermis, leading to hyperpigmentation of the surrounding skin and an increased inflammatory response [48, 54]. The solution is user friendly and can be applied with gauze or cotton tipped applicators to the desired area and is relatively inexpensive. Less hyperpigmentation and tattooing of the skin occur with a 10% ferrous sulfate solution when applied to the skin for 1-2 hours postoperatively [48]. Another caustic agent that has a better side-effect profile than others is aluminum chloride. This solution can be applied with a cotton-tipped applicator after shave biopsies and has been shown to be very effective [48].

## 13. Noncaustic Hemostatic Agents

This group of hemostatic agents can be a helpful addition to electrocoagulation, minimizing the amount of electrocoagulation needed during the procedure. These are beneficial alternatives to patients with a bleeding diathesis despite use of electrocoagulation and decrease thermal injury to the surrounding tissues. This section is going to focus on various subsets of noncaustic hemostatic agents. A majority of these agents enhance the patient's own clotting system, so if the patient has a hereditary or acquired deficiency in the clotting cascade, these agents are unlikely to be beneficial (see Table 5).

Physical noncaustic agents work to provide a structural meshwork that aids in platelet aggregation and coagulation [48, 52]. An example of a physical agent is the gelatin sponge. Gelatin sponges have been used for hemostasis after

TABLE 5: Hemostatic agents.

| Hemostatic agent | Product information | Mechanism of action | Potential side effects |
|---|---|---|---|
| *Caustic agents* | | | |
| Zinc chloride (Moh's paste) | Paste that can be applied topically. Used infrequently, but is effective in providing hemostasis to metastatic cutaneous wounds [53]. | Precipitates proteins causing coagulation of small vessels [48]. Left on for up to 48 hours. | Can be very painful and irritating to the patient [53]. |
| Ferric subsulfate (Monsel's solution) | Solution can be applied with a cotton tipped applicator or gauze pad [48, 54]. | Precipitates proteins intravascularly and oxidizes tissues. Less expensive, more accessible, and easy to apply [48, 54]. | Being used less due to intradermal ferruginous deposits causing tattooing of the skin after use [48, 54]. |
| Aluminum chloride | Solution can be applied with a cotton tipped applicator after shave biopsy [48]. | Precipitates proteins causing coagulation of vessels [48]. Easily accessible and easy to apply. | Can be painful and irritating to the patient [48]. |
| *Non-caustic agents* | | | |
| Gelatin (Gelfoam, Surgifoam) Gelfoam Plus (Gelatin combined with human thrombin) | Comes in a sterile powder or sponge. Porcine derived [48]. | The gelatin is able to absorb more than 45x its weight, providing a matrix for the clotting cascade in addition to providing a physical barrier. Absorbed by the body in 4–6 weeks [48, 55, 56]. | Can interfere with healing of wound edges, generally not recommended for use in skin incisions. Can facilitate bacterial growth leading to infection or leading to foreign body reactions when left in the tissue. Can increase in size leading to compression of surrounding structures, including nerve damage. When combined with thrombin can lead to allergic/anaphylactic reactions [48, 55]. |
| Polyethylene glycol Hydrogel (CoSeal) | Liquid composed of two PEG polymers that polymerize and cross-link in the tissue [57, 58]. | Increases platelet adherence, providing quick hemostasis [57]. | Swells up to 4x its size potentially causing damage to the surrounding tissues [58]. |
| Microporous polysaccharide spheres (Arista) | Comes in a white powder that is 100% plant based. Formed by cross-linking of purified plant starch [52, 58, 59]. | Dehydrates the blood, concentrating RBC's, platelets, proteins, promoting adherence to the gel matrix. Also causes a physical barrier in the tissue [52, 58, 59]. | Causes immediate swelling, has the potential to cause damage to surrounding structures. Use cautiously in diabetics due to potential to increase glucose load [58]. |
| Microfibrillar collagen (Avitene, Helistat) | Bovine collagen formed into flour, sheets, or sponges [48]. | Collagen framework promotes platelet aggregation and coagulation cascade [48]. Physically acts to tamponade the vessels and provide a meshwork for the fibrinolytic cascade to occur. Becomes gelatinous in 24–48 hrs and is absorbed by the body by 1–6 weeks. Relatively inexpensive [48]. | Side effects are rare. Allergic and foreign body reactions have occurred [48]. |
| Cellulose (Surgicel, Oxycel) | Oxidized cellulose arranged into sheets, gauze, or smaller strips. Can durably be placed in the tissue [48, 60]. | Forms an eschar in body in <60 seconds, due to the polymers dehydrating the blood and the potassium salt binding to the positively charged red blood cells [48, 52]. | Can cause granulomatous reactions and should be used carefully in closed spaces due to increased risk of swelling in the tissues, can cause compression of surrounding structures [60]. |
| Pro QR powder | Combination of a hydrophilic polymer and potassium salt packaged into a powder [48, 51]. Available over the counter, relatively inexpensive and easy to apply. | | Few side effects reported. |
| Thrombin (Thrombin-JMI, Recothrom, Evithrom, Floseal) | Can be bovine derived or human recombinant thrombin. Comes in a powder or solution. Floseal is composed of a gelatin matrix and thrombin and comes in two separate compartments that are not mixed until time of use [48, 60]. | Promotes body's physiologic clotting cascade by actively converting fibrinogen into fibrin. Should not be used in patients that have decreased fibrinogen levels [48, 57, 60]. | Bovine thrombin has been shown to cause coagulopathy weeks after use, due to antibodies forming against factor V. Human thrombin although cleansed thoroughly, has the potential to transmit viruses [48, 57, 60]. |

TABLE 5: Continued.

| Hemostatic agent | Product information | Mechanism of action | Potential side effects |
|---|---|---|---|
| Fibrin sealant (Tisseal, Crosseal, Evicel) | Human and bovine derived forms. Can be formed from autologous plasma or pooled from donors. Also comes in an aerosolized form [5]. Entails different methods of preparation depending on the product. Can be frozen in premixed form for up to two years, can be heated, and stirred for 20 minutes prior to use [48, 60]. Can also be sprayed directly to the area in the aerosolized form [5]. | Comes in a two compartment syringe with one compartment containing fibrinogen, factor XIII, fibronectin, and fibrinolysis inhibitors (aprotinin), and in the other is thrombin and calcium chloride [5, 48, 60]. When combined, thrombin becomes activated and activates the clotting cascade and enhances conversion of fibrinogen to fibrin. Absorbed from the body within 5–10 days [48]. Very effective in patients with coagulopathies. | Pooled donor plasma and older sealants containing bovine derived aprotinin increased the potential to cause hypersensitivity reactions and to transmit infectious diseases such as prion-related diseases [5, 58]. |
| Octyl-2-cyanoacrylate (Dermabond) | Comes as a topical liquid adhesive best used for smaller lacerations. May have some antibacterial properties. Good in pediatric population and people with cognitive deficits who cannot tolerate/understand stitch removal. Moderately expensive [47–49]. | Polymerization creates a physical barrier, tamponading the vessels [47–49]. | Small risk for inflammatory reactions and fibrosis [48]. |

Abbreviations: PEG: polyethylene glycol.

punch biopsies of the skin and may be more effective in areas such as cartilage or periosteum, which have a harder time forming granulation tissue [48]. One study showed that wounds treated with gelatin sponges and left to heal by secondary intention led to increased granulation tissue formation and an overall better appearance of the wound [55]. Absorbable gelatin sponges soaked in aluminum chloride have also been shown to provide quick hemostasis after nail punch biopsies when left in the wound for two weeks [56]. Another physical agent, polyethylene glycol hydrogel, is a synthetic, biodegradable hemostat that polymerizes quickly, providing hemostasis in less than 60 seconds. Caution should be taken with closed wounds because it can swell up to four times its own size, potentially leading to surrounding tissue damage [57, 58]. Another physical agent, collagen, has been shown to be a superior hemostat to other products, because not only platelets adhere more readily to the collagen matrix, but also they are stimulated to degranulate enhancing platelet aggregation [57]. This product is less effective in patients with thrombocytopenia [58]. The product is bovine derived, with the potential to cause allergic and foreign body reactions. Other hemostatic agents containing oxidized cellulose (Surgicel or Oxycel), arranged into sheets or gauze, can be durably placed into bleeding tissues, causing hemostasis by tamponading vessels and by providing a physical meshwork for the clotting cascade to occur [48, 51]. Although relatively inexpensive and easy to use, they can potentially cause granulomatous reactions and increased swelling tissues [48, 60]. Two more physical agents, Urgent QR powder and microporous polysaccharide hemispheres, can be sprinkled topically on wounds to enhance hemostasis. Urgent QR powder is a hydrophilic polymer combined with potassium salt, used only on wounds left open to heal by secondary intention, because of the body's inability to metabolize the substance [52]. It hemostatically forms an eschar in the body in less than a minute, due to the polymers dehydrating the blood and the potassium salt binding to the positively charged red blood cells [48, 52]. It is sold over the counter and is less expensive than some of the other hemostatic agents [52]. Another physical agent, composed of purified potato starch powder, is microporous polysaccharide hemispheres. This agent can be degraded by enzymes in the body (alpha-amylase and pyrase), allowing use in closed wounds [52]. It accelerates the clotting process, by dehydrating the blood, causing concentration of the platelets and clotting factors [52, 58, 59]. This product can be sprinkled topically as a powder or incorporated into wound dressings. This agent has been shown to be less hemostatically effective and more expensive than electrocoagulation but is a good alternative in individuals that have contraindication to electrocoagulation [59]. This product should be used cautiously in diabetics, because it has the potential to increase glucose loads [58].

Physiologic agents are other hemostatic agents, which potentiate the body's own physiologic clotting mechanisms. For example, thrombin products have been created to enhance the fibrinolytic cascade and the final conversion of fibrinogen into fibrin. Topical bovine thrombin and human recombinant thrombin have been shown to be effective hemostatic agents in areas where there is diffuse bleeding (the specific vessel cannot be identified) and from direct bleeding from bone [61]. Studies have shown an increased risk for postoperative coagulopathies with bovine-derived thrombin, because antibodies formed against the thrombin are cross-reactive against human factor V [48, 57, 61]. Human recombinant thrombin has less antigenic effects, decreasing the risk for developing a postoperative coagulopathy, but carries a small risk for viral transmission to the patient [48, 57, 58, 61].

Another class of hemostatic agents gaining in popularity is the fibrin sealants. Whereas other products may rely on the patient's own platelet and clotting factors for hemostatic activation, fibrin sealants do not. This may be beneficial in situations where the patient has an inherited or acquired coagulation abnormality [62]. In order to be activated, the two compartments full of thrombin and fibrinogen must be mixed together (which can lead to clotting, if mixed prematurely) [48, 62]. When combined, thrombin (from one compartment) converts fibrinogen (from the other compartment) into insoluble fibrin in the presence of calcium [5, 48]. The amount of thrombin contained in the fibrin sealant is thought to contribute to the rapidity of clot formation, whereas the amount of fibrinogen contributes to the mechanical strength of the clot [58]. A 2009 Cochrane review showed that fibrin sealants lead to an average reduction of blood loss of 161 mL per procedure and argued that the benefits of using the product must outweigh the potential side effects of its use [5]. Potential side effects of fibrin sealants are infectious disease transmission, hypersensitivity reactions, and neurotoxicity [5, 48]. The newest fibrin sealant, Evicel, is human derived and does not contain tranexamic acid, decreasing the risk for neurotoxicity with use [58]. Newer fibrin sealant formulations are derived from autologous plasma or from pooled plasma donors, leading to decreased hypersensitivity reactions with the autologous sealants [5, 58].

The authors recommend intraoperative hemostasis that is done with precision via electrosurgery as the mainstay of hemostasis in routine cutaneous surgeries. For smaller biopsies, where electrosurgery is not necessary, aluminum chloride is cheap and easily accessible and should also be considered as a mainstay. For postoperative bleeding complications, the other measures discussed in this section can be considered if physical hemostatic techniques (manual pressure) are inadequate.

## 14. Postoperative Recommendations and Complications

Patients that have increased intraoperative bleeding are at greater risk for postoperative bleeding complications, with complications most likely to occur within the first 48 hours following the procedure [10, 63]. A pressure dressing should be applied to the operative area for at least 24 hours post-operatively to ensure adequate compression of the tissues. The typical wound dressing normally consists of a topical antibiotic ointment, a Telfa pad cut to conform to the operative area, and a layer of gauze secured and compressed to the skin by adhesive tape [64]. It is generally recommended

TABLE 6: Postoperative recommendations.

| Postoperative recommendations | |
|---|---|
| (i) A pressure wound dressing should be applied for at least 24 hours, providing adequate compression to the tissues [10, 63].<br>(ii) Activity should be limited during the first 48 hours due to the increased risk for bleeding complications. Small blood vessels are vulnerable to rupture with minor activity. Strenuous activity should be limited until the wound regains tensile strength (up to 2 weeks for facial/neck wounds and up to 6 weeks for lower extremity wounds) [10].<br>(iii) Elevation of the operative area within the first 24 hours of the operation is important to decrease the amount of gravity and pressure on the tissues. For procedures of the face, scalp, or neck, placing pillows underneath the head and neck areas while lying down can help to alleviate pressure [64]. | (i) If bleeding is apparent, ice and cool compresses can be applied to the surgical area to vasoconstrict the blood vessels and decrease bleeding [64].<br>(ii) Manual compression can be applied externally to the wound area for up to 20 minutes to control minor bleeding.<br>(iii) If the gauze and current wound dressing appear to be saturated in blood, a clean dressing should be applied to the area to allow for better absorption and compression of the tissues.<br>(iv) If the patient begins to experience throbbing pain, increased pressure sensation, or heavy bleeding that is uncontrollable, they should return to the office immediately for further intervention and treatment [63]. |

TABLE 7: Hematoma management.

| Early hematoma formation | Late hematoma formation |
|---|---|
| (i) Reopen the wound and localize the bleeding site.<br>(ii) Achieve hemostasis by electrocoagulation/ligation of the affected vessels or by application of topical hemostatic agents.<br>(iii) If bleeding cannot be adequately controlled, place a drain into the wound for up to 24 hours.<br>(iv) Resuture the site and apply the appropriate pressure dressing. | (i) If small, may only require observation.<br>(ii) If large and within the first week, evacuate the area and leave open to heal by secondary intention [63].<br>(iii) If not discovered until late (weeks to months later), aspirate the area with a 16–18 gauge needle; [63, 65]. |

that patients avoid minor activity during the first 24 hours, allowing the vessels to remain coagulated, and to keep the wound site elevated for edema prevention. For procedures of the face, scalp, or neck, placing pillows underneath the head and neck areas while lying down can help to alleviate pressure and edema. Strenuous activity and heavy lifting should remain limited during the first month following the operation because the wound has only 40–50% of its tensile strength [64]. It is important to discuss with the patient that mild bleeding is anticipated, and if the patient starts to exhibit signs of increased bleeding, pressure and ice should be applied to the wound dressing for up to 20 minutes [63, 64]. Also, if the patient's wound dressing appears saturated with blood, it should be removed and a clean dressing should be applied to allow for better absorption and compression of the tissues. If the patient continues to have increased bleeding, the patient should return to the office for reevaluation. Alcohol ingestion is generally not recommended during the first week postoperatively due to ethanol's vasodilatory effects on the blood vessels leading to increased risk for bleeding (see Table 6).

Hematomas are most likely to occur within the first 24–72 hours postoperatively and can present with increased pressure sensation, throbbing pain, ecchymosis, and fluctuation of the tissues [10, 63]. Hematomas can form slowly due to continuous bleeding of smaller blood vessels into the newly closed wound or can expand rapidly when involving larger vessels.

Early recognition of a rapidly expanding hematoma is important. Usually a hematoma is easily evaluated and diagnosed clinically as an expansile fluctuant mass under a recent surgical site that is accompanied by the characteristic expansile ecchymosis on the skin surface. If a hematoma is suspected clinically, the wound should be reopened and the affected vessels should be localized and treated with suture ligation or electrocoagulation. If bleeding continues despite prior attempts at coagulation, a drain can be placed in addition to other topical hemostatic agents [7, 10]. The drain should not be left for more than 24 hours, because of an increased risk for infection if left longer [65]. When hemostasis is achieved, all of the layers of the wound should be resutured closed and a clean pressure dressing should be reapplied.

Hematomas become increasingly gelatinous and firm over time with the formation of clots. Patients who delay seeking treatment during the first week or who develop a hematoma very gradually can undergo observation or have their wound evacuated and left open to heal by secondary intention [63]. Weeks to months later, hematomas undergo liquefactive necrosis and resorption. During this stage, the hematoma can be aspirated and drained with a 16–18 gauge needle [63, 65]. Because hematomas are a nidus for bacteria, prophylactic antibiotics should be given early for infection prevention [7, 10]. If rapidly expanding hematomas are not controlled, they can lead to further complications such as wound dehiscence and skin graft necrosis (see Table 7 and Figure 4).

## 15. Summary

Hemostasis is an important concept to consider when performing dermatologic surgery. With careful attention paid to

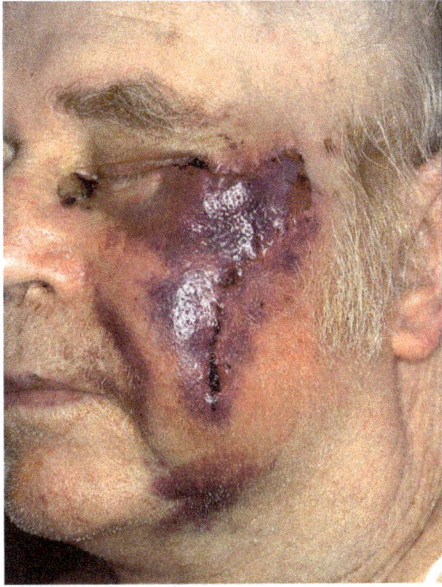

FIGURE 4: Acute hematoma formation following dermatologic surgery.

the preoperative evaluation, the patient's comorbidities and risk factors for bleeding, proper intraoperative hemostasis technique, and postprocedure monitoring, wound care, and education, many bleeding complications can be avoided or attended to promptly and effectively. During the procedure, many different hemostatic modalities are available, with electrocoagulation being among the most effective and commonly used. Many other methods of hemostasis can be used in conjunction with electrocoagulation with the optimal goal of minimizing blood loss. Postoperative complications due to increased bleeding include hematoma formation, skin or flap necrosis, and graft necrosis. Early evaluation of hematoma formation can help prevent the development of further complications such as infection, wound dehiscence, and skin graft necrosis.

## Conflict of Interests

The authors have no conflict of interests.

## References

[1] J. S. Bordeaux, K. J. Martires, D. Goldberg, S. F. Pattee, P. Fu, and M. E. Maloney, "Prospective evaluation of dermatologic surgery complications including patients on multiple antiplatelet and anticoagulant medications," *Journal of the American Academy of Dermatology*, vol. 65, no. 3, pp. 576–583, 2011.

[2] M. L. Diethorn and L. M. Weld, "Physiologic mechanisms of hemostasis and fibrinolysis," *The Journal of cardiovascular nursing*, vol. 4, no. 1, pp. 1–10, 1989.

[3] M. H. Kroll and A. I. Schafer, "Biochemical mechanisms of platelet activation," *Blood*, vol. 74, no. 4, pp. 1181–1195, 1989.

[4] J. H. Morrissey, "Tissue factor: an enzyme cofactor and a true receptor," *Thrombosis and Haemostasis*, vol. 86, no. 1, pp. 66–74, 2001.

[5] P. A. Carless, D. A. Henry, and D. M. Anthony, "Fibrin sealant use for minimising peri-operative allogeneic blood transfusion," *Cochrane Database of Systematic Reviews*, no. 2, p. CD004171, 2003.

[6] J. J. Pisano, J. S. Finlayson, and M. P. Peyton, "Cross-link in fibrin polymerized by factor XIII: $\varepsilon$-($\gamma$-glutamyl) lysine," *Science*, vol. 160, no. 3830, pp. 892–893, 1968.

[7] E. A. Hurst, S. S. Yu, R. C. Grekin, and I. M. Neuhaus, "Bleeding complications in dermatologic surgery," *Seminars in Cutaneous Medicine and Surgery*, vol. 26, no. 4, pp. 189–195, 2007.

[8] J. E. Lane, E. M. O'Brien, and D. E. Kent, "Optimization of thermocautery in excisional dermatologic surgery," *Dermatologic Surgery*, vol. 32, no. 5, pp. 669–675, 2006.

[9] D. J. Fader and T. M. Johnson, "Medical issues and emergencies in the dermatology office," *Journal of the American Academy of Dermatology*, vol. 36, no. 1, pp. 1–16, 1997.

[10] R. K. Roenigk, J. L. Ratz, and H. H. Roenigk, *Roenigk's Dermatologic Surgery: Current Techniques in Procedural Dermatology*, Informa Healthcare, New York, NY, USA, 2007.

[11] B. Katzung, S. Masters, and A. Trevor, *Basic and Clinical Pharmacology*, McGraw-Hill, New York, NY, USA, 2009.

[12] L. C. Stewart and J. A. A. Langtry, "Clopidogrel: mechanisms of action and review of the evidence relating to use during skin surgery procedures," *Clinical and Experimental Dermatology*, vol. 35, no. 4, pp. 341–345, 2010.

[13] R. H. Cook-Norris, J. D. Michaels, A. L. Weaver et al., "Complications of cutaneous surgery in patients taking clopidogrel-containing anticoagulation," *Journal of the American Academy of Dermatology*, vol. 65, no. 3, pp. 584–591, 2011.

[14] S. Syed, B. B. Adams, W. Liao, M. Pipitone, and H. Gloster, "A prospective assessment of bleeding and international normalized ratio in warfarin-anticoagulated patients having cutaneous surgery," *Journal of the American Academy of Dermatology*, vol. 51, no. 6, pp. 955–957, 2004.

[15] A. Ah-Weng, S. Natarajan, S. Velangi, and J. A. A. Langtry, "Preoperative monitoring of warfarin in cutaneous surgery," *British Journal of Dermatology*, vol. 149, no. 2, pp. 386–389, 2003.

[16] P. Bassas, R. Bartralot, and V. García-Patos, "Anticoagulation and antiplatelet therapy in dermatology," *Actas Dermo-Sifiliograficas*, vol. 100, no. 1, pp. 7–16, 2009.

[17] M. Alam, L. H. Goldberg, and S. J. Salasche, "Serious adverse vascular events associated with perioperative interruption of antiplatelet and anticoagulant therapy," *Dermatologic Surgery*, vol. 28, no. 11, pp. 992–998, 2002.

[18] C. C. Otley, "Continuation of medically necessary aspirin and warfarin during cutaneous surgery," *Mayo Clinic Proceedings*, vol. 78, no. 11, pp. 1392–1396, 2003.

[19] A. Y. Kirkorian, B. L. Moore, J. Siskind, and E. S. Marmur, "Perioperative management of anticoagulant therapy during cutaneous surgery: 2005 survey of mohs surgeons," *Dermatologic Surgery*, vol. 33, no. 10, pp. 1189–1197, 2007.

[20] K. G. Lewis and R. G. Dufresne Jr., "A meta-analysis of complications attributed to anticoagulation among patients following cutaneous surgery," *Dermatologic Surgery*, vol. 34, no. 2, pp. 160–164, 2008.

[21] H. M. Gloster Jr. and J. Twersky, "Surgical Pearl: the use of the CoaguChek S system for the preoperative evaluation of patients taking warfarin," *Journal of the American Academy of Dermatology*, vol. 50, no. 3, pp. 439–441, 2004.

[22] M. B. Chu, R. B. Turner, and D. A. Kriegel, "Patients with drug-eluting stents and management of their anticoagulant therapy

in cutaneous surgery," *Journal of the American Academy of Dermatology*, vol. 64, no. 3, pp. 553–558, 2011.

[23] D. G. Rizik and K. J. Klassen, "Assessing the landscape of stent thrombosis: the drug-eluting versus bare-metal stent controversy," *American Journal of Cardiology*, vol. 102, no. 9, pp. 4J–11J, 2008.

[24] S. C. Collins and R. G. Dufresne Jr., "Dietary supplements in the setting of Mohs surgery," *Dermatologic Surgery*, vol. 28, no. 6, pp. 447–452, 2002.

[25] P. M. Barnes, B. Bloom, and R. L. Nahin, "Complementary and alternative medicine use among adults and children: United States, 2007," *National Health Statistics Reports*, no. 12, pp. 1–23, 2009.

[26] S. M. Dinehart and L. Henry, "Dietary supplements: altered coagulation and effects on bruising," *Dermatologic Surgery*, vol. 31, no. 7, pp. 819–826, 2005.

[27] J. Heller, J. S. Gabbay, K. Ghadjar et al., "Top-10 list of herbal and supplemental medicines used by cosmetic patients: What the plastic surgeon needs to know," *Plastic and Reconstructive Surgery*, vol. 117, no. 2, pp. 436–445, 2006.

[28] M. J. Stanger, L. A. Thompson, A. J. Young, and H. R. Lieberman, "Anticoagulant activity of select dietary supplements," *Nutrition Reviews*, vol. 70, no. 2, pp. 107–117, 2012.

[29] A. J. Kellermann and C. Kloft, "Is there a risk of bleeding associated with standardized Ginkgo biloba extract therapy? A systematic review and meta-analysis," *Pharmacotherapy*, vol. 31, no. 5, pp. 490–502, 2011.

[30] C. K. Kepler, R. C. Huang, D. Meredith, J.-H. Kim, and A. K. Sharma, "Omega-3 and fish oil supplements do not cause increased bleeding during spinal decompression surgery," *Journal of Spinal Disorders & Techniques*, vol. 25, no. 3, pp. 129–132, 2011.

[31] R. E. Taylor and P. M. Blatt, "Clinical evaluation of the patient with bruising and bleeding," *Journal of the American Academy of Dermatology*, vol. 4, no. 3, pp. 348–368, 1981.

[32] H. K. Lee, Y. J. Kim, J. U. Jeong, J. S. Park, H. S. Chi, and S. B. Kim, "Desmopressin improves platelet dysfunction measured by in vitro closure time in uremic patients," *Nephron Clinical Practice*, vol. 114, no. 4, pp. c248–c252, 2010.

[33] D. E. Bernstein, L. Jeffers, E. Erhardtsen et al., "Recombinant factor VIIa corrects prothrombin time in cirrhotic patients: a preliminary study," *Gastroenterology*, vol. 113, no. 6, pp. 1930–1937, 1997.

[34] S. R. Peterson and A. K. Joseph, "Inherited bleeding disorders in dermatologic surgery," *Dermatologic Surgery*, vol. 27, no. 10, pp. 885–889, 2001.

[35] B. Firoz, N. Davis, and L. H. Goldberg, "Local anesthesia using buffered 0.5% lidocaine with 1:200,000 epinephrine for tumors of the digits treated with Mohs micrographic surgery," *Journal of the American Academy of Dermatology*, vol. 61, no. 4, pp. 639–643, 2009.

[36] P. Davila and I. Garcia-Doval, "Tumescent anesthesia in dermatologic surgery," *Actas Dermo-Sifiliograficas*, vol. 103, no. 4, pp. 285–287, 2012.

[37] J. A. Klein, "Tumescent technique for regional anesthesia permits lidocaine doses of 35 mg/kg for liposuction," *Journal of Dermatologic Surgery and Oncology*, vol. 16, no. 3, pp. 248–263, 1990.

[38] D. Balducci, O. Morandi, S. Mazzetti, M. Tonni, A. Becchetti, and R. Pancaldi, "Ambulatory saphenectomy: 80 operated cases using tumescent anesthesia," *Chirurgia Italiana*, vol. 54, no. 1, pp. 77–82, 2002.

[39] D. G. Ferris, S. Saxena, B. L. Hainer, J. R. Searle, J. L. Powell, and J. N. Gay, "Gynecologic and dermatologic electrosurgical units: a comparative review," *Journal of Family Practice*, vol. 39, no. 2, pp. 160–169, 1994.

[40] B. Bergdahl and B. Stenquist, "An automatic computerized bipolar coagulator for dermatologic surgery," *Journal of Dermatologic Surgery and Oncology*, vol. 19, no. 3, pp. 225–227, 1993.

[41] R. Hambley, P. A. Hebda, E. Abell, B. A. Cohen, and B. V. Jegasothy, "Wound healing of skin incisions produced by ultrasonically vibrating knife, scalpel, electrosurgery, and carbon dioxide laser," *Journal of Dermatologic Surgery and Oncology*, vol. 14, no. 11, pp. 1213–1217, 1988.

[42] W. S. Sawchuk, P. J. Weber, D. R. Lowy, and L. M. Dzubow, "Infectious papillomavirus in the vapor of warts treated with carbon dioxide laser or electrocoagulation: detection and protection," *Journal of the American Academy of Dermatology*, vol. 21, no. 1, pp. 41–49, 1989.

[43] K. Nouri and C. J. Ballard, "Cotton-tipped applicators used in surgery of the nose," *Dermatologic Surgery*, vol. 31, no. 11, pp. 1440–1441, 2005.

[44] I. Amir, E. S. Marmur, and D. A. Kriegel, "Bloodless nasal alar surgery: another innovative use of the chalazion clamp," *Dermatologic Surgery*, vol. 35, no. 5, pp. 843–844, 2009.

[45] E. Cigna, E. M. Buccheri, C. Monarca, and N. Scuderi, "Hemostasis in skin surgery," *Aesthetic Plastic Surgery*, vol. 32, no. 4, p. 702, 2008.

[46] A. B. Aksakal and E. Adişen, "Method for facilitating the application of digital tourniquets," *Dermatologic Surgery*, vol. 35, no. 9, p. 1389, 2009.

[47] D. M. Toriumi and A. A. Bagal, "Cyanoacrylate tissue adhesives for skin closure in the outpatient setting," *Otolaryngologic Clinics of North America*, vol. 35, no. 1, pp. 103–118, 2002.

[48] M. D. Palm and J. S. Altman, "Topical hemostatic agents: a review," *Dermatologic Surgery*, vol. 34, no. 4, pp. 431–445, 2008.

[49] W. H. Eaglstein, T. P. Sullivan, P. A. Giordano, and B. M. Miskin, "A liquid adhesive bandage for the treatment of minor cuts and abrasions," *Dermatologic Surgery*, vol. 28, no. 3, pp. 263–267, 2002.

[50] A. A. Ingraffea, "Use of a preliminary horizontal mattress suture on scalp biopsies to achieve rapid hemostasis," *Dermatologic Surgery*, vol. 36, no. 8, p. 1312, 2010.

[51] P. R. Cohen, P. T. Martinelli, K. E. Schulze, and B. R. Nelson, "The cuticular purse string suture: a modified purse string suture for the partial closure of round postoperative wounds," *International Journal of Dermatology*, vol. 46, no. 7, pp. 746–753, 2007.

[52] J. Ho and G. Hruza, "Hydrophilic polymers with potassium salt and microporous polysaccharides for use as hemostatic agents," *Dermatologic Surgery*, vol. 33, no. 12, pp. 1430–1433, 2007.

[53] M. Kakimoto, H. Tokita, T. Okamura, and K. Yoshino, "A chemical hemostatic technique for bleeding from malignant wounds," *Journal of Palliative Medicine*, vol. 13, no. 1, pp. 11–13, 2010.

[54] R. B. Armstrong, J. Nichols, and J. Pachance, "Punch biopsy wounds treated with Monsel's solution or a collagen matrix. A comparison of healing," *Archives of Dermatology*, vol. 122, no. 5, pp. 546–549, 1986.

[55] P. P. Rullan, C. Vallbona, J. M. Rullan, J. N. Mansbridge, and V. B. Morhenn, "Use of gelatin sponges in Mohs micrographic surgery defects and staged melanoma excisions: a novel approach to secondary wound healing," *Journal of Drugs in Dermatology*, vol. 10, no. 1, pp. 68–73, 2011.

[56] C. Hwa, O. I. Kovich, and J. A. Stein, "Achieving hemostasis after nail biopsy using absorbable gelatin sponge saturated in aluminum chloride," *Dermatologic Surgery*, vol. 37, no. 3, pp. 368–369, 2011.

[57] F. I. Broekema, W. Van Oeveren, J. Zuidema, S. H. Visscher, and R. R. M. Bos, "In vitro analysis of polyurethane foam as a topical hemostatic agent," *Journal of Materials Science*, vol. 22, no. 4, pp. 1081–1086, 2011.

[58] S. Dhillon, M. T. De Boer, E. N. Papacharalabous, and M. Schwartz, "Fibrin sealant (Evicel [quixil/crosseal]): a review of its use as supportive treatment for haemostasis in surgery," *Drugs*, vol. 71, no. 14, pp. 1893–1915, 2011.

[59] S. R. Tan and W. D. Tope, "Effectiveness of microporous polysaccharide hemospheres for achieving hemostasis in Mohs micrographic surgery," *Dermatologic Surgery*, vol. 30, no. 6, pp. 908–914, 2004.

[60] M. A. Schreiber and D. J. Neveleff, "Achieving hemostasis with topical hemostats: making clinically and economically appropriate decisions in the surgical and trauma settings," *AORN Journal*, vol. 94, no. 5, pp. S1–S20, 2011.

[61] W. C. Chapman, N. Singla, Y. Genyk et al., "A phase 3, randomized, double-blind comparative study of the efficacy and safety of topical recombinant human thrombin and bovine thrombin in surgical hemostasis," *Journal of the American College of Surgeons*, vol. 205, no. 2, pp. 256–265, 2007.

[62] L. K. Krishnan, M. Mohanty, P. R. Umashankar, and A. Vijayan Lal, "Comparative evaluation of absorbable hemostats: advantages of fibrin-based sheets," *Biomaterials*, vol. 25, no. 24, pp. 5557–5563, 2004.

[63] A. Delaney, S. Diamantis, and V. J. Marks, "Complications of tissue ischemia in dermatologic surgery," *Dermatologic Therapy*, vol. 24, no. 6, pp. 551–557, 2011.

[64] C. Y. Cho and J. S. Lo, "Dressing the part," *Dermatologic Clinics*, vol. 16, no. 1, pp. 25–47, 1998.

[65] S. J. Salasche, "Acute surgical complications: cause, prevention, and treatment," *Journal of the American Academy of Dermatology*, vol. 15, no. 6, pp. 1163–1185, 1986.

# 19

# The Incidence and Risk Factors for Lower Limb Skin Graft Failure

**Sumeet Reddy, Falah El-Haddawi, Michael Fancourt, Glenn Farrant, William Gilkison, Nigel Henderson, Stephen Kyle, and Damien Mosquera**

*Department of General Surgery, Taranaki Base Hospital, Private Bag 2016, New Plymouth 4342, New Zealand*

Correspondence should be addressed to Sumeet Reddy; sumeetkreddy@gmail.com

Academic Editor: Masutaka Furue

Lower limb skin grafts are thought to have higher failure rates than skin grafts in other sites of the body. Currently, there is a paucity of literature on specific factors associated with lower limb skin graft failure. We present a series of 70 lower limb skin grafts in 50 patients with outcomes at 6 weeks. One-third of lower limb skin grafts went on to fail with increased BMI, peripheral vascular disease, and immunosuppressant medication use identified as significant risk factors.

## 1. Introduction

The use of skin grafts to aid in the healing of wounds was first described by the ancient Indians over 2,500 years ago [1]. Although operative techniques have evolved over time, the principles of successful grafting have remained the same. Intrinsic and extrinsic factors unique to each patient can be the difference between success and failure [2]. This is especially apparent in the lower limb, where skin grafts have higher failure and complication rates than in other areas of the body [3, 4]. Currently, there is a paucity of research focused on factors contributing to lower limb skin graft failure and this may in part explain the heterogeneity with which clinicians manage patients requiring lower limb skin grafts [5]. The aim of this study was to determine the incidence of failure of lower limb skin grafts and to identify contributing factors.

## 2. Methods

A prospective observational study of all consecutive patients requiring lower limb skin grafts operated on between December 2012 and December 2013 was undertaken. Skin grafts were performed using well-established techniques. All operations were performed under general or regional anaesthetic with prophylactic antibiotics. Split thickness skin grafts (STSG) were harvested using an air dermatome (Zimmer, Warsaw, IN, USA) and full thickness grafts (FTSG) were harvested using a scalpel with subcutaneous tissue removed prior to application. STSG were typically meshed prior to application and grafts were fixed with sutures, staples, or Dermabond (Johnson & Johnson, Ethicon Inc., Somerville, NJ, USA). Cuticerin (Smith & Nephew, London, UK) was applied over the graft with either a standard sponge bolster or negative pressure dressing (PICO TM, Smith & Nephew, London, UK). Patients were then either admitted to hospital for a 3–7-day period of bed rest with low molecular weight heparin or discharged with immediate mobilisation at the discretion of the surgeon. Grafts were reviewed at 2 and 6 weeks postoperatively. A skin was deemed successful if greater than 80% graft take has occurred on clinical examination. Data was entered into Microsoft Excel (Microsoft Corp., Redmond, WA, USA). Statistical analysis was done with SPSS 21 (Chicago, IL, USA). Normal distribution for statistical analysis was assumed with a parametric $t$-test and fisher's exact univariate analysis was used to determine significance.

## 3. Results

In total, 70 skin grafts were performed on 51 patients; 14 patients had multiple grafts performed. Baseline demographic and comorbidity data is shown in Table 1, the median

TABLE 1: Baseline factors of patients having lower limb skin grafts, data presented as (*n*, %) unless otherwise stated.

| | *n* = 51 |
|---|---|
| Age: median (range) | 79 years old (56–94 years old) |
| Patients having multiple grafts | 14 (28%) |
| Sex (male : female) | 22 : 29 |
| ASA: median | 2.5 |
| BMI: median (range) | 30 (20–69) |
| Venous insufficiency | 25 (49%) |
| Ischemic heart disease | 25 (49%) |
| Diabetes | 11 (22%) |
| Peripheral vascular disease | 11 (22%) |
| Smoking | 9 (18%) |
| Continued on anticoagulation/antiplatelet agent | 10 (20%) |
| Immunosuppressant medication | 4 (8%) |

TABLE 2: Operative details of lower limb skin grafts, data presented as (*n*, %) unless otherwise stated.

| | *n* = 70 |
|---|---|
| Indication | |
| (i) Cancer | 60 (86%) |
| (ii) Trauma | 8 (11%) |
| (iii) Ulcer | 2 (3%) |
| Elective case | 59 (84%) |
| Surface area of graft: median (range) | 0. 98 cm$^2$ (0.12–8.8 cm$^2$) |
| Type of graft | |
| (i) Split thickness | 64 (91%) |
| (ii) Full thickness | 6 (9%) |
| Type of dressing | |
| (i) Vacuum | 49 (70%) |
| (ii) Sponge | 21 (30%) |
| Management | |
| (i) Bed rest | 48 (69%) |
| (ii) Immediate mobilization | 22 (31%) |

age of the participants was 79 (range: 56–94 years old), and the majority of patients were female (57%, *n* = 29). The median BMI was 30 (range: 20–69), and nearly half of the patients had venous insufficiency and ischemic heart disease. There were also a high proportion of patients on immunosuppressant medication (8%, *n* = 4), and 11 patients (22%) had diabetes and peripheral vascular disease (PVD).

Elective surgery was performed in the vast majority of grafts (Table 2) and the main indication for surgery was skin cancer treatment. Over 2/3 of the grafts had placement of negative pressure dressing and placed on bed rest. The overall success rates of the grafts were 94%, 76%, and 67% at first inspection, 2 weeks, and 6 weeks, respectively. 17 grafts (24%) developed infection requiring antibiotics and 6 grafts (9%) developed a hematoma or seroma.

Bed rest and negative pressure dressing did not appear to be associated with increased graft success. The factors associated with graft failure were PVD, increased BMI, and use of immunosuppressant medications (Table 3). All failed skin grafts have gone onto to heal by secondary intention and no patients have required revision skin grafting procedures.

## 4. Discussion

In our experience, one-third of lower limb skin grafts failed at 6 weeks. Literature has reported rates of failure in lower limbs grafts of between 0 and 33% [6]. However, these rates are in a heterogeneous population with a variety of different indications, operative techniques, and followup. In addition to PVD and immunosuppressant use, we found increased BMI to be strongly associated with skin graft failure. The association of increased BMI and skin graft failure has not been described before. Penington and Morrison had identified waist to hip ratio to be associated with FTSG failure in the head and neck region in 14 patients [7]. Obese individuals are at increased risk of wound complications including wound infection, dehiscence, hematoma, and seroma formation [8]. Local and cellular factors including reduced microperfusion and decreased tissue oxygenation have been thought to play a part in this [7, 8]. Studies to explore specific mechanisms and impact of obesity as independent risk factor for poor operative outcome are still a much needed area for future research.

In our study, there was no difference in graft success rates between STSG and FTSG. To our knowledge, no study has directly compared outcomes between STSG and FTSG in the lower limb. A prospective study randomised 68 patients undergoing elective operations requiring radial forearm free flaps into receiving STSG or FTSG to the radial forearm free flap donor site [9]. No difference in outcomes was seen between the two groups, although patients with STSG required significantly more wound dressing changes compared to those who had FTSG. FTSG are thought to be superior to STSG in terms of cosmesis and decreased donor site complications [1]. However, STSG remain the most common method of skin coverage in grafting of the lower limbs owing to better scar quality than healing by secondary intention, ease of use, and ability to expand coverage through meshing [10]. The wound defects in the lower limb are often too large to be closed primarily and local flap repair can be difficult to achieve especially in elderly populations. It is also simpler to undertake revision surgery and oncological surveillance in patients who have had skin graft repairs compared to those with local flap repairs [10].

No difference in outcomes or complications was seen between patients placed on bed rest and those immediately mobilised. The vast majority of patients requiring lower limb grafts were placed on bed rest by the operating surgeon in our study. Bed rest is still widely used throughout the world despite an increasing body of evidence showing no significant benefit in outcomes [11]. Its popularity may be partly due to the clinical observation of decreased tissue oedema and perceived less graft disruption with limb elevation and bed rest, especially in this population with high rates of venous insufficiency. Similarly, no benefit in graft success rate was

TABLE 3: Analysis of success grafts versus failed grafts, data presented as ($n$, %) unless otherwise stated.

| | Graft success ($n = 48$) | Failure ($n = 22$) | $P$ value |
|---|---|---|---|
| Age (median) | 79 years old | 78 years old | 0.908 |
| Sex (male : female) | 21 : 27 | 8 : 14 | 0.753 |
| Venous insufficiency | 25 (52%) | 15 (60%) | 0.547 |
| Ischemic heart disease | 24 (50%) | 13 (59%) | 0.702 |
| Diabetes | 11 (23%) | 8 (36%) | 0.374 |
| Peripheral vascular disease | 20 (42%) | 16 (73%) | 0.030 |
| Smoking | 7 (15%) | 5 (23%) | 0.605 |
| BMI (median) | 30 | 42 | 0.007 |
| Bed rest | 32 (67%) | 16 (73%) | 0.829 |
| Vacuum dressing | 30 (63%) | 19 (86%) | 0.093 |
| Split thickness skin graft | 44 (92%) | 20 (91%) | 0.999 |
| Immunosuppressants | 1 (2%) | 5 (22%) | 0.020 |
| Acute operations | 7 (14.5%) | 4 (18%) | 0.951 |
| Graft size (median) | 0.94 cm$^2$ | 1.28 cm$^2$ | 0.331 |

seen with the use of negative pressure dressings; a recent Cochrane review found no evidence to support or refute the effectiveness of commercial negative pressure dressing to improve healing rates of skin grafts [12].

## 5. Conclusion

Lower limb skin grafts have high failure rates. Increased BMI, immunosuppressant use, and PVD appear to be significant risk factors associated with graft failure. Knowledge of these factors is important in preoperative assessment to identify patients at increased risk of postoperative complications. A larger prospective trial assessing the comparative effectiveness of different strategies aimed at minimising complications of lower limbs is needed.

## Conflict of Interests

The authors declare that there is no conflict of interests regarding the publication of this paper.

## References

[1] D. Ratner, "Skin grafting: from here to there," *Dermatologic Clinics*, vol. 16, no. 1, pp. 75–90, 1998.

[2] J. Southwell-Keely and J. Vandervord, "Mobilisation versus bed rest after skin grafting pretibial lacerations: a meta-analysis," *Plastic Surgery International*, vol. 2012, Article ID 207452, 6 pages, 2012.

[3] N. J. Henderson, M. Fancourt, W. Gilkison, S. Kyle, and D. Mosquera, "Skin grafts: a rural general surgical perspective," *ANZ Journal of Surgery*, vol. 79, no. 5, pp. 362–366, 2009.

[4] S. Paradela, S. Pita-Fernández, C. Peña et al., "Complications of ambulatory major dermatological surgery in patients older than 85 years," *Journal of the European Academy of Dermatology and Venereology*, vol. 24, no. 10, pp. 1207–1213, 2010.

[5] S. H. Wood and V. C. Lees, "A prospective investigation of the healing of grafted pretibial wounds with early and late

mobilisation," *British Journal of Plastic Surgery*, vol. 47, no. 2, pp. 127–131, 1994.

[6] T. O. Smith, "When should patients begin ambulating following lower limb split skin graft surgery? A systematic review," *Physiotherapy*, vol. 92, no. 3, pp. 135–145, 2006.

[7] A. J. Penington and W. A. Morrison, "Skin graft failure is predicted by waist-hip ratio: a marker for metabolic syndrome," *ANZ Journal of Surgery*, vol. 77, no. 3, pp. 118–120, 2007.

[8] J. A. Wilson and J. J. Clark, "Obesity: impediment to postsurgical wound healing," *Advances in Skin & Wound Care*, vol. 17, no. 8, pp. 426–435, 2004.

[9] A. J. Sidebottom, L. Stevens, M. Moore et al., "Repair of the radial free flap donor site with full or partial thickness skin grafts: a prospective randomised controlled trial," *International Journal of Oral and Maxillofacial Surgery*, vol. 29, no. 3, pp. 194–197, 2000.

[10] K. Rao, O. Tillo, and M. Dalal, "Full thickness skin graft cover for lower limb defects following excision of cutaneous lesions," *Dermatology Online Journal*, vol. 14, no. 2, article 4, 2008.

[11] B. Luczak, J. Ha, and R. Gurfinkel, "Effect of early and late mobilisation on split skin graft outcome," *Australasian Journal of Dermatology*, vol. 53, no. 1, pp. 19–21, 2012.

[12] J. Webster, P. Scuffham, K. L. Sherriff, M. Stankiewicz, and W. P. Chaboyer, "Negative pressure wound therapy for skin grafts and surgical wounds healing by primary intention," *Cochrane Database of Systematic Reviews*, vol. 4, Article ID CD009261, 2012.

# 20

# Sporotrichosis: An Overview and Therapeutic Options

**Vikram K. Mahajan**

*Department of Dermatology, Venereology & Leprosy, Dr. R. P. Govt. Medical College, Kangra, Tanda, Himachal Pradesh 176001, India*

Correspondence should be addressed to Vikram K. Mahajan; vkmahajan1@gmail.com

Academic Editor: Craig G. Burkhart

Sporotrichosis is a chronic granulomatous mycotic infection caused by *Sporothrix schenckii*, a common saprophyte of soil, decaying wood, hay, and sphagnum moss, that is endemic in tropical/subtropical areas. The recent phylogenetic studies have delineated the geographic distribution of multiple distinct *Sporothrix* species causing sporotrichosis. It characteristically involves the skin and subcutaneous tissue following traumatic inoculation of the pathogen. After a variable incubation period, progressively enlarging papulo-nodule at the inoculation site develops that may ulcerate (fixed cutaneous sporotrichosis) or multiple nodules appear proximally along lymphatics (lymphocutaneous sporotrichosis). Osteoarticular sporotrichosis or primary pulmonary sporotrichosis are rare and occur from direct inoculation or inhalation of conidia, respectively. Disseminated cutaneous sporotrichosis or involvement of multiple visceral organs, particularly the central nervous system, occurs most commonly in persons with immunosuppression. Saturated solution of potassium iodide remains a first line treatment choice for uncomplicated cutaneous sporotrichosis in resource poor countries but itraconazole is currently used/recommended for the treatment of all forms of sporotrichosis. Terbinafine has been observed to be effective in the treatment of cutaneous sporotrichosis. Amphotericin B is used initially for the treatment of severe, systemic disease, during pregnancy and in immunosuppressed patients until recovery, then followed by itraconazole for the rest of the therapy.

## 1. Introduction

Deep mycoses involving the skin and/or subcutaneous tissue (subcutaneous mycoses), fascial planes and bones, and/or various organs systems (deep mycoses) account for almost 1% of the total mycoses cases. In most instances of sub cutaneous mycoses, infection occurs following traumatic implantation of the etiologic fungi that are saprophytes to the soil and plant detritus. Although once considered endemic in tropical countries, these opportunistic infections are being increasingly observed across populations following accidental exposure to pathogen especially among returning travelers/workers. Current era of immunosuppression due to HIV infection, immunosuppressive therapy for cancers, autoimmune diseases, or organ transplantation has further contributed towards their increased prevalence. While chromoblastomycosis and phaeohyphomycosis, mycetomas, subcutaneous zygomycosis (entomophthoromycosis and mucormycosis), hyalohyphomycosis, and lobomycosis have limited area-specific presence, sporotrichosis, a subcutaneous mycotic infection from *Sporothrix schenckii*

species complex, perhaps remains the most reported subcutaneous mycosis worldwide. The heterogeneous morphology of lesions (nodules, plaques, noduloulcerative, ulcerative, nodulocystic or warty lesions, discharging sinuses, and subcutaneous swellings or masses) often makes the clinical diagnosis difficult particularly in nonendemic areas leading to delayed treatment and protracted clinical course causing significant morbidity and impact on public health. In majority, treatment becomes imperative as spontaneous resolution occurs as an exception [1]. Extracutaneous sporotrichosis is also an emerging mycosis in HIV infected patients [2, 3]. This paper presents an overview of sporotrichosis and therapeutic options.

## 2. Epidemiology

This chronic granulomatous subcutaneous mycotic infection is caused by *Sporothrix schenckii* species complex, a common saprophyte of soil, decaying wood, hay, and sphagnum moss. Recent molecular studies have demonstrated that *S. schenckii* is a complex of at least six clinicoepidemiologically important species with significant differences in geographical distribution, biochemical properties (dextrose, sucrose, and raffinose assimilation), degree of virulence, different disease patterns, and response to therapy. These include *S. albicans*, *S. brasiliensis* (in Brazil), *S. mexicana* (in Mexico), *S. globosa* (in UK, Spain, Italy, China, Japan, USA, and India), and *S. schenckii* sensu stricto [4–9]. Hence, the nomenclature "*Sporothrix schenckii* species complex" is preferred to earlier "*Sporothrix schenckii*" that was used to describe the strains from all over the world. According to Marimon et al. [7] human infections are mainly associated with *S. schenckii* sensu stricto, *Sporothrix brasiliensis*, and *Sporothrix globosa* while *Sporothrix mexicana* have only been identified among isolates of environmental origin with occasional exception [8, 10]. Henceforth, the nomenclature "*Sporothrix schenckii*" is used to represent the "*Sporothrix schenckii* species complex."

Sporotrichosis occurs worldwide with focal areas of hyperendemicity. It is particularly common in tropical/subtropical areas and temperate zones with warm and humid climate favoring the growth of saprophytic fungus but large outbreaks have occurred in other parts as well [11, 12]. Its worldwide incidence is unknown but Japan, China, Australia, Central and South America (Mexico, Brazil, Colombia, and Peru), and India (along the Sub-Himalayan region) account for most frequent occurrences [13–16]. Approximately, one case occur per 1000 people in Peru and in US 200–250 cases (1-2 cases per million) occur annually.

No age, gender, or race is spared of this infection as its occurrence depends upon the fungus in the environment and the portal of entry. The preponderance of males in most reported cases is attributed to their higher exposure risk than gender susceptibility. The traumatic inoculation is the obvious reason that exposed body parts, the extremities in particular, are involved most frequently; the upper limbs are affected twice as commonly as the lower limbs and involvement is infrequent [14, 17, 18].

The disease is almost endemic in rural areas and professionals handling plants or plant material such as farmers, gardeners, florists, foresters, and nursery workers are particularly at higher risk. The majority of these patients are between 20 and 50 years of age; the most active years of life when the individual is probably exposed maximally to injuries [14]. *S. schenckii* gains entry into the skin by traumatic implantation from contaminated thorns, hay stalks, barbs, soil, splinters, and bizarre/roadside injuries leading to cutaneous infection [14]. However, only 10–62% of patients recall any history of trauma as it is usually innocuous, occurs few weeks earlier, and is mostly forgotten [1, 14]. Although animals are not significant source of infection in humans, zoonotic transmission has been reported from insect bites, fish handling, and bites of cats, birds, dogs, rats, reptiles, and horses [19, 20]. Cats have been found to be important vehicle in dissemination of *S. schenckii* in a long-lasting epidemic of sporotrichosis in Brazil diagnosed by isolation of *S. schenckii* (*S. brasiliensis* in 97% isolates) from different types of samples, both from humans and from feline, indicating the emergence of another set of at-risk personnel [20–24]. Human-to-human spread, mostly from wound contamination from infected dressings or indigenous/herbal topical medication, interestingly remains underestimated [14, 25].

## 3. Clinical Presentations

Its exact incubation period remains unknown and may range from a few days to a few months, the average being 3 weeks [26]. The skin and the surrounding lymphatics are involved primarily leading to development of a small, indurated, progressively enlarging papulo-nodule at the inoculation site that may ulcerate (sporotrichotic chancre) without causing systemic symptoms. It may remain as such, or develops multiple lesions. Thereafter, sporotrichosis is presented in three main clinical types: lymphocutaneous, fixed cutaneous, and multifocal or disseminated cutaneous sporotrichosis. Extracutaneous or systemic sporotrichosis occurs from hematogenous spread from the primary inoculation site, the lymph node, or more usually from pulmonary disease in immunosuppressed patients. In children clinical profile is almost similar but facial involvement is more frequent accounting for 40–60% or as high 97% in some series [13, 17, 27]. It is also interesting to know that Brazilian isolates present a distinct clinical picture with immune manifestations (erythema multiforme), disseminated cutaneous lesions, and atypical forms [28, 29]. Such a varied disease spectrum has been attributed to factors like the mode of inoculation, the size and depth of the traumatic inoculum, the host immunity (fixed cutaneous sporotrichosis is considered to occur in patients with certain immunity against the fungus), and the virulence and thermotolerance of the fungus (the strains growing best at 35°C purportedly cause fixed cutaneous sporotrichosis and strains that grow both at 35°C and 37°C have been implicated for lymphocutaneous and extracutaneous disease) [12, 15, 30, 31]. However, the concept of thermosensitive strains of *S. schenckii* causing different clinical forms of the disease remains unsubstantiated [32]. Similarly, whether climate influences predominance of one or the other form also needs validation [33, 34].

*3.1. Lymphocutaneous Sporotrichosis.* It is the most common variety and accounts for 70–80% of the cases of cutaneous sporotrichosis [15, 35]. The extremities are affected most frequently. A noduloulcerative lesion (sporotrichotic chancre) at inoculation site and a string of similar nodules along the proximal lymphatics, with or without transient satellite adenopathy, characterizes this form (Figure 1). These secondary lesions appearing along lymphatics have varied morphology of erythematous papules, nodules, or plaques, having smooth or warty surface, and may soften and ulcerate discharging seropurulent material. They are mostly asymptomatic, may itch or become painful, and have indolent clinical course similar to that of the primary lesions.

*3.2. Fixed Cutaneous Sporotrichosis.* It occurs less commonly and is characterized by localized lesions at the inoculation site (Figure 2). Facial involvement occurs more frequently in fixed cutaneous sporotrichosis than in lymphocutaneous variety. The lesions are asymptomatic, erythematous, papules,

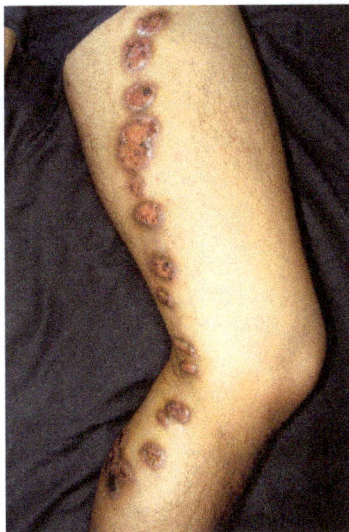

FIGURE 1: Lymphocutaneous sporotrichosis. Noduloulcerative lesions appear along the lymphatics proximal to the initial inoculation injury site.

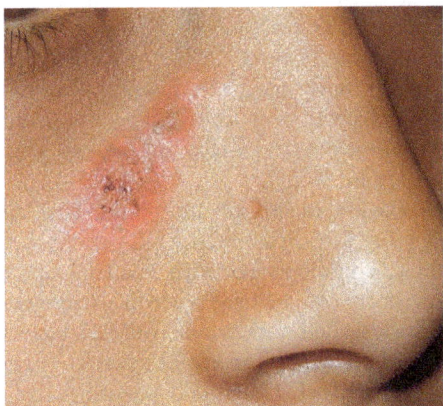

FIGURE 2: Fixed cutaneous sporotrichosis. A crusted/verrucous plaque develops at inoculation site, seen here over face of a child.

papulopustules, nodules, or verrucous plaques and occasionally nonhealing ulcers or small abscesses. The lesions may resemble keratoacanthoma, facial cellulitis, pyoderma gangrenosum, prurigo nodularis, soft tissue sarcoma, basal cell carcinoma, erysipeloid, or rosacea [14, 36, 37]. This form is considered to occur usually among hosts having high resistance wherein minimal lesions may subside spontaneously or persist exceptionally if not treated, and responds better to treatment [15, 38].

*3.3. Multifocal or Disseminated Cutaneous Sporotrichosis.* This rarely described variety means ≥3 lesions involving 2 different anatomical sites implies cutaneous dissemination following multiple traumatic implantations of the fungus or rarely from hematogenous spread in individuals apparently having no predisposing factors for immunosuppression [15, 39, 40].

*3.4. Extracutaneous Sporotrichosis.* This form of the disease usually occurs in the setting of immunosuppression as from alcoholism, diabetes, AIDS, underlying malignancy, use of corticosteroids, or other immunosuppressive drugs [1, 41, 42]. Although sinusitis, pulmonary, ocular or central nervous system disease, meningitis, and endophthalmitis are the usual manifestations, osteoarticular sporotrichosis remains the most common systemic manifestation both in immunocompetent and in immunocompromised individuals that is often confused with other chronic inflammatory arthritis until destruction of adjacent bones or draining sinuses develop [14, 43–45]. Cutaneous lesions are uncommon in osteoarticular sporotrichosis and it usually begins as monoarticular disease without systemic illness. The pain is usually less severe than the bacterial arthritis but functional impairment may become severe in untreated cases. Sporotrichotic osteoarthritis usually affects knee, wrist, elbow, and ankle joints in order of frequency manifesting initially with tenosynovitis, joint effusion, bursitis, and synovial cyst formation [44]. Extensive destructive changes often occur in the affected joints because of delayed diagnosis that is very common owing to lack of clinical suspicion. Radiographs of involved joint usually show soft tissue swelling and osteoporosis of contiguous bones or show no abnormality. Parasynovial swelling, subchondral erosions, and narrowing of joint space are uncommon.

Pulmonary disease from inhalation of conidia is rare and characterized by cough, low-grade fever, weight loss, mediastinal lymphadenitis, cavitation mimicking tuberculosis, fibrosis, and rarely massive hemoptysis [46, 47]. Apical lesions resembling pulmonary tuberculosis may occur in 85% of these cases [1]. Most patients usually have underlying severe chronic obstructive pulmonary disease and may present with subacute/chronic pneumonia. Involvement of central nervous system/meningeal in immunocompromised patients usually has subtle changes in mental status as the only symptom.

## 4. Diagnosis

Clinical suspicion is the key for early diagnosis and cutaneous lesions need to be differentiated from cutaneous tuberculosis, cutaneous leishmaniasis, nocardiosis, chromoblastomycosis, blastomycosis, paracoccidioidomycosis, and atypical mycobacteriosis [15, 16, 48]. Ulcerating lesions can mimic pyoderma gangrenosum [49].

Direct smear examination of pus or biopsy specimen for causative fungus is not diagnostic because of paucity of fungal cells. Fine needle aspiration cytology from a lesion, particularly in extracutaneous or disseminated forms, may occasionally show epithelioid cell granuloma, asteroid bodies, and/or yeast cells and cigar shaped bodies when stained with periodic acid-Schiff (PAS) or Gomori-methenamine silver (GMS) stains [1, 14, 50]. Civila et al. [51] could demonstrate asteroid bodies of *S. schenckii* in almost 86% cases comprising 36 patients of lymphocutaneous and 6 patients of fixed cutaneous sporotrichosis; nearly 95% of these cases also yielded positive cultures. However, the sensitivity/specificity of direct microscopic examination of tissue sample remains understudied as most researchers consider it unhelpful diagnostic tool due to paucity of fungal cells. The culture of *S. schenckii* in artificial media remains gold standard in diagnosis. The animal inoculation studies are usually not needed for diagnosis.

*4.1. Histopathology.* Histopathology is usually nonspecific and mimics other granulomatous diseases (deep fungal infections, cutaneous tuberculosis, leprosy, sarcoidosis, and foreign body granulomas). The histologic features varies from acute on chronic inflammation with characteristic zonation to chronic epithelioid cell granuloma with foreign body or Langhans' giant cells at both ends and nonspecific chronic granulomatous inflammatory cell infiltration of the dermis in the middle of the spectrum [14]. The major histopathologic features of fixed cutaneous sporotrichosis include central ulceration of epidermis, hyperkeratosis at the edge, acanthosis, and epidermal hyperplasia that may vary to the extent of pseudoepitheliomatous hyperplasia. Neutrophilic abscesses may be seen in the dermis and/or epidermis. There is usually dense cellular infiltrate comprising lymphocytes plasma cells and variable number of epithelioid histiocytes, giant cells, and eosinophils (mixed granulomatous cellular infiltrate) in upper- and middermis with or without fibro-capillary proliferation [52, 53]. Nodules of lymphocutaneous sporotrichosis characteristically show 3 concentric zones; the central necrotic zone contains amorphous debris and polymorphonuclear leukocytes (zone of chronic suppuration); the middle tuberculoid zone is composed of epithelioid cells, giant cells (predominantly Langhans' type), and the outer zone comprising numerous plasma cells, lymphocytes, and fibroblasts with prominent capillary hyperplasia and proliferation (syphiloid zone) [14, 52]. However, this zonation becomes indistinct in older lesions. The fungal elements, when present, are visualized within these zones in PAS or GMS stained histologic sections. They appear globose, budding yeast-like cells measuring $3-8\,\mu m$ in diameter (in 84% cases), cigar shaped cells sized $1-2 \times 4-5\,\mu m$ (in 33% cases) or oval to round or single budding forms of the yeast within the cytoplasm of giant cells or in the centre of asteroid bodies [1, 17, 54]. Asteroid bodies, sized $15-35\,\mu m$ in diameter, are usually seen in 40–85% of chronic sporotrichosis cases as extracellular and within the abscesses [1, 16, 17, 54]. Although observed more frequently in the lymphocutaneous variety, they do not differ morphologically from those seen in fixed cutaneous sporotrichosis. Their demonstration by direct immunofluorescence and specific immunohistochemical techniques is considered more sensitive and specific [55, 56]. Splendore-Hoeppli phenomenon, wherein one of the several fungal elements enveloped by an eosinophilic material radiating centrifugally in a sunburst fashion with its central portion reacting immunohistochemically with an anti-*Sporothrix schenckii* antibody, perhaps represents an immunologic interaction between the host and the pathogen [50–52]. However, the presence of asteroid bodies or Splendore-Hoeppli phenomenon is not pathognomonic and may be observed often in other granulomatous and/or infectious diseases as well; at best, they can aid in the diagnosis [51].

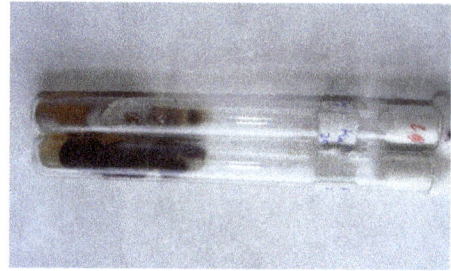

FIGURE 3: *Sporothrix schenckii* colony on Sabouraud's glucose agar (SDA) at $25°C$. Initial cream color turns brown black as it matures.

*4.2. Culture and Identification of Causative Fungus.* The various *Sporothrix* species appear similar in morphology, but only *S. schenckii* is pathogenic to humans. *S. schenckii* can be grown from skin biopsy or other clinical samples (sputum, pus, synovial fluid/biopsy, bone drainage/biopsy, and cerebrospinal fluid) on Sabouraud's glucose agar (SDA), brain heart infusion agar, or Mycosel at $25°C$ and the growth is visible in 3–5 days to 2 weeks [1]. Incubation of cultures at $37°C$ in blood glucose-cysteine agar or brain-heart infusion broth will produce its yeast form. The initial cream-colored colonies grown on SDA at $25°C$ are smooth and moist but turn brown/black after a few weeks due to melanin production that protects it from phagocytosis and killing by human monocytes and macrophages and extracellular proteinases (Figure 3) [57].

Microscopically, in lactophenol cotton blue mounts, *S. schenckii* appears as delicate branching septate hyphae with slender, short, conidiophores with tapering tips and surrounding pyriform conidia in a flower-like arrangement or as individual thick-walled, dark brown conidia attached directly to the hypha often in dense sleeve-like pattern (Figure 4(a)). In practice, S. schenckii is usually identified by its characteristic colony morphology, microscopic appearance and temperature dimorphism that is, its ability to exist as a mold at $25°C$ (room temperature) and as yeast at $37°C$ (in host tissues) (Figure 4(b)) [1, 58].

*4.3. Intradermal Testing, Molecular and Other Diagnostic Techniques.* The diagnostic value of all these tests is not reliable for diagnosis of sporotrichosis in view of significant variations in their specificity and sensitivity. Moreover, these tests remain to be of limited value in view of their unavailability for routine diagnostic use. Nevertheless, they are useful to raise a diagnostic suspicion prompting more aggressive diagnostic workup.

The diagnostic significance of intradermal tests to detect delayed hypersensitivity using sporotrichin or peptide-rhamnomannan (PRM) antigen remains ambiguous. They are negative in severe or disseminated sporotrichosis cases and are often positive in cured patients or in healthy people living in endemic areas [14, 15].

Analysis of antibody responses by immunoblotting and enzyme-linked immunosorbent assay (ELISA), agglutination, compliment-fixation tests, immunohistochemical,

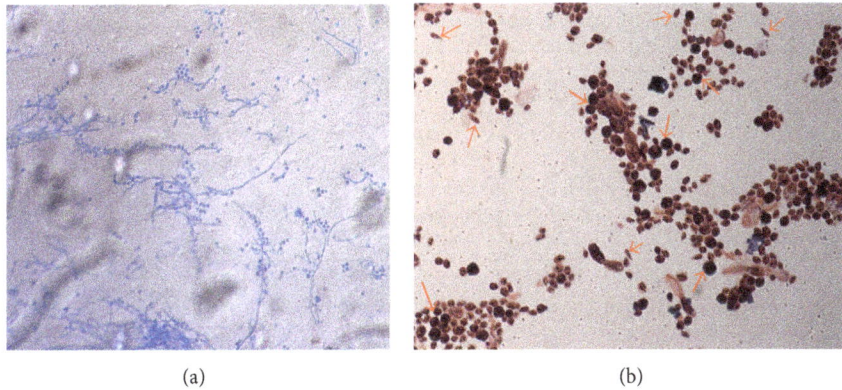

(a)                                              (b)

FIGURE 4: (a) *Sporothrix schenckii* from culture on SDA at 25°C. Seen here is delicate branching, mold form with pyriform conidia in characteristic flower-like arrangement or sleeve-like pattern (stain-lactophenol cotton blue ×40). (b) Yeast phase of *Sporothrix schenckii* isolate from culture on brain heart infusion agar at 37°C. Budding yeast cells (thick arrows) and cigar shaped yeast cells (thin arrows) interspersed between spores (Grams' stain, ×100) are seen here.

immunofluorescence, immunodiffusion, and immunoelectrophoresis techniques and detection of *S. schenckii* by polymerase chain reaction (PCR) or polymerase chain reaction-restriction fragment length polymorphism (PCR-RFLP) of calmodulin gene are useful in diagnosing rarer extracutaneous and disseminated forms [15, 59–61]. For instance, cerebrospinal fluid (CSF) antibody titers higher than serum antibody titers may be indicative of sporotrichotic meningitis. The ELISA has a reported sensitivity of 90% with 86% overall efficacy when tested against sera obtained from patients with any form of sporotrichosis [62]. Restriction fragment length polymorphism (RFLP) analysis of mitochondrial DNA is reportedly useful for identification, taxonomy, typing, and epidemiology of *S. Schenckii* [63]. Serological testing using antigenic fraction of the *S. schenckii* that binds concanavalin-A represents a more recent diagnostic tool [64].

*4.4. Imaging Studies.* Routine radio-imaging studies are usually not needed for the diagnosis of sporotrichosis unless specific systemic involvement is suspected. For instance, conventional X-rays or CT scan for the chest (pulmonary sporotrichosis) or other involved areas (osteoarticular sporotrichosis) will be supportive in the management but not specifically diagnostic of sporotrichosis.

# 5. Treatment Options

Spontaneous resolution is extremely rare and majority of the patients will require treatment. There are no well-controlled studies for the treatment of sporotrichosis and various treatment schedules recommended by Infectious Diseases Society of America are empirical and primarily based on case reports, retrospective reviews, and nonrandomized trials (Table 1) [65]. Low cost, ease of administration, safety profile, and the site of infection (localized or disseminated) often dictate the choice of therapy. Severe and systemic infection will require treatment that is more aggressive despite concern for drug-associated toxicities. Resolution of active infection and eradication of *S. Schenckii* from tissues remain the desired outcome of all treatments. The duration of 3–6 months for

treatment of sporotrichosis remains arbitrary but any treatment must be continued for at least a period of 4 to 6 weeks after complete clinical remission to achieve mycological cure. Although treatment is prolonged and expensive, complete recovery without scarring is expected in cutaneous sporotrichosis following appropriate therapy. However, compromised pulmonary functions in pulmonary disease, severe disability from chronic osteoarticular sporotrichosis, or occasional scarring may result [36, 47, 66]. Patients with immunosuppression usually require life-long suppressive therapy.

Until recently and before the availability/approval of itraconazole, saturated solution of potassium iodide had been the standard treatment since the time it was introduced in 19th century and yet remains a first choice to treat uncomplicated disease in resource poor countries.

*5.1. Saturated Solution of Potassium Iodide.* Saturated solution of potassium iodide (SSKI) administered orally remains the low cost, first choice of the treatment for uncomplicated cutaneous sporotrichosis especially when high cost of itraconazole is precluding. However, it is not effective in extracutaneous form of sporotrichosis. The exact mechanism of its action against *S. Schenckii* remains poorly elucidated. Possibly, it inhibits granuloma formation through some immunologic and nonimmunologic mechanisms thereby exposing the fungus to the host defenses or other antifungal agents used concurrently [67]. However, it does not appear to increase monocyte or neutrophil killing of *S. Schenckii*. Interestingly, *S. Schenckii* can grow when plated with 10% SSKI suggesting that it has no fungistatic or fungicidal activity. It has been suggested that it gets converted to iodine *in-vivo* by myeloperoxidase, a hydrogen peroxide system of polymorphonuclear cells, and exerts its cidal effect as has been demonstrated from its inhibitory effect on germination of cells and their direct destruction on ultrastructure examination of *S. Schenckii* exposed to iodine-potassium-iodine solution [68].

SSKI is the most extensively used mode of treatment in both fixed cutaneous and lymphocutaneous sporotrichosis across countries especially from developing world where

TABLE 1: Recommendations by Infectious Diseases Society of America for Sporotrichosis Treatment[*].

| Sr. number | Clinical manifestations | Preferred treatment [dose] | Alternative treatment | Remarks |
|---|---|---|---|---|
| 1 | Uncomplicated cutaneous sporotrichosis | Itraconazole [200 mg/day] | Itraconazole [200 mg b.i.d.] or terbinafine [500 mg b.i.d.] or SSKI [increasing doses] or fluconazole [400–800 mg/day] or local hyperthermia | Treatment for 2–4 weeks after lesions have resolved |
| 2 | Osteoarticular sporotrichosis | Itraconazole [200 mg twice daily (b.i.d.)] | Liposomal amphotericin B (3–5 mg/kg/day) or deoxycholate amphotericin B [0.7–1 mg/kg/day] until resolution | Switching to itraconazole after resolution and treatment for a total of 12 months |
| 3 | Pulmonary sporotrichosis | Liposomal amphotericin B [3–5 mg/kg/day] and then itraconazole [200 mg b.i.d.] | Deoxycholate amphotericin B [0.7–1 mg/kg/day] until recovery and then itraconazole [200 mg b.i.d.] | Treating less severe disease with itraconazole. Treatment for at least 12 months |
| 4 | Meningeal sporotrichosis | Liposomal Amphotericin B [3–5 mg/kg/day] and then itraconazole [200 mg b.i.d.] | Deoxycholate amphotericin B [0.7–1 mg/kg/day] until recovery and then itraconazole [200 mg b.i.d.] | Length of therapy with amphotericin B is not established. Treatment for 4–6 weeks and total of 12 months. Suppressive therapy with itraconazole is needed |
| 5 | Disseminated sporotrichosis | Liposomal amphotericin B [3–5 mg/kg/day] and then itraconazole [200 mg b.i.d.] | Deoxycholate amphotericin B [0.7–1 mg/kg/day] until recovery and then Itraconazole [200 mg b.i.d.] | Treatment with amphotericin B until objective improvement and for at least 12 months. Suppressive therapy with itraconazole is needed |
| 6 | Sporotrichosis in pregnant women | Treating only severe sporotrichosis with liposomal amphotericin B [3–5 mg/kg/day] or deoxycholate amphotericin B [0.7–1 mg/kg/day]. Treatment with local hyperthermia [approx. 45°C] for uncomplicated cutaneous sporotrichosis | | Preferably, defer treatment for uncomplicated cases |
| 7 | Sporotrichosis in children | Itraconazole [6–10 mg/kg/d or maximum of 400 mg/day] for mild disease, deoxycholate amphotericin B [0.7–1 mg/kg/day] for severe disease | SSKI with increasing doses equivalent to half the adult dose for a duration as in adults | Treating severe disease with an amphotericin B formulation |

[*]Modified after Kauffman et al. [65].

most cases occur and that too is without specific treatment trials. Failure of therapy unrelated to compliance is reported exceptionally [69, 70] and most reports delineate its efficacy to an extent that a favorable therapeutic response is considered nearly diagnostic in the absence of mycologic support [1, 13, 14, 17, 18, 39, 58, 71, 72]. It has been found effective even in cases not responding to itraconazole [73, 74]. However, no specific recommendations/guidelines or treatment schedules are available. SSKI, containing 1 g/mL of potassium iodide, is usually prescribed in a starting dose of 5 drops (using a standard eye dropper) three times a day (t.i.d.), taken orally mixed with fruit juice or milk to mask its unpalatable taste. The dose is increased daily by 5 drops t.i.d. up to a maximum dose of 30 to 40 drops t.i.d. until complete healing. The response becomes evident within 2 weeks and healing occurs in 4–32 weeks [14, 72]. However, this schedule remains incomprehensive particularly for patients working outdoors

for long hours resulting in poor compliance. Cabezas et al. [75] compared the safety and efficacy of once-daily versus 3-times daily dosing in a randomized nonblinded clinical trial on 57 pediatric patients with culture confirmed fixed cutaneous or lymphocutaneous sporotrichosis. The starting dose of SSKI 150 mg/day was increased to maximum of 160 mg/day in both groups. Although, adverse events were higher (61% versus 42%) with once-daily dose, the cure rates were comparable in both groups.

Adverse effects such as metallic taste, flu-like syndrome, excessive lacrimation, gastrointestinal upsets, parotid swelling, acneiform or papulopustular eruptions, exacerbation of dermatitis herpetiformis, and lesional pain and inflammation in rare instances may lead to noncompliance in as high as 60% cases but rarely need discontinuation of treatment [13, 15, 17, 39]. Metallic taste signifies threshold of maximum tolerable dose and the dosage is adjusted at a lower level. Hypothyroidism or hyperthyroidism, iododerma, cardiac irritability, vasculitis, pustular psoriasis, pulmonary edema, urticaria and angioedema, myalgia, lymphadenopathy, and eosinophilia are some potential adverse reactions [14, 76]. Hypothyroidism associated with SSKI therapy is usually precipitated in patients already having defective (partial) autoregulation mechanism (as from Hashimoto's thyroiditis, surgery, or radioactive iodide therapy for Graves' disease) that maintains thyroid hormone synthesis. Thyroid gland stops producing thyroid hormone by negative feedback mechanism when excess quantities of iodine exist (Wolff-Chaikoff effect). Inbuilt autoregulation mechanism maintains a storage pool of organic iodine in the thyroid gland and ensures that it produces enough thyroid hormone for the patient to remain euthyroid (escape phenomenon) [76]. In the complete absence of autoregulation mechanism (as in patients from areas of iodine deficiency having long-standing goiter) due to presence of autonomous thyroid foci the thyroid synthesizes excess thyroid hormone leading to thyrotoxicosis (Jod-Basedow disease). However, unless preexisting thyroid disease is suspected baseline thyroid function studies are not required as the therapeutic effect usually occurs in few weeks and within the period of "escape phenomenon." Discontinuation of SSKI will usually restore normal thyroid functioning within a month in case of iatrogenic hypothyroidism. Patients taking angiotensin-converting enzyme inhibitors, potassium-sparing diuretics, or with renal impairment may develop potassium toxicity and need careful monitoring during SSKI therapy. SSKI is currently pregnancy category D drug. Therapy with SSKI should not be reinstituted in patients developing "flu-like syndrome"/hypersensitivity to SSKI as they will suffer adverse reactions even at low doses.

### 5.2. Azoles (Itraconazole, Fluconazole, and Ketoconazole).
All azoles inhibit cytochrome P450 enzyme system and concomitant administration of drugs metabolized by this enzyme system (digoxin, warfarin, phenytoin, carbamazepine, phenobarbitone, rifampicin, cisapride, astemizole, triazolam, midazolam, lovastatin/simvastatin, H-2 antagonists, and oral hypoglycemic agents) remains contraindicated because of potential serious toxicities. They are also contraindicated in pregnancy and hypersensitivity to azoles.

*Itraconazole*, the oral antifungal agent from azoles, in a dose of 100–200 mg daily is effective and well-tolerated and has largely replaced SSKI and amphotericin B with its 90–100% efficacy rates in cutaneous as well as extracutaneous sporotrichosis [77]. It inhibits enzyme cytochrome P450 lanosterol 14$\alpha$-demethylase that converts lanosterol to ergosterol, the main sterol in fungal cell wall. Its minimum inhibitory concentration (MIC) of 0.1–1.0 mg/L for the yeast form is well achieved with the recommended therapeutic doses and has concentration in stratum corneum that is nearly 10-fold higher than the plasma levels. Itraconazole is also used in pulse regimens as it persists in the stratum corneum for 3-4 weeks (for 6–12 months in nails) after discontinuation. Despite its high cost it has become the drug of choice for treating both cutaneous (fixed and lymphocutaneous) and osteoarticular varieties of sporotrichosis

with success rates varying between 90 and 100% (60%–80% for osteoarticular sporotrichosis) [60, 75]. It is administered orally in a dose of 200–400 mg/day (minimum dose 200 mg/day) for a period of 3 to 6 months (1 year for osteoarticular and disseminated forms) as per current guidelines from Infectious Diseases Society of America (IDSA) [65]. Adequate response without recurrences or adverse effects has been observed in both fixed and lymphocutaneous sporotrichosis even at 100 mg daily given for a mean duration of 18 weeks but higher doses between 150 and 200 mg daily are generally favored [26, 78, 79]. It is an acceptable alternative in patients who are intolerant to SSKI or when itraconazole is easily available/affordable despite reported relapses or therapeutic failure [73, 74, 79]. Fixed cutaneous variety responds at lesser duration than lymphocutaneous form. However, higher doses are generally recommended for poor responders or relapsed cases but are associated with adverse drug reactions [80]. Bonifaz et al. [81] by using oral itraconazole 400 mg/day for one week with a 3-week break (pulse therapy) achieved clinical and mycological cure in their 4 of 5 patients with cutaneous sporotrichosis (one of four patient with lymphocutaneous variety was lost to follow-up, and one patient had fixed cutaneous sporotrichosis). Thereafter, the drug was administered as pulses until clinical and mycological cure that was achieved after 2 (for fixed cutaneous variety) to 5 pulses. Song et al. [82] further compared oral itraconazole pulse therapy (200 mg b.i.d. for 1 week and off for 3 weeks, average pulses 2.65 $\pm$ 0.81) with daily dosing (100 mg b.i.d., mean duration 2.80 $\pm$ 2.33 months) in prospective, randomized, evaluator blinded study comprising 25 patients with cutaneous sporotrichosis in each group. Although more patients receiving continuous therapy showed cure (95.8%) than those receiving pulse therapy (81.8%) at 48 weeks, the results were not statistically significant. However, not many studies are available on this mode of treatment for making any recommendation. It was moderately effective in osteoarticular sporotrichosis with a cure rate of 73% in a small series of 11 patients who had relapsed after initial cure [75]. However, all 6 patients of osteoarticular sporotrichosis responded to itraconazole in another study [83]. Nevertheless, relapses have occurred 1–7 months after treatment duration of 6–18 months or even after repeated treatment with itraconazole [79]. Nausea and epigastric pain, hypercholesterolemia or hypertriglyceridemia, altered liver function tests (rarely serious hepatotoxicity), headache, and peripheral edema are some of its reported adverse effects observed more frequently with higher doses. Variable therapeutic outcome is another limitation for its use. No dosage adjustment is usually needed in patients with hepatorenal dysfunction.

*Fluconazole* is a synthetic broad-spectrum bistriazole antifungal agent that selectively inhibits fungal cytochrome P-450 that is necessary for sterol C-14 alpha-demethylation to ergosterol, an essential for fungal cytoplasmic membrane integrity. This leads to abnormal permeability, membrane bound enzyme activity, and coordination of chitin synthesis. Used orally alone or in combination with SSKI, fluconazole provides another useful therapeutic option. It has been used to treat both fixed and lymphocutaneous sporotrichosis in doses between 150 mg once a week and 200 mg daily [84, 85]. However, higher doses between 400 and 600 mg/day are generally recommended especially for treating visceral and osteoarticular sporotrichosis but the response generally remains poor [36, 72, 86, 87]. Prolonged therapy with doses of 400–800 mg/day given for several months has been associated with alopecia [86]. Nausea, vomiting and diarrhea, abdomen pain, headache, and abnormal liver enzymes observed commonly rarely necessitate discontinuation of treatment. It is contraindicated in pregnancy because of its teratogenic potential [88]. As the experience with fluconazole therapy in sporotrichosis is limited, it remains a second-line treatment option for patients intolerant to itraconazole for being moderately effective.

Response to *Ketoconazole* remains discouraging and it is not recommended to treat sporotrichosis [14, 79, 89]. Sharkey-Mathis et al. [79] observed complete failure of treatment with ketoconazole at doses as high as 400–600 mg given daily for 7–9 months. Apart from low efficacy, even lower than fluconazole, hepatotoxicity is another limitation for its use.

*5.3. Allylamines (Terbinafine).* Terbinafine is another alternative agent to treat cutaneous or lymphocutaneous sporotrichosis that is unresponsive to itraconazole or when itraconazole is not tolerated. It is well absorbed following oral administration, has low binding to microsomal cytochrome P450 enzyme, and has no effect on bioavailability of other drugs metabolized by this enzyme system. Being highly lipophilic its antifungal activity is maintained from adipose tissue depots few weeks after discontinuation of treatment. It inhibits ergosterol synthesis by inhibiting squalene epoxidase for exerting its fungicidal effect. It is effective against most dermatophytes, *Aspergillus* species, blastomycosis, histoplasmosis, and *Scopulariopsis brevicaulis* and other fungi including *S. schenckii*. It has a long half-life and has been shown to have good *in vitro* activity against *S. schenckii* (MIC range of 0.007–0.5 μg/mL) [90]. However, there is no consensus for optimal dosage and duration schedule for terbinafine. It has been used alone or in combination with SSKI to treat few patients in doses ranging from 125 to 1000 mg/day given for 4–37 weeks to achieve clinical cure in small series or case reports [90, 91]. Francesconi et al. [90] achieved cure with terbinafine 250 mg daily without recurrences in 96% of 50 patients with cutaneous sporotrichosis being on simultaneous treatment for other comorbidities like hypertension, diabetes mellitus, dyslipidemias, arrhythmia, and so forth. Its efficacy in a dose of 250 mg/day is reportedly comparable with itraconazole 100 mg/day (92.7% versus 92%) administered for mean duration of 11.5 and 11.8 weeks, respectively [92]. However, terbinafine regimens using higher doses have shown superior efficacy. Terbinafine 500 mg b.i.d. administered for a mean of 13.9±6.7 weeks cured 87% of 35 patients as compared to 52% of 28 patients receiving 250 mg b.i.d. for a mean of 17.7 ± 5.8 weeks in a multicenter, double blind, randomized clinical trial [93]. It is currently a pregnancy category B drug.

*5.4. Polyenes (Amphotericin B).* Amphotericin B (deoxycholate), a lipophilic polyene macrolide antibiotics synthesized from *Streptomyces nodosus*, is available mainly for intravenous or topical use as an antifungal agent. It binds to ergosterol or other sterols in the fungal cytoplasmic membrane causing mechanical interruption enhancing permeability of fungal cell membrane for monovalent ions (sodium, potassium) and other molecules and cell death. However, its main fungicidal activity has been attributed to its ability to cause autooxidation of the cytoplasmic membrane and release of lethal free radicals. It is safe during pregnancy and is a drug of choice for treating severely recalcitrant and disseminated cutaneous and/or pulmonary/meningeal sporotrichosis or HIV-associated disease. It may also be indicated in patients with extensive osteoarticular sporotrichosis or who are not responding to adequate itraconazole therapy but its intraarticular use is considered unwarranted [75]. After initial 1 mg intravenous testing dose, the recommended adult dose of 0.25 mg/kg/day is increased to achieve the targeted dose of 2–3 gm [26]. Fever, chills, headache, malaise, and vomiting that may occur during drug administration can be ameliorated by premedication with sedatives, antipyretics, and corticosteroids. Hypokalemia, hypomagnesemia, nephrotoxicity, and reversible normochromic normocytic anemia are common adverse effect and require regular once-weekly monitoring. Cardiovascular and bone marrow toxicity occurs rarely [26]. Availability of new lipid formulations of amphotericin B has improved its safety profile by delivering higher concentrations of the drug and decreased nephrotoxicity. It is usually used in a dose of 3–5 mg/kg of lipid formulation or 0.7 to 1.0 mg/kg/day of amphotericin B deoxycholate depending upon the severity of the disease [65]. Although there are no guidelines in view of variable therapeutic response from amphotericin B, it is usually recommended in the initial phase of therapy, until a favorable response is achieved, followed by itraconazole for rest of the treatment course [65].

*5.5. Flucytosine.* This synthetic fluorinated pyrimidine acts synergistically with amphotericin B to reduce its dose to lessen its toxicity. Amphotericin B enhances permeability of fungal cell wall and facilitates penetration of flucytosine. Its deamination occurs within fungal cells to fluorouracil that disrupts fungal RNA and DNA metabolism. The usual dose is 50–150 mg/kg/day given four times daily for 6–12 weeks [26]. Cure has been achieved for disseminated sporotrichosis of skin and bone with a combination of amphotericin B (4.8 gm) and 5-fluorocytosine (8 gm/day, 100 mg/kg/day) in 6 months [94]. However, its use is no longer recommended due to serious adverse reactions (gastrointestinal intolerance, bone marrow toxicity, and photosensitivity) and availability of better alternatives.

*5.6. Newer Antifungals.* The use of posaconazole or ravuconazole in patients with sporotrichosis remains understudied. Posaconazole has shown good activity against all the five species of *S. schenckii* complex and activity of ravuconazole is limited to only against *S. brasiliensis* in *in vitro* studies [83]. Echinocandins has shown no activity against *S. schenckii* and voriconazole is not recommended for treatment of sporotrichosis due to its limited *in vitro* activity against *Sporothrix* spp. [95–97].

*5.7. Antifungal Susceptibility Profile.* The variability in therapeutic efficacy and *in vitro* activity demonstrated in different studies is attributed to the fact that *S. schenckii* is a complex of different species. For instance, itraconazole has shown good *in vitro* activity against *S. brasiliensis* whereas the drug showed high minimum inhibitory concentrations when tested for the other species [95]. Terbinafine was the most active drug in *in vitro* studies as compared to itraconazole, ketoconazole, or posaconazole against human and animal isolates of *S. schenckii* while *S. brasiliensis* showed the best response to antifungals and *S. mexicana* had the worst response [95, 98]. *S. globosa* and *S. schenckii* were found to be itraconazole-resistant strains while terbinafine was the most active drug, followed by ketoconazole and itraconazole, and fluconazole and voriconazole were less effective in a recent *in vitro* study from Brazil [99]. In a similar study from Sao Paulo (Brazil), itraconazole and posaconazole were moderately effective against *S. schenckii* and *S. brasiliensis* while flucytosine, caspofungin, and fluconazole showed no *in vitro* antifungal activity against any of *Sporothrix* species (*S. schenckii*, *S. brasiliensis*, and *S. mexicana*) in another study [100]. Posaconazole has shown efficacy for *S. brasiliensis* and *S. schenckii* sensu stricto infections in experimental murine models [101]. Voriconazole had not shown antifungal activity against *S. brasiliensis* and had only fungistatic effect in mice infected with *S. schenckii* sensu stricto [102].

*5.8. Thermotherapy.* Temperatures above 38.5°C are detrimental to the growth of *Sporothrix* and directly damage the pathogen and, in addition, local hyperthermia is considered to enhance intracellular killing capability of neutrophils [103]. The daily application of local heat (42°-43°C) to the lesion for weeks using heat compresses or hand held pocket warmer, infrared or far infrared heater is recommended for treating small lesions in fixed cutaneous variety or cutaneous sporotrichosis in pregnant women pending specific therapy. Its reported cure rate is 71% among 14 patients in a study by using different modes of thermotherapy but in general its efficacy remains largely unevaluated [65, 71, 104]. Nonetheless, it can best be combined with SSKI or itraconazole for adjunctive benefit. The heat is usually applied for 15–60 minutes several times daily until the lesions heal or specific therapy is instituted [71].

*5.9. Surgical Interventions.* Surgical excision is usually not recommended, as it is not unusual for the disease to get destabilized and disseminate following minor trauma such as biopsy procedure [36]. However, invasive procedures are required for obtaining clinical samples such as full-thickness skin or bone biopsy, arthrocentesis for synovial tissue biopsy, or bronchoscopy with bronchoalveolar lavage for culture and transbronchial biopsy to establish laboratory diagnosis. Similarly, surgical therapy sometimes becomes unavoidable as in the management of osteoarticular sporotrichosis along with antimicrobial therapy for eradication of infection as

for any other bone and joint infections. Joint damage can be minimized by appropriate drainage of infected joints or debridement of sequestrum but arthrodesis may be needed when joint destruction ensues [66]. Combination of surgical resection of the involved lung segment and amphotericin B is considered better than either mode used alone for pulmonary sporotrichosis [65]. Nevertheless, surgical excision/debridement as a sole therapy is neither effective nor recommended and it will always be prudent to combine surgical procedures with appropriate drug therapy for better therapeutic outcome.

*5.10. Treatment of Sporotrichosis in Pregnant Women and Children.* SSKI is currently pregnancy category D drug and remains contraindicated in pregnant/lactating women for possible development of neonatal hypothyroidism and/or thyromegaly unless benefits outweigh the risks. Terbinafine is not approved for use in pregnancy and azoles must be avoided. Local hyperthermia can be used to treat cutaneous sporotrichosis that does not require urgent therapy. However, for sporotrichosis that must be treated during pregnancy, liposomal amphotericin B (3–5 mg/kg/day) can be used. As there is no risk of worsening of sporotrichosis or its dissemination to the fetus, treatment is best delayed in pregnant patients. Cases of sporotrichosis in children have been reported less frequently than in adults. Nevertheless, they are not uncommon. Pediatric patients with sporotrichosis can be treated with an equivalent to half the adult dose of SSKI, up to a maximum of 15 drops thrice daily or itraconazole 6–10 mg/kg/day (max 400 mg/d) for 3-4 months as in adults [14, 27]. Most clinicians prefer itraconazole as their first choice of treatment in children for convenient once a day dosing. SSKI, itraconazole, and terbinafine have been used successfully to treat sporotrichosis in infants aged <10 months [105]. However, availability of pediatric formulations of antifungal agents remains a limitation. Local heat therapy is another useful option for limited cutaneous disease in children.

*5.11. Treatment of Sporotrichosis in Patients with Immunosuppression or HIV Disease.* Predisposing conditions responsible for immunosuppression like diabetes mellitus, chronic alcoholism, myeloproliferative disorders, immunosuppressive therapy for organ transplant, autoimmune disorders, or cancers, prolonged treatment with systemic corticosteroids and HIV infection have been implicated for extracutaneous sporotrichosis, an opportunistic form of infection. Cutaneous lesions are usually multiple and widespread. Cutaneous dissemination with or without systemic involvement can occur in patients with AIDS. Extracutaneous sporotrichosis in the form of invasive sinusitis, ocular sporotrichosis, pulmonary infection, osteoarthritis, and spread to central nervous system has been documented [2, 3, 106]. Immunocompromised patients having dissemination of infection to central nervous system/meninges usually manifest with subtle changes in mental status as the only symptom. Liposomal amphotericin B in recommended doses is the drug of first choice in these patients and they will need suppressive therapy with oral itraconazole 200 mg/d for life after the clinical cure, as eradication of the pathogen may not be possible at all.

## 6. Comments

Cutaneous and subcutaneous involvement in sporotrichosis is more common than disseminated forms and can be treated readily, if the cost is not precluding, with oral itraconazole 200 mg/d for 2–4 weeks after all lesions have healed usually for 3–6 months. Patients not responding to this regimen should get either oral itraconazole 200 mg twice daily, oral terbinafine 500 mg twice daily, or SSKI in standard dosing schedule. The osteoarticular, visceral, and disseminated forms of sporotrichosis are uncommon and occur more often in patients with immunosuppression and are difficult to treat. Oral itraconazole 200 mg twice daily for at least 12 months is generally recommended for osteoarticular sporotrichosis and less-severe disease. Liposomal amphotericin B (3–5 mg/kg/day) can be used for initial therapy with subsequent switch to oral itraconazole for severe or life-threatening pulmonary sporotrichosis, meningeal sporotrichosis, and disseminated sporotrichosis. Upon clinical stabilization, therapy can be changed to oral itraconazole 200 mg twice daily for a minimum of 12 months.

Recent concept that *S. schenckii* is a complex of different phylogenic species with different geographic distribution, virulence, and *in vitro* susceptibility to antifungal agents has helped in understanding variability of therapeutic response observed across antimicrobial agents. This perhaps will form the basis for future research particularly in therapeutics that remains under studied and lacks well-designed controlled clinical trials. The possibility of yeast form of *S. schenckii* being more susceptible to various antifungal agents also needs to be explored further [107]. Infectious Diseases Society of America currently recommends itraconazole as first line treatment for subcutaneous sporotrichosis. However, SSKI still forms the preferred treatment in most developing countries where major chunk of the disease occurs. Thus, improved formulations of SSKI that are more palatable, have simplified administration regimen, and have improved compliance are highly desirable. The observed improved efficacy of itraconazole in combination with SSKI versus either drug used alone in phaeohyphomycosis requires evaluation in the treatment of sporotrichosis as well [108]. The possible efficacy of topical eberconazole and topical formulations of amphotericin B in cutaneous sporotrichosis, as in case of cutaneous leishmaniasis, too needs assessment [107, 109, 110]. There also remains a scope for new therapies that can cure the disease in shorter period of time and treat the disseminated forms effectively. Inhibition of melanin formation that protects the fungus from body's immune system can perhaps be another target for development of new therapeutic agents and requires further research. As early diagnosis remains a challenge for the treating physicians, development of new diagnostic tools with shorter turnaround time than culture is another area for future researchers. Patient education for preventive aspects for minimizing the risk and counseling for protracted, prolonged treatment will benefit in the long-term.

## Conflict of Interests

The author declares that there is no conflict of interests regarding the publication of this paper.

## References

[1] R. Morris-Jones, "Sporotrichosis," *Clinical and Experimental Dermatology*, vol. 27, no. 6, pp. 427–431, 2002.

[2] J. A. Al-Tawfiq and K. K. Wools, "Disseminated sporotrichosis and Sporothrix schenckii fungemia as the initial presentation of human immunodeficiency virus infection," *Clinical Infectious Diseases*, vol. 26, no. 6, pp. 1403–1406, 1998.

[3] F. M. Durden and B. Elewski, "Fungal infections in HIV-infected patients," *Seminars in Cutaneous Medicine and Surgery*, vol. 16, no. 3, pp. 200–212, 1997.

[4] M. C. G. Galhardo, R. M. Z. de Oliveira, A. C. F. do Valle et al., "Molecular epidemiology and antifungal susceptibility patterns of *Sporothrix schenckii* isolates from a cat-transmitted epidemic of sporotrichosis in Rio de Janeiro, Brazil," *Medical Mycology*, vol. 46, no. 2, pp. 141–151, 2008.

[5] X. Liu, C. Lian, L. Jin, L. An, G. Yang, and X. Lin, "Characterization of *Sporothrix schenckii* by random amplification of polymorphic DNA assay," *Chinese Medical Journal*, vol. 116, no. 2, pp. 239–242, 2003.

[6] R. Marimon, J. Gené, J. Cano, L. Trilles, M. D. S. Lazéra, and J. Guarro, "Molecular phylogeny of *Sporothrix schenckii*," *Journal of Clinical Microbiology*, vol. 44, no. 9, pp. 3251–3256, 2006.

[7] R. Marimon, J. Cano, J. Gené, D. A. Sutton, M. Kawasaki, and J. Guarro, "Sporothrix brasiliensis, *S. globosa*, and *S. mexicana*, three new Sporothrix species of clinical interest," *Journal of Clinical Microbiology*, vol. 45, no. 10, pp. 3198–3206, 2007.

[8] I. Arrillaga-Moncrieff, J. Capilla, E. Mayayo et al., "Different virulence levels of the species of Sporothrix in a murine model," *Clinical Microbiology and Infection*, vol. 15, no. 7, pp. 651–655, 2009.

[9] H. F. Vismer and P. R. Hull, "Prevalence, epidemiology and geographical distribution of *Sporothrix schenckii* infections in Gauteng, South Africa," *Mycopathologia*, vol. 137, no. 3, pp. 137–143, 1997.

[10] N. M. Dias, M. M. E. Oliveira, M. A. Portela, C. Santos, R. M. Zancope-Oliveira, and N. Lima, "Sporotrichosis caused by *Sporothrix mexicana*, Portugal," *Emerging Infectious Diseases*, vol. 17, no. 10, pp. 1975–1976, 2011.

[11] D. Quintal, "Sporotrichosis infection on mines of the Witwatersrand," *Journal of Cutaneous Medicine and Surgery*, vol. 4, no. 1, pp. 51–54, 2000.

[12] D. M. Dixon, I. F. Salkin, R. A. Duncan et al., "Isolation and characterization of *Sporothrix schenckii* from clinical and environmental sources associated with the largest U.S. epidemic of sporotrichosis," *Journal of Clinical Microbiology*, vol. 29, no. 6, pp. 1106–1113, 1991.

[13] M. Itoh, S. Okamoto, and H. Kariya, "Survey of 200 cases of sporotrichosis," *Dermatologica*, vol. 172, no. 4, pp. 209–213, 1986.

[14] V. K. Mahajan, N. L. Sharma, R. C. Sharma, M. L. Gupta, G. Garg, and A. K. Kanga, "Cutaneous sporotrichosis in Himachal Pradesh, India," *Mycoses*, vol. 48, no. 1, pp. 25–31, 2005.

[15] A. P. Gonçalves, "Sporotrichosis," in *Clinical Tropical Dermatology*, O. Canizare and R. Harman, Eds., pp. 88–93, Blackwell Scientific Publications, Cambridge, Mass, USA, 1992.

[16] T. De Araujo, A. C. Marques, and F. Kerdel, "Sporotrichosis," *International Journal of Dermatology*, vol. 40, no. 12, pp. 737–742, 2001.

[17] A. C. M. da Rosa, M. L. Scroferneker, R. Vettorato, R. L. Gervini, G. Vettorato, and A. Weber, "Epidemiology of sporotrichosis: a study of 304 cases in Brazil," *Journal of the American Academy of Dermatology*, vol. 52, no. 3, pp. 451–459, 2005.

[18] N. L. Sharma, R. C. Sharma, M. L. Gupta, P. Singh, and N. Gupta, "Sporotrichosis: study of 22 cases from himachal pradesh," *Indian Journal of Dermatology, Venereology and Leprology*, vol. 56, no. 4, pp. 296–298, 1990.

[19] R. N. Fleury, P. R. Taborda, A. K. Gupta et al., "Zoonotic sporotrichosis. Transmission to humans by infected domestic cat scratching: report of four cases in São Paulo, Brazil," *International Journal of Dermatology*, vol. 40, no. 5, pp. 318–322, 2001.

[20] K. D. Reed, F. M. Moore, G. E. Geiger, and M. E. Stemper, "Zoonotic transmission of sporotrichosis: case report and review," *Clinical Infectious Diseases*, vol. 16, no. 3, pp. 384–387, 1993.

[21] R. S. Reis, R. Almeida-Paes, M. D. M. Muniz et al., "Molecular characterisation of *Sporothrix schenckii* isolates from humans and cats involved in the sporotrichosis epidemic in Rio de Janeiro, Brazil," *Memórias do Instituto Oswaldo Cruz*, vol. 104, no. 5, pp. 769–774, 2009.

[22] M. Bastos de Lima Barros, A. de Oliveira Schubach, M. C. Gutierrez Galhardo et al., "Sporotrichosis with widespread cutaneous lesions: report of 24 cases related to transmission by domestic cats in Rio de Janeiro, Brazil," *International Journal of Dermatology*, vol. 42, no. 9, pp. 677–681, 2003.

[23] A. Falqueto, S. B. Maifrede, and M. A. Ribeiro, "Unusual clinical presentation of sporotrichosis in three members of one family," *International Journal of Dermatology*, vol. 51, no. 4, pp. 434–438, 2012.

[24] A. M. Rodrigues, M. de Melo Teixeira, G. S. de Hoog et al., "Phylogenetic analysis reveals a high prevalence of *Sporothrix brasiliensis* in feline sporotrichosis outbreaks," *PLoS Neglected Tropical Diseases*, vol. 7, no. 6, Article ID e2281, 2013.

[25] B. P. Nusbaum, N. Gulbas, and S. N. Horwitz, "Sporotrichosis acquired from a cat," *Journal of the American Academy of Dermatology*, vol. 8, no. 3, pp. 386–391, 1983.

[26] M. G. Mercurio and B. E. Elewski, "Therapy of sporotrichosis," *Seminars in Dermatology*, vol. 12, no. 4, pp. 285–289, 1993.

[27] A. Bonifaz, A. Saúl, V. Paredes-Solis et al., "Sporotrichosis in childhood: clinical and therapeutic experience in 25 patients," *Pediatric Dermatology*, vol. 24, no. 4, pp. 369–372, 2007.

[28] M. C. Gutierrez-Galhardo, M. B. L. Barros, A. O. Schubach et al., "Erythema multiforme associated with sporotrichosis," *Journal of the European Academy of Dermatology and Venereology*, vol. 19, no. 4, pp. 507–509, 2005.

[29] A. Schubach, M. B. de Lima Barros, T. M. P. Schubach et al., "Primary conjunctival sporotrichosis: two cases from a zoonotic epidemic in Rio de Janeiro, Brazil," *Cornea*, vol. 24, no. 4, pp. 491–493, 2005.

[30] K. J. Kwon-Chung, "Comparison of isolates of *Sporothrix schenckii* obtained from fixed cutaneous lesions with isolates from other types of lesions," *Journal of Infectious Diseases*, vol. 139, no. 4, pp. 424–431, 1979.

[31] A. H. Verner and B. E. Werner, "Sporotrichosis in man and animal," *International Journal of Dermatology*, vol. 33, no. 10, pp. 692–700, 1994.

[32] M. B. de Albornoz, M. Mendoza, and E. D. de Torres, "Growth temperatures of isolates of *Sporothrix schenckii* from disseminated and fixed cutaneous lesions of sporotrichosis," *Mycopathologia*, vol. 95, no. 2, pp. 81–83, 1986.

[33] I. A. C. Diaz, "Epidemiology of sporotrichosis in Latin America," *Mycopathologia*, vol. 108, no. 2, pp. 113–116, 1989.

[34] J. E. Mackinnon, "Regional peculiarities of some deep mycoses," *Mycopathologia et Mycologia Applicata*, vol. 46, no. 3, pp. 249–265, 1972.

[35] E. S. Rafal and J. E. Rasmussen, "An unusual presentation of fixed cutaneous sporotrichosis: a case report and review of the literature," *Journal of the American Academy of Dermatology*, vol. 25, no. 5, pp. 928–932, 1991.

[36] N. L. Sharma, K. I. S. Mehta, V. K. Mahajan, A. K. Kanga, V. C. Sharma, and G. R. Tegta, "Cutaneous sporotrichosis of face: polymorphism and reactivation after intralesional triamcinolone," *Indian Journal of Dermatology, Venereology and Leprology*, vol. 73, no. 3, pp. 188–190, 2007.

[37] V. K. Mahajan, N. L. Sharma, V. Shanker, P. Gupta, and K. Mardi, "Cutaneous sporotrichosis: unusual clinical presentations," *Indian Journal of Dermatology, Venereology and Leprology*, vol. 76, no. 3, pp. 276–280, 2010.

[38] S. K. Rathi, M. Ramam, and C. Rajendran, "Localized cutaneous sporotrichosis lasting for 10 years," *Indian Journal of Dermatology, Venereology and Leprology*, vol. 69, no. 3, pp. 239–240, 2003.

[39] P. G. Pappas, I. Tellez, A. E. Deep, D. Nolasco, W. Holgado, and B. Bustamante, "Sporotrichosis in Peru: description of an area of hyperendemicity," *Clinical Infectious Diseases*, vol. 30, no. 1, pp. 65–70, 2000.

[40] M. B. de Lima Barros, A. de Oliveira Schubach, M. C. G. Galhardo et al., "Sporotrichosis with widespread cutaneous lesions: report of 24 cases related to transmission by domestic cats in Rio de Janeiro, Brazil," *International Journal of Dermatology*, vol. 42, no. 9, pp. 677–681, 2003.

[41] P. C. Janes and R. J. Mann, "Extracutaneous sporotrichosis," *Journal of Hand Surgery*, vol. 12, no. 3, pp. 441–445, 1987.

[42] R. W. Steele, P. B. Cannady Jr., W. L. Moore Jr., and L. O. Gentry, "Skin test and blastogenic responses to *Sporotrichum schenckii*," *The Journal of Clinical Investigation*, vol. 57, no. 1, pp. 155–160, 1976.

[43] M. Morgan and R. Reves, "Invasive sinusitis due to *Sporothrix schenckii* in a patient with AIDS," *Clinical Infectious Diseases*, vol. 23, no. 6, pp. 1319–1320, 1996.

[44] A. Gordhan, P. K. Ramdial, N. Morar, S. D. Moodley, and J. Aboobaker, "Disseminated cutaneous sporotrichosis: a marker of osteoarticular sporotrichosis masquerading as gout," *International Journal of Dermatology*, vol. 40, no. 11, pp. 717–719, 2001.

[45] D. Vieira-Dias, C. M. Sena, F. Oréfice, M. A. G. Tanure, and J. S. Hamdan, "Ocular and concomitant cutaneous sporotrichosis," *Mycoses*, vol. 40, no. 5-6, pp. 197–201, 1997.

[46] B. A. Davis, "Sporotrichosis," *Dermatologic Clinics*, vol. 14, no. 1, pp. 69–76, 1996.

[47] E. F. Haponik, M. K. Hill, and C. C. Craighead, "Pulmonary sporotrichosis with massive hemoptysis," *The American Journal of the Medical Sciences*, vol. 297, no. 4, pp. 251–253, 1989.

[48] R. C. Sharma and N. L. Sharma, "Sporotrichoid reactions to mycobacterial infections," *Indian Journal of Dermatology, Venereology and Leprology*, vol. 60, no. 5, pp. 283–285, 1994.

[49] D. R. Byrd, R. A. El-Azhary, L. E. Gibson, and G. D. Roberts, "Sporotrichosis masquerading as pyoderma gangrenosum: case report and review of 19 cases of sporotrichosis," *Journal of the

*European Academy of Dermatology and Venereology*, vol. 15, no. 6, pp. 581–584, 2001.

[50] P. Zaharopoulos, "Fine needle aspiration cytologic diagnosis of lymphocutaneous sporotrichosis: a case report," *Diagnostic Cytopathology*, vol. 20, no. 2, pp. 74–77, 1999.

[51] E. S. Civila, J. Bonasse, I. A. Conti-Díaz, and R. A. Vignale, "Importance of the direct fresh examination in the diagnosis of cutaneous sporotrichosis," *International Journal of Dermatology*, vol. 43, no. 11, pp. 808–810, 2004.

[52] B. C. Hirsh and W. C. Johnson, "Pathology of granulomatous diseases. Mixed inflammatory granulomas," *International Journal of Dermatology*, vol. 23, no. 9, pp. 585–597, 1984.

[53] J. W. Rippon, "Sporotrichosis," in *Medical Mycology: The Pathogenic Fungi and the Pathogenic Actinomycetes*, J. W. Rippon, Ed., pp. 325–352, WB Saunders, Philadelphia, Pa, USA, 3rd edition, 1988.

[54] G. Rodríguez and L. Sarmiento, "The asteroid bodies of Sporothrix schenckii," *The American Journal of Dermatopathology*, vol. 20, pp. 246–249, 1998.

[55] W. Kaplan and M. S. Ivens, "Fluorescent antibody staining of *Sporotrichum schenckii* in cultures and clinical materials," *The Journal of Investigative Dermatology*, vol. 35, pp. 151–159, 1960.

[56] A. R. Irizarry-Rovira, L. Kaufman, J. A. Christian et al., "Diagnosis of sporotrichosis in a donkey using direct fluorescein-labeled antibody testing," *Journal of Veterinary Diagnostic Investigation*, vol. 12, no. 2, pp. 180–183, 2000.

[57] R. Romero-Martinez, M. Wheeler, A. Guerrero-Plata, G. Rico, and H. Torres-Guerrero, "Biosynthesis and functions of melanin in *Sporothrix schenckii*," *Infection and Immunity*, vol. 68, no. 6, pp. 3696–3703, 2000.

[58] C. A. Kauffman, "Sporotrichosis," *Clinical Infectious Diseases*, vol. 29, no. 2, pp. 231–237, 1999.

[59] E. N. Scott and H. G. Muchmore, "Immunoblot analysis of antibody responses to *Sporothrix schenckii*," *Journal of Clinical Microbiology*, vol. 27, no. 2, pp. 300–304, 1989.

[60] S. Hu, W.-H. Chung, S.-I. Hung et al., "Detection of *Sporothrix schenckii* in clinical samples by a nested PCR assay," *Journal of Clinical Microbiology*, vol. 41, no. 4, pp. 1414–1418, 2003.

[61] A. M. Rodrigues, G. S. de Hoog, and Z. P. de Camargo, "Genotyping species of the Sporothrix schenckii complex by PCR-RFLP of calmodulin," *Diagnostic Microbiology and Infectious Disease*, vol. 78, no. 4, pp. 383–387, 2014.

[62] C. Toriello, L. C. Arjona-Rosado, M. L. Diaz-Gomez, and M. L. Taylor, "Efficiency of crude and purified fungal antigens in serodiagnosis to discriminate mycotic from other respiratory diseases," *Mycoses*, vol. 34, no. 3-4, pp. 133–140, 1991.

[63] R. Arenas, "Sporotrichosis," in *Topley & Wilson's Microbiology & Microbial Infections: Medical Mycology*, W. G. Merz and R. J. Hay, Eds., pp. 367–384, ASM Press, Washington, DC, USA, 10th edition, 2005.

[64] Y. P. Loureiro and B. Lopes, "Concanavalin A-binding cell wall antigens of *Sporothrix schenckii*: a serological study," *Medical Mycology*, vol. 38, no. 1, pp. 1–7, 2000.

[65] C. A. Kauffman, B. Bustamante, S. W. Chapman, and P. G. Pappas, "Clinical practice guidelines for the management of sporotrichosis: 2007 update by the Infectious Diseases Society of America," *Clinical Infectious Diseases*, vol. 45, no. 10, pp. 1255–1265, 2007.

[66] R. S. Purvis, D. G. Diven, R. D. Drechsel, J. H. Calhoun, and S. K. Tyring, "Sporotrichosis presenting as arthritis and subcutaneous nodules," *Journal of the American Academy of Dermatology*, vol. 28, no. 5, pp. 879–884, 1993.

[67] B. Coskun, Y. Saral, N. Akpolat, A. Ataseven, and D. Çiçek, "Sporotrichosis successfully treated with terbinafine and potassium iodide: case report and review of the literature," *Mycopathologia*, vol. 158, no. 1, pp. 53–56, 2004.

[68] M. Hiruma and S. Kagawa, "Ultrastructure of *Sporothrix schenckii* treated with iodine-potassium iodide solution," *Mycopathologia*, vol. 97, no. 2, pp. 121–127, 1987.

[69] N. L. Sharma, V. K. Mahajan, N. Verma, and S. Thakur, "Cutaneous sporotrichosis: an unusual clinico-pathologic and therapeutic presentation," *Mycoses*, vol. 46, no. 11-12, pp. 515–518, 2003.

[70] L. F. Ray and E. M. Rockwood, "Sporotrichosis: report of a case which was resistant to treatment," *Archives of Dermatology and Syphilology*, vol. 46, no. 2, pp. 211–217, 1942.

[71] C. A. Kauffman, "Old and new therapies for sporotrichosis," *Clinical Infectious Diseases*, vol. 21, no. 4, pp. 981–985, 1995.

[72] V. K. Sharma, S. Kaur, B. Kumar et al., "Sporotrichosis in North Western India," *Indian Journal of Dermatology, Venereology and Leprology*, vol. 54, no. 3, pp. 142–147, 1988.

[73] K. Sandhu and S. Gupta, "Potassium iodide remains the most effective therapy for cutaneous sporotrichosis," *Journal of Dermatological Treatment*, vol. 14, no. 4, pp. 200–202, 2003.

[74] H. Fujii, M. Tanioka, M. Yonezawa et al., "A case of atypical sporotrichosis with multifocal cutaneous ulcers," *Clinical and Experimental Dermatology*, vol. 33, no. 2, pp. 135–138, 2008.

[75] C. Cabezas, B. Bustamante, W. Holgado, and R. E. Begue, "Treatment of cutaneous sporotrichosis with one daily dose of potassium iodide," *Pediatric Infectious Disease Journal*, vol. 15, no. 4, pp. 352–354, 1996.

[76] J. B. Sterling and W. R. Heymann, "Potassium iodide in dermatology: a 19th century drug for the 21st century—uses, pharmacology, adverse effects, and contraindications," *Journal of the American Academy of Dermatology*, vol. 43, no. 4, pp. 691–697, 2000.

[77] C. A. Kauffman, R. Hajjeh, and S. W. Chapman, "Practice guidelines for the management of patients with sporotrichosis," *Clinical Infectious Diseases*, vol. 30, no. 4, pp. 684–687, 2000.

[78] A. Restrepo, J. Robledo, I. Gomez, A. M. Tabares, and R. Gutiérrez, "Itraconazole therapy in lymphangitic and cutaneous sporotrichosis," *Archives of Dermatology*, vol. 122, no. 4, pp. 413–417, 1986.

[79] P. K. Sharkey-Mathis, C. A. Kauffman, J. R. Graybill et al., "Treatment of sporotrichosis with itraconazole," *American Journal of Medicine*, vol. 95, no. 3, pp. 279–285, 1993.

[80] M. B. de Lima Barros, A. O. Schubach, R. de Vasconcellos Carvalhaes de Oliveira, E. B. Martins, J. L. Teixeira, and B. Wanke, "Treatment of cutaneous sporotrichosis with itraconazole—study of 645 patients," *Clinical Infectious Diseases*, vol. 52, no. 12, pp. e200–e206, 2011.

[81] A. Bonifaz, L. Fierro, A. Saúl, and R. M. Ponce, "Cutaneous sporotrichosis. Intermittent treatment (pulses) with itraconazole," *European Journal of Dermatology*, vol. 18, pp. 1–4, 2008.

[82] Y. Song, S.-X. Zhong, L. Yao et al., "Efficacy and safety of itraconazole pulses vs. continuous regimen in cutaneous sporotrichosis," *Journal of the European Academy of Dermatology and Venereology*, vol. 25, no. 3, pp. 302–305, 2011.

[83] R. E. Winn, J. Anderson, J. Piper, N. E. Aronson, and J. Pluss, "Systemic sporotrichosis treated with itraconazole," *Clinical Infectious Diseases*, vol. 17, no. 2, pp. 210–217, 1993.

[84] S. Z. Ghodsi, S. Shams, Z. Naraghi et al., "An unusual case of cutaneous sporotrichosis and its response to weekly fluconazole," *Mycoses*, vol. 43, pp. 75–77, 2000.

[85] L. G. M. Castro, W. Belda Jr., L. C. Cuce, S. A. P. Sampaio, and D. A. Stevens, "Successful treatment of sporotrichosis with oral fluconazole: a report of three cases," *British Journal of Dermatology*, vol. 128, no. 3, pp. 352–356, 1993.

[86] C. A. Kauffman, P. G. Pappas, D. S. McKinsey et al., "Treatment of lymphocutaneous and visceral sporotrichosis with fluconazole," *Clinical Infectious Diseases*, vol. 22, no. 1, pp. 46–50, 1996.

[87] M. Diaz, R. Negroni, F. Montero-Gei et al., "A Pan-American 5-year study of fluconazole therapy for deep mycoses in the immunocompetent host," *Clinical Infectious Diseases*, vol. 14, supplement 1, pp. S68–S76, 1992.

[88] T. J. Pursley, I. K. Blomquist, J. Abraham, H. F. Andersen, and J. A. Bartley, "Fluconazole-induced congenital anomalies in three infants," *Clinical Infectious Diseases*, vol. 22, no. 2, pp. 336–340, 1996.

[89] W. E. Dismukes, A. M. Stamm, J. R. Graybill et al., "Treatment of systemic mycoses with ketoconazole: emphasis on toxicity and clinical response in 52 patients. National institute of allergy and infectious diseases collaborative antifungal study," *Annals of Internal Medicine*, vol. 98, no. 1, pp. 13–20, 1983.

[90] G. Francesconi, A. Valle, S. Passos, R. Reis, and M. Galhardo, "Terbinafine (250 mg/day): an effective and safe treatment of cutaneous sporotrichosis," *Journal of the European Academy of Dermatology and Venereology*, vol. 23, no. 11, pp. 1273–1276, 2009.

[91] P. R. Hull and H. F. Vismer, "Treatment of cutaneous sporotrichosis with terbinafine," *British Journal of Dermatology*, vol. 126, supplement 39, pp. 51–55, 1992.

[92] G. Francesconi, A. C. F. do Valle, S. L. Passos et al., "Comparative study of 250 mg/day terbinafine and 100 mg/day itraconazole for the treatment of cutaneous sporotrichosis," *Mycopathologia*, vol. 171, no. 5, pp. 349–354, 2011.

[93] S. W. Chapman, P. Pappas, C. Kauffmann et al., "Comparative evaluation of the efficacy and safety of two doses of terbinafine (500 and 1000 mg day$^{-1}$) in the treatment of cutaneous or lymphocutaneous sporotrichosis," *Mycoses*, vol. 47, no. 1-2, pp. 62–68, 2004.

[94] W. B. Shelley and P. A. Sica Jr., "Disseminate sporotrichosis of skin and bone cured with 5-fluorocytosine: photosensitivity as a complication," *Journal of the American Academy of Dermatology*, vol. 8, no. 2, pp. 229–235, 1983.

[95] R. Marimon, C. Serena, J. Gené, J. Cano, and J. Guarro, "In vitro antifungal susceptibilities of five species of *Sporothrix*," *Antimicrobial Agents and Chemotherapy*, vol. 52, no. 2, pp. 732–734, 2008.

[96] B. Bustamante and P. E. Campos, "Sporotrichosis treatment: overview and update," *Current Fungal Infection Reports*, vol. 5, no. 1, pp. 42–48, 2011.

[97] P. G. Pappas, "The role of azoles in the treatment of invasive mycoses: review of the infectious diseases society of America guidelines," *Current Opinion in Infectious Diseases*, vol. 24, supplement 2, pp. S1–S13, 2011.

[98] L. M. Kohler, P. C. F. Monteiro, R. C. Hahn, and J. S. Hamdan, "In vitro susceptibilities of isolates of *Sporothrix schenckii* to itraconazole and terbinafine," *Journal of Clinical Microbiology*, vol. 42, no. 9, pp. 4319–4320, 2004.

[99] C. D. O. Stopiglia, C. M. Magagnin, M. R. Castrillón et al., "Antifungal susceptibilities and identification of species of the *Sporothrix schenckii* complex isolated in Brazil," *Medical Mycology*, vol. 52, no. 1, pp. 56–64, 2014.

[100] A. M. Rodrigues, G. S. de Hoog, D. de Cássia Pires et al., "Genetic diversity and antifungal susceptibility profiles in causative agents of sporotrichosis," *BMC Infectious Diseases*, vol. 14, no. 1, article 219, 2014.

[101] F. Fernández-Silva, J. Capilla, E. Mayayo, and J. Guarro, "Efficacy of posaconazole in murine experimental sporotrichosis," *Antimicrobial Agents and Chemotherapy*, vol. 56, no. 5, pp. 2273–2277, 2012.

[102] F. Fernández-Silva, J. Capilla, E. Mayayo, and J. Guarro, "Modest efficacy of voriconazole against murine infections by *Sporothrix schenckii* and lack of efficacy against *Sporothrix brasiliensis*," *Mycoses*, vol. 57, no. 2, pp. 121–124, 2014.

[103] C. B. Doherty, S. D. Doherty, and T. Rosen, "Thermotherapy in dermatologic infections," *Journal of the American Academy of Dermatology*, vol. 62, no. 6, pp. 909–927, 2010.

[104] M. Hiruma, A. Kawada, H. Noguchi, A. Ishibashi, and I. A. C. Diaz, "Hyperthermic treatment of sporotrichosis: experimental use of infrared and far infrared rays," *Mycoses*, vol. 35, no. 11-12, pp. 293–299, 1992.

[105] Y. Song, L. Yao, S.-X. Zhong, Y.-P. Tian, Y.-Y. Liu, and S.-S. Li, "Infant sporotrichosis in northeast China: a report of 15 cases," *International Journal of Dermatology*, vol. 50, no. 5, pp. 522–529, 2011.

[106] M. M. Rocha, T. Dassin, R. Lira, E. L. Lima, L. C. Severo, and A. T. Londero, "Sporotrichosis in patient with AIDS: report of a case and review," *Revista Iberoamericana de Micologia*, vol. 18, no. 3, pp. 133–136, 2001.

[107] L. Trilles, B. Fernández-Torres, M. dos Santos Lazéra et al., "In vitro antifungal susceptibilities of *Sporothrix schenckii* in two growth phases," *Antimicrobial Agents and Chemotherapy*, vol. 49, no. 9, pp. 3952–3954, 2005.

[108] V. K. Mahajan, P. S. Chauhan, K. S. Mehta, C. Abhinav, V. Sharma, and K. Thakur, "Subcutaneous phaeohyphomycosis of the face presenting as rhinoentomophthoramycosis," *International Journal of Dermatology*, vol. 52, no. 9, pp. 1105–1108, 2013.

[109] A. Zvulunov, E. Cagnano, S. Frankenburg, Y. Barenholz, and D. Vardy, "Topical treatment of persistent cutaneous leishmaniasis with ethanolic lipid amphotericin B," *Pediatric Infectious Disease Journal*, vol. 22, no. 6, pp. 567–569, 2003.

[110] V. K. Mahajan, K. S. Mehta, P. S. Chauhan, M. Gupta, R. Sharma, and R. Rawat, "Fixed cutaneous sporotrichosis treated with topical amphotericin B and heat therapy in an immune suppressed patient," *Medical Mycology Case Reports*, in press.

# 21

# Epidermal Growth Factor Receptor Inhibitors: A Review of Cutaneous Adverse Events and Management

**K. Chanprapaph, V. Vachiramon, and P. Rattanakaemakorn**

*Division of Dermatology, Faculty of Medicine Ramathibodi Hospital, Mahidol University, 270 Rama VI Road, Rajthevi, Bangkok 10400, Thailand*

Correspondence should be addressed to K. Chanprapaph; kumutnartp@hotmail.com

Academic Editor: Masutaka Furue

Epidermal growth factor inhibitors (EGFRI), the first targeted cancer therapy, are currently an essential treatment for many advance-stage epithelial cancers. These agents have the superior ability to target cancers cells and better safety profile compared to conventional chemotherapies. However, cutaneous adverse events are common due to the interference of epidermal growth factor receptor (EGFR) signaling in the skin. Cutaneous toxicities lead to poor compliance, drug cessation, and psychosocial discomfort. This paper summarizes the current knowledge concerning the presentation and management of skin toxicity from EGFRI. The common dermatologic adverse events are papulopustules and xerosis. Less common findings are paronychia, regulatory abnormalities of hair growth, maculopapular rash, mucositis, and postinflammatory hyperpigmentation. Radiation enhances EGFRI rash due to synergistic toxicity. There is a positive correlation between the occurrence and severity of cutaneous adverse effects and tumor response. To date, prophylactic systemic tetracycline and tetracycline class antibiotics have proven to be the most effective treatment regime.

## 1. Introduction

New chemotherapeutic agents have been developed with increased understanding of the pathogenesis of malignant tumors. Treatments of many epithelial cancers have focused on attacking specific inhibitors of oncologic molecules. These agents have improved ability to target cancers cells and enhance safety profile compared to conventional chemotherapies. Despite the benefits, targeted chemotherapies have enormous skin adverse events, which may lead to poor adherence, dose interruption, and discontinuation of these therapeutic regimens. Moreover, psychosocial discomfort leading to reduction in the quality of life can frequently occur. However, the presence and severity of cutaneous toxicity has shown to have positive correlation with patient survival and could be a surrogate marker for tumor response, especially for the epidermal growth factor receptor inhibitors (EGFRI). Optimum management is essential and will allow enabling patients to remain on these life prolonging therapies.

This paper summarizes the current knowledge concerning the presentation and management of skin toxicity from targeted chemotherapy, giving emphasis on the single-targeted inhibitor, EGFRI. It is based on published article from Medline database. The reports on prevalence and severity of skin side effects are based on prospective and retrospective studies and clinical reviews. The management of targeted chemotherapy which induced skin toxicity can be divided into prophylactic and treatment measures. Prophylactic treatments are reviewed under the consensus of few randomized control trials. However, as far as specific treatment for cutaneous toxicity is concerned, evidence based treatments are lacking and recommendations from weaker sources, for example, uncontrolled trials and expert recommendations, have been utilized.

## 2. Epidermal Growth Factor Receptor Inhibitors

Human epithelial cancer cells are distinguished by the functional activities of growth factors and their receptor, mainly of the epidermal growth factor receptor (EGFR) family.

It belongs to a family receptor named tyrosine kinase. Overexpression of EGFR promotes gene amplification and mutation consequence in cell proliferation, survival, invasion, metastasis, and tumor induced neoangiogenesis [1]. EGFR inhibitor was the first agent developed as a target cancer therapy. Two classes of EGFR inhibitors are in current use: the monoclonal antibodies (cetuximab, panitumumab, and matuzumab) that target the extracellular ligand-binding domain and small-molecule tyrosine kinase inhibitors (gefitinib, erlotinib, lapatinib, and afatinib) which target intracellular domain [1, 2]. EGFR inhibitors have been approved for the treatment of metastatic non-small-cell lung cancer, colorectal cancer, pancreatic cancer, and squamous cell carcinoma of the head and neck [1]. When the expression of EGFR is decreased, inhibition of downstream signaling occurs in malignant tumor cells. This results in inhibition of metastasis, growth, proliferation, differentiation, and angiogenesis and causing apoptosis of cancer cells [2].

Unlike conventional chemotherapy that generally targets rapidly dividing cells by interfering with DNA and RNA synthesis, EGFR inhibitors have favorable systemic adverse events. However, EGFR is crucial for the normal development and physiology of the skin. It is highly expressed in the epidermis especially in the basal cell layer, the outer root sheath of hair follicles, and the sebaceous epithelium. It is also moderately expressed in the eccrine epithelium and dendritic antigen-presenting cells. Therefore, clinically distinct patterns of cutaneous toxicity of EGFR inhibitors can be observed from alteration of the normal function of these structures. Cutaneous eruptions are considered as drug class-specific. Wide range dermatologic adverse events can be found. The common findings are papulopustules and xerosis. Less common side effects are paronychia, regulatory abnormalities of hair growth, maculopapular rash, mucositis, and postinflammatory hyperpigmentation.

## 3. Clinical Findings of Dermatologic Adverse Events

The earliest and most common cutaneous adverse events occurring from 50 to 100% of the reported clinical trials are papulopustular rash, sometimes referred to as acneform eruption [3–6]. They usually develop within the first weeks of treatment and can occur as early as 2 days and as late as 6 weeks after EGFR inhibitors have commenced [7].

Typical presentations comprise erythematous follicular centered papules, pustules with absence comedones. Lesions can be painful and pruritic [8].

Because EGFRs are highly expressed in sebaceous epithelium, eruptions are generally presented in seborrheic areas involving the scalp, face, neck, chest, and upper back (Figure 1). Involvement of the extremities, lower back, abdomen, and buttocks can also occur. Periorbital region and the palms and soles are usually spared [9].

The pathogenesis behind EGFRI induced papulopustules is marked alterations in growth, differentiation of the epidermis leading to altered corneocyte terminal differentiation. Compact orthokeratosis and dyskeratosis of the epidermis

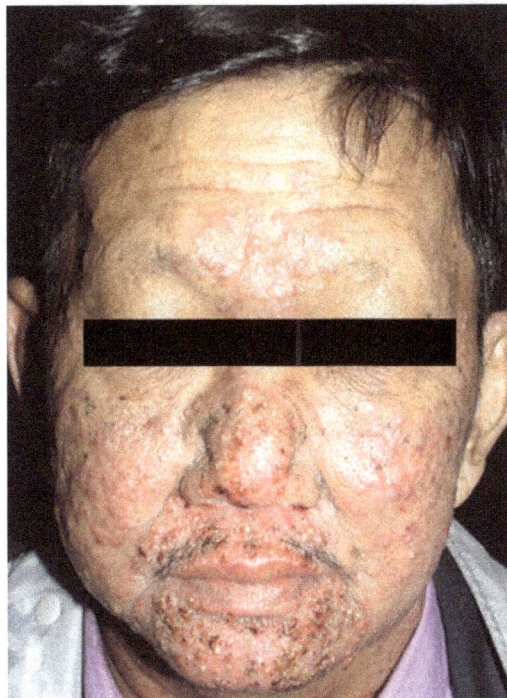

FIGURE 1: Papulopustular eruption. A 52-year-old man with non-small-cell lung carcinoma stage IV developed papulopustules 6 days after erlotinib was commenced.

can be seen in both the affected and unaffected skin [10]. Other major changes are damages of the sebaceous glands and follicular infundibula which generate cytokine release as well as inflammatory cell infiltration in periappendageal areas. Dermal neutrophilic suppurative infiltrations without evidence of infections are seen at the onset of papulopustular rash [7, 10]. The initial reaction is considered as sterile folliculitis, supporting that microorganisms are not the major cause of folliculitis. However, through time, presence of secondary infection may occur from compromised epidermal barrier. Retrospective studies and case series have shown some evidence of dermatologic infection, mainly bacterial, at sites previously affected by dermatologic toxicity for EGFRI [11–13]. This enhances the value of antibiotic treatment, as well as routine bacterial cultures on papulopustular rashes.

Papulopustular eruptions associated with monoclonal antibodies tend to be more severe and widespread compared to small-molecule tyrosine kinase inhibitors [14]. Regardless of the offending agent, lesions will decrease in intensity over several weeks but persist as mild erythema and follicular papules throughout the course of treatment [15, 16].

Xerosis is the second most common cutaneous adverse event from EFFRI, occurring from over 35% in most reports. It has also shown to be the leading skin adverse event in a few reports, prevalence of approximately 50% to 100% [17, 18]. Older patients with prior exposure to cytotoxic agents leading to alteration in skin barrier are prone to develop dry skin. Xerosis presents as dry, itchy, scaly patches which may progress to painful fissuring and xerotic eczema. It may take place at sites where papulopustules have developed; however,

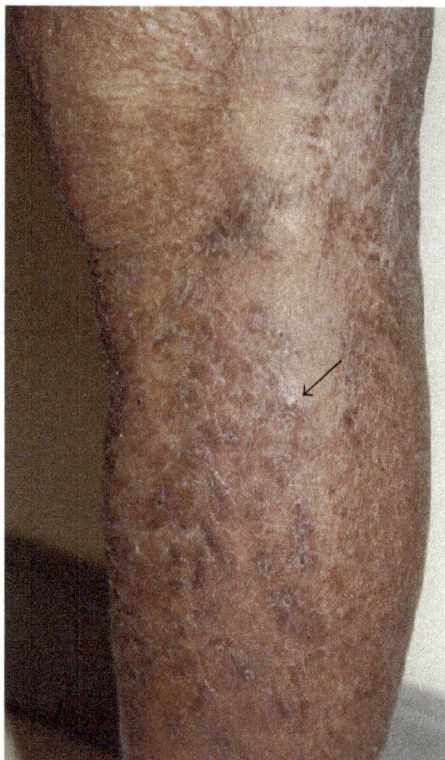

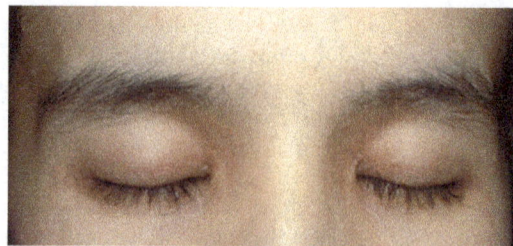

FIGURE 3: Trichomegaly. Trichomegaly developed in a 40-year-old woman, 3 months preceding erlotinib. Notice the wavy, curly, and aberrant elongation of the eyelashes.

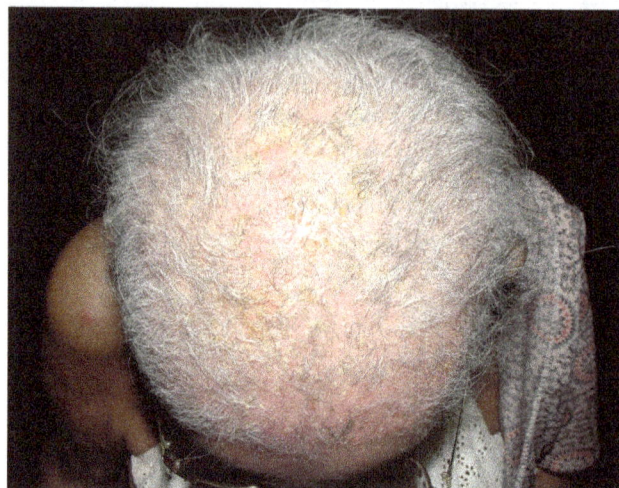

FIGURE 2: Xerosis. Ill-defined dried scaly patch with mild erythema on the left leg, occurring 3 weeks following gefitinib. Notice scattered pustules, showing evidence that xerosis took place where papulopustules have developed.

FIGURE 4: Scalp pustule and scaring alopecia. A 78-year-old woman developed follicular centered pustular eruption on the scalp and scaring alopecia after 3 months of erlotinib.

more widespread involvement usually occurs (Figure 2) [7, 8].

Paronychia is a less common side effect described in 5–20% [17–20]. It usually presents as painful periungual inflammation. Paronychia, which involves many fingers and toes, is particularly disturbing when the finger nails are affected [7]. In severe cases, ingrown nail, periungual absess, and pyogenic granuloma-like lesions can occur. Paronychia usually develops later, approximately after 1-2 months. The pathogenesis remains unclear, but it is proposed that EGFRI may directly inhibit keratinocytes in the nail matrix [7]. Infection is not the main culprit of paronychia, as Staphylococcus aureus was cultured in a few patients and they were unresponsive to antistaphylococcal antibiotics [21].

Regulatory abnormalities of the hair growth can infrequently occur. Hair overgrowth such as trichomegaly and hypertrichosis have been described, the former being more relevant clinically. Trichomegaly usually develops 2–5 months after initiating EGFRI. It is relatively rare but can have significant esthetic damage. Eyelashes will appear wavy, curly, and aberrant (Figure 3). This may lead to corneal irritation and ultimately ulceration. The pathogenesis is hypothesized to be from increased terminal differentiation from EGFR inhibition [7].

Follicular pustules may infrequently occur [22]. Extensive scalp pustules may lead to scaring alopecia (Figure 4). Hair loss both scarring and nonscarring inflammatory alopecia have also been reported [23, 24]. The precise mechanism for

inflammatory hair loss is unclear but may possibly reflect severe endpoint of the follicular papulopustular eruptions [24]. Hair curling and rigidity and hair repigmentation or depigmentation have been reported [25].

Other less common cutaneous sides are maculopapular rash, mucositis, and postinflammatory hyperpigmentation [7, 17].

## 4. Severity Grading System

There are many proposed criteria to grade the severity of cutaneous toxicity from EGFRI. By far the most commonly used one is the system developed by the US National Cancer Institute in the catalog of common toxicity criteria (NCI-CTC version 4.0) Grade 1: papules and/or pustules covering <10% of the body-surface area (BSA) with or without symptoms of pruritis or tenderness, Grade 2: papules and/or pustules covering 10–30% of the BSA with or without symptoms of pruritis or tenderness; with psychosocial impact, Grade 3: papules and/or pustules covering >30% of the BSA with or without symptoms of pruritis or tenderness; limiting self-care activities of daily living, associated with local superinfection with oral antibiotics indicated, Grade 4: covering any percentage of the BSA with or without symptoms of pruritis or tenderness; associated with extensive super-infection with intravenous antibiotics indicate; life-threatening consequences, and Grade 5: Death [26].

## 5. Skin Toxicity and Tumor Response

Evidence has revealed that tumor response and patient survival have improved in the present and increased severity rash from EGFR inhibitors [27]. Cutaneous toxicity is currently considered as a surrogate marker for tumor response as well as overall survival [28]. Moreover, patients experiencing multiple cutaneous toxicity had better therapeutic outcome compared to single skin adverse event [17]. Frequency and severity of skin rashes are dose dependent [29]. Therefore, gradual dose increment until the skin eruptions appears is a strategy to maximize efficacy of EGFR inhibitors.

## 6. The Effect of EGFRI and Concurrent Ionized Radiation

Patient receiving EGFRI have advance stage carcinoma and frequently require radiation in addition to chemotherapy. The effect of concurrent ionized radiation and EGFRI can be categorized into early and late phase. Initially, when EGFRI is commenced in the same period as radiation compared to radiation alone, the ratio for radiation dermatitis as well as EGFRI side effects increases. EGFRI eruption occurs predominantly in the irradiated areas (Figure 5). These agents have synergistic cytotoxicity as well as therapeutic response. Radiation upregulates EGFR in the normal skin; hence, the presence of EGFRI rash accelerates [30–33]. These cutaneous side effects may also lead to treatment interruption. Late actions of EGFR inhibitors and ionized radiation are totally different from the early phases of enhance cutaneous side effects. With prolong irradiation there is absence of skin toxicity to EGFR inhibitors in the preirradiated area. This is due to the fact that radiation induces depletion of basal layer stem cells by apoptosis. Moreover, late chronic radiation causes loss of hair follicles and sebaceous glands by TGF-beta mediated fibrosis [34].

## 7. Management of EGFRI Induced Skin Toxicity

The management of EGFRI which induce skin toxicity can be categorized into prophylaxis and reactive treatment. There are several well-designed randomized control trials (RCT) on agents that could possibly prevent or alleviate symptoms of cutaneous toxicities given prior to EGFRI. However, there are only a few uncontrolled trials, case series, and case reports for reactive treatment of EGFRI-associated dermatologic adverse event.

## 8. Prophylactic Treatment

*8.1. Antibiotics: Tetracycline and Tetracycline-Class.* To date, there are 4 published randomized control and 1 meta-analysis

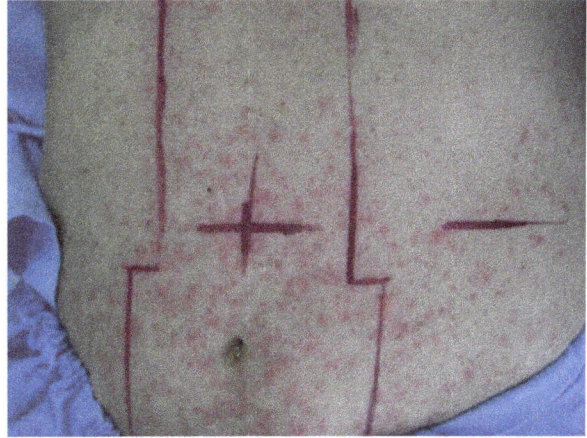

FIGURE 5: Papulopustules on irradiated area. A 65-year-old-man with non-small-cell lung cancer stage IV and cauda equina syndrome was admitted for radiation. Erlotinib was given 7 days ago. After 2 days of radiotherapy he developed papulopustular eruption predominantly on the irradiation field.

on the use of antibiotics, all comprising tetracycline and the tetracycline-class (Table 1).

The first published clinical trial on the prophylaxis of EGFRI induced papulopustule was done by Scope et al. This was a randomized double-blinded trial on prophylactic oral minocycline and topical tazarotene for papulopustules from cetuximab. The group of patients who received minocycline showed benefit initially, during weeks 1 to 4, with less development of facial lesions and lower itch severity. After the 1st month this advantage was no longer evident [35]. Another randomized control trial by Jatoi et al. compared the efficacy of prophylactic oral tetracycline versus placebo on the incidence and severity of rash from EGFRIs. The presence of rash was the same in the 2 groups. However, the severity was significantly lower in the tetracycline group during the first 4 weeks of treatment [36].

Lacouture et al. published a trial on patients receiving panitumumab-containing therapy. Participants were randomly assigned to receive either prophylactic or reactive treatment. Prophylactic treatment comprised using skin moisturizers, sunscreen, 1% hydrocortisone cream, and doxycycline. The reactive treatment meant any kind of treatment necessary following skin side effects. The results revealed that their prophylactic regimen (doxycycline arm) could decrease the incidence of ≥2 grade skin toxicity compared to the reactive treatment [37].

Deplanque et al. conducted a large randomized clinical trial to access the effect of doxycycline in reducing the incidence and severity of erlotinib-induced folliculitis during 4 months of treatment. The results showed that the incidence and severity of folliculitis were significantly less in the doxycycline arm compared to placebo. Moreover, doxycycline was associated with decrease in severity of other cutaneous adverse events [38].

A meta-analysis on antibiotic as a prophylactic regimen for skin rash concluded that antibiotics did not reduce the incidence of rash from EGFRI. However, the relative risk for

TABLE 1: Summery of oral antibiotic in the prevention of EGFRI-induced skin toxicity.

| Author Year | EGFRI agent | Patients (n) | Antibiotic | Objective | Results | Quality of life |
|---|---|---|---|---|---|---|
| Scope et al. 2007 [35] | Cetuximab | 48 | Minocycline | To decrease or prevent skin toxicity | Lower facial lesion count with minocycline (P value 0.05) | Lower itch severity |
| Jatoi et al. 2008 [36] | Multiple | 61 | Tetracycline | To prevent or decrease grade ≥2 rash | No difference in rash incidence (70% versus 76% P value 0.61) Significant lower grade ≥2 rash (17% versus 55%, P value 0.04) | Less burning and irritation with tetracycline |
| Laouture et al. 2010 [37] | Panitumumab | 95 | Doxycycline (plus skin moisturizer, sunscreen, and topical steroid) as prophylactic regimen | To decrease grade ≥2 toxicity | Lower incidence of grade ≥2 toxicity in prophylactic regimen (29 versus 62%, OR, 0.3; 95% CL, 0.1 to 0.6) | More improvement of DLQI in prophylactic group |
| Deplaque et al. 2010 [38]. | Erlotinib | 147 | Doxycycline | To prevent or decrease severity of folliculitis | No difference in folliculitis incidence (68% versus 82%, P value = 0.055). Significant decrease in severity P < 0.001 Lower incidence of grade ≥2 folliculitis in doxycycline arm (39% versus 82%) | NA |

All are RCTs.
DLQI: Dermatologic Life Quality Index. NA: not assessed.

severity of rash was reduced by 42% to 47% with the use of antibiotics [39].

## 9. Topical Treatments

Up until now, there have been several control trials on the prophylactic use of topical agents, one for pimecrolimus, one for tazarotene, and one for sunscreen. There has also been one uncontrolled trial for the preventive measures of topical vitamin K1 for EGFRI rashes (Table 2).

The preventive effect of tazarotene was evaluated in parallel to minocycline for patients receiving cetuximab by Scope et al. Tazarotene was allocated randomly to apply on either the left or right side of the face. This study showed that tazarotene caused significant irritation and gave no benefit in preventing the rash. The rash was even assessed as more severe in the tazarotene side in 10% of the patients. Therefore, this agent is not recommended [35].

Scope et al. conducted a haft face study to evaluate whether pimecrolimus could reduce acne-like eruption as well as rash severity induced by cetuximab. After 2 weeks, lesion counts were significantly less in the pimecrolimus treated side. This benefit was maintained to week 5. However, there was a trend towards lesion decrement on both sides. Moreover, no significant difference in rash severity and

patient assessment of symptoms was observed. Therefore, pimecrolimus did not achieve significant clinical benefit [40].

Vitamin K, a phosphatase inhibitor, and one of the most potent EGFR activators, was evaluated as another prophylactic agent in patients receiving cetuximab combined with chemotherapy. This was an uncontrolled study on Vitamin K1 analog. Vitamin K1 cream had shown to prevent high grade cutaneous side effect. None of the patients developed Grade 3 or 4 toxicity which should normally develop in 20% of patient receiving cetuximab [41].

The effectiveness of sunscreen in the prevention EGFRI induced rash was conducted by Jatoi et al. Patients receiving various types of EGFRIs were randomly assigned to receive either twice daily sun protecting factor 60 sunscreen or placebo for 4 weeks. There was no significant difference in rash severity or patient-reported outcome in both groups. Moreover, application of sunscreen did not cause improvement in the quality of life [42].

## 10. Reactive Treatment of Skin Toxicity

Despite vast publications on expert experience regarding the optimal treatment of EGFRI induced skin toxicity, they are mainly based on a few small studies and anecdotal reports.

TABLE 2: Summery of topical treatment in the prevention of EGFRI-induced skin toxicity.

| Author Year | Type of study | EGFRI agent | Patients (n) | Topical agent | Objective | Results | Quality of life |
|---|---|---|---|---|---|---|---|
| Scope et al. 2007 [35] | RCT | Cetuximab | 48 | Tazarotene applied to half of the face | To decrease or prevent skin toxicity | No difference in the two groups | 32.6% discontinued tazarotene due to significant irritation |
| Ocvirk et al. 2008 [41] | Uncontrolled trial | Cetuximab | 43 | Vitamin K1 cream | To decrease or prevent skin toxicity | 65% developed skin toxicity, limited to merely grade 1 and 2 | NA |
| Scope et al. 2009 [40] | RCT | Cetuximab | 24 | Pimecrolimus applied to half of the face | To decrease or prevent skin toxicity | Decrease lesion count in pimecrolimus treated side $P$ value < 0.001 in week 2 $P$ value = 0.02 in week 5 | NA |
| Jatoi et al. 2010 [42] | RCT | Multiple | 110 | Sunscreen with SPF of 60 | To decrease or prevent skin toxicity | No difference in rash incidence (72% versus 80% $P = 1.00$) or severity | No difference in quality of life |

NA: not assessed.

Therefore, evidence-based treatment recommendations are lacking.

Kanazawa et al. tested the effect of aspirin on the management of skin toxicity from gefitinib. In this study, gefitinib was given solely for the first 2 years in the first group. Then in the following 2 years, gefitinib was administered concomitantly with low dose aspirin (100 mg per day) in the second group. While there was no difference in therapeutic response in the two groups, the frequency of rash was significantly higher in the nonaspirin group [43].

Wong et al. evaluated the effect of Regenecare gel composing 2% lidocaine, aloe vera, marine collagen, and sodium alginate on skin toxicity induced by various types of EGFRIs. Regenecare gel was applied to the right side of the face for 1 week and later applied to the entire face. There was a significant improvement in itchiness. However, the authors did not provide any information about its impact on skin toxicity [44].

Vitamin K1 cream was administered as the management of cutaneous side effects from EGFRI in several uncontrolled studies. The first was a study by Ocvirk and Rebersek. Vitamin K1 cream was given twice daily to patients treated with cetuximab in combination with other chemotherapies after the first document of skin toxicity. All patients had improvement of cutaneous toxicity with downstaging in rash of at least one grade in 18 days [45]. Pinto et al. conducted another study where vitamin K1 cream was applied at the first onset of Grade ≥2 rash on patients receiving cetuximab or panitumumab. Oral tetracycline was also given in conjunction to vitamin K1 in 39.4% of the patients. 36.4% of the patients showed decrease in skin rash from Grade 0 to 1, 39.4% showed unchanged grading, and the rest had increase in grading to Grade 3. Good rash associated symptoms were obtained in the majority of patients [46].

The effectiveness of topical nadifloxacin cream and prednicarbate cream on acneform eruptions from cetuximab was evaluated by Katzer et al. This was an uncontrolled, open labeled study where nadifloxacin and prednicarbate cream were applied once daily on the skin lesions. The authors reported significant improvement in papules, pustules, and erythema at all-time points of evaluation [47].

Anecdotal reports of the success of retinoids on cutaneous toxicity from EGFRI have been published. Acetretin has been reported to improve erlotinib induced papulopustules [48]. Oral isotretinoin was a successful treatment for acneform skin lesions associated with cetuximab [49]. Application of adapalene reduced severe acneform eruptions from cetuximab [50].

Taking published trials into account, prophylactic systemic tetracycline and tetracycline class antibiotics have proven to be most effective. Avoidance of prolong sun exposure and application of sunscreen along with moisturizing cream and gentle cleansers, although lacking evidence, should still be considered as general patient recommendations.

## 11. Conclusions

In the era where administration of targeted monotherapeutic agents was increasingly popular, EGFRI have shown to have enormous cutaneous toxicity. It is important for physicians and dermatologist to recognize the wide variety of skin adverse events as well as give best possible treatment. Prophylactic measures give promising results, particularly oral tetracycline and tetracycline class antibiotics. Standard studies-based therapies are lacking. Optimizing management will continue to gain importance because it will allow these patients to remain on this life-saving targeted chemotherapy.

## Conflict of Interests

The authors declare that there is no conflict of interests regarding the publication of this paper.

## Acknowledgment

The authors thank Dr. Patcha Pongcharoen for some valuable clinical photography.

## References

[1] F. Ciardiello and G. Tortora, "EGFR antagonists in cancer treatment," *The New England Journal of Medicine*, vol. 358, no. 11, pp. 1160–1174, 2008.

[2] P. M. Harari, G. W. Allen, and J. A. Bonner, "Biology of interactions: antiepidermal growth factor receptor agents," *Journal of Clinical Oncology*, vol. 25, no. 26, pp. 4057–4065, 2007.

[3] B. Burtness, M. A. Goldwasser, W. Flood, B. Mattar, and A. A. Forastiere, "Phase III randomized trial of cisplatin plus placebo compared with cisplatin plus cetuximab in metastatic/recurrent head and neck cancer: an eastern cooperative oncology group study," *Journal of Clinical Oncology*, vol. 23, no. 34, pp. 8646–8654, 2005.

[4] D. Cunningham, Y. Humblet, S. Siena et al., "Cetuximab monotherapy and cetuximab plus irinotecan in irinotecan-refractory metastatic colorectal cancer," *The New England Journal of Medicine*, vol. 351, no. 4, pp. 337–345, 2004.

[5] M. Fakih and M. Vincent, "Adverse events associated with anti-EGFR therapies for the treatment of metastatic colorectal cancer," *Current Oncology*, vol. 17, supplement 1, pp. S18–S30, 2010.

[6] E. Molinari, J. de Quatrebarbes, T. André, and S. Aractingi, "Cetuximab-induced acne," *Dermatology*, vol. 211, no. 4, pp. 330–333, 2005.

[7] J. C. Hu, P. Sadeghi, L. C. Pinter-Brown, S. Yashar, and M. W. Chiu, "Cutaneous side effects of epidermal growth factor receptor inhibitors: clinical presentation, pathogenesis, and management," *Journal of the American Academy of Dermatology*, vol. 56, no. 2, pp. 317–326, 2007.

[8] M. E. Lacouture and S. E. Lai, "The PRIDE (Papulopustules and/or paronychia, Regulatory abnormalities of hair growth, Itching, and Dryness due to Epidermal growth factor receptor inhibitors) syndrome," *British Journal of Dermatology*, vol. 155, no. 4, pp. 852–854, 2006.

[9] B. Belloni, N. Schonewolf, S. Rozati, S. M. Goldinger, and R. Dummer, "Cutaneous drug eruptions associated with the use of new oncological drugs," *Chemical Immunology and Allergy*, vol. 97, pp. 191–202, 2012.

[10] E. Guttman-Yassky, A. Mita, M. de Jonge et al., "Characterisation of the cutaneous pathology in non-small cell lung cancer (NSCLC) patients treated with the EGFR tyrosine kinase inhibitor erlotinib," *European Journal of Cancer*, vol. 46, no. 11, pp. 2010–2019, 2010.

[11] R. E. Eilers, M. Gandhi, J. D. Patel et al., "Dermatologic infections in cancer patients treated with epidermal growth factor receptor inhibitor therapy," *Journal of the National Cancer Institute*, vol. 102, no. 1, pp. 47–53, 2010.

[12] S. H. Kardaun and K. F. van Duinen, "Erlotinib-induced florid acneiform rash complicated by extensive impetiginization," *Clinical and Experimental Dermatology*, vol. 33, no. 1, pp. 46–49, 2008.

[13] H. K. Lord, E. Junor, and J. Ironside, "Cetuximab is effective, but more toxic than reported in the Bonner trial," *Clinical Oncology*, vol. 20, no. 1, p. 96, 2008.

[14] W. Jacot, D. Bessis, E. Jorda et al., "Acneiform eruption induced by epidermal growth factor receptor inhibitors in patients with solid tumours," *British Journal of Dermatology*, vol. 151, no. 1, pp. 238–241, 2004.

[15] S. E. Abdullah, M. Haigentz Jr., and B. Piperdi, "Dermatologic toxicities from monoclonal antibodies and tyrosine kinase inhibitors against EGFR: pathophysiology and management," *Chemotherapy Research and Practice*, vol. 2012, Article ID 351210, 10 pages, 2012.

[16] R. Gutzmer, A. Wollenberg, S. Ugurel, B. Homey, A. Ganser, and A. Kapp, "Cutaneous side effects of new antitumor drugs: clinical features and management," *Deutsches Ärzteblatt International*, vol. 109, no. 8, pp. 133–140, 2012.

[17] K. Chanprapaph, P. Pongcharoen, and V. Vachiramon, "Cutaneous adverse events of epidermal growth factor receptor inhibitors: a review of 99 cases," *Division of Dermatology, Faculty of Medicine, Ramathibodi Hospital, Mahidol University*. In press.

[18] A. Osio, C. Mateus, J.-C. Soria et al., "Cutaneous side-effects in patients on long-term treatment with epidermal growth factor receptor inhibitors," *British Journal of Dermatology*, vol. 161, no. 3, pp. 515–521, 2009.

[19] K. W. Boucher, K. Davidson, B. Mirakhur, J. Goldberg, and W. R. Heymann, "Paronychia induced by cetuximab, an antiepidermal growth factor receptor antibody," *Journal of the American Academy of Dermatology*, vol. 47, no. 4, pp. 632–633, 2002.

[20] T. Dainichi, M. Tanaka, N. Tsuruta, M. Furue, and K. Noda, "Development of multiple paronychia and periungual granulation in patients treated with gefitinib, an inhibitor of epidermal growth factor receptor," *Dermatology*, vol. 207, no. 3, pp. 324–325, 2003.

[21] G.-C. Chang, T.-Y. Yang, K.-C. Chen, M.-C. Yin, R.-C. Wang, and Y.-C. Lin, "Complications of therapy in cancer patients: case 1. Paronychia and skin hyperpigmentation induced by gefitinib in advanced non-small-cell lung cancer," *Journal of Clinical Oncology*, vol. 22, no. 22, pp. 4646–4648, 2004.

[22] H. Y. Chiu and H. C. Chiu, "Scalp pustules in a patient receiving chemotherapy," *The Journal of the American Medical Association*, vol. 310, no. 10, pp. 1068–1069, 2013.

[23] J. C. Donovan, D. M. Ghazarian, and J. C. Shaw, "Scarring alopecia associated with use of the epidermal growth factor receptor inhibitor gefitinib," *Archives of Dermatology*, vol. 144, no. 11, pp. 1524–1525, 2008.

[24] J. E. Graves, B. F. Jones, A. C. Lind, and M. P. Heffernan, "Nonscarring inflammatory alopecia associated with the epidermal growth factor receptor inhibitor gefitinib," *Journal of the American Academy of Dermatology*, vol. 55, no. 2, pp. 349–353, 2006.

[25] Y. P. Cheng, H. J. Chen, and H. C. Chiu, "Erlotinib-induced hair repigmentation," *International Journal of Dermatology*, vol. 53, no. 1, pp. e55–e57, 2014.

[26] "Common Terminology Criteria for Adverse Events (CTCAE) v4.0," US Department of Health and Human Services. National Institute of Health. National Cancer Institute, 2009, http://evs.nci.nih.gov/ftp1/CTCAE/CTCAE_4.03_2010-06-14_QuickReference_5x7.pdf.

[27] R. Pérez-Soler, A. Chachoua, L. A. Hammond et al., "Determinants of tumor response and survival with erlotinib in patients with non-small-cell lung cancer," *Journal of Clinical Oncology*, vol. 22, no. 16, pp. 3238–3247, 2004.

[28] H. B. Liu, Y. Wu, T. F. Lv et al., "Skin rash could predict the response to EGFR tyrosine kinase inhibitor and the prognosis for patients with non small cell lung cancer: a systematic review

and meta-analysis," *PLoS ONE*, vol. 8, no. 1, Article ID e55128, 2013.

[29] C. A. Perez, H. Song, L. E. Raez et al., "Phase II study of gefitinib adaptive dose escalation to skin toxicity in recurrent or metastatic squamous cell carcinoma of the head and neck," *Oral Oncology*, vol. 48, no. 9, pp. 887–892, 2012.

[30] J. A. Bonner, P. M. Harari, J. Giralt et al., "Radiotherapy plus cetuximab for squamous-cell carcinoma of the head and neck," *The New England Journal of Medicine*, vol. 354, no. 6, pp. 567–578, 2006.

[31] J. A. Bonner, P. M. Harari, J. Giralt et al., "Radiotherapy plus cetuximab for locoregionally advanced head and neck cancer: 5-year survival data from a phase 3 randomised trial, and relation between cetuximab-induced rash and survival," *The Lancet Oncology*, vol. 11, no. 1, pp. 21–28, 2010.

[32] C. Giro, B. Berger, E. Bölke et al., "High rate of severe radiation dermatitis during radiation therapy with concurrent cetuximab in head and neck cancer: results of a survey in EORTC institutes," *Radiotherapy and Oncology*, vol. 90, no. 2, pp. 166–171, 2009.

[33] A. Tejwani, S. Wu, Y. Jia, M. Agulnik, L. Millender, and M. E. Lacouture, "Increased risk of high-grade dermatologic toxicities with radiation plus epidermal growth factor receptor inhibitor therapy," *Cancer*, vol. 115, no. 6, pp. 1286–1299, 2009.

[34] T. Li and R. Perez-Soler, "Skin toxicities associated with epidermal growth factor receptor inhibitors," *Targeted Oncology*, vol. 4, no. 2, pp. 107–119, 2009.

[35] A. Scope, A. L. C. Agero, S. W. Dusza et al., "Randomized double-blind trial of prophylactic oral minocycline and topical tazarotene for cetuximab-associated acne-like eruption," *Journal of Clinical Oncology*, vol. 25, no. 34, pp. 5390–5396, 2007.

[36] A. Jatoi, K. Rowland, J. A. Sloan et al., "Tetracycline to prevent epidermal growth factor receptor inhibitor-induced skin rashes: results of a placebo-controlled trial from the North Central Cancer Treatment Group (N03CB)," *Cancer*, vol. 113, no. 4, pp. 847–853, 2008.

[37] M. E. Lacouture, E. P. Mitchell, B. Piperdi et al., "Skin toxicity evaluation protocol with Panitumumab (STEPP), a phase II, open-label, randomized trial evaluating the impact of a preemptive skin treatment regimen on skin toxicities and quality of life in patients with metastatic colorectal cancer," *Journal of Clinical Oncology*, vol. 28, no. 8, pp. 1351–1357, 2010.

[38] G. Deplanque, J. Chavaillon, A. Vergnenegre et al., "CYTAR: a randomized clinical trial evaluating the preventive effect of doxycycline on erlotinibinduced folliculitis in non-small cell lung cancer patients," *Journal of Clinical Oncology*, vol. 28, abstract 9019, 2010.

[39] J. Ocvirk, S. Heeger, P. McCloud, and R. D. Hofheinz, "A review of the treatment options for skin rash induced by EGFR-targeted therapies: evidence from randomized clinical trials and a meta-analysis," *Radiology and Oncology*, vol. 47, no. 2, pp. 166–175, 2013.

[40] A. Scope, J. A. Lieb, S. W. Dusza et al., "A prospective randomized trial of topical pimecrolimus for cetuximab-associated acnelike eruption," *Journal of the American Academy of Dermatology*, vol. 61, no. 4, pp. 614–620, 2009.

[41] J. Ocvirk and M. Rebersek, "Treatment of cetuximab-associated cutaneous side effects using topical aplication oh vitamin K1 cream," *Journal of Clinical Oncology*, vol. 27, supplement, Article ID e15087, 2009.

[42] A. Jatoi, A. Thrower, J. A. Sloan et al., "Does sunscreen prevent epidermal growth factor receptor (EGFR) inhibitor-induced rash? Results of a placebo-controlled trial from the north central cancer treatment group (N05C4)," *Oncologist*, vol. 15, no. 9, pp. 1016–1022, 2010.

[43] S. Kanazawa, K. Yamaguchi, Y. Kinoshita, M. Muramatsu, Y. Komiyama, and S. Nomura, "Aspirin reduces adverse effects of gefitinib," *Anti-Cancer Drugs*, vol. 17, no. 4, pp. 423–427, 2006.

[44] S. Wong, K. Osann, A. Lindgren, T. Byun, and M. Mummaneni, "Pilot cross-over study to evaluate Regenecare topical gel in patients with epidermal growth factor receptor (HER1/EGFR) inhibitors-induced skin toxicity: the final analysis," *Journal of Clinical Oncology*, vol. 26, Article ID 20507, 2008.

[45] J. Ocvirk and M. Rebersek, "Management of cutaneous side effects of cetuximab therapy with vitamin K1 crème," *Radiology and Oncology*, vol. 42, no. 4, pp. 215–224, 2008.

[46] C. Pinto, C. Barone, A. Martoni, P. di Tullio, F. di Fabio, and A. Cassano, "Vitamin K1 cream in the management of skin rash during anti-EGFR monocloncal antibody (mAb) treatment in patients with metastatic cancer: first analysis of an observational Italian study," *Journal of Clinical Oncology*, vol. 29, abstract 594, 2011.

[47] K. Katzer, J. Tietze, E. Klein, V. Heinemann, T. Ruzicka, and A. Wollenberg, "Topical therapy with nadifloxacin cream and prednicarbate cream improves acneiform eruptions caused by the EGFR-inhibitor cetuximab—a report of 29 patients," *European Journal of Dermatology*, vol. 20, no. 1, pp. 82–84, 2010.

[48] R. G. Pomerantz, R. E. Chirinos, L. D. Falo Jr., and L. J. Geskin, "Acitretin for treatment of EGFR inhibitor-induced cutaneous toxic effects," *Archives of Dermatology*, vol. 144, no. 7, pp. 949–950, 2008.

[49] R. Gutzmer, T. Werfel, R. Mao, A. Kapp, and J. Elsner, "Successful treatment with oral isotretinoin of acneiform skin lesions associated with cetuximab therapy," *British Journal of Dermatology*, vol. 153, no. 4, pp. 849–851, 2005.

[50] K. Taguchi, A. Fukunaga, T. Okuno, and C. Nishigori, "Successful treatment with adapalene of cetuximab-induced acneiform eruptions," *The Journal of Dermatology*, vol. 39, no. 9, pp. 792–794, 2012.

# 22

# Zinc Therapy in Dermatology: A Review

**Mrinal Gupta, Vikram K. Mahajan, Karaninder S. Mehta, and Pushpinder S. Chauhan**

*Department of Dermatology, Venereology & Leprosy, Dr. R. P. Govt. Medical College, Kangra (Tanda), Himachal Pradesh 176001, India*

Correspondence should be addressed to Vikram K. Mahajan; vkmahajan1@gmail.com

Academic Editor: Craig G. Burkhart

Zinc, both in elemental or in its salt forms, has been used as a therapeutic modality for centuries. Topical preparations like zinc oxide, calamine, or zinc pyrithione have been in use as photoprotecting, soothing agents or as active ingredient of antidandruff shampoos. Its use has expanded manifold over the years for a number of dermatological conditions including infections (leishmaniasis, warts), inflammatory dermatoses (acne vulgaris, rosacea), pigmentary disorders (melasma), and neoplasias (basal cell carcinoma). Although the role of oral zinc is well-established in human zinc deficiency syndromes including acrodermatitis enteropathica, it is only in recent years that importance of zinc as a micronutrient essential for infant growth and development has been recognized. The paper reviews various dermatological uses of zinc.

## 1. Introduction

Zinc, a divalent cation, is an essential micronutrient for humans and its importance can be gauged from the fact that it is an essential component of more than 300 metalloenzymes and over 2000 transcription factors that are needed for regulation of lipid, protein and nucleic acid metabolism, and gene transcription. It is involved in gene transcription at various levels, via participation in histone deacetylation reactions and via factors possessing the zinc-finger motifs [1]. An important family of zinc-finger proteins is the steroid or thyroid hormone receptors that bind hormones and facilitate their wide range of effects. Zinc also plays an important role in maintaining the proper reproductive function, immune status, and wound repair via regulation of DNA and RNA polymerases, thymidine kinase, and ribonuclease. It maintains macrophage and neutrophil functions, natural killer cell activity, and complement activity. It activates natural killer cells and phagocytic function of granulocytes and stabilizes the plasma subcellular membranes especially the lysosomes. It inhibits the expression of integrins by keratinocytes and modulates the production of TNF-$\alpha$ and IL-6 and reduces the production of inflammatory mediators like nitric oxide. It is also proposed that it is toll-like receptors mediated regulation of zinc homeostasis which influences dendritic cell function and immune processes [2]. Zinc also possesses antioxidant property and has been found useful in preventing UV-induced damage and reducing the incidence of malignancies. It has also been demonstrated to possess antiandrogenic properties as it causes modulation of 5$\alpha$-reductase type 1 and 2 activity [1, 3, 4].

## 2. Zinc Physiology and Zinc Deficiency States

It will be prudent to revisit the physiological aspects of zinc metabolism before discussing zinc deficiency states. Briefly, an average adult weighing 70 kg has a body zinc content of 1.4–2.3 gm, the highest tissue concentration (>500 $\mu$g/g dry weight) being in the prostate, seminal fluid, uveal tissue, and skin. While about half of the total body zinc is in the bones, the skin contains nearly 6% of total body zinc. As movement of zinc across various tissues is limited and there is no storage depot, the continuous external supply of zinc is important for metabolic needs, growth, and tissue repair. The recommended daily allowance of zinc for an average adult male is 11 mg and the requirement increases from 8 mg/d to up to 12 mg/d in females during pregnancy and lactation. Animal foods like meat, eggs, fish, and oysters are rich in zinc. Although cereals and legumes contain moderate amount of zinc, only 20–40% of the ingested metal is absorbed. Its absorption is hampered by the presence of phytates, calcium, and phosphates while chelating agents like EDTA and animal proteins increase its absorption from gut. Zinc is mainly absorbed from proximal jejunum and distal duodenum and is perhaps facilitated by the presence of low molecular weight zinc binding ligands. It is excreted mainly through feces and in small amounts in urine and sweat.

Zinc deficiency is a common problem with an estimated 1/3rd of world population suffering from zinc deficiency and is highly prevalent in Southeast Asia, sub-Saharan Africa, and other developing countries [5]. Zinc deficiency can be from inadequate dietary intake and poor absorption or because of increased loss. Endemic zinc deficiency occurring in rural Iran, Egypt, and Turkey has been attributed to eating whole grain bread with high fibre and phytate contents that render zinc nearly unabsorbable. Poor-socioeconomic status, protein calorie malnutrition, protein restricted and vegetarian diets, anorexia nervosa, exclusive parenteral nutrition, chronic gastrointestinal diseases, hookworm infestation and malabsorption syndromes, pancreatic insufficiency, chronic renal failure or malignancies, infants on formula milk with low zinc or parenteral alimentation, and acrodermatitis enteropathica are some of the predisposing factors for poor availability and/or absorption of zinc.

## 3. Hypozincemia of Infancy

Zinc is now well-recognized micronutrient essential for infant growth and development and is a standard component in parenteral nutrition for infants with low birth weight or chronic gastrointestinal dysfunction. Some researchers have differentiated hypozincemia of infancy in three categories: type-1 or classic acrodermatitis enteropathica is a rare genetic disorder of zinc deficiency because of mutations in zinc transporter genes, type-2 or due to defective secretion of zinc in mother's milk, and type-3 or hypozincemia in preterm infants on prolonged parenteral alimentation. Type-1 or classic acrodermatitis enteropathica is autosomal recessive disorder while type-2 hypozincemia is perhaps inherited as an autosomal recessive or x-linked disorder. Type-3 or hypozincemia in preterm infants is temporary and occurs from deficient low body reserves due to prematurity or parenteral nutrition deficient in zinc. The clinical manifestations are mainly due to low zinc levels and are similar in all three types and improvement is usually rapid on initiation of zinc therapy.

## 4. Acrodermatitis Enteropathica

Acrodermatitis enteropathica is a rare disease with an estimated prevalence of 1 in 500000 people in Denmark. The exact cause of poor zinc absorption is poorly understood but picnolic acid, a tryptophan derivative, has been implicated as the deficient ligand. The onset of symptoms is usually seen around 4–6 weeks after weaning or even earlier in infant not on breast milk. The infant becomes irritable and withdrawn and develops photophobia. Anorexia, pica, growth impairment, hypogonadism, impaired taste and smell, night blindness, and neuropsychiatric symptoms (mood changes, tremors, dysarthria, and jitteriness) eventuate in untreated cases. Cutaneous changes include periorificial and acral

dermatitis (some lesions are burn like, oozy, or psoriasiform) localized around mouth, cheeks, ears, nostrils, buttocks, anus, dorsal skin of hands, feet, fingers, toes, and heels, paronychia, nail dystrophy, and hair loss. Delayed wound healing, angular stomatitis, conjunctivitis, blepharitis, increased susceptibility to infection, and growth retardation may also be seen. Low serum alkaline phosphatase and zinc levels (<50 $\mu$g%) are diagnostic and will improve after zinc therapy but hypoalbuminemia does not necessarily indicate zinc deficiency. Treatment with oral zinc (2-3 mg/kg/day) will cure all clinical manifestations within 1-2 weeks and needs to be continued up to adulthood for continuous supplementation and favorable long-term prognosis.

## 5. Zinc Therapy in Dermatology

Zinc, elemental or in its various forms (salts), has been used as a therapeutic modality for centuries. Topical preparations like zinc oxide, calamine, or zinc pyrithione have been in use as photoprotecting, soothing agents or as active ingredient of antidandruff shampoos. Its use has also expanded manifold over the years for a number of dermatological conditions including infections (warts, leishmaniasis), inflammatory dermatoses (acne vulgaris, rosacea), pigmentary disorders (melasma), and neoplasias (basal cell carcinoma). Although the role of oral zinc is well-established in human zinc deficiency syndromes including acrodermatitis enteropathica, it is only in recent years that importance of zinc as a micronutrient essential for infant growth and development has been recognized. We review here various therapeutic uses of both topical and oral zinc in dermatology clinical practice (Table 1).

## 6. Infections

Zinc, alone or as an adjuvant, has been found useful in many dermatological infections owing to its modulating actions on macrophage and neutrophil functions, natural killer cell/phagocytic activity, and various inflammatory cytokines.

*6.1. Warts.* Warts are a common dermatological human papilloma virus infection with numerous available treatment modalities. Over the years, various destructive procedures performed accurately have remained the only effective remedy for common warts. Zinc can be a useful topical or oral treatment modality in common warts as many studies have demonstrated efficacy of both oral and topical zinc in treating warts without significant adverse effects. Sharquie et al. [6] studied the efficacy of topical zinc sulphate in viral warts. In their pilot clinical trial 10 patients with plane warts were treated with 10% zinc sulphate solution applied thrice daily for a period of 4 weeks. They observed complete clearance in 80% patients. The authors also reported results of double blind clinical trial in the same study comprising 50 patients with common warts and 40 patients with plane warts treated with topical 10% and 5% zinc sulphate solution applied thrice daily for 4 weeks while distilled water was used as a control [6]. Complete clearance of plane warts was seen in 85.7% and 42.8% cases from topical 10% and 5%

TABLE 1: Therapeutic uses of systemic and topical zinc.

| Disease | Route of administration | Efficacy | Reference number |
|---|---|---|---|
| Warts | Topical | Efficacious as 5%, 10% zinc sulphate lotion, 20% zinc oxide paste, and 2% intralesional zinc sulphate injection. | [6, 7, 11] |
| | Oral | 10 mg/kg/day oral zinc sulphate for 2 months was an effective modality for recalcitrant warts. | [9, 10] |
| Cutaneous leishmaniasis | Intralesional | Clinical cure with 2% intralesional zinc sulphate was comparable to meglumine antimoniate. | [12] |
| | Oral | Oral zinc sulphate in doses of 2.5, 5, and 10 mg/kg/day for 45 days was an effective and safe treatment option. | [13] |
| Leprosy | Oral | Rapid clinical improvement in leprosy lesions and erythema nodosum leprosum seen on addition of oral zinc along with MDT. | [15, 16] |
| Herpes genitalis | Topical | Topical 1%, 2%, and 4% zinc sulphate for 3 months was effective in treating and preventing recurrences of herpes genitalis. | [18] |
| Dermatophytoses | Topical | 20% zinc-undecylenate powder applied twice daily for 4 weeks showed clinical improvement in tinea pedis. | [19] |
| Bromhidrosis | Topical | Topical 15% zinc sulphate solution was efficacious in management of bromhidrosis and foot malodour. | [20, 21] |
| Pityriasis versicolor | Topical | Topical 15% zinc sulphate solution applied once daily for 3 weeks was effective in pityriasis versicolor. | [22] |
| Acne vulgaris | Topical | Topical 5% zinc sulphate was effective in mild to moderate acne. | [34, 36] |
| | Oral | Oral zinc sulphate and zinc gluconate were useful in moderate to severe acne. | [37–40] |
| Rosacea | Oral | Oral zinc sulphate 100 mg thrice a day was effective in rosacea after 3 months of therapy. | [48] |
| Hidradenitis suppurativa | Oral | Oral zinc gluconate 90 mg/day showed significant clinical improvement. | [50] |
| Psoriasis and psoriatic arthritis | Topical | Topical 0.25% zinc pyrithione applied twice daily was found useful in plaque psoriasis. | [52] |
| | Oral | Oral zinc sulphate was efficacious in psoriatic arthritis. | [53] |
| Eczemas | Topical | Zinc oxide paste and zinc sulphate were effective in diaper dermatitis and hand eczemas. | [57] |
| Ulcers | Topical | Topical zinc oxide paste induced rapid healing of vascular and leprosy ulcers. | [60–62] |
| | Oral | No role of systemic zinc sulphate noted in leg ulcers. | [59] |
| Behcet's disease and oral aphthae | Oral | Oral zinc sulphate 100 mg/day was an effective in oral aphthosis and Behcet's disease. | [63, 64] |
| Alopecia areata | Oral | 5 mg/kg/day of oral zinc sulphate induced significant hair growth after 6 months of therapy. | [68] |
| Oral lichen planus | Topical | 0.2% zinc mouthwash with fluocinolone was effective in oral lichen planus. | [72] |
| Xeroderma pigmentosum | Topical | 20% zinc sulphate solution applied twice daily cleared the solar keratoses and small malignancies. | [73] |
| Actinic keratoses | Topical | 25% zinc sulphate solution applied twice daily for 12 weeks cleared majority of the lesions. | [74] |
| Basal cell carcinoma | Intralesional | Intralesional 2% zinc gluconate was efficacious in basal cell carcinoma. | [75] |
| Vitiligo | Oral | Oral zinc sulphate showed moderate efficacy when given as an adjuvant with topical steroids. | [78] |
| Melasma | Topical | 10% zinc sulphate solution applied twice daily for 3 months showed significant reduction in MASI score. | [79] |
| Keloids | Topical | Locally applied zinc tape showed significant clearing and reduction in relapses of keloids. | [82, 83] |
| Antiageing | Topical | 0.1% copper-zinc malonate cream applied twice daily for 8 weeks showed significant reduction of wrinkles. | [84] |

zinc sulphate solution, respectively, while complete clearance was also seen in 11% and 5% of patients with common warts using 10% and 5% zinc sulphate solution, respectively, which was statistically insignificant. Khattar et al. [7] observed that topical 20% zinc oxide was more effective than ointment containing salicylic acid (15%) and lactic acid (15%) for the treatment of warts in a randomized double-blind controlled trial of 44 patients. A complete cure was observed after 3 months in 50% patients with common warts in zinc oxide group as compared to 42% in the other group. Oral zinc sulphate (10 mg/kg/day) given for 2 months in common warts also resulted in complete clearance in 61% patients in one month and 87% after two months of therapy in a placebo controlled trial by Al-Gurairi et al. [8], whereas clearance rate was 50% with the same dose of oral zinc sulphate after 2 months in an open-label clinical study by Mun et al. [9]. Oral zinc (10 mg/kg/day) has been reported to clear recalcitrant warts in a patient with epidermodysplasia verruciformis in 12 weeks [10]. Intralesional 2% zinc sulphate too has been found to induce clearance of warts [11]. Topical or oral zinc can be a useful therapeutic modality for warts especially in children wherein painful physical treatment options have limited usefulness.

### 6.2. Cutaneous Leishmaniasis.

Cutaneous leishmaniasis is a major health problem that causes significant morbidity due to long clinical course and residual scarring. It is caused by parasites of *Leishmania* spp. It occurs worldwide especially in countries having tropical climatic conditions and is significant problem among returning travelers. It has been estimated that 1.5 million new cases of cutaneous leishmaniasis occur annually with majority of them being reported in Brazil, Iran, and Afghanistan. New endemic foci too are being recognized world over in recent years. Although pentavalent antimonials remain the drug of choice despite concerns for cardiac and renal toxicity, search for safer and effective alternative drugs continues. Many other agents including zinc have been tried with variable success. Zinc, both intralesionally and orally, has been found effective in the management of cutaneous leishmaniasis. Iraji et al. [12], in a prospective, double blind, case-control clinical study, observed a comparable response rate with intralesional 2% zinc sulphate and meglumine antimoniate after six weeks of therapy. Sharquie et al. [13] used oral zinc sulphate in doses of 2.5, 5, and 10 mg/kg/day for 45 days among 104 patients with cutaneous leishmaniasis and observed cure rates of 83.9%, 93.1%, and 96.9% for the 2.5 mg/kg, 5 mg/kg, and 10 mg/kg treatment groups, respectively, without significant adverse effects. Although low cost and better safety profile of oral zinc sulphate as compared to antimonials appears attractively advantageous, inconsistent outcome remains a limiting factor for its solo use.

### 6.3. Leprosy.

Leprosy is a chronic infection of skin and peripheral nerves caused by *Mycobacterium leprae*. Almost 4 million people have been affected by leprosy and nearly 250,000 new cases are still being detected annually throughout the world. WHO recommended multidrug therapy (MDT) which has been the mainstay of treatment for leprosy and in reducing its prevalence to near elimination levels. However, lepra reactions and nerve damage cause significant morbidity among patients affected with leprosy. Apart from well-established treatment with systemic corticosteroids and thalidomide, and many anti-inflammatory and immunomodulator drugs, oral zinc has been found useful in the management of lepra reactions owing to its immunostimulatory properties. Zinc is found to stimulate production of IL-2 and induces a shift from Th2 to Th1 response. It has also been demonstrated to decrease the serum levels of TNF-$\alpha$ and inhibit the TNF-$\alpha$ induced apoptosis of peripheral blood mononuclear cells that helps in controlling the disease activity and reactional states [14]. In a study comprising patients of recurrent erythema nodosum leprosum additionally receiving zinc, the steroids could be tapered off completely and the duration and severity of reaction were also reduced [15]. Addition of oral zinc to antileprosy treatment too has been shown to improve therapeutic outcome. Oral zinc when given as an adjuvant to dapsone in lepromatous leprosy induced rapid lepromin conversion and bacterial clearance in the patients as compared to the control group. The clinical improvement was also faster in patients receiving zinc as an adjuvant along with standard MDT [16]. Oral zinc perhaps makes an adjuvant of choice in leprosy treatment.

### 6.4. Herpes Genitalis.

Herpes genitalis, caused by Herpes simplex virus (HSV) 1 and 2, is characterized by a high rate of recurrences. *In vivo* use of zinc acetate gel has been found effective in preventing sexual transmission of HSV-2 and HIV infections [17]. Mahajan et al. [18] used zinc sulphate as 1%, 2%, and 4% topically in three groups of 30 patients each with herpes genitalis for a period of 3 months and observed that higher concentrations were more effective in treating as well as preventing recurrences. However, not many studies are available for making any recommendations.

### 6.5. Dermatophytoses.

Dermatophytoses are a diverse array of disorders involving the skin, hair, and nails. Antifungals agents like azoles and allylamines, both topical and systemic, form the mainstay of treatment. Of late, emergence of resistance to these agents is being observed in clinical practice when a need for different/additional treatment modalities is being felt. Zinc in combination with 2% undecylenic acid has been tried for the treatment of dermatophytoses. Chretien et al. [19] in a randomized control trial in 151 patients of tinea pedis studied the efficacy of a powder containing 20% zinc-undecylenate, 2% undecylenic acid, and a placebo powder. After a study period of 4 weeks, a negative culture and a negative KOH examination were seen in 88% and 80% as compared to 17% and 49% in placebo group. Clinical improvement in the form of decreased erythema, scaling, and itching was also significantly more in the former group.

### 6.6. Bromhidrosis.

Bromhidrosis is a common disorder characterized by foul smelling sweat. A strong odor is usually associated with increased bacterial flora, usually of *Corynebacterium* sp. Topical antibacterials and antiperspirants are the treatment of choice along with maintenance of good hygiene. Owing to its antibacterial action, topical zinc sulphate has been tried and found effective in the management of axillary bromhidrosis and plantar malodor [20, 21]. Sharquie et al. [21] in a single blinded placebo controlled therapeutic trial studied the efficacy of 15% zinc sulphate solution for foot malodor. Zinc sulfate solution 15% was applied to sole and toe-webs once daily for two weeks and three times per week for next two weeks followed by single application weekly as maintenance after clearance of odor for two months. Fifty-eight patients received zinc sulphate solution while other 50 patients received a placebo solution. Thirty-five of the 50 (70%) patients who completed the study showed complete clearance of foot odor as compared to only 1 (2%) subject in placebo group and the difference was statistically significant.

*6.7. Pityriasis Versicolor.* Pityriasis versicolor is a common fungal disorder presenting as truncal hypopigmented scaly macules. It is a common condition in tropics and may affect up to 40% of the population. Azole antifungals, like itraconazole and ketoconazole, both in topical and systemic formulations, form the mainstay of treatment. Zinc pyrithione 1% is a proven treatment modality for pityriasis versicolor owing to its anti-inflammatory action and direct cytotoxic action on *Pityrosporum ovale*. Topical zinc sulphate too has been used for the management of pityriasis versicolor. Sharquie et al. [22] observed complete clinical and mycological cure after 3 weeks' treatment with once daily application of 15% topical zinc sulphate in their single blinded placebo controlled study comprising 30 patients with pityriasis versicolor while no patient in placebo group showed any response.

# 7. Inflammatory Dermatoses

The anti-inflammatory properties of zinc have been the reasons for its use in many common inflammatory dermatoses like acne, rosacea, eczemas, and ulcers and wounds of varied etiology.

*7.1. Acne Vulgaris.* Acne vulgaris is the most common disorder among the adolescent age group affecting 90–95% of the midteen population. A large variety of topical and systemic agents is used for their management. Oral and topical antibiotics and/or retinoids are the commonly used therapies. A chronic persistent clinical course along with the emergence of resistance to common antibiotics has led to trial of numerous novel agents in acne management. Zinc has been used extensively both topically and systemically for the management of acne vulgaris since the time its favorable effect on acne was recognized by Michaelsson in a patient of acrodermatitis enteropathica and subsequent studies demonstrated low serum zinc in acne patients [23–28]. Although topical zinc sulfate was not effective and caused significant local irritation, the efficacy of topical antiacne medications containing zinc acetate or octoate with or without erythromycin is either equal or superior to erythromycin, tetracycline, or clindamycin used alone in reducing the severity of acne and the number of lesions [29–33]. Contrarily, Sharquie et al. [34] observed beneficial effect of topical 5% zinc sulfate in a single-blinded randomized study in 47 patients with mild acne

vulgaris comparing it with topical 2% tea lotion. Although zinc appears to enhance the topical absorption of erythromycin in a study, the onset of action of erythromycin with zinc acetate applied twice daily was slower than benzoyl peroxide with clindamycin phosphate used once daily while overall efficacy and adverse effects were similar in another study [35, 36]. Oral zinc sulfate is reportedly more effective in the treatment of severe acne than for the treatment of mild to moderate acne but nausea, vomiting, and diarrhea occur frequently [37–40]. Similarly, oral zinc gluconate has been found useful in managing inflammatory acne but the initial loading dose is not beneficial [41–43]. However, acne treatment with zinc salts appears to be equal or less effective compared with systemic tetracyclines (minocycline, oxytetracycline) [40, 42, 44]. Recently a methionine bound zinc complex with antioxidants has been tried and found useful in managing mild to moderate acne vulgaris [45]. Zinc, with or without nicotinamide, is also another emerging alternate acne treatment to reduce possible adverse effects of antibiotics and in view of *Propionibacterium acnes* strains developing resistance to conventional antibiotics [46]. The exact mechanism of zinc in acne treatment remains poorly elucidated and is considered to act directly on microbial inflammatory equilibrium and facilitate antibiotic absorption when used in combination. Topical zinc alone as well as in combination with other agents is effective perhaps because of its anti-inflammatory activity and ability to reduce *P. acnes* counts by inhibition of *P. acnes* lipases and free fatty acid levels [37]. Another proposed mechanism for the benefit of zinc in acne is suppression of sebum production by its antiandrogenic activity [47].

*7.2. Rosacea, Hidradenitis Suppurativa, Acne Conglobata, and Folliculitis Decalvans.* Rosacea is a chronic disorder characterized by frequent flushing, erythema, and telangiectasia, interspersed by episodes of inflammation during which swelling, papules, and pustules are seen. A number of drugs, which include antibiotics (tetracyclines, metronidazole), immunosuppressants (calcineurin inhibitors-tacrolimus, pimecrolimus), retinoids, and vascular lasers, are the commonly used treatments. Oral zinc sulphate was found useful in the management of rosacea by Sharquie et al. [48]. They used zinc sulphate 100 mg thrice daily in 25 patients of rosacea in a double blind randomized control trial and observed a statistically significant decrease in disease activity after three months of therapy without any serious adverse effects. However, Bamford et al. [49] observed no significant improvement with oral zinc therapy in another randomized control trial. The antioxidant and anti-inflammatory properties of zinc have been postulated to be useful in the management of rosacea. The anti-inflammatory and antioxidant actions of zinc have also been utilized for the management of other follicular occlusion disorders like hidradenitis suppurativa, acne conglobata, and folliculitis decalvans as well. Brocard et al. [50] observed clinical response without significant side effects in all 22 patients of hidradenitis suppurativa when treated with zinc gluconate 90 mg/day. Similarly, Kobayashi et al. [51] reported complete cure of acne conglobata and dissecting cellulitis with oral zinc sulphate. However, overall benefit of zinc in these disorders remains understudied.

*7.3. Psoriasis and Psoriatic Arthritis.* Psoriasis is a common disorder affecting nearly 2-3% of general population with joint involvement being a common disabling complication. A large armamentarium of drugs ranging from time tested modalities like coal tar and phototherapy, methotrexate, and retinoids to newer "biological" modalities are being currently used. However, the chronically relapsing nature of the disease has always compelled the researchers to look for novel and safe therapies. Zinc has been tried for the management of psoriasis and psoriatic arthritis. Sadeghian et al. [52] found topical 0.25% zinc pyrithione cream, applied twice daily, effective for localized plaque psoriasis in a randomized double-blind controlled trial. The benefit was attributed to antiproliferative effect of zinc pyrithione. Oral zinc sulphate was found effective for psoriatic arthritis by Clemmensen et al. [53] in a double blind crossover trial versus placebo in 24 patients of psoriatic arthritis. However, oral zinc sulphate did not produce clinically significant improvement as a treatment modality for plaque psoriasis [54].

*7.4. Eczemas.* Eczemas comprise a diverse group of dermatoses with variable etiology and clinical manifestations and constitute significant proportion of all dermatological diseases with an estimated prevalence of 18 cases per 1000 US population. Contact dermatitis of occupational origin is by far the most common form of eczema and hand eczema accounts for majority of the cases. Depending upon the principal causative factors, the eczema may be endogenous eczema (atopic dermatitis, seborrhoeic dermatitis, discoid or nummular eczema, and asteatotic eczema) or exogenous or contact eczema (allergic or irritant contact dermatitis, photoallergic contact dermatitis). However, the clinical presentation of eczema may be modified by regional variation in skin structure and function such as in case of hand eczema. Apart from removal of the etiological agent, use of immunosuppressants like corticosteroids and calcineurin inhibitors form the mainstay of treatment. Zinc has anti-inflammatory properties and increases reepithelialization supporting its use for treating eczemas. Zinc oxide paste has been used for the treatment of diaper dermatitis since long. Although it is less effective as compared to other treatment modalities like topical corticosteroids, it is a useful soothing and antipruritic agent [55, 56]. A statistically significant improvement was observed with a combination cream containing zinc sulphate (2.5%) and clobetasol (0.05%) over plain clobetasol (0.05%) cream in 47 patients of chronic hand eczema in a double-blind, right to left, prospective clinical trial by Faghihi et al. [57]. Topical zinc oxide for its strong antioxidant and antibacterial action has been also used in treating atopic dermatitis, a chronic inflammatory eczematous dermatosis characterized by the impairment of the skin-barrier function, increased oxidative cellular stress, and bacterial colonization. Zinc oxide impregnated textiles have been tried *in vivo* for the management of atopic dermatitis in a study and a significant improvement was observed in the disease severity, pruritus, and subjective sleep in patients who wore zinc oxide-impregnated textiles than in control group [58]. These zinc oxide-functionalized textiles could be the upcoming treatment modality of choice for atopic dermatitis for future.

*7.5. Ulcers and Wounds.* Ulcers of variable etiology are a common presentation in the dermatology outpatients with an estimated community prevalence of 0.2%. Ulcer management is a challenging task for the treating physician as poor response to treatment is frequent in a sizeable proportion of cases due to the persistence of underlying etiological factors. Zinc, both oral and topical, for its healing properties has been used for a long time for the management of ulcers and wounds of varied etiology. Although oral zinc sulphate was initially reported to enhance the healing of arterial/venous leg ulcers, recent systematic reviews and meta-analysis have found no statistically significant response [59]. However, topical preparations containing zinc oxide have been used in the management of arterial and venous leg ulcers, pressure ulcers, and diabetic foot ulcers. The reported response rate was 83% in a study on efficacy of topical zinc oxide paste in both arterial and venous ulcers [60]. Usefulness of zinc iontophoresis has been demonstrated in ischemic skin ulcers as well [61]. Sehgal et al. [62] used phenytoin sodium, zinc oxide paste in 40 leprosy patients with trophic ulcers. After 4 weeks of daily therapy, 55% patients showed complete clearance of the ulcers while 82.5% showed development of granulation tissue. This therapeutically beneficial effect of zinc in chronic cutaneous ulcers is attributed to its anti-inflammatory and antibacterial properties and its ability to enhance reepithelialization. However, there is not enough scientific evidence to make any recommendations for its use in chronic leg ulcers [59, 63].

*7.6. Behcet's Disease and Oral Aphthosis.* Behcet's disease is a vasculopathic condition characterized by recurrent episodes of oral and genital ulcerations with positive pathergy test. Oral aphthae are another troublesome condition of obscure etiology characterized by recurrent painful oral ulcerations particularly in adolescents. Several treatment modalities including corticosteroids and immunosuppressants have been used with variable results. Sharquie et al. [64] in a randomized, controlled, double-blind crossover trial comprising 30 subjects found oral zinc sulphate, 100 mg given thrice daily for three months, to be an effective treatment modality for Behcet's disease without any major adverse effects. They also found oral zinc sulphate (100 mg thrice daily) useful in the treatment of recurrent oral aphthae in another double-blind placebo controlled study of 15 patients [65]. Zinc sulphate had both therapeutic and prophylactic action as it also reduced the relapse rate in recurrent aphthae.

*7.7. Necrolytic Migratory Erythema (NME).* It is a dermatosis which is usually associated with an underlying pancreatic tumor especially glucagonoma. However, many cases have been described without any underlying pancreatic malignancy. Zinc deficiency is considered a possible reason among many pathogenic hypotheses put forth for this unusual entity as both acrodermatitis enteropathica (inherited zinc deficiency) and acquired zinc deficiency have a striking clinicopathological similarity with necrolytic migratory erythema. It has been also observed that patients of NME have low serum zinc levels and the most consistent improvement is noted with zinc sulfate 440 mg/day [66]. Even in patients with normal serum zinc levels, zinc supplementation leads to clinical improvement of NME [67].

## 8. Disorders of Hair and Mucosa

*8.1. Alopecias.* Androgenetic alopecia is a common disorder with an estimated 90% of males above the age of 20 years having some degree of frontal recession. Drugs like minoxidil and finasteride and surgical modalities like hair transplantation form the mainstay of treatment. Zinc has been found to possess antiandrogen action and it modulates 5α-reductase type 1 and 2 activity [3]. Although it was less effective as compared to topical 5% minoxidil lotion, a considerable hair growth was observed with topical zinc pyrithione 1% solution in androgenic alopecia in a randomized, investigator-blinded, parallel-group clinical study [68]. Alopecia areata is another common autoimmune disorder with numerous treatment modalities but none is being universally effective. Sharquie et al. [69] in a randomized placebo-controlled, double-blinded crossover study used zinc sulphate in a dose of 5 mg/kg/day in three divided doses for a period of six months and observed a visible clinical response in 62% of patients with alopecia areata. However, there is overall paucity of relevant literature.

*8.2. Erosive Pustular Dermatosis of Scalp.* It is another rare chronic disease manifesting with extensive pustular lesions, erosions, and crusting of the scalp, leading ultimately to scarring alopecia. Response to therapy has been variable with different treatments including topical or systemic antibiotics, oral isotretinoin, or dapsone. Ikeda et al. [70] found oral zinc sulphate to be a safe and effective treatment modality for this uncommon entity.

*8.3. Seborrhoeic Dermatitis.* Seborrhoeic dermatitis is a common entity with an estimated prevalence of 1–3% in the general population. Zinc pyrithione 1% in a shampoo base is a proven treatment modality for seborrhoeic dermatitis and is an active ingredient, mostly in combination with ketoconazole, of several antidandruff shampoos available over the counter or on prescription. It possesses cytotoxic activity against *Pityrosporum ovale* and has antiproliferative action as well which are considered responsible for its clinical efficacy. It also prevents recurrence of flaking, itching, and irritation associated with dandruff and its antifungal activity has been attributed to its ability to disrupt fungal membrane transport by blocking the proton pump that energizes the transport mechanism. However, a combination of zinc pyrithione and ketoconazole is more effective than either agent used alone. Zinc pyrithione 1% in a shampoo base has been found to cause significant reduction in scaling and inflammation but its response was less when compared with 1% ketoconazole [71, 72].

*8.4. Mucosal (Oral) Lichen Planus.* Lichen planus is a chronic inflammatory disease of skin and mucous membranes. Despite plethora of medications, corticosteroids, retinoids, dapsone, and immunosuppressants, a definite cure for lichen planus remains unknown. Mehdipour et al. [73] compared the efficacy of 0.2% zinc mouthwash in combination with fluocinolone with a plain fluocinolone mouthwash in 20 patients of erosive lichen planus. It was observed that pain, irritation, and lesion surface area decreased in both groups. However, decrease in surface area with zinc mouthwash plus fluocinolone was statistically more significant than that with fluocinolone alone.

## 9. Premalignant and Malignant Dermatoses

Zinc in high concentration has been found to possess a direct cytotoxic effect and is well known to induce apoptosis of malignant cells and tissue necrosis. This property of zinc has been utilized for its use in premalignant and malignant conditions of skin like xeroderma pigmentosa, actinic keratosis, and basal cell carcinoma. Topical therapy with zinc sulfate solution has been found to have both therapeutic and prophylactic role in patients with xeroderma pigmentosa. Sharquie et al. [74] studied the effect of 20% topical zinc sulphate in 19 patients with xeroderma pigmentosa. Improvement in all types of skin lesions, including softening and lightening of the skin color, and clearance of solar keratosis and small malignancies were observed in 15 patients who continued the study during monthly followup over a follow-up period of 2 years. There was no exacerbation of old lesions or no development of new malignancy. Actinic keratosis, a premalignant condition resulting from proliferation of aberrant epidermal keratinocytes, occurs primarily on sun-exposed skin. Many therapeutic modalities including curettage and cautery, topical agents like 5-fluorouracil, imiquimod (5%) cream, and 3% diclofenac gel, are used for its treatment. Sharquie et al. [75] observed a statistically significant response in the form of clearance of lesions with 25% topical zinc sulphate applied twice daily over the lesions for 12 weeks in 14 of 18 patients. They also observed significant improvement in all 100 lesions of basal cell carcinoma with intralesional 2% zinc gluconate solution without any significant adverse effects in another open-label case interventional study [76]. These beneficial effects of zinc in xeroderma pigmentosa or actinic keratosis are attributable to enhanced wound healing, antioxidant action, sunscreen property, enhanced DNA repair, improved immunity, and accelerated apoptosis of malignant cells [74].

## 10. Pigmentary Disorders

Topical zinc has been used for both vitiligo and melasma. Vitiligo is a common depigmenting disorder with variable etiology seen in about 0.1%–2% of the population. As vitiligo patients have been found to have significant low serum zinc levels than normal controls, zinc was postulated to play a role in the management of vitiligo [77, 78]. Yaghoobi et al. [79] in a randomized control trial compared the efficacy of topical steroids alone with the combination of topical steroids and oral zinc sulphate in 15 patients each. An appreciable but statistically insignificant clinical response was observed in 24.7% patients in oral zinc-topical corticosteroid group after four months of therapy as compared to 21.43% in the topical corticosteroid group. Zinc possesses significant antiapoptotic and antioxidant activity and along with other micronutrients like copper and manganese also postulated to play an important role in melanogenesis.

Melasma, a common pigmentary dermatosis, causes significant psychological stress due to cosmetic morbidity in affected patients. It affects all races with a predilection for Hispanics and Asians and accounts for 0.25 to 4% of the patients seen in dermatology practice in Southeast Asia. Genetic predisposition, pregnancy, oral contraceptives, endocrine dysfunction, hormone treatments, or exposure to UV light have been implicated frequently in its pathogenesis. Clinically, it presents in three distinct patterns of centrofacial, malar, and mandibular pigmentation observed in 55–75%, 24–43%, and 1.5–2% patients, respectively, across studies. A large number of treatment modalities have been tried for the treatment of melasma ranging from depigmenting agents like hydroquinone to lasers. Topical zinc sulphate has also been tried in the management of melasma owing to its peeling and sunscreen properties. Sharquie et al. [80] reported a significant reduction in MASI (melasma area and severity index) scores in 14 melasma patients after three months of therapy with 10% topical zinc sulphate without any significant adverse effects. However, this mode of treatment did not find much favor as results could not be reproduced in other studies and no statistically significant improvement was seen with topical zinc therapy [81, 82]. Moreover, it is not cosmetically elegant and acceptability remains poor. Nevertheless, zinc oxide, in micronized forms, remains a common ingredient of most sunscreens used for treatment of melasma.

## 11. Miscellaneous Dermatoses

*11.1. Scars and Keloids.* Hypertrophic scars and keloids of any origin are associated with considerable disfigurement. Propensity for recurrences seen with keloids is associated with significant psychological morbidity. Treatment with intralesional corticosteroids, topical silicon gel sheets, surgery, and other physical treatment modalities including lasers and cryotherapy have their own advantages and disadvantages. The beneficial effect of topical zinc in the treatment of keloids in few studies has been attributed to its ability to inhibit lysyl oxidase and stimulate collagenase that leads to decreased production and increased degradation of collagen. Söderberg et al. [83] reported a clinical response in 23 of the 41 patients with keloids after six months of application of a zinc tape. Similarly, Moshref [84] reported a complete clearance of keloids with a very low rate of recurrence in 34% patients with the use of a zinc tape. However, few well-designed studies remain desirable for acceptance of this low cost treatment for this highly distressing condition.

*11.2. Antiageing.* Mahoney et al. [85] evaluated the effects of a bi-metal, 0.1% copper-zinc malonate, containing cream on elastin biosynthesis and elastic tissue accumulation in 21 female patients with photoaged facial skin. After 8 weeks of therapy, significant elastic fiber regeneration was seen in the papillary dermis leading to effacement of wrinkles. The combined photoprotective and elastic regenerative properties of zinc could be used for the development of effective antiageing therapies.

*11.3. Pruritus.* Calamine lotion contains zinc oxide or zinc carbonate and is used frequently for symptomatic relief in pruritus because of its soothing properties. Zinc also inhibits mast cell degranulation and thereby reduces the secretion of histamine, an important mediator of inflammatory response and an inducer of itch, thereby making it a useful treatment option in pruritic conditions [86].

*11.4. Prevention of Photodamage and Skin Cancers.* Zinc oxide is widely used as a broad spectrum physical sunscreen. Its advantage lies in its low cost and an excellent safety profile. It has been used alone and in combination with other physical (titanium oxide) or chemical sunscreen agents. Recently microfine and nano-sized zinc oxide has become available which provides better cosmetic appeal and photoprotection than traditional zinc oxide preparations. Zinc oxide provides protection against UV-A1 (340–380) superior to titanium oxide providing better spectrum protection [87].

## 12. Comments

Zinc is an important micronutrient required for the normal function of skin. The daily allowance of elemental zinc in infants with zinc deficiency is usually 3 mg/d for first 6 months and 5 mg/d for second six months. Subsequently, zinc may be supplemented as 10 mg/d during 1–10 years, 15 mg/d for adolescents and adults, and 20–25 mg/d during pregnancy and lactation. For therapeutic purpose zinc is administered orally or parenterally as zinc sulfate (22.5 mg of elemental zinc/100 mg), zinc acetate (30 mg elemental zinc/100 mg), or zinc oxide (80 mg elemental zinc/100 mg). The recommended doses for elemental zinc are 0.5–1 mg/kg/day in divided doses in children and 15–30 mg/day in adults. Gastrointestinal upsets with bloody diarrhea may occur sometimes after ingestion of zinc sulfate beyond recommended doses. Therapeutically, zinc can be used, both topically and in systemic form, for a large number of dermatological disorders. Its efficacy in treating acne perhaps remains the most studied despite varied results. However, it should not substitute the treatment with proven first line therapeutic modalities as most of the studies showing efficacy of zinc are small case series or have small sample size. Interestingly, systemic zinc as a therapeutic modality does not find much favor despite many dermatological conditions shown responding to it. Perhaps more experimental and clinical evidence in the form of appropriately blinded randomized control trials and case-control studies for the treatment of various dermatoses is needed to determine the efficacy of this low cost mode of treatment and compare it with the established treatment modalities. Only after adequate studies for its efficacy and safety, the treatment guidelines or recommendations for zinc therapy can be made. Nevertheless, it can best be used as an adjuvant to established treatment modalities.

## Conflict of Interests

The authors declare that there is no conflict of interests regarding the publication of this paper.

# References

[1] Y. B. Nitzan and A. D. Cohen, "Zinc in skin pathology and care," *Journal of Dermatological Treatment*, vol. 17, no. 4, pp. 205–210, 2006.

[2] H. Kitamura, H. Morikawa, H. Kamon et al., "Toll-like receptor-mediated regulation of zinc homeostasis influences dendritic cell function," *Nature Immunology*, vol. 7, no. 9, pp. 971–977, 2006.

[3] A. Brocard, A. Knol, A. Khammari, and B. Dréno, "Hidradenitis suppurativa and zinc: a new therapeutic approach—a pilot study," *Dermatology*, vol. 214, no. 4, pp. 325–327, 2007.

[4] N. L. Sharma, "Zinc, an update," *Indian Journal of Dermatology, Venereology and Leprology*, vol. 51, pp. 305–308, 1985.

[5] H. K. Bangash and A. Sethi, "Zinc and skin health: an overview," in *Handbook of Diet, Nutrition and the Skin*, vol. 2 of *Human Health Handbooks no. 1*, pp. 178–195, Wageningen Academic, 2012.

[6] K. E. Sharquie, A. A. Khorsheed, and A. A. Al-Nuaimy, "Topical zinc sulphate solution for treatment of viral warts," *Saudi Medical Journal*, vol. 28, no. 9, pp. 1418–1421, 2007.

[7] J. A. Khattar, U. M. Musharrafieh, H. Tamim, and G. N. Hamadeh, "Topical zinc oxide vs salicylic acid-lactic acid combination in the treatment of warts," *International Journal of Dermatology*, vol. 46, no. 4, pp. 427–430, 2007.

[8] F. T. Al-Gurairi, M. Al-Waiz, and K. E. Sharquie, "Oral zinc sulphate in the treatment of recalcitrant viral warts: randomized placebo-controlled clinical trial," *British Journal of Dermatology*, vol. 146, no. 3, pp. 423–431, 2002.

[9] J. H. Mun, S. H. Kim, D. S. Jung et al., "Oral zinc sulfate treatment for viral warts: an open-label study," *Journal of Dermatology*, vol. 38, pp. 541–545, 2011.

[10] S. Sharma, K. D. Barman, R. Sarkar, M. Manjhi, and V. K. Garg, "Efficacy of oral zinc therapy in epidermodysplasia verruciformis with squamous cell carcinoma," *Indian Dermatology*, vol. 5, pp. 55–58, 2014.

[11] K. A. Sharquine and A. A. Al-Nuaimy, "Treatment of viral warts by intralesional injection of zinc sulphate," *Annals of Saudi Medicine*, vol. 22, no. 1-2, pp. 26–28, 2002.

[12] F. Iraji, A. Vali, A. Asilian, M. A. Shahtalebi, and A. Z. Momeni, "Comparison of intralesionally injected zinc sulfate with meglumine antimoniate in the treatment of acute cutaneous leishmaniasis," *Dermatology*, vol. 209, no. 1, pp. 46–49, 2004.

[13] K. E. Sharquie, R. A. Najim, I. B. Farjou, and D. J. Al-Timimi, "Oral zinc sulphate in the treatment of acute cutaneous leishmaniasis," *Clinical and Experimental Dermatology*, vol. 26, no. 1, pp. 21–26, 2001.

[14] A. Gupta, V. K. Sharma, H. Vohra, and N. K. Ganguly, "Inhibition of apoptosis by ionomycin and zinc in peripheral blood mononuclear cells (PBMC) of leprosy patients," *FEMS Immunology and Medical Microbiology*, vol. 24, pp. 49–55, 1999.

[15] N. K. Mathur, R. A. Bumb, and H. N. Mangal, "Oral zinc in recurrent erythema nodosum leprosum reaction," *Leprosy In India*, vol. 55, no. 3, pp. 547–552, 1983.

[16] N. K. Mathur, R. A. Bumb, H. N. Mangal, and M. L. Sharma, "Oral zinc as an adjunct to dapsone in lepromatous leprosy," *International Journal of Leprosy*, vol. 52, no. 3, pp. 331–338, 1984.

[17] J. A. Fernández-Romero, C. J. Abraham, A. Rodriguez et al., "Zinc acetate/carrageenan gels exhibit potent activity in vivo against high-dose herpes simplex virus 2 vaginal and rectal challenge," *Antimicrobial Agents and Chemotherapy*, vol. 56, no. 1, pp. 358–368, 2012.

[18] B. B. Mahajan, M. Dhawan, and R. Singh, "Herpes genitalis—topical an alternative therapeutic modality," *Indian Journal of Sexually Transmitted Diseases*, vol. 34, pp. 32–34, 2013.

[19] J. H. Chretien, J. G. Esswein, L. M. Sharpe, J. J. Kiely, and F. E. Lyddon, "Efficacy of undecylenic acid-zinc undecylenate powder in culture positive tinea pedis," *International Journal of Dermatology*, vol. 19, no. 1, pp. 51–54, 1980.

[20] M. D. Scribner, "Zinc sulfate and axillary perspiration odor," *Archives of Dermatology*, vol. 113, no. 9, article 1302, 1977.

[21] K. E. Sharquie, A. A. Noaimi, and S. D. Hameed, "Topical 15% zinc sulfate solution is an effective therapy for feet odor," *Journal of Cosmetics, Dermatological Sciences and Applications*, vol. 3, pp. 203–208, 2013.

[22] K. E. Sharquie, W. S. Al-Dori, I. K. Sharquie, and A. A. Al-Nuaimy, "Treatment of pityriasis versicolor with topical 15% zinc sulfate solution," *Iraqi Journalof Community Medicine*, vol. 21, pp. 61–63, 2008.

[23] G. Michaelsson, "Zinc therapy in acrodermatitis enteropathica," *Acta Dermato—Venereologica*, vol. 54, no. 5, pp. 377–381, 1974.

[24] B. Dreno, D. Moyse, M. Alirezai et al., "Multicenter randomized comparative double-blind controlled clinical trial of the safety and efficacy of zinc gluconate versus minocycline hydrochloride in the treatment of inflammatory acne vulgaris," *Dermatology*, vol. 203, no. 2, pp. 135–140, 2001.

[25] L. Hillström, L. Pettersson, L. Hellbe, A. Kjellin, C. G. Leczinsky, and C. Nordwall, "Comparison of oral treatment with zinc sulphate and placebo in acne vulgaris," *British Journal of Dermatology*, vol. 97, no. 6, pp. 681–684, 1977.

[26] K. Goransson, S. Liden, and L. Odsell, "Oral zinc in acne vulgaris: a clinical and methodological study," *Acta Dermato-Venereologica*, vol. 58, no. 5, pp. 443–448, 1978.

[27] K. Verma, A. Saini, and S. Dhamija, "Oral zinc sulfate therapy in acne vulgaris: a double-blind trial," *Acta Dermato-Venereologica*, vol. 60, no. 4, pp. 337–340, 1980.

[28] S. Lidén, K. Göransson, and L. Odsell, "Clinical evaluation in acne," *Acta Dermato—Venereologica*, vol. 89, pp. 47–52, 1980.

[29] R. J. Cochran, S. B. Tucker, and S. A. Flannigan, "Topical zinc therapy for acne vulgaris," *International Journal of Dermatology*, vol. 24, no. 3, pp. 188–190, 1985.

[30] C. L. Feucht, B. S. Allen, D. K. Chalker, and J. G. Smith Jr., "Topical erythromycin with zinc in acne. A double-blind controlled study," *Journal of the American Academy of Dermatology*, vol. 3, no. 5, pp. 483–491, 1980.

[31] L. Habbema, B. Koopmans, H. E. Menke, S. Doornweerd, and K. De Boulle, "A 4% erythromycin and zinc combination (Zineryt) versus 2% erythromycin (Eryderm) in acne vulgaris: a randomized, double-blind comparative study," *British Journal of Dermatology*, vol. 121, no. 4, pp. 497–502, 1989.

[32] L. Schachner, W. Eaglestein, C. Kittles, and P. Mertz, "Topical erythromycin and zinc therapy for acne," *Journal of the American Academy of Dermatology*, vol. 22, no. 2, part 1, pp. 253–260, 1990.

[33] L. Schachner, A. Pestana, and C. Kittles, "A clinical trial comparing the safety and efficacy of a topical erythromycin-zinc formulation with a topical clindamycin formulation," *Journal of the American Academy of Dermatology*, vol. 22, no. 3, pp. 489–495, 1990.

[34] K. E. Sharquie, A. A. Noaimi, and M. M. Al-Salih, "Topical therapy of acne vulgaris using 2% tea lotion in comparison with 5% zinc sulphate solution," *Saudi Medical Journal*, vol. 29, no. 12, pp. 1757–1761, 2008.

[35] E. J. van Hoogdalem, I. J. Terpstm, and A. L. M. Baven, "Evaluation of the effect of zinc acetate on the stratum corneum penetration kinetics of erythromycin in healthy male volunteers," *Skin Pharmacology*, vol. 9, no. 2, pp. 104–110, 1996.

[36] A. Langner, R. Sheehan-Dare, and A. Layton, "A randomized, single-blind comparison of topical clindamycin + benzoyl peroxide (Duac) and erythromycin + zinc acetate (Zineryt) in the treatment of mild to moderate facial acne vulgaris," *Journal of the European Academy of Dermatology and Venereology*, vol. 21, no. 3, pp. 311–319, 2007.

[37] Y. S. Bae, N. D. Hill, Y. Bibi, J. Dreiher, and A. D. Cohen, "Innovative uses for zinc in dermatology," *Dermatologic Clinics*, vol. 28, no. 3, pp. 587–597, 2010.

[38] L. Orris, A. R. Shalita, D. Sibulkin, S. J. London, and E. H. Gans, "Oral zinc therapy of acne. Absorption and clinical effect.," *Archives of Dermatology*, vol. 114, no. 7, pp. 1018–1020, 1978.

[39] V. M. Weimar, S. C. Puhl, W. H. Smith, and J. E. TenBroeke, "Zinc sulfate in acne vulgaris," *Archives of Dermatology*, vol. 114, no. 12, pp. 1776–1778, 1978.

[40] W. J. Cunliffe, "Unacceptable side-effects of oral zinc sulphate in the treatment of acne vulgaris.," *British Journal of Dermatology*, vol. 101, article 363, 1979.

[41] B. Dreno, P. Amblard, P. Agache, S. Sirot, and P. Litoux, "Low doses of zinc gluconate for inflammatory acne," *Acta Dermato-Venereologica*, vol. 69, no. 6, pp. 541–543, 1989.

[42] B. Dréno, D. Moyse, M. Alirezai et al., "Multicenter randomized comparative double-blind controlled clinical trial of the safety and efficacy of zinc gluconate versus minocycline hydrochloride in the treatment of inflammatory acne vulgaris," *Dermatology*, vol. 203, no. 2, pp. 135–140, 2001.

[43] J. Meynadier, "Efficacy and safety study of two zinc gluconate regimens in the treatment of inflammatory acne," *European Journal of Dermatology*, vol. 10, no. 4, pp. 269–273, 2000.

[44] G. Michaelsson, L. Juhlin, and K. Ljunghall, "A double blind study of the effect of zinc and oxytetracycline in acne vulgaris," *British Journal of Dermatology*, vol. 97, no. 5, pp. 561–566, 1977.

[45] K. Sardana and V. K. Garg, "An observational study of methionine-bound antioxidants for mild to moderate vulgaris," *Dermatology and Therapy*, vol. 23, pp. 411–418, 2010.

[46] K. A. James, C. N. Burkhart, and D. S. Morrell, "Emerging drugs for acne," *Expert Opinion on Emerging Drugs*, vol. 14, no. 4, pp. 649–659, 2009.

[47] C. Pierard-Franchimont, V. Goffin, J. N. Visser, H. Jacoby, and G. E. Pierard, "A double blind controlled evaluation of the sebosuppressive activity of topical erythromycin-zinc complex," *European Journal of Clinical Pharmacology*, vol. 49, no. 1-2, pp. 57–60, 1995.

[48] K. E. Sharquie, R. A. Najim, and H. N. Al-Salman, "Oral zinc sulfate in the treatment of rosacea: a double-blind, placebo-controlled study," *International Journal of Dermatology*, vol. 45, no. 7, pp. 857–861, 2006.

[49] J. T. Bamford, C. E. Gessert, I. V. Haller, K. Kruger, and B. P. Johnson, "Randomized, double-blind trial of 220mg zinc sulfate twice daily in the treatment of rosacea," *International Journal of Dermatology*, vol. 51, pp. 459–462, 2012.

[50] A. Brocard, A. C. Knol, A. Khammari, and B. Dréno, "Hidradenitis suppurativa and zinc: a new therapeutic approach. A pilot study," *Dermatology*, vol. 214, no. 4, pp. 325–327, 2007.

[51] H. Kobayashi, S. Aiba, and H. Tagami, "Successful treatment of dissecting cellulitis and acne conglobata with oral zinc," *British Journal of Dermatology*, vol. 141, no. 6, pp. 1137–1138, 1999.

[52] G. Sadeghian, H. Ziaei, and M. A. Nilforoushzadeh, "Treatment of localized psoriasis with a topical formulation of zinc pyrithione," *Acta Dermatovenerologica Alpina, Pannonica et Adriatica*, vol. 20, no. 4, pp. 187–190, 2011.

[53] O. J. Clemmensen, J. Siggaard-Andersen, A. M. Worm, D. Stahl, F. Frost, and I. Bloch, "Psoriatic arthritis treated with oral zinc sulphate," *British Journal of Dermatology*, vol. 103, no. 4, pp. 411–415, 1980.

[54] N. P. Burrows, A. J. Turnbull, N. A. Punchard, R. P. H. Thompson, and R. R. Jones, "A trial of oral zinc supplementation in psoriasis," *Cutis*, vol. 54, no. 2, pp. 117–118, 1994.

[55] A. B. G. Landsdown, "Zinc in the healing wound," *The Lancet*, vol. 347, no. 9003, pp. 706–707, 1996.

[56] S. Baldwin, M. R. Odio, S. L. Haines, R. J. O'Connor, J. S. Englehart, and A. T. Lane, "Skin benefits from continuous topical administration of a zinc oxide/petrolatum formulation by a novel disposable diaper," *Journal of the European Academy of Dermatology and Venereology*, vol. 15, supplement 1, pp. 5–11, 2001.

[57] G. Faghihi, F. Iraji, A. Shahingohar, and A. H. Saidat, "The efficacy of "0.05% Clobetasol + 2.5% zinc sulphate" cream versus "0.05% Clobetasol alone" cream in the treatment of the chronic hand eczema: a double-blind study," *Journal of the European Academy of Dermatology and Venereology*, vol. 22, no. 5, pp. 531–536, 2008.

[58] C. Wiegand, U. C. Hipler, S. Boldt, J. Strehle, and U. Wollina, "Skin-protective effects of a zinc oxide-functionalized textile and its relevance for atopic dermatitis," *Clinical, Cosmetic and Investigational Dermatology*, vol. 6, pp. 115–121, 2013.

[59] E. A. J. Wilkinson, "Oral zinc for arterial and venous leg ulcers," *Cochrane Database of Systematic Reviews*, vol. 8, Article ID CD001273, 2012.

[60] H. E. Strömberg and M. S. Ågren, "Topical zinc oxide treatment improves arterial and venous leg ulcers," *British Journal of Dermatology*, vol. 111, pp. 461–468, 1984.

[61] M. C. Cornwall, "Zinc iontophoresis to treat ischemic skin ulcers," *Physical Therapy*, vol. 61, no. 3, pp. 359–360, 1981.

[62] V. N. Sehgal, P. V. S. Prasad, P. K. Kaviarasan, and D. Rajan, "Trophic skin ulceration in leprosy: evaluation of the efficacy of topical phenytoin sodium zinc oxide paste," *International Journal of Dermatology*, vol. 53, no. 7, pp. 873–878, 2014.

[63] E. A. J. Wilkinson and C. I. Hawke, "Does oral zinc aid the healing of chronic leg ulcers? A systematic literature review," *Archives of Dermatology*, vol. 134, no. 12, pp. 1556–1560, 1998.

[64] K. E. Sharquie, R. A. Najim, W. S. Al-Dori, and R. K. Al-Hayani, "Oral zinc sulfate in the treatment of Behcet's disease: a double blind cross-over study," *Journal of Dermatology*, vol. 33, no. 8, pp. 541–546, 2006.

[65] K. E. Sharquie, R. A. Najim, R. K. Al-Hayani, A. A. Al-Nuaimy, and D. M. Maroof, "The therapeutic and prophylactic role of oral zinc sulfate in management of recurrent aphthous stomatitis (ras) in comparison with dapsone," *Saudi Medical Journal*, vol. 29, no. 5, pp. 734–738, 2008.

[66] S. A. Sinclair and N. J. Reynolds, "Necrolytic migratory erythema and zinc deficiency," *The British Journal of Dermatology*, vol. 136, no. 5, pp. 783–785, 1997.

[67] U. Patel, A. Loyd, R. Patel, S. Meehan, and R. Kundu, "Necrolytic acral erythema," *Dermatology*, vol. 16, no. 11, p. 15, 2010.

[68] R. S. Berger, J. L. Fu, K. A. Smiles et al., "The effects of minoxidil, 1% pyrithione zinc and a combination of both on hair density: a randomized controlled trial," *British Journal of Dermatology*, vol. 149, no. 2, pp. 354–362, 2003.

[69] K. E. Sharquie, A. A. Noaimi, and E. R. Shwail, "Oral zinc sulphate in treatment of alopecia areata," *Journal of Clinical and Experimental Dermatology Research*, vol. 3, p. 150, 2012.

[70] M. Ikeda, J. Arata, and H. Isaka, "Erosive pustular dermatosis of the scalp successfully treated with oral zinc sulphate.," *British Journal of Dermatology*, vol. 106, no. 6, pp. 742–743, 1982.

[71] R. Marks, A. D. Pearse, and A. P. Walker, "The effects of a shampoo containing zinc pyrithione on the control of dandruff," *British Journal of Dermatology*, vol. 112, no. 4, pp. 415–422, 1985.

[72] C. Piérard-Franchimont, V. Goffin, J. Decroix, and G. E. Piérard, "A multicenter randomized trial of ketoconazole 2% and zinc pyrithione 1% shampoos in severe dandruff and seborrheic dermatitis," *Skin Pharmacology and Applied Skin Physiology*, vol. 15, no. 6, pp. 434–441, 2002.

[73] M. Mehdipour, A. Taghavi Zenouz, A. Bahramian, J. Yazdani, F. Pouralibaba, and K. Sadr, "Comparison of the effect of mouthwashes with and without fluocinolone on the healing process of erosive oral planus," *Journal of Dental Research, Dental Clinics, Dental Prospects*, vol. 4, pp. 25–28, 2010.

[74] K. E. Sharquie, A. A. Noaimi, and N. O. Kadir, "Topical therapy of xeroderma pigmentosa with 20% zinc sulfate solution," *Iraqi Journal of Postgraduate Medicine*, vol. 7, pp. 231–237, 2008.

[75] K. E. Sharquie, S. A. Al-Mashhadani, A. A. Noaimi, and A. A. Hasan, "Topical zinc sulphate (25%) solution: a new therapy for actinic keratosis," *Journal of Cutaneous and Aesthetic Surgery*, vol. 5, p. 53, 2012.

[76] K. E. Sharquie, A. A. Al-Nuaimy, and F. A. Al-Shimary, "New intralesional therapy for basal cell carcinoma by 2% zinc sulphate solution," *Saudi Medical Journal*, vol. 26, no. 2, pp. 359–361, 2005.

[77] P. Shameer, P. V. S. Prasad, and P. K. Kaviarasan, "Serum zinc level in vitiligo: a case control study," *Indian Journal of Dermatology, Venereology and Leprology*, vol. 71, no. 3, pp. 206–207, 2005.

[78] N. Bagherani, R. Yaghoobi, and M. Omidian, "Hypothesis: Zinc can be effective in treatment of vitiligo," *Indian Journal of Dermatology*, vol. 56, no. 5, pp. 480–484, 2011.

[79] R. Yaghoobi, M. Omidian, and N. Bagherani, "Comparison of therapeutic efficacy of topical corticosteroid and oral zinc sulfate-topical corticosteroid combination in the treatment of vitiligo patients: a clinical trial," *BMC Dermatology*, vol. 11, article 7, 2011.

[80] K. E. Sharquie, S. A. Al-Mashhadani, and H. A. Salman, "Topical 10% zinc sulfate solution for treatment of melasma," *Dermatologic Surgery*, vol. 34, no. 10, pp. 1346–1349, 2008.

[81] A. Yousefi, Z. Khani Khoozani, S. Zakerzadeh Forooshani, N. Omrani, A. M. Moini, and Y. Eskandari, "Is topical zinc effective in the treatment of melasma? A double-blind randomized comparative study," *Dermatologic Surgery*, vol. 40, no. 1, pp. 33–37, 2014.

[82] F. Iraji, N. Tagmirriahi, and K. Gavidnia, "Comparison between the efficacy of 10% zinc sulfate solution with 4% hydroquinone cream on improvement of melasma," *Advanced Biomedical Research*, vol. 1, article 39, 2012.

[83] T. Söderberg, G. Hallmans, and L. Bartholdson, "Treatment of keloids and hypertrophic scars with adhesive zinc tape," *Scandinavian Journal of Plastic and Reconstructive Surgery and Hand Surgery*, vol. 16, no. 3, pp. 261–266, 1982.

[84] S. Moshref, "Topical zinc oxide adhesive tape for keloid management," *The Egyptian Journal of Surgery*, vol. 25, pp. 169–177, 2006.

[85] M. G. Mahoney, D. Brennan, B. Starcher et al., "Extracellular matrix in cutaneous ageing: the effects of 0.1% copper-zinc malonate-containing cream on elastin biosynthesis," *Experimental Dermatology*, vol. 18, no. 3, pp. 205–211, 2009.

[86] G. Marone, M. Columbo, A. de Paulis, R. Cirillo, R. Giugliano, and M. Condorelli, "Physiological concentrations of zinc inhibit the release of histamine from human basophils and lung mast cells," *Agents and Actions*, vol. 18, no. 1-2, pp. 103–106, 1986.

[87] S. R. Pinnell, D. Fairhurst, R. Gillies, M. A. Mitchnick, and N. Kollias, "Microfine zinc oxide is a superior sunscreen ingredient to microfine titanium dioxide," *Dermatologic Surgery*, vol. 26, no. 4, pp. 309–314, 2000.

# 23

# *Mycobacterium ulcerans* Disease with Unusual Sites Not to Be Ignored

**Sangaré Abdoulaye, Kourouma Sarah Hamdan, Kouassi Yao Isidore, Ecra Elidjé Joseph, Kaloga Mamadou, and Gbery Ildevert Patrice**

*Department of Dermatology of the University Teaching Hospital of Treichville, Riviera, BP 408 Cidex 03 Abidjan, Cote d'Ivoire*

Correspondence should be addressed to Sangaré Abdoulaye; sang_abdoulaye@yahoo.fr

Academic Editor: H. Honigsmann

*Objective.* The usual preferential site of BU is in the limbs. In our experience, we noticed atypical and often misleading sites which pose serious issues for the diagnosis and often for the treatment. *Methods.* This is a retrospective study conducted over a period of ten years of BU treatment at the Department of Dermatology of the University Teaching Hospital of Treichville (Abidjan, Côte d'Ivoire). We included in this study all BU cases with atypical site diagnosed clinically and confirmed either by the histology, by smear, or by PCR. *Results.* Epidemiologically, the age of patients ranged from 3 to 72 years with a median age of 14.2 years. Children aged less than 15 years were affected in almost 80% of case. The clinical table was dominated by ulcerated forms in 82.1% of cases. The unusual topography mostly observed was that of the torso (thorax, back, and abdomen) in 76.8% of cases. *Conclusion.* BU is an endemic disease in Côte d'Ivoire where it constitutes a serious public health issue. Several years following its first cases, BU still is little known. This dermatosis may present atypical misleading clinical aspects which must be ignored.

## 1. Introduction

*Mycobacterium ulcerans* (MU) also known as Buruli ulcer (BU) named after the District of Uganda where an epidemic occurred in the 1960s is mycobacteriosis [1]. This disease believed to be mysterious by many parents is characterized by preulcerative lesions leading in the long term to major chronic cutaneous deterioration often associated to definitive disabilities [2]. In Côte d'Ivoire, Buruli ulcer which is the second mycobacteriosis after tuberculosis constitutes an emerging endemic. This is the reason why the government initiated, since 1998, the National Programme of Fight against Mycobacterium Ulcers (PNUM) in Côte d'Ivoire.

Its preferential site in 9 out of 10 cases is in lower limbs [3, 4]. However, in our experience, we observed some unusual sites. So the purpose of this study is to contribute to a better understanding of them.

The specific objectives of this study are to determine sociodemographic characteristics and to describe clinical and topographical aspects of such unusual sites.

## 2. Patients and Method

This is a retrospective, cross-sectional, and descriptive study related to BU cases observed over a period of ten years (i.e., from 2003 to 2013). This study was conducted in the Dermatology Department of the University Teaching Hospital of Treichville which is the reference centre for cutaneous pathologies in Abidjan and served as the head office of the PNUM.

We included patients, irrespective of their gender and age, who over the study period developed an unusual (atypical) ulcer or a nodule clinically evoking *Mycobacterium ulcerans*.

We considered, as the usual or typical site of BU, any ulcer that is found on the limbs and more specifically on lower limbs.

However, any site, other than the limb, is said to be unusual, atypical, or misleading. The subject matter of this study is unusual sites.

The BU was diagnosed on the basis of clinical and paraclinical arguments.

With regard to clinical aspects, we considered the existence of the following:

(i) manifestations which evoke the inception of a BU: nodule, oedema, and infiltrated plate,

(ii) at latter stage, the characteristic ulceration with its thickened, devitalized, and peeled edges, surpassing the base.

With regard to paraclinical aspects, there should be at least the result of one of the following examinations:

(i) the histology of a nodule, an oedema, or an infiltrated plate with Ziehl-Neelsen stain;

(ii) the smear conducted from the exudates of the ulceration edges with Ziehl-Neelsen stain;

(iii) the PCR (polymerase chain reaction) conducted on the exudate.

Cutaneous biopsies were conducted at the Department of Dermatology and plates were read in the anatomic pathology laboratory of the same University Teaching Hospital. The smear and PCR were conducted by the "Institut Pasteur of Côte d'Ivoire."

The histology was revelatory of a BU case if an infiltrate of lymphocyte, histiocytosis, and hypodermic necrosis were found or if AFB (acid-alcohol-fast Bacilli) were revealed by the Ziehl-Neelsen stain method.

With regard to smear, a positive Ziehl-Neelsen stain was considered as a potential BU case. However, when the Ziehl-Neelsen stain was negative, a PCR (polymerase chain reaction) was conducted on the sampling in order to confirm the diagnosis.

The smear and histology are less expensive but they have an average sensibility. Moreover, such examinations have a poor specificity and do not permit discriminating mycobacteria.

With regard to PCR, its sensibility and specificity are above 90%.

On the basis of clinical and paraclinical arguments, we collected in all 213 BU records comprising classic sites as well as unusual sites.

We did not include in this study all the incomplete records which had no paraclinical data.

## 3. Results

*3.1. Overall Incidence of BU during the Study Period.* During the study period, we recorded in the whole department 42495 patients who came for consultation for various dermatosis. Of the whole population who came for consultation in our department over the study period, we observed 213 BU cases, that is, an overall incidence of 0.5%.

*3.2. Sociodemographic Characteristics of Atypical BU (Table 1)*

*3.2.1. Incidence of BU with Atypical Site.* Of the 213 cases of BU collected, we observed 39 cases of BU with atypical site (i.e., 18.3%) and 174 cases of BU found on the limbs (81.6%).

TABLE 1: Epidemiological and clinical characteristics of atypical forms.

| Parameters | Numbers (N) | Percentage (%) |
|---|---|---|
| Incidences of atypical site | | |
| Sites on the limbs | 174 | 81.6 |
| Atypical sites | **39** | **18.3** |
| Sociodemographic characteristics | | |
| Age | | |
| < or = 15 years | **31** | **79.5** |
| >15 | 08 | 20.5 |
| Sex | | |
| Female | **28** | **71.7** |
| Male | 11 | 28.3 |
| Residence | | |
| Swampy zones | **30** | **77** |
| Far | 09 | 23 |
| Clinical aspects | | |
| Ulcerated forms | **32** | **82.1** |
| Edematous forms | 04 | 10.2 |
| Nodular forms | 03 | 7.7 |
| Topographic aspects | | |
| Thorax | **12** | **30.7** |
| Abdomen | **10** | **25.6** |
| Back | **08** | **20.5** |
| Face | 06 | 15.3 |
| Genitals | 03 | 7.7 |

*3.2.2. Age of Patients with BU of Atypical Site.* The age of patients ranged from 3 to 72 years. The mean age was 14.2 years. Children aged less than 15 years were affected in almost 80% of the cases.

*3.2.3. Gender of Patients with BU of Atypical Site.* We observed a female predominance of 71.7%. The sex ratio was 2.5.

*3.3. Clinical Characteristics of BU Cases with Atypical Site.* Clinical forms of atypical site were dominated by ulcerated forms (82.1%).

*3.4. Topographical Aspects of BU with Atypical Site.* Sites on the torso (thorax, abdomen, and back) were the most frequent forms (76.8%).

## 4. Discussion

BU is a mycobacteriosis which rages under the form of endemic foci in our country to the extent that, in 1995, the Ivorian government set up a National Programme of Fight against Mycobacterium Ulcers (PNUM). Unlike its usual sites in the limbs which are well documented, atypical sites are not. As a matter of fact, they are misleading forms whose diagnosis and treatment are difficult and should not be ignored by practitioners; they are likely to threaten the functional prognosis and survival in some cases. Such forms in our study had a hospital incidence of 18.3%.

Sociodemographic characteristics of misleading forms are similar to usual forms of BU. BU with atypical sites affects, like its classic form, mostly children. In 79.5% of the cases, atypical forms were observed in children aged less than 15 years. The BU predominance in this target is observed in various studies [5–7]. It was related to a deficit of immunity in those children [8]. The factor accounting for that situation is the absence of specific vaccine protection against MU and the antituberculosis vaccination, BCG (Bacilli Calmette-Guerin), offers only a transitional protection which subsides from 6 months to 1 year [9, 10]. Moreover, games or fishing, by those children near waters, exposes them to cutaneous microtrauma which favours the penetration of MU in the body [11].

In our study, females patients were the most affected people. The epidemiological profile classically shows that the BU affects the children without distinction of sex. This ascendancy of females in this study would be of recruitment bias.

They represent 71.7% of patients. As a matter of fact, women, in our traditions, are in charge of household chores which are mainly laundry and dishes. These chores are also conducted near stretch of water and swamps in 77% of the cases (please refer to Table 1).

Our country, Côte d'Ivoire, is a country with limited resources. The minimum wage is $120. Due to poverty, only few households have access to drinking water. As a result, many families are obliged to use swamp water for the needs of their household. Though the BU transmission mode is not clearly identified, one knows that contact with those stagnant waters is a major factor in the outbreak of the disease [12]. As a matter of fact, a PCR conducted enabled us to discover freshwater bugs of the like of *Naucoris* and *Diplonychus* on the roots of some aquatic plants which might shelter MU [1].

In our experience, patients are barely consulted at the inception which is oedema (10.2%) and nodule (7.7%). However, when the disease is diagnosed at this stage, the treatment is less complex and the prognosis is better [13]. However, in 82.1% of the cases, patients go to hospital at the ulcerative stage which is the severest form, the most dilapidating, with at times a risk of incapacitating scares in children [14]. This negligence of diseases can be explained by poverty. As a matter of fact, due to economic reasons, those patients undertake self-medication at the inception of the pathology. They would only go to health centres, after several weeks or months when their treatments have failed or when the case has developed into some complications. As well, those unusual sites of BU are sometimes very misleading and give rise to misdiagnosis and delays in the efficient treatment, given that it is ignored by many practitioners. This is the reason of our vehement advice to our colleagues in endemic zones to undertake in case of doubt the incisional biopsy of any nodule in order to conduct histological examination and, at the ulceration stage, conduct wound edge swabbing in view

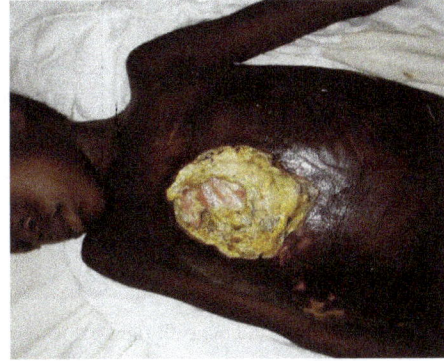

FIGURE 1: Thoracic BU revealing the ribs of an 8-year-old girl.

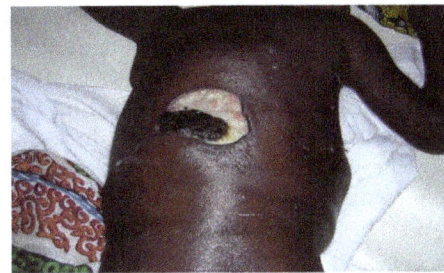

FIGURE 2: BU of the back.

of conducting a PCR which would allow for early diagnosis of BU within 48 hours [15, 16].

Histology and smear are examinations with an average sensibility and a poor specificity. The poor performance of these examinations could actually induce a bias of recruitment by omitting confirmed cases of BU or registering false cases. However given that these tests are less expensive and easy to carry out, they permit defining probable cases of BU in endemic zones like ours, according to the WHO [17].

However, the PCR has quite a good sensibility and its specificity is above 90%. In the event of a positive result, it allows the confirmation of BU cases [17]. But its high cost prevents its use as a routine examination.

With regard to topography, BU may affect any part of the human body but limbs remain its predilection site [18–20]. Unusual topographic aspects observed were predominantly in the torso (thorax, abdomen, and back) in 76.8% (Figures 1 and 2). There are severe forms which could threaten survival due to pneumothorax type complications or pleurisy which go along with them in some cases [21].

Apart from these predominant forms found on the torso, the study revealed moreover facial affections of up to 15.3% (Figure 3). These forms located on the face, in addition to presenting diagnostic difficulties, pose a problem with regard to their surgical treatment given their proximity to the eyes. The functional prognostic of these forms is related to the likeliness of extension of BU to the eyes as it was observed with some patients.

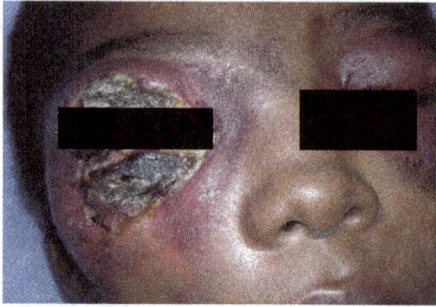

FIGURE 3: Facial BU above and beneath right palpebral fissure.

## 5. Conclusion

BU is an endemic disease in Côte d'Ivoire where it constitutes a serious public health issue. Several years following its first description by Mac Callum, BU remains understudied. As a matter of fact, in addition to its mode of transmission which is yet to be elucidated, this dermatosis may clinically present atypical and misleading aspects likely to threaten survival. Future researches could help for a better understanding of the various unknown aspects of this disease.

## Abbreviations

AFB:    Acid-alcohol-fast Bacilli
BCG:    Bacilli Calmette-Guerin
MU:    *Mycobacterium ulcerans*
PCR:    Polymerase chain reaction
PNUM: National Programme of Fight against
       Mycobacterium Ulcers
B.U:    Buruli ulcers.

## Conflict of Interests

The authors declare that there is no conflict of interests regarding the publication of this paper.

## References

[1] J. M. Kanga, E. D. Kacou, K. Kouame et al., "Buruli ulcer: epidemiological, clinical and therapeutic aspects in Côte d'Ivoire," *Medecine Tropicale*, vol. 64, no. 3, pp. 238–242, 2004.

[2] R. Josse, A. Guedenon, H. Darie, S. Anagonou, F. Portaels, and W. M. Meyers, "Mycobacterium ulcerans skin infection: Buruli ulcers," *Medecine Tropicale*, vol. 55, no. 4, pp. 363–373, 1995.

[3] L. S. B. Manou, F. Portaels, M. Eddyani, A. U. Book, K. Vandelannoote, and B. C. de Jong, "*Mycobacterium ulcerans* disease (Buruli ulcer) in Gabon: 2005–2011," *Medecine et Sante Tropicales*, vol. 23, no. 4, pp. 450–457, 2013.

[4] K. Kollie, Y. A. Amoako, J. Ake et al., "Buruli ulcer in Liberia, 2012," *Emerging Infectious Diseases*, vol. 20, no. 3, pp. 494–496, 2014.

[5] B. Saka, D. E. Landoh, B. Kobara et al., "Profile of Buruli ulcer treated at the national reference centre of Togo: a study of 119 cases," *Bulletin de la Societe de Pathologie Exotique*, vol. 106, no. 1, pp. 32–36, 2013.

[6] J. M. Kanga, D. E. Kacou, A. Sangaré, Y. Dabila, N. H. Asse, and S. Djakeaux, "Recurrence cases observed after surgical treatment of Buruli ulcer in Cote d'Ivoire," *Bulletin de la Societe de Pathologie Exotique*, vol. 96, no. 5, pp. 406–409, 2004.

[7] H. Darie, "Mycobacterium ulcerans infection: epidemiological, clinical and therapeutical aspects," *Bulletin de la Societe de Pathologie Exotique*, vol. 96, no. 5, pp. 368–371, 2004.

[8] J. M. Kanga, E. D. Kacou, K. Kouamé et al., "Fighting against Buruli ulcer: the Côte-d'Ivoire experience," *Bulletin de la Societe de Pathologie Exotique*, vol. 99, no. 1, pp. 34–38, 2006.

[9] A. Sangaré, E. Ecra, M. Kouyaté, C. Ahogo, and M. Kaloga, "Epidemiological profile of Buruli Ulcer in Abidjan," *Afrique Biomédicale*, vol. 11, no. 2, pp. 20–25, 2006.

[10] P. J. Converse, D. V. Almeida, E. L. Nuermberger, and J. H. Grosset, "BCG-mediated protection against *Mycobacterium ulcerans* infection in the mouse," *PLoS Neglected Tropical Diseases*, vol. 5, no. 3, article e985, 2011.

[11] M. W. Bratschi, M. T. Ruf, A. Andreoli et al., "Mycobacterium ulcerans persistence at a village water source of Buruli ulcer patients," *PLoS Neglected Tropical Diseases*, vol. 8, no. 3, Article ID e2756, 2014.

[12] K. H. Jacobsen and J. J. Padgett, "Risk factors for *Mycobacterium ulcerans* infection," *International Journal of Infectious Diseases*, vol. 14, no. 8, pp. e677–e681, 2010.

[13] E. Ecra, J. M. Kanga, I. D. Gbery et al., "Detection and treatment of early forms of Mycobacterium ulcerans infection in Ivory Coast," *Médecine tropicale : revue du Corps de santé colonial.*, vol. 65, no. 4, pp. 334–338, 2005.

[14] T. S. van Der Werf, W. T. A. van Der Graaf, J. W. Tappero, and K. Asiedu, "Mycobacterium ulcerans infection," *The Lancet*, vol. 354, no. 9183, pp. 1013–1018, 1999.

[15] A. Ménard, P. Couppié, D. Sainte-Marie, and R. Pradinaud, "Diagnosis of *Mycobacterium ulcerans* infection by PCR: about three cases observed in French Guiana," *Bulletin de la Societe de Pathologie Exotique*, vol. 96, no. 5, pp. 403–405, 2004.

[16] E. Ekaza, A. Kacou-N'Douba, N. C. Oniangué et al., "Contribution of genic amplification in the detection of *M. ulcerans* in exudates and in cutaneous biopsies in Côte d'Ivoire," *Bulletin de la Societe de Pathologie Exotique*, vol. 97, no. 2, pp. 95–96, 2004.

[17] http://www.who.int/buruli/laboratory/diagnosis/fr/.

[18] D. Ouattara, G. K. Aka, J. P. Meningaud, A. Sica, L. Kaba, and S. Gadegbeku, "Facial localizations of Buruli ulcers: two cases," *Revue de Stomatologie et de Chirurgie Maxillo-Faciale*, vol. 104, no. 4, pp. 231–234, 2003.

[19] M. Kondo, I. Kurokawa, Y. Ito, K. I. Yamanaka, T. Yamazaki, and H. Mizutani, "Leg ulcer caused by Mycobacterium ulcerans ssp. shinshuense infection," *International Journal of Dermatology*, vol. 48, no. 12, pp. 1330–1333, 2009.

[20] K. N'Guessan, P. Guié, P. Iovenitti, G. Carta, V. Loue, and V. Angoi, "Primitive breast localisation of Buruli ulcer in an endemic zone: a rare case," *Clinical and Experimental Obstetrics & Gynecology*, vol. 36, no. 4, pp. 265–267, 2009.

[21] E. J. Ecra, I. P. Gbery, B. R. Aka, A. Sangaré, K. kouamé, and L. Dion, "Ulcère de Buruli: à propos de deux cas thoraco-abdominaux associés à une pleurésie," *Médecine d'Afrique Noire*, vol. 48, no. 5, pp. 213–216, 2001.

# 24

# Expression of Maspin and Ezrin Proteins in Periocular Basal Cell Carcinoma

**Mansooreh Bagheri,**[1] **Masoomeh Eghtedari,**[2] **Mandana Bagheri,**[1]
**Bita Geramizadeh,**[3] **and Mohammadreza Talebnejad**[1]

[1]*Poostchi Ophthalmology Research Center, Shiraz University of Medical Sciences, Shiraz, Iran*
[2]*Ophthalmology Department, Shiraz University of Medical Sciences, Shiraz, Iran*
[3]*Pathology Department, Liver Transplant Research Center, Shiraz University of Medical Sciences, Shiraz, Iran*

Correspondence should be addressed to Mandana Bagheri; manbagheri@yahoo.com

Academic Editor: Jane M. Grant-Kels

*Background.* The aim of this study was to investigate maspin and ezrin expression in different subtypes of periocular basal cell carcinoma (BCC). *Methods.* Tissue samples from 43 patients with periocular BCC. Our cases were comprised of 10 morpheaform, 25 nodular, and 8 adenoid type BCCs. Immunohistochemical staining for maspin and ezrin was performed by Envision detection system. *Results.* There was no difference between different subtypes of BCC in maspin expression regarding positivity, intensity, and pattern of expression. Ezrin was expressed in all subtypes of BCC but the intensity was significantly higher in morpheaform BCC compared to nodular and adenoid types ($P < 0.001$ and $P = 0.012$, resp.); ninety percent of morpheaform samples showed strong ezrin intensity, while this strong intensity was only present in 25% and 12% of adenoid and nodular subtypes, respectively. There was no correlation between age, sex, or tumor margin involvement and expression of neither maspin nor ezrin. There was no correlation between maspin and ezrin expression except in nodular type, in which an inverse correlation was found ($P = 0.004$). *Conclusion.* Ezrin is expressed intensely in morpheaform BCC of periocular region. Further studies are needed to show the significance of this finding in prognosis of morpheaform BCC.

## 1. Introduction

Basal cell carcinoma (BCC) of the skin, the most frequent malignancy in human population, represents 20% of eyelid tumors and 90% of eyelid malignancies [1, 2]. BCC subtypes, including nodular, adenoid, superficial, micronodular, and morphoeic/infiltrative subtypes, have different clinical and morphological pictures [3].

Recently, various tumor biomarkers are identified which have great importance in predicting clinical behavior of the cancers [3], among them, maspin and ezrin may be involved in BCC pathogenesis. Maspin protein, a member of the serpin family of protease inhibitors, presents as a secreted, cytoplasmic, nuclear, or cell surface-associated protein [4, 5]. Maspin is the product of a tumor suppressor gene and is involved in apoptosis and inhibition of carcinoma invasion, metastasis,

and angiogenesis [4]. Its expression is downregulated during cancer progression [6].

Ezrin, a member of the ERM (ezrin-radixin-moesin) protein family, acts as linkers between the cell membrane and the actin cytoskeleton and is involved in several cellular functions, including cell adhesion to the extracellular matrix, cell-cell communication, signal transduction, and apoptosis [7, 8]. Ezrin has active role in regulating tumor growth and progression and metastatic dissemination of many cancers [9, 10].

Little is known about expression of maspin and ezrin biomarkers in periocular skin tumors. The aim of this work was to investigate maspin and ezrin expression in periocular BCC to throw light on their role in pathogenesis of this carcinoma by immunohistochemistry, together with correlating their expression with the clinicopathological features of the tumor.

## 2. Materials and Methods

Excised tissue samples, obtained from 43 patients with diagnosis of periorbital BCC, were retrieved from archive of Pathology Laboratory at Khalili Hospital, Shiraz University of Medical Sciences, during April 2011 to April 2012. All patients were diagnosed initially during this period and no patient received any treatment for their BCC prior to sample collection. Hematoxylin & eosin stained sections were examined under the light microscope for confirmation of the diagnosis and determination of BCC type and involvement of tumor margins. Metatypical carcinomas with squamous differentiation in histological evaluations were excluded. Tissue samples from pigmented BCC cases showed pathologic characteristics of nodular type, so they were assigned as nodular type. Five micrometer-thick sections were taken from paraffin-embedded tissue blocks and mounted on poly L lysine slides. Then sections were deparaffinized in xylene and rehydrated in descending grades of ethanol.

Immunohistochemical staining for maspin and ezrin was performed by Envision detection system. This is a 2-step procedure; the first step is incubation of the tissue with optimally diluted primary antibody (1/2000), and the second step is incubation of tissue with Envision reagents. Envision reagent is a peroxidase-conjugated polymer, which also carries antibodies to the rabbit or mouse immunoglobulins.

Maspin monoclonal primary antibody (mouse antihuman antibody, Santa Cruz Biotechnology Inc., Texas, USA) was raised against recombinant protein corresponding to N-terminal region of human maspin. Ezrin polyclonal primary antibody (rabbit antihuman antibody, Texas, Santa Cruz Biotechnology Inc., Texas, USA) was raised against C-terminus peptide of human ezrin. Maspin and ezrin antibodies were diluted to 1 : 2000 by TRIS-EDTA and citrate buffer, respectively. Antigen retrieval was done by boiling mounted tissue in TRIS-HCL buffer (pH 7.4). Then, primary antibody was employed and samples were kept overnight in 4°C.

Envision detection system consists of a dextran backbone coupled with peroxidase molecules and secondary antibody. The applied secondary antibodies (Cat number K5007, code number S3245 DAKO Cytomation) were mouse and rabbit IgG antibodies against maspin and ezrin, respectively. The substrate system was diaminobenzidine (DAB) chromogen. Mayer's hematoxylin was used as the counterstain. Prostatic glandular basal cells and duodenal mucosal tissue were used as the positive controls for maspin and ezrin, respectively. Normal skin was also used as positive control during staining for both maspin and ezrin. Negative control for staining of both maspin and ezrin was obtained by substitution of primary antibody with PBS in staining procedure.

Maspin immune reactivity was evaluated in tumoral tissue and adjacent epidermal layer as negative or positive, where the positivity was assigned as cytoplasmic and/or nuclear staining. Ezrin immunoreactivity was assessed in the tumor and adjacent epidermis and peritumoral lymphocytes (a reference of strong immunoreactivity). Cases

TABLE 1: Clinical and pathological data of different types of periocular BCC.

| | Morpheaform BCC ($n = 10$) | Nodular BCC ($n = 25$) | Adenoid BCC ($n = 8$) |
|---|---|---|---|
| Sex (M/F) | 5/5 | 11/14 | 5/3 |
| Age (mean ± SD) | 67.85 ± 19.13 | 62.5 ± 16.16 | 57.5 ± 17.57 |
| Age (range) | (26–95) | (31–85) | (26–85) |
| Involved surgical margin | 6 (60%) | 10 (40%) | 2 (25%) |

were assigned positive for ezrin expression when cytoplasmic positivity with or without membranous immunoreactivity was present. The intensity of maspin and ezrin expression was assigned as a score of 0–3 with 0 indicating no staining and 1 for weak, 2 for moderate, and 3 for strong staining. All slides were independently assessed by two pathologists.

*2.1. Statistical Analysis.* Results were analyzed by statistical package SPSS version 17 (SPSS Inc. Chicago, USA). Fisher's exact test and Spearman correlation coefficient were used to analyze data. $P$ value of $< 0.05$ was considered statistically significant. Kappa statistic was used to test interrater reliability.

## 3. Results

Our cases were comprised of 10 morpheaform, 25 nodular, and 8 adenoid type BCCs. No superficial, nodulocystic, and micronodular types were detected. All BCC samples along with control samples from normal skin showed diffuse cytoplasmic maspin expression in all epidermal layers. Clinical and pathological data of different types of periocular BCC are shown in Table 1. Maspin protein was expressed in 74.4% of samples. There was no significant difference between different types of BCC regarding maspin expression and intensity of staining ($P = 0.63$ and $0.82$, resp.). Pattern of maspin expression was not different in BCC subtypes. Table 2 shows maspin expression in different types of periocular BCC. Samples of negative, weak, and moderate maspin staining in tumoral cells are shown in Figure 1.

Ezrin protein was expressed in 93% of all samples. There was no significant difference between different types of BCC regarding ezrin expression while the intensity of staining was different among different types. Intensity of ezrin expression was significantly higher in morpheaform BCC compared to nodular and adenoid types ($P < 0.001$ and $P = 0.012$, resp.); ninety percent of morpheaform samples showed strong ezrin intensity, while this strong intensity was only present in 25% and 12% of adenoid and nodular subtypes, respectively. There was no significant difference between nodular and adenoid subtypes regarding ezrin intensity ($P = 0.66$). Ezrin expression among different types of periocular BCC is shown in Table 3. Figure 2 shows samples of weak, moderate, and strong ezrin expression in tumoral cells.

There was no correlation between ezrin and maspin expression regarding intensity in morpheaform and adenoid

TABLE 2: Maspin protein expression among different types of periocular BCC.

| | Morpheaform BCC ($n = 10$) | Nodular BCC ($n = 25$) | Adenoid BCC ($n = 8$) | Total ($n = 43$) | $P$ value |
|---|---|---|---|---|---|
| Positivity (%) | 8 (80) | 17 (68) | 7 (87.5) | 32 (74.4) | 0.63* |
| Intensity | | | | | 0.82* |
| Negative | 2 (20) | 8 (32) | 1 (12.5) | 11 (25.6) | |
| Weak (%) | 5 (50) | 8 (32) | 2 (25) | 15 (34.9) | |
| Moderate (%) | 3 (30) | 9 (36) | 5 (62.5) | 17 (39.5) | |
| Strong | 0 | 0 | 0 | 0 | |
| Pattern | | | | | |
| Cytoplasmic (%) | 5 (62.5) | 7 (41.2) | 1 (12.5) | 13 (40.6) | 0.25* |
| Cytoplasmic/nucleus (%) | 3 (37.5) | 10 (58.8) | 6 (62.5) | 19 (59.4) | 0.15* |

*Fisher's exact test.

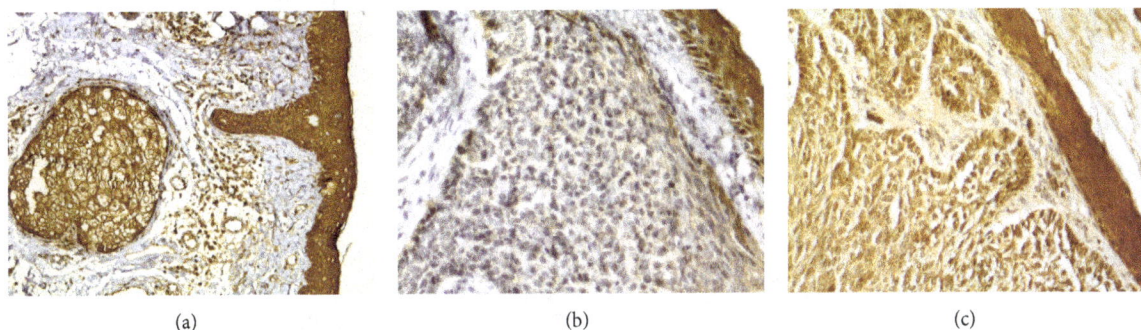

(a)                                    (b)                                    (c)

FIGURE 1: Maspin immunoreactivity in periocular basal cell carcinoma (immunohistochemical staining ×400 for (a), (b), and (c)): (a) strong maspin immunoreactivity in the epidermis and sebaceous gland in one of the control cases, (b) weak maspin immunoreactivity, and (c) moderate maspin immunoreactivity.

BCC types ($P = 0.20$ and $0.16$, resp.) but there was an inverse correlation between ezrin and maspin expression in nodular type ($P = 0.004$).

There was no correlation between age and expression of neither maspin ($P = 0.78$) nor ezrin ($P = 0.75$). We also did not find any significant correlation between margin involvement and maspin or ezrin expression ($P = 0.12$ and $0.058$, resp.).

Sex did not have significant association with neither maspin nor ezrin expression ($P$ value = 0.53 and 0.96, resp.). There was no significant association between sex and maspin and ezrin expression in any of the BCC subtypes.

We reached the Kappa value of 0.86 and 0.75 in maspin and ezrin assay for interrater reliability, respectively. Both values are in the range of almost perfect agreement. This finding means that the assay for maspin and ezrin was reproducible in this study.

## 4. Discussion

Identification of biomarkers, involved in the mechanisms of malignant cell transformation, is of great importance in predicting further clinical behavior of the cancer and has

prognostic value in diagnosis and treatment [3]. In this study, we evaluated the expression of maspin and ezrin in different types of periocular BCC. Micronodular, infiltrative, basosquamous, morpheaform, and mixed BCC subtypes are known to have aggressive histological characteristics and adenoid variant is believed to be the nonaggressive subtypes [11]. We excluded metatypical BCC cases due to their intermediate features with squamous cell carcinoma. We did not detect micronodular, nodulocystic, and superficial types in our cases, so we categorized the cases to three groups: morpheaform, nodular, and adenoid.

Maspin, a product of tumor suppressor gene, is thought to inhibit carcinoma invasion, metastasis, and angiogenesis [12]. However, both decrease and increase of the expression of maspin parallel tumor progression [12]. Positive maspin expression was identified in 74.4% of our cases. Our results are in agreement with the study done by Reis-Filho et al. [13] in which maspin expression in BCC was shown to be 87.5%. However, in the study done by Abdou et al. maspin expression in BCC was 48%, probably due to the presence of 3 metatypical cases [12]. In their study, 16% and 32% of BCC cases showed weak and moderate expression of maspin, respectively, and no cases had strong maspin expression

TABLE 3: Ezrin expression among different types of periocular BCC.

| Type | Morpheaform BCC ($n = 10$) | Nodular BCC ($n = 25$) | Adenoid BCC ($n = 8$) | Total ($n = 43$) | P value |
|---|---|---|---|---|---|
| Positivity (%) | 10 (100) | 23 (92) | 7 (87.5) | 40 (93) | 0.75* |
| Intensity | | | | | <0.001**#& |
| Weak (%) | 0 (0) | 15 (60) | 3 (37.5) | 18 (41.9) | |
| Moderate (%) | 1 (10) | 5 (20) | 2 (25) | 8 (18.6) | |
| Strong (%) | 9 (90) | 3 (12) | 2 (25) | 14 (32.5) | |

* Fisher's exact test.
# Intensity of ezrin expression was significantly higher in morpheaform BCC compared to nodular and adenoid types ($P < 0.001$ and $P = 0.012$, resp.).
& No significant difference between nodular and adenoid types ($P = 0.66$).

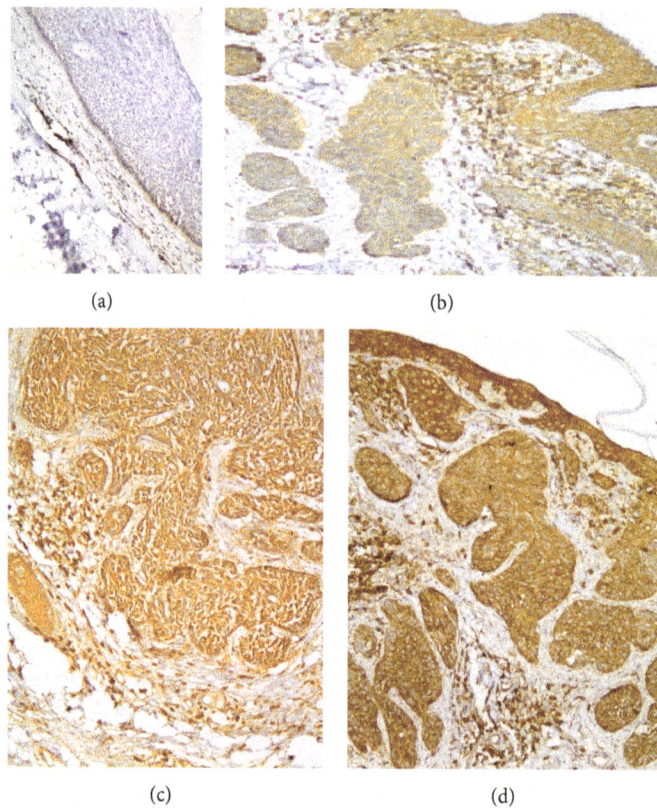

FIGURE 2: Ezrin immunoreactivity in periocular basal cell carcinoma (immunohistochemical staining ×200 for (a), ×100 for (b), ×200 for (c), and ×100 for (d)): (a) negative ezrin immunoreactivity, (b) weak ezrin immunoreactivity, (c) moderate ezrin immunoreactivity, and (d) strong ezrin immunoreactivity. Note strong immunoreactivity of tumor-associated lymphocytes and/or epidermis.

[12]. We also did not detect strong expression of maspin in any cases, and weak and moderate maspin expressions were found to be present in 34.9% and 39.5% of our cases.

Result of our study was not in favor of any difference between different types of BCC in maspin expression regarding positivity, intensity, and pattern of expression or any association with the age of patient. Also, we did not find any significant correlation between maspin expression and tumor margin involvement.

Maspin is predominantly a soluble cytoplasmic protein and its presence in the nucleus is due to passive diffusion through the nuclear membrane or due to chaperonage to

the nucleus [12]. Some studies have revealed that nuclear expression of maspin is associated with better prognosis in various tumors like breast cancer [14], non-small-cell carcinoma of the lung [15], and pancreatic ductal adenocarcinoma [16]. Maspin nuclear expression was also correlated with a lower recurrence rate and a longer disease-free interval after surgery of laryngeal squamous cell carcinoma [17].

We detected nuclear expression of maspin in 59.4% of all cases who expressed this marker and the remaining samples showed only cytoplasmic expression. However, in a study done by Abdou et al. only 33.3% of positive cases had nuclear expression of maspin [12]. The importance of our finding is to be verified since it was previously suggested that nuclear staining of maspin in cutaneous BCC has tumor suppressor role [12]. Abdou et al. detected significant association between nuclear expression of maspin with older age and adenoid variant in cutaneous BCC [12]. However, we did not find any association between nuclear expression of maspin with patient age and tumor margin involvement. We also did not detect any significant difference between adenoid, nodular, and morpheaform subtypes regarding nuclear and cytoplasmic expression of maspin.

Previous studies have shown that expression of ezrin, a member of the ERM (ezrin-radixin-moesin) cytoskeleton-associated protein family, is correlated with poor outcome in many types of human cancers [18]. For example, cytoplasmic expression of ezrin was associated with higher grade, hormonal-receptor negativity, and lymph-node metastases in breast cancer [19]. Ezrin expression was shown to be higher in squamous cell carcinoma compared with less aggressive tumors such as Bowen's disease, actinic keratosis, keratoacanthoma, and seborrheic keratosis [9]. Furthermore, ezrin expression was found to be correlated with metastasis, tumor thickness, progression, and invasion in primary melanomas of the skin [20]. Ezrin overexpression in gastrointestinal stromal tumors was associated with the nongastric location and decreased disease-free survival [10]. Ezrin was expressed in 93% of our cases. Our results are in agreement with previous studies in the fact that intensity of ezrin staining was significantly higher in more aggressive morpheaform BCC compared to adenoid and nodular types. There was no significant association between ezrin expression and patient's age or margin involvement by tumor.

To the best of our knowledge, no relationship between expression of maspin, as a tumor suppressor product, and ezrin, as a marker of tumor progression, has been reported in BCC. No significant association was found between maspin and ezrin expression except in nodular type. There was an inverse correlation between maspin and ezrin expression in this type of periocular tumor.

## 5. Conclusion

We can conclude that maspin is expressed in most cases of periocular BCC regardless of its subtype, while ezrin intensity was higher in morpheaform BCC compared to nodular and adenoid types. There was no association between maspin and ezrin expression except in nodular type, in which inverse correlation exists between maspin and ezrin expression. No correlation was found between maspin and ezrin expression and the age of patient and tumor margin involvement at the time of surgery.

The shortcoming of our study was the limited number of cases. Lack of significant correlation between margin involvement and maspin or ezrin expression had low power to detect clinical significance because of $P$ values near 0.05 ($P$ = 0.12 and 0.058, resp.). Furthermore, lack of data on clinical outcomes of our patients possibly affects the clinical utility of our results. More cases are needed to highlight the importance of expression of these two tumor markers

on diagnosis and outcome of patients with BCC. We also recommend comparison of periocular BCC cases with BCC in other parts of the body regarding maspin and ezrin expression, due to the fact that region of tumor origin may affect its biological and clinical features.

## Conflict of Interests

The authors have no relevant affiliations or financial involvement with any organizations or entity with a financial interest in or financial conflict with the subject matters or materials discussed in the paper.

## Acknowledgment

This work was supported by Grant no. 4180 from Poostchi Ophthalmology Research Center, Shiraz University of Medical Sciences, Shiraz, Iran.

## References

[1] J. Reifenberger, "Basal cell carcinoma. Molecular genetics and unusual clinical features," *Hautarzt*, vol. 58, no. 5, pp. 406–411, 2007.

[2] J. Allali, F. D'Hermies, and G. Renard, "Basal cell carcinomas of the eyelids," *Ophthalmologica*, vol. 219, no. 2, pp. 57–71, 2005.

[3] V. Bartoš, K. Adamicová, M. Kullová, and M. Péč, "Basal cell carcinoma of the skin—biological behaviour of the tumor and a review of the most important molecular predictors of disease progression in pathological practice," *Klinicka Onkologie*, vol. 24, no. 1, pp. 8–17, 2011.

[4] K. Kashima, N. Ohike, S. Mukai, M. Sato, M. Takahashi, and T. Morohoshi, "Expression of the tumor suppressor gene maspin and its significance in intraductal papillary mucinous neoplasms of the pancreas," *Hepatobiliary & Pancreatic Diseases International*, vol. 7, no. 1, pp. 86–90, 2008.

[5] J. Lockett, S. Yin, X. Li, Y. Meng, and S. Sheng, "Tumor suppressive maspin and epithelial homeostasis," *Journal of Cellular Biochemistry*, vol. 97, no. 4, pp. 651–660, 2006.

[6] M.-J. Lee, C.-H. Suh, and Z.-H. Li, "Clinicopathological significance of maspin expression in breast cancer," *Journal of Korean Medical Science*, vol. 21, no. 2, pp. 309–314, 2006.

[7] V. L. Bonilha, "Focus on Molecules: ezrin," *Experimental Eye Research*, vol. 84, no. 4, pp. 613–614, 2007.

[8] K. W. Hunter, "Ezrin, a key component in tumor metastasis," *Trends in Molecular Medicine*, vol. 10, no. 5, pp. 201–204, 2004.

[9] H.-R. Park, S. K. Min, K. Min et al., "Differential expression of ezrin in epithelial skin tumors: cytoplasmic ezrin immunoreactivity in squamous cell carcinoma," *International Journal of Dermatology*, vol. 49, no. 1, pp. 48–52, 2010.

[10] Y.-C. Wei, C.-F. Li, S.-C. Yu et al., "Ezrin overexpression in gastrointestinal stromal tumors: an independent adverse prognosticator associated with the non-gastric location," *Modern Pathology*, vol. 22, no. 10, pp. 1351–1360, 2009.

[11] R. S. Batra and L. C. Kelley, "Predictors of extensive subclinical spread in nonmelanoma skin cancer treated with Mohs micrographic surgery," *Archives of Dermatology*, vol. 138, no. 8, pp. 1043–1051, 2002.

[12] A. G. Abdou, A. H. Maraee, M. A. E. Shoeib, and A. M. Abo Saida, "Maspin expression in epithelial skin tumours: an immunohistochemical study," *Journal of Cutaneous and Aesthetic Surgery*, vol. 4, no. 2, pp. 111–117, 2011.

[13] J. S. Reis-Filho, B. Torio, A. Albergaria, and F. C. Schmitt, "Maspin expression in normal skin and usual cutaneous carcinomas," *Virchows Archiv*, vol. 441, no. 6, pp. 551–558, 2002.

[14] S. K. Mohsin, M. Zhang, G. M. Clark, and D. C. Allred, "Maspin expression in invasive breast cancer: association with other prognostic factors," *Journal of Pathology*, vol. 199, no. 4, pp. 432–435, 2003.

[15] F. Lonardo, X. Li, F. Siddiq et al., "Maspin nuclear localization is linked to favorable morphological features in pulmonary adenocarcinoma," *Lung Cancer*, vol. 51, no. 1, pp. 31–39, 2006.

[16] D. Cao, Q. Zhang, L. S.-F. Wu et al., "Prognostic significance of maspin in pancreatic ductal adenocarcinoma: tissue microarray analysis of 223 surgically resected cases," *Modern Pathology*, vol. 20, no. 5, pp. 570–578, 2007.

[17] G. Marioni, S. Blandamura, L. Giacomelli et al., "Nuclear expression of maspin is associated with a lower recurrence rate and a longer disease-free interval after surgery for squamous cell carcinoma of the larynx," *Histopathology*, vol. 46, no. 5, pp. 576–582, 2005.

[18] D. Okamura, M. Ohtsuka, F. Kimura et al., "Ezrin expression is associated with hepatocellular carcinoma possibly derived from progenitor cells and early recurrence after surgical resection," *Modern Pathology*, vol. 21, no. 7, pp. 847–855, 2008.

[19] D. Sarrió, S. M. Rodríguez-Pinilla, A. Dotor, F. Calero, D. Hardisson, and J. Palacios, "Abnormal ezrin localization is associated with clinicopathological features in invasive breast carcinomas," *Breast Cancer Research and Treatment*, vol. 98, no. 1, pp. 71–79, 2006.

[20] S. Ilmonen, A. Vaheri, S. Asko-Seljavaara, and O. Carpen, "Ezrin in primary cutaneous melanoma," *Modern Pathology*, vol. 18, no. 4, pp. 503–510, 2005.

# 25

# Skin Biopsy in the Context of Dermatological Diagnosis: A Retrospective Cohort Study

**Chrysovalantis Korfitis,[1] Stamatis Gregoriou,[2] Christina Antoniou,[3] Andreas D. Katsambas,[3] and Dimitris Rigopoulos[2]**

[1] *Department of Dermatology, Veterans Administration Hospital, 10-12 Monis Petraki Street, 11521 Athens, Greece*
[2] *Department of Dermatology, Attikon Hospital, 1 Rimini Street, Haidari, 12462 Athens, Greece*
[3] *Department of Dermatology, Andreas Sygros Hospital, 5 I. Dragoumi Street, 16121 Athens, Greece*

Correspondence should be addressed to Stamatis Gregoriou; stamgreg@yahoo.gr

Academic Editor: Lajos Kemeny

*Background.* Skin biopsy is an established method for allying the dermatologist in overcoming the diagnostic dilemmas which occur during consultations. However neither do all skin biopsies produce a conclusive diagnosis nor the dermatologists routinely perform this procedure to every patient they consult. The aim of this study was to investigate the favourable clinical diagnoses set by dermatologists when performing skin biopsy, the diagnoses reached by the dermatopathologists after microscopic examination, and the relationship between them and finally to comment on the instances that skin biopsy fails to fulfill the diagnostic task. *Methods.* Six thousand eight hundred and sixteen biopsy specimens were reviewed and descriptive statistics were performed. *Results.* The mean age of the patients was $54.58 \pm 0.26$ years, the most common site of biopsy was the head and neck (38.3%), the most frequently proposed clinical diagnoses included malignancies (19.28%), and the most prevalent pathological diagnosis was epitheliomas (21.9%). After microscopic examination, a specific histological diagnosis was proposed in 83.29% of the cases and a consensus between clinical and histological diagnoses was observed in 68% of them. *Conclusions.* Although there are cases that skin biopsy exhibits diagnostic inefficiency, it remains a valuable aid for the dermatology clinical practice.

## 1. Introduction

The management of skin diseases requires a pertinent diagnosis, which in many occasions constitutes an intricate process. Skin biopsy is an established diagnostic procedure which connects clinical diagnostic methodology with the invisible to the unaided eye microscopic field of skin pathology. Taking under consideration the potentials and limitations of optical microscopy and the indications of performing an invasive technique, dermatologists often rely on skin biopsy for enhancing their diagnostic abilities. The aim of this study was to investigate the favourable clinical diagnoses set by dermatologists when performing skin biopsy, the diagnoses reached by the dermatopathologists after microscopic examination, as well as the relationship between them, and finally to comment on the instances that skin biopsy fails to fulfill the diagnostic task.

## 2. Methods

Six thousand eight hundred and sixteen (6816) biopsies were reviewed which were included in 5941 histopathology report forms and were processed in the "Andreas Sygros" hospital during the years 2004–2006. Furthermore, a topographic anatomy coding system was developed along with an ad hoc coding system for skin diseases in order to meet the requirements of the study (data not shown). Each of the 5941 patients underwent at least one and at most seven skin biopsies at any session. The frequencies of the various sites of biopsy, the percentages of all clinical diagnoses proposed by the dermatologists, and the percentages of the histological diagnoses set by the dermatopathologists were calculated and statistical significance was evaluated.

Data were analyzed using PASW Statistics version 18 (SPSS Inc, Chicago IL). Descriptive statistics were applied including frequencies and percentages, as well as the chi-square test, both for one-way and contingency tables. The level of significance was set at less than 0.05.

## 3. Results

*3.1. Gender and Age.* Out of 5941 patients that underwent skin biopsy, 48.2% ($n = 2862$) were males and 51.8% ($n = 3075$) females, with $n = 4$ missing data. The mean age was $54.58 \pm 0.26$ and the median 57 years. The mean age for males was $56.54 \pm 0.37$ (median 60 years) and for females $52.79 \pm 0.36$ (median 54 years).

*3.2. Site of Biopsy.* The site of each biopsy was studied regarding both anatomic regions and specific locations. Regarding anatomic regions, the respective frequencies were found to be the head and neck 38.3% ($n = 2515$), the anterior and lateral tegument 14.3% ($n = 941$), the posterior tegument 12.3% ($n = 810$), the pelvis 6.9% ($n = 454$), the upper extremities 11.1% ($n = 729$), and the lower extremities 17.1% ($n = 1124$). Out of 6573 valid biopsy sites ($n = 243$ missing) the most common specific locations were the back 8.8% ($n = 579$), the scalp 5.9% ($n = 387$), the nose 3.3% ($n = 218$), and the abdomen 3.3% ($n = 217$). After performing the chi-square test, the differences in the frequencies were found statistically significant ($\chi^2 = 2434.521$, $P < 0.001$).

*3.3. Clinical Diagnoses.* In order to study the clinical diagnoses that were proposed by the dermatologists, 6733 out of 6816 biopsies (98.78%) were evaluated. There were 11194 valid specific diagnoses, divided in 367 different terms of skin diseases, after excluding clinical descriptions and intangible expressions (12579 in total, 13 of which referring to different tissue other than skin), producing a ratio of 1.66 proposed diagnoses per skin biopsy. No diagnosis at all was given in $n = 158$ cases (2.4%). A classification of 14 categories of all clinical diagnoses is presented in Figure 1. The respective frequencies were "malignant tumors" $n = 2158$ (19.28%), "papulosquamous dermatoses" $n = 1358$ (12.13%), and "nevi" $n = 1176$ (10.51%) including melanocytic nevi, congenital nevi, Spitz nevi, blue nevi, dysplastic nevi, junctional-compound-intradermal nevi, nonmelanocytic nevi, and epidermal nevi, all expressed forms of "dermatitis" $n = 941$ (8.4%) including dermatitis, contact dermatitis, acute or chronic dermatitis, dyshidrotic eczema, nummular eczema, atopic dermatitis, and seborrheic dermatitis; also, "connective tissue diseases" $n = 803$ (7.17%), noninfectious granulomas and "granulomatous diseases" $n = 389$ (3.48%), "immunobullous diseases" $n = 376$ (3.36%), "cutaneous infections" $n = 351$ (3.14%), "benign tumors" $n = 344$ (3.07%), "drug eruptions" $n = 314$ (2.8%), "vasculitides" $n = 230$ (2.06%), acne and "acneiform eruptions" $n = 119$ (1.06%), hemangiomas and "vascular malformations" $n = 118$ (1.05%), and miscellaneous dermatoses $n = 2517$ (22.49%). After applying the chi-square test, the differences in the frequencies were found statistically significant ($\chi^2 = 9396.640$, $P < 0.001$).

Out of the 367 different clinical expressions, the most common specific diagnoses were "basal cell carcinoma" 9.3%

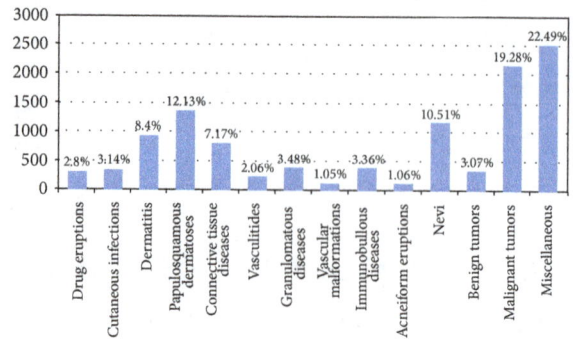

Figure 1: Bar chart of a classification of all the proposed clinical diagnoses.

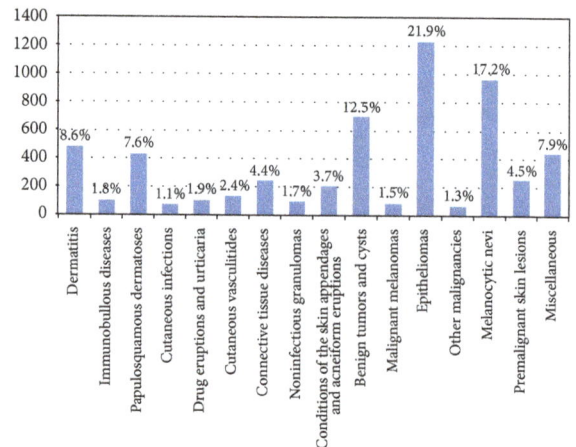

Figure 2: Bar chart of a classification of all the suggested histological diagnoses.

($n = 1037$), "melanocytic nevus" 7.9% ($n = 880$), "dermatitis" 6.1% ($n = 685$), "plaque psoriasis" 4.6% ($n = 515$), and "squamous cell carcinoma" 3.9% ($n = 436$).

*3.4. Histological Diagnoses.* The study of the histological diagnoses that were produced by the dermatopathologists included 6720 skin biopsies (6733 in total, excluding 13 other than skin) and their distinctive pathology that were previously diagnosed clinically by the dermatologists. Five thousand five hundred and ninety-seven (5597) specific histological diagnoses were suggested (83.29%), divided in 259 different terms of skin diseases. A classification of 16 categories of all histological diagnoses is presented in Figure 2. The frequencies and percentages were "epitheliomas" $n = 1224$ (21.9%) comprising basal cell carcinoma, squamous cell carcinoma, basosquamous carcinoma, collision tumors with any epithelioma as a component (e.g., with seborrheic keratosis), keratoacanthoma, fibroepithelioma, and lymphoepithelioma-like carcinoma of the skin, "melanocytic nevi" $n = 965$ (17.2%), "benign tumors and cysts" $n = 700$ (12.5%), "dermatitis" $n = 484$ (8.6%), "papulosquamous dermatoses" $n = 425$ (7.6%), "premalignant skin lesions" $n = 253$ (4.5%), "connective tissue diseases" $n = 244$ (4.4%), "conditions of the skin appendages and acneiform eruptions" $n = 205$

TABLE 1: Frequencies and percentages of a classification describing the relationship between clinical and histological diagnoses.

| Case | Frequency | Percentage |
|---|---|---|
| Case 1: one specific histological diagnosis inconsistent with the unspecified clinical diagnoses | 207 | 3.1 |
| Case 2: one specific histological diagnosis consistent with one specific clinical diagnosis | 2642 | 39.3 |
| Case 3: one specific histological diagnosis consistent with at least one clinical diagnosis regarding the disease category | 1668 | 24.8 |
| Case 4: one specific histological diagnosis inconsistent with the specific clinical diagnoses | 1080 | 16.1 |
| Case 5: no specific histological diagnosis without usable features inconsistent with the specific clinical diagnoses | 162 | 2.4 |
| Case 6: no specific histological diagnosis inconsistent with the unspecified clinical diagnoses | 25 | 0.4 |
| Case 7: no specific histological diagnosis but with usable features, inconsistent with the specific clinical diagnoses | 567 | 8.4 |
| Case 8: two or more specific histological diagnoses constituting subset of the proposed clinical diagnoses | 50 | 0.7 |
| Case 9: two or more specific histological diagnoses different from the proposed clinical diagnoses | 108 | 1.6 |
| Case 10: two or more specific histological diagnoses exhibiting partial overlap with the proposed clinical diagnoses | 211 | 3.1 |
| Total | 6720 | 100.0 |

(3.7%), "cutaneous vasculitides" $n = 135$ (2.4%), "drug eruptions and urticaria" $n = 106$ (1.9%), "immunobullous diseases" $n = 101$ (1.8%), "noninfectious granulomas" and granulomatous diseases $n = 99$ (1.7%), "malignant melanomas" $n = 84$ (1.5%), "other malignancies" besides melanomas and epitheliomas $n = 70$ (1.3%), "cutaneous infections" $n = 61$ (1.1%), and miscellaneous dermatoses $n = 441$ (7.9%). Performing the chi-square test, the differences in the frequencies were found statistically significant ($\chi^2 = 5150.109$, $P < 0.001$). Also, applying the test for contingency tables, the site of biopsy and histological diagnosis were found dependent ($\chi^2 = 2917.638$, $P < 0.001$) with the most important associations being between epitheliomas followed by conditions of the skin appendages in the head and neck region, cutaneous vasculitides on the lower extremities, melanocytic nevi on the posterior tegument, and dermatitis on the anterolateral tegument.

Among the 259 different expressions used by the dermatopathologists, the most common were "junctional, compound, and intradermal nevi" $n = 903$ (16.1%), "basal cell carcinoma" $n = 858$ (15.3%), and "squamous cell carcinoma" $n = 304$ (5.4%).

*3.5. Relationship between Clinical and Histological Diagnosis.* As mentioned before, 5597 specific histological diagnoses were proposed regarding the underlying pathology of 6720 skin biopsies. In the remaining cases, either a differential diagnosis was offered or no particular suggestion was made. In order to assess the relationship between clinical and histological diagnoses, a classification of ten cases that occurred was employed and for that purpose a separate evaluation was made. The observed frequencies and percentages along with the description of the ten cases are presented in Table 1. A specific histological diagnosis was provided in $n = 5597$ instances (83.3%), no specific histological diagnosis in $n = 754$ (11.2%), whereas two or more were proposed in $n = 369$

(5.5%) of the cases. Useful data orientating the dermatologist in establishing a final clinical diagnosis (cases 1–4 and 7–10 in Table 1) was provided in $n = 6533$ (97.2%) of all biopsies. Histological and clinical diagnoses were found substantially consistent (cases 2, 3, 8, and 10 in Table 1) in $n = 4571$ (68%) of instances. The dermatologists did not provide any specific clinical diagnosis (cases 1 and 6) in $n = 232$ (3.5%) of instances. Moreover, the lack of a specific clinical diagnosis combined with the absence of usable histological data (case 6 only) occurred in $n = 25$ (0.4%) of all cases. With the chi-square test the differences in the frequencies between the cases were found statistically significant ($\chi^2 = 10212.560$, $P < 0.001$). There was also a dependence of the relationship between clinical and histological diagnosis with the site of biopsy ($\chi^2 = 378.979$, $P < 0.001$), By interpreting the adjusted residuals, it was found that the correlation lied mostly between case 3 (as described in Table 1) and the biopsy site of the posterior tegument. Also between case 2 and the head and neck region, as well as case 7 and biopsies taken from the pelvis. Also the biopsies from head and neck and the anterolateral and posterior tegument showed a higher consistency between clinical and histological diagnosis.

In Table 1, cases 5 to 7 summarize $n = 754$ skin biopsies with no specific histological diagnosis. Possible reasons that resulted in this difficulty were extrapolated after reviewing the histopathology report forms and classifying the dermatopathologists' comments. Out of a total of 754 biopsies, $n = 91$ (12.1%) specimens were considered as destructed or inappropriate for microscopic examination and $n = 39$ (5.2%) were found of inadequate quantity, where in $n = 27$ (3.6%) the site of biopsy was regarded as not representative or adjacent to the examined lesion, in $n = 24$ (3.2%) the pathological features were altered due to previous treatment, in $n = 23$ (3.1%) optical microscopy with standard staining was considered as inappropriate for a specific diagnosis, and in $n = 16$ (2.1%) the examined lesion was identified as either not fully developed or resolved. The remaining 534 (70.8%) cases were documented as not pathognomonic and without exhibiting distinctive features.

## 4. Discussion

There are many occasions in which a clinician is challenged by a strenuous diagnostic problem. Skin biopsy constitutes a simple and inexpensive procedure performed in the dermatology setting which facilitates clinical decisions regarding diagnosis and treatment. Also, various studies consider histological confirmation as the standard for the correct diagnosis in dermatology as compared to the clinical evaluation, and the results produced in such manner are used in determining the epidemiological characteristics and patterns of skin diseases [1, 2]. Therefore, high diagnostic accuracy is pursued which relies upon the minimization of factors such as inappropriate choice of the lesion, poorly executed technique, unspecified clinical diagnosis and insufficient clinical information, faulty tissue fixation and processing, improper staining for specific diagnoses, or inadequate cooperation between the dermatologist and the dermatopathologist [3–5]. Furthermore, the diagnostic accuracy can be enhanced by using dermoscopy when selecting the site of biopsy [6] and additionally applying immunohistochemical staining and immunofluorescence techniques when appropriate [7, 8].

A few studies have been conducted in order to assess the diagnostic accuracy of skin diseases by physicians by comparing the clinical to the histological diagnosis. One of these studies measured the diagnostic yield of nondermatologists between 34% to 45% and that of dermatologists being 71% and 75% for inflammatory dermatoses or neoplasms and cysts, respectively [9]. Another study found 76.8% of pathological diagnoses to be consistent with the ones given by the dermatologists [10], whereas a third one measured a clinicopathological agreement of up to 92% with this success being attributed by the author to the close cooperation between the dermatologist and the pathologist [2]. In the present study, which was the largest of this kind to our knowledge, a 68% consistency of clinical and histological diagnoses was observed which is lesser than but in accord with the published data. Moreover, further data produced by this study comprise that a specific histological diagnosis was provided in 83.3% of all cases and usable information for the dermatologists was offered in 97.2% of all biopsies.

The data presented herein supports the empirically acquired knowledge of every dermatologist that although skin biopsy is performed for the diagnosis of a wide range of dermatoses, it is used predominantly for the determination of malignancies, mainly melanomas and epitheliomas, and also for inflammatory dermatoses such as dermatitis and psoriasis. Nevertheless, despite the high diagnostic usefulness of skin biopsy (97.2% in this study) with a diagnostic accuracy of 83.3%, there have been 11.2% of all instances lacking histological diagnosis. The possible reasons for this discrepancy have not been quantitatively assessed in the literature. Technically speaking, this could be attributed to several factors such as inadequate and inappropriate specimens, as previously analyzed. However, a number of $n = 25$ (0.4%) of all skin biopsies were lacking both clinical diagnosis and usable histological data. Also there were $n = 232$ (3.5%) without specific clinical diagnosis and $n = 158$ (2.4%) without any clinical description or diagnosis. Although these cases were infrequent, they would probably cause therapeutic problems. Hence, a closer cooperation between the dermatologist and the dermatopathologist is advisable.

## 5. Conclusion

Despite the fact that a plethora of modern techniques have been developed and utilized in the diagnosis of skin disease, dermatologists still rely vastly on biopsy for diagnostic purposes. As discussed in this study, there is a wide range of diseases that allow dermatologists to select skin biopsy in order to confirm their suspected diagnosis, and the histological perspective proves to be both helpful and reliable in the majority of cases. However, there are also limitations in this method and there are cases that the performance of a biopsy does not produce diagnostic results. As a consequence proper diagnosis is delayed and all imminent therapeutic decisions rely heavily upon the dermatologist's comprehension of the situation. Therefore an optimal use of the process is suggested with comprehensive descriptions and relevant diagnoses by the dermatologist along with a closer cooperation with the dermatopathologist performing clinicopathological correlation whenever possible.

## Conflict of Interests

The authors declare that there is no conflict of interests regarding the publication of this paper.

## References

[1] I. Ahnlide and M. Bjellerup, "Accuracy of clinical skin tumour diagnosis in a dermatological setting," *Acta Dermato-Venereologica*, vol. 93, no. 3, pp. 305–308, 2013.

[2] F. B. Yap, "Dermatopathology of 400 skin biopsies from Sarawak," *Indian Journal of Dermatology, Venereology and Leprology*, vol. 75, no. 5, pp. 518–519, 2009.

[3] U. Khopkar and B. Doshi, "Improving diagnostic yield of punch biopsies of the skin," *Indian Journal of Dermatology, Venereology and Leprology*, vol. 74, no. 5, pp. 527–531, 2008.

[4] R. Sleiman, M. Kurban, and O. Abbas, "Maximizing diagnostic outcomes of skin biopsy specimens," *International Journal of Dermatology*, vol. 52, no. 1, pp. 72–78, 2013.

[5] E. McInnes, "Artefacts in histopathology," *Comparative Clinical Pathology*, vol. 13, no. 3, pp. 100–108, 2005.

[6] L. Bomm, M. D. Benez, J. M. Maceira, I. C. Succi, and M. F. Scotelaro, "Biopsy guided by dermoscopy in cutaneous pigmented lesion—case report," *Anais Brasileiros de Dermatologia*, vol. 88, no. 1, pp. 125–127, 2013.

[7] J. Wasserman, J. Maddox, M. Racz, and V. Petronic-Rosic, "Update on immunohistochemical methods relevant to dermatopathology," *Archives of Pathology and Laboratory Medicine*, vol. 133, no. 7, pp. 1053–1061, 2009.

[8]  G. Pohla-Gubo and H. Hintner, "Direct and indirect immun-ofluorescence for the diagnosis of bullous autoimmune dis-eases," *Dermatologic Clinics*, vol. 29, no. 3, pp. 365–372, 2011.

[9]  K. Sellheyer and W. F. Bergfeld, "A retrospective biopsy study of the clinical diagnostic accuracy of common skin diseases by different specialties compared with dermatology," *Journal of the American Academy of Dermatology*, vol. 52, no. 5, pp. 823–830, 2005.

[10]  C. Aslan, F. Göktay, A. T. Mansur, I. E. Aydingöz, P. Güneş, and T. R. Ekmekçi, "Clinicopathological consistency in skin disorders: a retrospective study of 3949 pathological reports," *Journal of the American Academy of Dermatology*, vol. 66, no. 3, pp. 393–400, 2012.

# 26

# High Frequency of Symptomatic Zinc Deficiency in Infants in Northern Ethiopia

**Federica Dassoni,**[1,2,3] **Zerihun Abebe,**[1] **Federica Ricceri,**[4] **Aldo Morrone,**[5] **Cristiana Albertin,**[6] **and Bernard Naafs**[7]

[1]*Ayder Referral Hospital, Mekelle, Ethiopia*
[2]*INMP Istituto Nazionale per la Promozione della Salute delle Popolazioni Migranti ed il Contrasto delle Malattie della Povertà,*
 *Via di San Gallicano 25, 00153 Roma, Italy*
[3]*Unità Operativa di Dermatologia, Università di Milano, I.R.C.C.S. Fondazione Ca' Granda Ospedale Maggiore Policlinico,*
 *20122 Milano, Italy*
[4]*Dipartimento di Chirurgia e Medicina Traslazionale, Sezione di Dermatologia, Università degli Studi di Firenze,*
 *Viale Michelangelo 41, 50125 Firenze, Italy*
[5]*Ospedale S. Camillo Forlanini, Piazza Carlo Forlanini 1, 00151 Rome, Italy*
[6]*Dipartimento di Dermatologia, Università di Padova, Via Mocenigo 8, 35127 Padova, Italy*
[7]*Stitching Tropen Dermatologie, Gracht 15, 8485KN15 Munnekeburen Friesland, The Netherlands*

Correspondence should be addressed to Federica Dassoni; federica.dx@gmail.com

Academic Editor: Jag Bhawan

*Background*. Zinc deficiency occurs in infants when its demand exceeds its supply. It presents with cutaneous signs which, in severe cases, are associated with diarrhea, alopecia, and irritability. Genetic and acquired forms of zinc deficiency have been reported and often overlap clinical features. Malnutrition, prematurity, malabsorption syndromes, and burns may cause an increased demand for zinc. *Methods*. Cases of acquired transient infantile zinc deficiency (TIZD) observed during a period of 3 years at Ayder Referral Hospital of Mekelle, Northern Ethiopia, are reported here. Since no sophisticated tests were available at our center, the diagnosis was based on the clinical signs and prompt response to oral zinc supplementation. *Results*. We observed 18 cases of TIZD at our center. All patients were full-term and breastfeeding infants with no relevant associated diseases. *Conclusions*. In this region, a high incidence of this condition is observed. We could not rule out whether heterozygosity for the genetic mutation was present or that the disease was caused by a nutritional deficiency in the mothers or more probably because both the factors coexisted together. However, further studies are necessary to better understand the causes of the increased incidence of this disease in Northern Ethiopia.

## 1. Introduction

Zinc deficiency occurs in infants when its demand exceeds its supply. It presents with cutaneous signs which, in severe cases, are associated with diarrhea, alopecia, and irritability. Genetic and acquired forms of zinc deficiency have been described and often have overlapping clinical features. However, they usually differ in their time of presentation [1]. The genetic form of the disease, idiopathic acrodermatitis enteropathica (AE), is a rare autosomal recessive disease characterized by acral and periorificial dermatitis and low serum zinc levels [2]. The mutation occurs in the SLC39A4 gene, an intestinal zinc transporter. Since breast milk is thought to facilitate zinc absorption, it appears after the interruption of breast feeding and requires an unending zinc supplementation in most cases.

Transient infantile zinc deficiency (TIZD) is a disease clinically indistinguishable from idiopathic AE, though with different pathologic mechanisms. It occurs during the first 6 months of life, usually in infants with increased zinc requirements and/or inadequate diet concentrations of zinc. Malnutrition, prematurity, total parenteral nutrition, and burns may cause an increased demand for zinc. The supply of zinc to the growing child is reduced in congenital malabsorption syndromes. Nevertheless, zinc deficiency in healthy, full-term, breast-fed infants is also seen [3–11]. These deficiencies were related to low zinc levels in the maternal milk [12]. Heterozygosity for mutation of the gene SLC30A2 may be found in these cases [2–5]. This is known as transient neonatal zinc deficiency (TNZD).

Cutaneous lesions are observed in all the affected children, while more rarely they may be accompanied by diarrhea, irritability, alopecia, low grade fever, and conjunctivitis. Zinc deficiency is rapidly eliminated after treating the patients with oral zinc supplement, with prompt improvement in the clinical signs and symptoms.

The cases of transient infantile zinc deficiency (TIZD) observed during a 3-year period in Tigray region of Northern Ethiopia are reported here. Our observations indicate that this is a relatively frequent disease as compared with that in the other reports [8–14]. Diagnosis was based on clinical presentation and prompt response to oral zinc supplementation. To our knowledge, this is the first report on zinc deficiency encountered in patients at our center in Northern Ethiopia.

The aim of our report is to make the reader aware of the high presence of this rare and life threatening condition in Ethiopia, where it is often misdiagnosed by general doctors. It is therefore important to recognize and treat it properly. We hope further studies will lead to a better understanding of the causes of its high incidence.

## 2. Case Reports

We encountered 18 cases of symptomatic zinc deficiency at the Italian Dermatological Center of Ayder Hospital, Mekelle, Northern Ethiopia, from January 2008 to January 2011.

All the cases reported here showed typical clinical features of zinc deficiency of varying severity and duration. Patients were not severely malnourished and did not have evidence of growth retardation. One patient was moderately malnourished (underweight).

During a period of 3 years (January 2008 to January 2011), we encountered a total of 18 infants (11 females and 7 males, F : M = 1 : 0.6) aged 4 to 20 months with clinical skin features of acrodermatitis enteropathica. Lesions were symmetrical, well defined, erythematous, and often with ulcerations or erosions secondary to blisters, in some cases with overlying brown crusts. They were located on the periorificial areas (perianal, genital, nasal, ocular, and perioral), the limbs (mostly the lower limbs), the extremities, and in some cases the nape and the scalp (Figures 1 and 2).

One child presented with poliosis which underwent complete repigmentation after therapy with zinc supplement.

All children were totally or partially breast fed. Some of them were referred late to our facility by other health facilities after they had received systemic antibiotics without improvement with already widespread lesions. None of them had signs or symptoms of diarrhea, irritability, severe growth failure, or burns. Their general condition was good, except for that only child affected by moderate malnutrition.

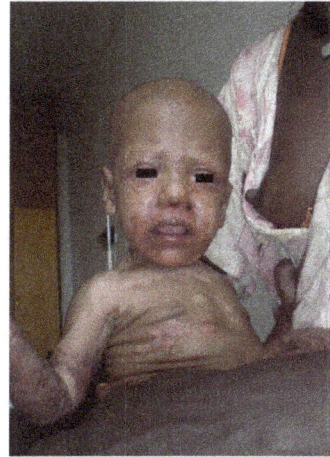

FIGURE 1: Periorificial lesions on face in an extensive case.

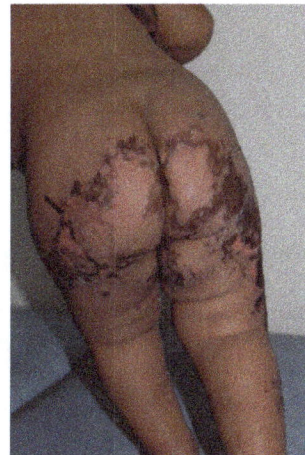

FIGURE 2: Lesions on buttocks. Marked margins, erosions, and brown crusts.

Whether they were of normal birth weight and gestational age remained unknown. However, none of them reported any history of prematurity. Moreover, since they were living in rural villages with scanty health facilities, they were not likely to be significantly preterm unless they had a history of admission to the referral hospital.

Cutaneous manifestations were mostly moderate to severe and with ulceration or erosions (Table 1).

All of them showed a good and prompt improvement after short course of oral zinc supplement (3 mg/kg/day for 2-3 months). None of the patients had relapse of the lesions after discontinuing the treatment. For this reason, our diagnosis was transient neonatal zinc deficiency (TNZD).

Zinc levels in the patient's and mother's blood and in the mother's milk could not be measured, and mutation screening of the SLC30A2 gene could not be performed because of the lack of diagnostic facilities in this region of Ethiopia. However, all the mothers were in good general health and had no cutaneous manifestations.

One patient had positive family history for the same disease (one brother). We are not able to demonstrate whether

TABLE 1: Mean features of the patients.

|  | Age (m)* | Sex | Severity of disease** | Ulcerations/erosions | Associated problems |
|---|---|---|---|---|---|
| 1 | 5 | F | Moderate | Yes | |
| 2 | 7 | F | Severe | Yes | White hair or poliosis |
| 3 | 6 | F | Mild/moderate | No | |
| 4 | 4 | M | Moderate | Yes | |
| 5 | 8 | M | Mild | Yes | Polydactyly |
| 6 | 14 | M | Moderate | Yes | |
| 7 | 10 | F | Severe and spread | No | |
| 8 | 6 | M | Moderate | Yes | Chromosomal anomaly |
| 9 | 18 | F | Moderate | Yes | |
| 10 | 12 | F | Moderate | Yes | Conjunctivitis, history of affected brother |
| 11 | 16 | F | Severe | Yes | Scabies, underweight |
| 12 | 5 | F | Severe | Yes | |
| 13 | 8 | F | Severe | Yes | |
| 14 | 10 | F | Mild | Yes | |
| 15 | 5 | F | Moderate | Yes | |
| 16 | 20 | M | Moderate | No | |
| 17 | 4 | M | Mild | Yes | |
| 18 | 6 | M | Moderate | No | |

*(m): months. **Mild: less than 10% BSA involved. Moderate: 10 to 30% BSA involved. Severe: more than 30% BSA involved. BSA = body surface area.

other brothers/sisters presented mild signs of the disease; these were not reported by the mothers.

One patient presented with an unusual "facies" characterized by hypertelorism, prominent ears, and slightly small sized head, making us think of an associated chromosomal anomaly which was not possible to diagnose as there were no facilities for chromosome mapping.

One patient also had polydactyly, a common congenital defect encountered in this region.

One patient presented with associated scabies, which is also a highly prevalent disease in this region.

## 3. Discussion

Transient neonatal zinc deficiency (TNZD) is mainly observed in breast-fed infants and does not reoccur after weaning [4]. We think that the number of cases observed in Northern Ethiopia is very high as other reports in the literature are mostly single-case or two-case reports [2, 3, 6–12]. Taking into account the cases observed in full-term infants, to our knowledge only 15 cases have been reported since 1985 from different countries [1–3, 5–15]; it is therefore considered a rare disease.

Most of the previously reported cases in premature and also full-term infants were associated with low zinc levels in the maternal milk, although in some cases maternal zinc level was normal.

A low zinc level in the maternal milk is an important cofactor. Breast milk may be low in zinc because of a rare abnormality of zinc secretion by the mammary gland [16]. This may be the cause of symptomatic zinc deficiency, which is more severe and more common in premature infants because of the increased zinc requirements in this

group. Symptomatic zinc deficiency can also appear from a combination of the SLC39A4 mutation in the infant and low milk zinc concentration from the mother who has the same heterozygous mutation [2].

All our patients had an excellent clinical improvement and discontinued the treatment after 2-3 months with no relapses. This indicates the diagnosis of TNZD and made us exclude AE, which requires lifelong treatment. Breast feeding, partial or total, was also a supporting factor for the diagnosis.

Zinc deficiency may also be secondary to a poor intestinal absorption or an increased urinary and intestinal secretion [13]. Disorders of intestinal malabsorption are other possible etiologic factors. None of the children reported here had clinical evidence of intestinal disease. It was not possible to measure urinary zinc levels. In our patients, we were not able to demonstrate any increased demand for zinc or any decreased ability of zinc storage. In fact, none of them was evidently preterm, had burns, had parenteral nutrition, or had any other evident reason to require increased zinc supplementation.

We could not rule out whether mother and child presented heterozygosity for a SLC39A4 or SLC30A2 gene mutation or whether the clinical features could be due to a dietary zinc deficiency of the mothers and/or increased zinc requirements of the infants. All the mothers were asymptomatic and had no skin abnormalities. As reported in previous studies from different regions of Ethiopia [17–19], they could also probably have a primary dietary asymptomatic zinc deficiency.

Since sophisticated diagnostic techniques are not generally available in developing countries, our diagnosis was clinical and confirmed by the prompt and remarkable healing of the lesions after treatment with oral zinc supplement.

Most probably, an association of both heterozygosity for SLC30A2 gene mutation and dietary zinc deficiency in the mothers was contributing to the clinical manifestations in the infants.

Zinc is essential for growth, as it is involved in the development of the immune system, the muscles, and the bones, as well as the skin. In developing countries, diets often do not contain zinc in sufficient quantity or of sufficient bioavailability [18, 19]. Dietary zinc deficiency, as well as other nutritional deficiencies, has been reported from different regions of Ethiopia, affecting both pregnant women and children, although association with cutaneous signs has not been reported. Low levels of zinc in breast milk in Ethiopian mothers were reported in different studies [19–22], although there is no evidence of its association with clinical manifestations in children.

Most of the observed infants presented with signs of moderate or severe skin manifestations (14/18) and with ulcerations or erosions (14/18). This is probably due to the delayed access to our center. Beyond the difficult access to health facilities in rural areas of developing countries, some of our patients were previously treated at other health centers/hospitals with systemic or local antibiotics and only referred to us when no improvement was achieved.

Children were otherwise in good general health, except one case affected by moderate malnutrition.

We observed a preponderance of female infants affected (11 out of 18), although this is not statistically significant given the small number of patients. We could not identify a specific biological or cultural/behavioral reason which could explain the higher number of females affected.

Further studies are necessary to understand the causes of the increased incidence of TNZD in this population and to confirm the preponderance of female affected patients.

Transient neonatal zinc deficiency is a life threatening disease, often misdiagnosed by rural health workers and general doctors in Northern Ethiopia. Many of the reported patients were in fact in advanced stage conditions. If not diagnosed and treated properly, TNZD may have severe consequences on the child's growth. Keeping in mind the presence of the disease in the region is essential to recognize its clinical features and to give the correct treatment, as specific diagnostic tests are often not available in developing countries. Health workers should be made aware of the presence of the disease in order to refer to hospital all those patients who do not respond to first line therapy.

## Conflict of Interests

The authors declare that there is no conflict of interests regarding the publication of this paper.

## References

[1] E. C. Haliasos, P. Litwack, L. Kristal, and A. Chawla, "Acquired zinc deficiency in full-term newborns from decreased zinc content in breast milk," Cutis, vol. 79, no. 6, pp. 425–428, 2007.

[2] N. El Fékih, K. Monia, S. Schmitt, I. Dorbani, S. Küry, and M. R. Kamoun, "Transient symptomatic zinc deficiency in a breast-fed infant: relevance of a genetic study," Nutrition, vol. 27, no. 10, pp. 1087–1089, 2011.

[3] M. C. Miletta, A. Bieri, K. Kernland et al., "Transient neonatal zinc deficiency caused by a heterozygous G87R mutation in the zinc transporter ZnT-2 (SLC30A2) gene in the mother highlighting the importance of $Zn^{2+}$ for normal growth and development," International Journal of Endocrinology, vol. 2013, Article ID 259189, 8 pages, 2013.

[4] N. Itsumura, Y. Inamo, F. Okazaki et al., "Compound heterozygous mutations in SLC30A2/ZnT2 results in low milk zinc concentrations: a novel mechanism for zinc deficiency in a breast-fed infant," PLoS ONE, vol. 8, no. 5, Article ID e64045, 2013.

[5] I. Lasry, Y. A. Seo, H. Ityel et al., "A dominant negative heterozygous G87R mutation in the zinc transporter, ZnT-2 (SLC30A2), results in transient neonatal zinc deficiency," The Journal of Biological Chemistry, vol. 287, no. 35, pp. 29348–29361, 2012.

[6] A. M. E. Bye, A. Goodfellow, and D. J. Atherton, "Transient zinc deficiency in a full-term breast-fed infant of normal birth weight," Pediatric Dermatology, vol. 2, no. 4, pp. 308–311, 1985.

[7] Y. Kuramoto, Y. Igarashi, S. Kato, and H. Tagami, "Acquired zinc deficiency in two breast-fed mature infants," Acta Dermato-Venereologica, vol. 66, no. 4, pp. 359–361, 1986.

[8] L. J. Roberts, C. F. Shadwick, and P. R. Bergstresser, "Zinc deficiency in two full-term breast-fed infants," Journal of the American Academy of Dermatology, vol. 16, no. 2, pp. 301–304, 1987.

[9] M. T. Glover and D. J. Atherton, "Transient zinc deficiency in two full-term breast-fed siblings associated with low maternal breast milk zinc concentration," Pediatric Dermatology, vol. 5, no. 1, pp. 10–13, 1988.

[10] M. G. Lee, K. T. Hong, and J. J. Kim, "Transient symptomatic zinc deficiency in a full-term breast-fed infant," Journal of the American Academy of Dermatology, vol. 23, no. 2, part 2, pp. 375–379, 1990.

[11] A. J. Mancini and W. W. Tunnessen Jr., "Picture of the month. Acrodermatitis enteropathica-like rash in a breast-fed, full-term infant with zinc deficiency," Archives of Pediatrics and Adolescent Medicine, vol. 152, no. 12, pp. 1239–1240, 1998.

[12] U. K. Singh and R. K. Sinha, "Symptomatic zinc deficiency in a breast fed full term infant," The Indian Journal of Pediatrics, vol. 61, no. 3, pp. 307–308, 1994.

[13] J. Stevens and L. Lubitz, "Symptomatic zinc deficiency in breast-fed term and premature infants," Journal of Paediatrics and Child Health, vol. 34, no. 1, pp. 97–100, 1998.

[14] S. C. Murthy, M. M. Udagani, A. V. Badakali, and B. C. Yelameli, "Symptomatic zinc deficiency in a full-term breast-fed infant," Dermatology Online Journal, vol. 16, no. 6, article 3, 2010.

[15] S. Coelho, B. Fernandes, F. Rodrigues, J. P. Reis, A. Moreno, and A. Figueiredo, "Transient zinc deficiency in a breast fed, premature infant," European Journal of Dermatology, vol. 16, no. 2, pp. 193–195, 2006.

[16] A. W. Zimmerman, K. M. Hambidge, M. L. Lepow, R. D. Greenberg, M. L. Stover, and C. E. Casey, "Acrodermatitis in breast-fed premature infants: evidence for a defect of mammary zinc secretion," Pediatrics, vol. 69, no. 2, pp. 176–183, 1982.

[17] R. S. Gibson, "Zinc supplementation for infants," The Lancet, vol. 355, no. 9220, pp. 2008–2009, 2000.

[18] S. Gebremedhin, F. Enquselassie, and M. Umeta, "Prevalence of prenatal zinc deficiency and its association with socio-demographic, dietary and health care related factors in Rural Sidama, Southern Ethiopia: a cross-sectional study," *BMC Public Health*, vol. 11, article 898, 2011.

[19] M. Umeta, C. E. West, H. Verhoef, J. Haidar, and J. G. A. J. Hautvast, "Factors associated with stunting in infants aged 5–11 months in the Dodota-Sire District, Rural Ethiopia," *Journal of Nutrition*, vol. 133, no. 4, pp. 1064–1069, 2003.

[20] A. Kassu, T. Yabutani, A. Mulu, B. Tessema, and F. Ota, "Serum zinc, copper, selenium, calcium, and magnesium levels in pregnant and non-pregnant women in Gondar, Northwest Ethiopia," *Biological Trace Element Research*, vol. 122, no. 2, pp. 97–106, 2008.

[21] J. Haidar, M. Umeta, and W. Kogi-Makau, "Effect of iron supplementation on serum zinc status of lactating women in Addis Ababa, Ethiopia," *East African Medical Journal*, vol. 82, no. 7, pp. 349–352, 2005.

[22] R. S. Gibson, Y. Abebe, S. Stabler et al., "Zinc, gravida, infection, and iron, but not vitamin B-12 or folate status, predict hemoglobin during pregnancy in Southern Ethiopia," *Journal of Nutrition*, vol. 138, no. 3, pp. 581–586, 2008.

# 27

# Propranolol in Treatment of Huge and Complicated Infantile Hemangiomas in Egyptian Children

**Basheir A. Hassan[1] and Khalid S. Shreef[2]**

[1] Pediatrics Department, Faculty of Medicine, Zagazig University, Zagazig 44519, Egypt
[2] Surgery Department, Faculty of Medicine, Zagazig University, Zagazig 44519, Egypt

Correspondence should be addressed to Basheir A. Hassan; alzahar2005@yahoo.com

Academic Editor: Giuseppe Argenziano

*Background.* Infantile hemangiomas (IHs) are the most common benign tumours of infancy. Propranolol has recently been reported to be a highly effective treatment for IHs. This study aimed to evaluate the efficacy and side effects of propranolol for treatment of complicated cases of IHs. *Patients and Methods.* This prospective clinical study included 30 children with huge or complicated IHs; their ages ranged from 2 months to 1 year. They were treated by oral propranolol. Treatment outcomes were clinically evaluated. *Results.* Superficial cutaneous hemangiomas began to respond to propranolol therapy within one to two weeks after the onset of treatment. The mean treatment period that was needed for the occurrence of complete resolution was 9.4 months. Treatment with propranolol was well tolerated and had few side effects. No rebound growth of the tumors was noted when propranolol dosing stopped except in one case. *Conclusion.* Propranolol is a promising treatment for IHs without obvious side effects. However, further studies with longer follow-up periods are needed.

## 1. Introduction

Infantile hemangiomas (IHs) are the most common benign tumors of infancy affecting 1% to 2.6% of newborns and up to 10% of children in the age of one. The incidence is higher in girls and premature infants. The majority of lesions involve the skin and subcutaneous tissues and eventually resolve spontaneously without complications [1–4].

However, about 20% of IHs are extremely disfiguring and destructive to normal tissue and may even be life threatening [5]. A central characteristic of most IHs is a predictable life cycle. The initial proliferative phase lasts 6 to 10 months, during which the tumor grows rapidly because of excessive vascular endothelial cells (ECs). This is followed by an involution phase, spanning up to 7 years. Normal involution is thought to occur via cell senility and eventual apoptosis [5–7].

Ulceration is the most common complication and occurs most often toward the end of the growth phase [8]. However, in some IHs, ulceration precedes proliferation and is actually the presenting clinical sign of IHs [8, 9]. This early ulceration suggests that it may not simply be a response to rapid growth or tensile stress on the overlying skin but other causes such as local tissue hypoxia may play a role [10, 11].

Lesions can be subtyped as localized (which originate from a focal point), segmental (which follow a geographic distribution), indeterminate, and multifocal (8 or more noncontiguous lesions) [12].

Approximately 80% of IHs are found on the face and neck, favoring the anterior cheek, forehead, and preauricular area [5, 12]. The remaining IHs are found in decreasing order on the trunk, lower extremities, and upper extremities and occasionally on mucosal surfaces.

Facial IHs were divided according to embryological segments as suggested by Haggstrom et al. [13] as follows: frontonasal, frontotemporal, maxillary, and mandibular.

Corticosteroids, interferon-alfa, vincristine, laser therapy, and topical imiquimod are used in the treatment of IHs [5]. Surgical excision had also been reported to be effective.

Recently, the use of propranolol, a nonselective beta blocker, has been described in the treatment of IHs, with a spectacular efficacy in all cases [3]. Proposed mechanisms of the action of propranolol on hemangiomas include control of hypoxic stress with upregulated HIF-1a, apoptosis induction,

TABLE 1: Demographic and clinical data of study population variable.

| | |
|---|---|
| Total number of patients | **30 (100%)** |
| Preterm | **22 (73.3%)** |
| Fullterm | **8 (26.6%)** |
| Age at initiation of treatment (month), | |
| Mean ± SD | **3.7 ± 2.5** |
| Gender, n (%) | |
| Male | **9 (30%)** |
| Female | **21** (70%) |
| Type, n (%) | |
| Localized | **18** (60%) |
| Segmental | **9** (30%) |
| Multifocal | **3 (10%)** |
| Location of IH, n (%) | |
| Facial Segments: | |
| Frontotemporal (seg.1) | 3 (10%) |
| Maxillary (seg.2) | 5 (16.6%) |
| Mandibular (seg.3) | 8 (26.6%) |
| Frontonasal (seg.4) | 2 (6.6%) |
| Other locations: | |
| Trunk | 8 (26.6%) |
| Extremities | 3 (10%) |
| Neck | 1 (3.3%) |
| Duration of treatment till resolution (month), | **9.4 ± 2.6** |
| Mean (range) | (6–14) |
| Side effects of treatment, n (%) | |
| Tachypnea | **2 (6.6%)** |
| Hypoglycemia | **1 (3.3%)** |
| Cold extrmities | **1 (3.3%)** |
| Constipation | **2 (6.6%)** |

and decreased production of endothelial vascular and fibroblastic growth factors [3].

So, our study aimed to describe the efficacy of propranolol in 30 children with IHs and the adverse effects related to this therapy.

## 2. Patients and Methods

This prospective clinical study was carried out at the Pediatric Department and Pediatric Surgery Unit, Zagazig University Hospitals, Egypt, during the period from April 2010 to September 2012.

The patients were included in the study according to the following inclusion criteria: eyelid involvement with ocular risk of occlusion or compression, airway obstruction, large IHs with considerable aesthetic derangement or ulceration, and all rapidly proliferating hemangiomas with functional deficit and/or disfigurement.

Exclusion criteria included history of hypoglycemia, asthma or bronchospasm, patients with known cardiac abnormalities, and patients with PHACES (posterior fossa

malformations, hemangioma, arterial anomalies, cardiac defects, eye abnormalities, and sternal clefts) syndrome.

All infants were subjected to full history taking and thorough clinical examination which included complete cardiac examination, electrocardiography, and echocardiography. As most of our patients included in this study had segmental IHs in the face, a cerebral magnetic resonance imaging/magnetic resonance angiography (MRI/MRA), electrocardiography, and echocardiography were carried out in these patients before initiating therapy to rule out PHACES syndrome.

All patients were admitted to hospital during the first two days of treatment for monitoring of blood pressure, heart rate, and serum glucose level one to three times a day; measurements were taken before and 2 hours after each dose of propranolol. At the first week, the dose of propranolol was 1 mg/kg/day and then increased to full dosage (1.5 mg/kg/12 hours). The full dosage was maintained during the whole period of the study. A treatment period of at least 12 weeks was scheduled, which could be further expanded if the patient required more time to achieve the resolution of the problem that had led to initiation of propranolol therapy. Propranolol was withdrawn gradually over a period of at least 4 weeks.

Follow-up visits were scheduled every 2 weeks in the outpatient clinic for further physical examination of IH and monitoring of ECG, blood pressure, and heart rate. During the treatment period, the progressive effect of propranolol therapy was measured by comparing the diameters and colors in the front and lateral photos of every patient that were taken before treatment and at every follow-up visit.

Informed written consents for propranolol treatment and use of the patients' photographs were obtained prior to inclusion in the study from the children's guardians. The study protocol was approved by the Pediatric Ethical Committee in Zagazig University.

## 3. Results

Thirty patients (21 females, 9 males) (their ages ranged from 2 months to 1 year) with different sites of IHs were treated with propranolol. Demographic data, types, locations of hemangiomas, duration, and side effects of treatment of these patients are summarized in Table 1.

The mean age for starting propranolol treatment was 3.7 months (ranged from 2 to 12 months). IHs were seen more commonly in preterm than full-term babies (73.3% versus 26.6%) with female predominance (70%).

The appearance of hemangiomas occurred after the age of one month in 23 (76.6%) patients. Eighteen (60%) patients had localized hemangiomas; 9 (30%) patients had segmental lesions while 3 (10%) patients had multifocal lesion.

The anatomical sites of hemangiomas were shown in Table 1.

Twelve (40%) patients had impairment of vision, hearing, and/or difficult swallowing. Three (10%) patients had painful ulceration in the face and two (6.6%) patients had disfiguring hemangioma in the face.

Superficial cutaneous hemangiomas started to respond to propranolol therapy within one to two weeks after the onset of

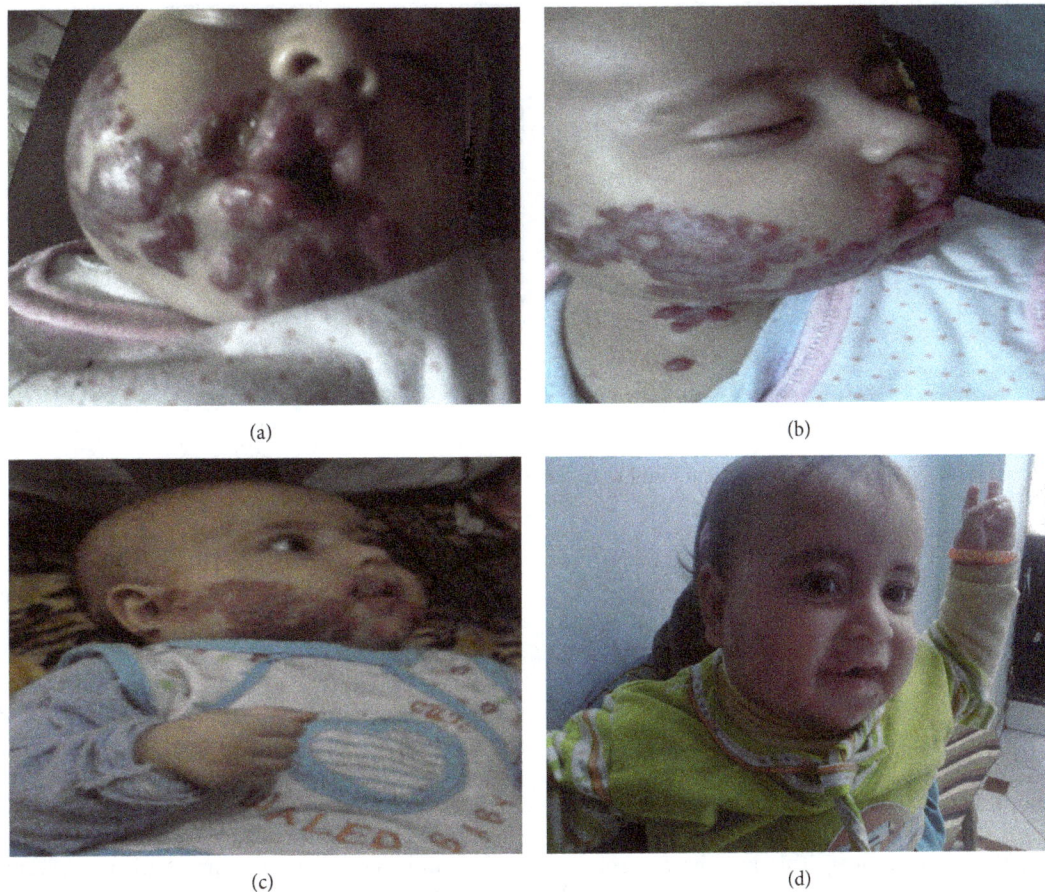

FIGURE 1: Hemangioma in patient number 1. Before treatment (a), one week (b), one month (c), and six months after treatment (d).

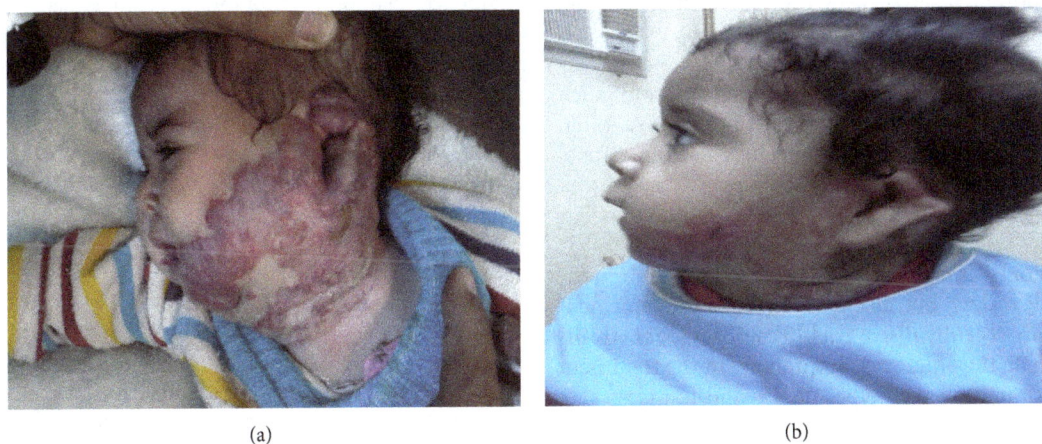

FIGURE 2: Hemangioma in patient number 10. Before treatment (a) and 8 months after treatment (b).

treatment. They began to change from intense red to purple with softening and continued to improve until they became nearly flat with significantly diminished color, together with regression of the tumor size (Figures 1, 2, and 3).

The ulcerated IHs experienced a reduction in severity similar to nonulcerated hemangiomas, and ulceration was completely resolved in all patients within 2–8 weeks of treatment.

The treatment period that was needed for the occurrence of complete resolution ranged from 6 to 14 months (mean 9.4). After resolution, the treatment was withdrawn gradually over a period of at least 4 weeks.

Regarding propranolol-associated side effects, 2 (6.6%) patients had a wheezy chest and tachypnea at 2 weeks after treatment and one (3.3%) patient developed hypoglycemia at 1 month after treatment. Cold extremities were found in

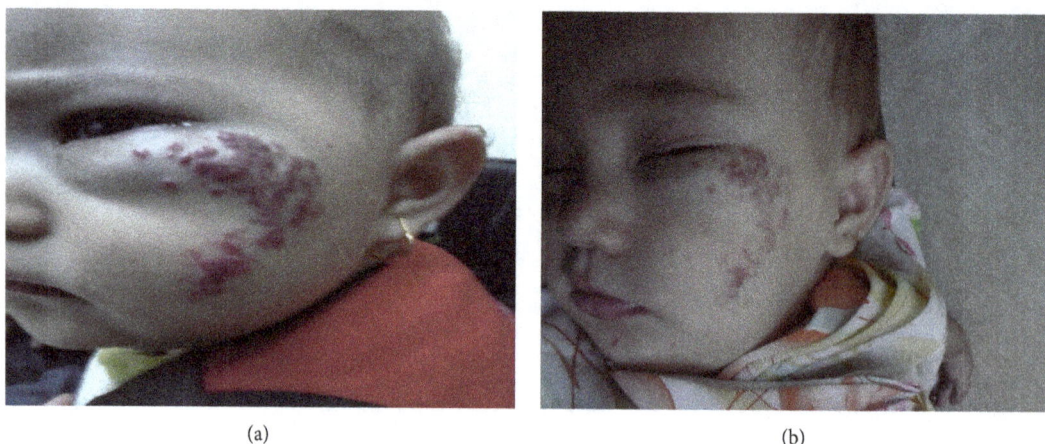

(a)                                                                (b)

FIGURE 3: Hemangioma in patient number 11. Before treatment (a) and 8 months after treatment (b).

one (3.3%) patient and constipation developed in 2 patients (6.6%).

No rebound growth of the tumors was noted after the stoppage of treatment except in one case with complicated left retroorbital hemangioma with lagophthalmos and proptosis.

## 4. Discussion

Most hemangiomas are relatively small and pose only minor clinical problems, but approximately 20% become clinically significant and require treatment. This may be a result of their aggressive growth and/or their location close to vital structures that they can invade, impairing the function and thus threatening the child's life; large hemangiomas in the area of the mouth, nose, or eyes prevent normal feeding, respiration, or vision [1, 14].

Ulceration, hemorrhage, infection, and high output cardiac failure may complicate IHs. Even apart from such clinically problematic situations, hemangiomas are often disfiguring and can have significant psychological/emotional impact on the affected child. This causes many parents to seek treatment rather than wait for the natural involution to occur [15].

Propranolol hydrochloride has been used in children for a variety of disorders, but its effectiveness in the treatment of IHs was only recently discovered [3]. So we designed this study to evaluate the efficacy of propranolol in the treatment of huge and/or complicated types of IHs and to assess side effects related to this therapy.

In our study, there was a predominance of female and premature infants among the patients. These results were consistent with that of Hsu et al.'s study [16].

In our study, the mean duration of therapy was 9.4 months. In the literature, duration of therapy varies from 2 to 10 months. Hogeling and his colleagues stated that IHs significantly dropped in volume, redness, and elevation from the skin with a six-month course of propranolol [17]. Bertrand et al., in their study, stated that all patients treated with propranolol had good to excellent improvement at 6 months and the mean duration of treatment was 10.6 months (range 7–13 months) [18].

The drug appeared to be safe with no significant hypotension, hypoglycemia, or bradycardia among our patients. This efficacy and safety have been observed in other studies as demonstrated in a recent systematic literature review summarizing the effectiveness and adverse effects of propranolol in the treatment of IHs [19]. Lawley et al. reported two cases who received propranolol in the recommended dosage; one experienced severe hypotension and the other experienced severe hypoglycemia [20]. Other authors have reported similar cases [21, 22]. Buckmiller [23] observed gastroesophageal reflux and somnolence in some patients. Adverse effects of propranolol have also been reported, including hypotension, bradycardia, bronchospasm, and hypoglycemia [24].

In conclusion, this study contributes to the growing evidence that oral propranolol is an efficacious and safe treatment for IHs, with a careful dosing and monitoring regimen. Nevertheless, further studies and longer followup are needed.

## Conflict of Interests

The authors declare that there is no conflict of interests.

## References

[1] P. D. Martinez, N. A. Fein, L. M. Boon, and J. B. Mulliken, "Not all hemangiomas look like strawberries: uncommon presentations of the most common tumor of infancy," *Pediatric Dermatology*, vol. 12, no. 1, pp. 1–6, 1995.

[2] C. Kilcline and I. J. Frieden, "Infantile hemangiomas: how common are they? A systematic review of the medical literature," *Pediatric Dermatology*, vol. 25, no. 2, pp. 168–173, 2008.

[3] C. Léauté-Labrèze, E. Dumas de la Roque, T. Hubiche, F. Boralevi, J.-B. Thambo, and A. Taïeb, "Propranolol for severe hemangiomas of infancy," *The New England Journal of Medicine*, vol. 358, no. 24, pp. 2649–2651, 2008.

[4] J. Li, X. Chen, S. Zhao et al., "Demographic and clinical characteristics and risk factors for infantile hemangioma: a Chinese case-control study," *Archives of Dermatology*, vol. 147, no. 9, pp. 1049–1056, 2011.

[5] E. Boye, M. Jinnin, and B. R. Olsen, "Infantile hemangioma: challenges, new insights, and therapeutic promise," *Journal of Craniofacial Surgery*, vol. 20, no. 1, pp. 678–684, 2009.

[6] K.-Y. Suh and I. J. Frieden, "Infantile hemangiomas with minimal or arrested growth: a retrospective case series," *Archives of Dermatology*, vol. 146, no. 9, pp. 971–976, 2010.

[7] S. L. Chamlin, A. N. Haggstrom, B. A. Drolet et al., "Multicenter prospective study of ulcerated hemangiomas," *Journal of Pediatrics*, vol. 151, no. 6, pp. 684–689, 2007.

[8] M. G. Liang, I. J. Frieden, J. C. Shaw, and J. Knispel, "Perineal ulcerations as the presenting manifestation of hemangioma," *Archives of Dermatology*, vol. 138, no. 1, pp. 126–127, 2002.

[9] J. Knispel and J. C. Shaw, "Nonhealing perianal ulcer," *Archives of Dermatology*, vol. 137, no. 3, pp. 365–370, 2001.

[10] D. R. Wright, D. C. Russi, A. J. Mancini, and S. L. Chamlin, "The nasal crease sign in segmental facial hemangioma-an early sign of cartilage destruction," *Pediatric Dermatology*, vol. 24, no. 3, pp. 241–245, 2007.

[11] D. W. Metry, A. N. Haggstrom, B. A. Drolet et al., "A prospective study of PHACE syndrome in infantile hemangiomas: demographic features, clinical findings, and complications," *American Journal of Medical Genetics*, vol. 140, no. 9, pp. 975–986, 2006.

[12] K. G. Chiller, D. Passaro, and I. J. Frieden, "Hemangiomas of infancy: clinical characteristics, morphologic subtypes, and their relationship to race, ethnicity, and sex," *Archives of Dermatology*, vol. 138, no. 12, pp. 1567–1576, 2002.

[13] A. N. Haggstrom, E. J. Lammer, R. A. Schneider, R. Marcucio, and I. J. Frieden, "Patterns of infantile hemangiomas: new clues to hemangioma pathogenesis and embryonic facial development," *Pediatrics*, vol. 117, no. 3, pp. 698–703, 2006.

[14] J. B. Mulliken, S. J. Fishman, and P. E. Burrows, "Vascular anomalies," in *Vascular Anomalies*, S. A. Wells and L. L. Creswell, Eds., pp. 517–584, Mosby, St. Louis, Mo, USA, 2000.

[15] D. J. Atherton, "Infantile haemangiomas," *Early Human Development*, vol. 82, no. 12, pp. 789–795, 2006.

[16] T. C. Hsu, J. D. Wang, C. H. Chen et al., "Treatment with propranolol for infantile hemangioma in 13 Taiwanese newborns and young infants," *Pediatrics & Neonatology*, vol. 53, no. 2, pp. 125–132, 2012.

[17] M. Hogeling, S. Adams, and O. Wargon, "A randomized controlled trial of propranolol for infantile hemangiomas," *Pediatrics*, vol. 128, no. 2, pp. e259–e266, 2011.

[18] J. Bertrand, C. McCuaig, J. Dubois, A. Hatami, S. Ondrejchak, and J. Powell, "Propranolol versus prednisone in the treatment of infantile hemangiomas: a retrospective comparative study," *Pediatric Dermatology*, vol. 28, no. 6, pp. 649–654, 2011.

[19] A. L. Marqueling, V. Oza, and I. J. Frieden, "Propranolol and infantile hemangiomas four years later: a systematic review," *Pediatric Dermatology*, vol. 30, no. 2, pp. 182–191, 2013.

[20] L. P. Lawley, E. Siegfried, and J. L. Todd, "Propranolol treatment for hemangioma of infancy: risks and recommendations," *Pediatric Dermatology*, vol. 26, no. 5, pp. 610–614, 2009.

[21] K. E. Holland, I. J. Frieden, P. C. Frommelt, A. J. Mancini, D. Wyatt, and B. A. Drolet, "Hypoglycemia in children taking propranolol for the treatment of infantile hemangioma," *Archives of Dermatology*, vol. 146, no. 7, pp. 775–778, 2010.

[22] E. Bonifazi, A. Acquafredda, A. Milano, O. Montagna, and N. Laforgia, "Severe hypoglycemia during successful treatment of diffuse hemangiomatosis with propranolol," *Pediatric Dermatology*, vol. 27, no. 2, pp. 195–196, 2010.

[23] L. M. Buckmiller, "Propranolol treatment for infantile hemangiomas," *Current Opinion in Otolaryngology and Head and Neck Surgery*, vol. 17, no. 6, pp. 458–459, 2009.

[24] E. C. Siegfried, W. J. Keenan, and S. Al-Jureidini, "More on propranolol for hemangiomas of infancy," *The New England Journal of Medicine*, vol. 359, no. 26, pp. 2846–2847, 2008.

# 28

# IL-1RN VNTR Polymorphism in Adult Dermatomyositis and Systemic Lupus Erythematosus

**Zornitsa Kamenarska,**[1] **Gyulnas Dzhebir,**[1] **Maria Hristova,**[2] **Alexey Savov,**[3] **Anton Vinkov,**[4] **Radka Kaneva,**[1] **Vanio Mitev,**[1] **and Lyubomir Dourmishev**[5]

[1] *Molecular Medicine Center and Department of Medical Chemistry and Biochemistry, Medical University-Sofia, 2 Zdrave Street, 1431 Sofia, Bulgaria*

[2] *Department of Clinical Laboratory and Clinical Immunology and Department of Nephrology, Medical University-Sofia, 1 Georgi Sofijski Street, 1431 Sofia, Bulgaria*

[3] *National Genetic Laboratory, Maichin Dom Hospital, 2 Zdrave Street, 1431 Sofia, Bulgaria*

[4] *28 Diagnostic and Consultative Center-Sofia, 1 Iliya Beshkov Street, 1592 Sofia, Bulgaria*

[5] *Department of Dermatology and Venereology, Medical University-Sofia, 1 Georgi Sofijski Street, 1431 Sofia, Bulgaria*

Correspondence should be addressed to Zornitsa Kamenarska; kamenarska@yahoo.com

Academic Editor: Elizabeth Helen Kemp

Polymorphisms in the cytokine genes and their natural antagonists are thought to influence the predisposition to dermatomyositis (DM) and systemic lupus erythematosus (SLE). A variable number tandem repeat (VNTR) polymorphism of 86 bp in intron 2 of the interleukin-1 receptor antagonist (IL-1RN) gene leads to the existence of five different alleles which cause differences in the production of both IL-1RA (interleukin-1 receptor antagonist) and IL-1$\beta$. The aim of this case-control study was to investigate the association between the IL-1RN VNTR polymorphism and the susceptibility to DM and SLE in Bulgarian patients. Altogether 91 patients, 55 with SLE and 36 with DM, as well as 112 unrelated healthy controls, were included in this study. Only three alleles were identified in both patients and controls ((1) four repeats, (2) two repeats, and (3) five repeats). The IL-1RN*2 allele ($P = 0.02$, OR 2.5, and 95% CI 1.2–5.4) and the 1/2+2/2 genotypes were found prevalent among the SLE patients ($P = 0.05$, OR 2.6, and 95% CI 1–6.3). No association was found between this polymorphism and the ACR criteria for SLE as well as with the susceptibility to DM. Our results indicate that the IL-1RN VNTR polymorphism might play a role in the susceptibility of SLE but not DM.

## 1. Introduction

Dermatomyositis (DM) and systemic lupus erythematosus (SLE) are diseases of unknown etiology. However, the dysregulation of cytokine production or action is thought to have an important role in their development [1].

Interleukin-1$\alpha$ (IL-1$\alpha$) and interleukin-1$\beta$ (IL-1$\beta$) are proinflammatory cytokines which belong to the IL-1 family. The interleukin-1 receptor antagonist (IL-1RA) is a naturally occurring competitive inhibitor of IL-1. The dysregulation of IL-1 production caused by IL-1RA leads to abnormal inflammatory activity which results in subsequent tissue damage commonly observed in the pathogenesis of SLE and DM. The interleukin-1 receptor antagonist (IL-1RN) gene is polymorphic, resulting in quantitative differences in both IL-1RA and IL-1$\beta$ production. A tandem repeat sequence of 86 base pairs in length was described in intron 2 of the IL-1RN gene [2]. The number of times this sequence is repeated varies from 2 to 6. The most common is allele 1 (four repeats) followed by allele 2 (2 repeats). The other three alleles are rare, found in less than 1% in most populations. IL-1RN*2 allele was found associated with increased IL-1RA production in vitro [3]. The serum levels of IL-1RA were found significantly higher in lupus [4] and DM [5, 6] patients than in controls.

TABLE 1: Demographic and clinical data.

| Disease | | DM | | SLE |
| --- | --- | --- | --- | --- |
| Demographic parameters | Female/male | 23/13 | Female/male | 46/9 |
| | Age, mean ± SD years | 52 ± 14.7 | Age, mean ± SD years | 40 ± 12.4 |
| Clinical parameters | | | Malar rash | 34 (61.8%) |
| | | | Discoid rash | 11 (20.0%) |
| | Cutaneous disease | 27 (78.8%) | Arthritis | 37 (67.3%) |
| | Muscle weakness | 28 (78.8%) | Oral ulcer | 4 (7.3%) |
| | Elevated muscle enzymes | 19 (54.6%) | Photosensitivity | 31 (56.4%) |
| | EMG findings | 20 (54.6%) | Serositis | 11 (20.0%) |
| | Photosensitivity | 21 (60.6%) | Renal disease | 55 (100%) |
| | Autoantibodies | 9 (18.2%) | Neurological disease | 12 (22.2%) |
| | | | Haematological disease | 20 (36.4%) |
| | | | Immunological disease | 34 (61.8%) |
| | | | ANA | 39 (70.9%) |

SD: standard deviation, EMG: electromyography, and ANA: antinuclear antibodies.

The higher IL-1RA levels could serve as predictive biomarker for renal involvement in SLE [7] and positively correlated with PM/DM disease activity [8, 9].

The objective of our study was to determine whether the IL-1RN VNTR polymorphism is a risk factor for the development of adult DM and SLE in Bulgarian patients and to define its contribution to the increased risk.

## 2. Materials and Methods

*2.1. Patient Population.* Thirty-six patients with dermatomyositis who met the criteria of Bohan and Peter [10, 11] and Targoff et al. [12] and fifty-five with systemic lupus erythematosus who met the American College of Rheumatology (ACR) criteria were included in this study. Only patients with definite or probable disease were included. The clinical and demographic data are presented in Table 1. In the DM group, 23 patients were female and 13 male. The mean age was 52 with a range of 18–82 years. In the SLE group, 46 were female and 9 male. The mean age was 40 with a range of 15–78 years. The patients have been followed for a mean of 10 years at the Department of Dermatology and Venereology, Medical University-Sofia, at the Department of Nephrology, Medical University-Sofia, and at the Department of Nephrology, Ministry of Interior Hospital-Sofia.

The control group consisted of 112 anonymous healthy volunteers who did not show any clinical or laboratory signs of autoimmune skin diseases, as well as kinship with patients suffering from autoimmune skin diseases. They were randomly selected from the Biobank of the Molecular Medicine Center and the National Genetic Laboratory as to match the patients in age, gender, and ethnicity.

*2.2. Genetic Analysis.* The scientific investigation presented in this paper has been carried out in accordance with The Code of Ethics of the World Medical Association (Declaration of Helsinki) for experiments involving humans. The study was approved by the local ethics committee at the Medical University-Sofia. All participants signed an informed consent and venous blood was drawn for DNA isolation. Genomic DNA was extracted from the peripheral blood with the Chemagen DNA purification kit, using Chemagic Magnetic Separation Module I (Chemagen AG).

The analysis of IL-1RN 86 bp repeat polymorphism was performed as previously described by Tarlow et al. [2]. Standard primer pairs were used (5′-CTCAGCAACACTCCTAT; 3′-TCCTGGTCTGCAGGTAA). Amplification was performed under the following conditions: denaturing step at 95°C for 10 minutes, 35 cycles of 95°C for 60 seconds, 59°C for 60 seconds, 72°C for 60 seconds, and 1 cycle of extension at 72°C for 10 minutes. The products were visualized on a 3% agarose gel stained with ethidium bromide.

*2.3. Statistical Analysis.* Allele and genotype frequencies were compared between DM and SLE cases and controls, using Fisher's exact test to calculate $P$ values for $2 \times 2$ tables. Where significant, data were expressed as $P$ value, odds ratios (OR) with exact 95% confidence intervals (CI).

## 3. Results

The observed allele and genotype frequencies of the IL-1RN VNTR polymorphism among the patients with DM, SLE, and the healthy controls are summarized in Table 2.

Only three alleles were detected among the Bulgarian population: 1 (four repeats), 2 (two repeats), and 3 (five repeats). The IL-1RN*2 allele ($P = 0.02$, OR 2.5, and 95% CI 1.2–5.4) and the 12 + 22 genotypes ($P = 0.05$, OR 2.6, and 95% CI 1–6.3) were found associated with SLE (Table 2).

No association was found between that polymorphism and DM as well as with the clinical manifestations of the two diseases (Table 3).

## 4. Discussion

The majority of the studies relating IL-1RN gene polymorphisms to disease susceptibility have dealt with patients with autoimmune diseases or disorders associated with chronic inflammation [13].

TABLE 2: Genotype and allele frequencies of the IL-1RN VNTR polymorphism among patients with DM, SLE, and controls.

| Genotype N: number of patients | DM N = 36 | SLE N = 55 | Controls N = 112 |
|---|---|---|---|
| Genotypes | | | |
| 1/1 | 33 (91.7%) | 41 (74.6%) | 96 (85.7%) |
| 1/2 | 0 (0.0%) | 8 (14.5%) | 9 (8.0%) |
| 2/2 | 1 (2.8%) | 4 (7.3%) | 2 (1.8%) |
| 1/3 | 2 (5.6) | 1 (1.8%) | 4 (3.6%) |
| 2/3 | 0 (0.0%) | 0 (0.0%) | 1 (0.9%) |
| 3/3 | 0 (0.0%) | 1 (1.8%) | 0 (0.0%) |
| P value | NS* | **12 + 22, P = 0.05** | |
| Alleles | | | |
| 1 | 68 (94.4%) | 91 (82.7%) | 205 (91.5%) |
| 2 | 2 (2.8%) | 16 (14.6%) | 14 (6.3%) |
| 3 | 2 (2.8%) | 3 (2.7%) | 5 (2.2%) |
| P value | NS | **2, P = 0.02** | |

*NS: not significant.

TABLE 3: Comparison between the genotypes and the ACR criteria for SLE.

| Genotype | 1/1 (n = 41) | 1/2 (n = 8) | 2/2 (n = 4) | 1/3 (n = 1) | 3/3 (n = 1) | P value |
|---|---|---|---|---|---|---|
| Malar rash | 28 (68.3%) | 4 (50.0%) | 2 (50.0%) | 0 (0.0%) | 0 (0.0%) | NS* |
| Discoid rash | 7 (17.1%) | 3 (37.5%) | 1 (25.0%) | 0 (0.0%) | 0 (0.0%) | NS |
| Photosensitivity | 23 (57.1%) | 5 (61.5%) | 2 (50.0%) | 1 (100.0%) | 0 (0.0%) | NS |
| Oral ulcer | 3 (7.3%) | 1 (12.5%) | 0 (0.0%) | 0 (0.0%) | 0 (0.0%) | NS |
| Arthritis | 29 (70.7%) | 5 (62.5%) | 2 (50.0%) | 0 (0.0%) | 1 (100.0%) | NS |
| Serositis | 10 (24.4%) | 1 (12.5%) | 0 (0.0%) | 0 (0.0%) | 0 (0.0%) | NS |
| Renal disease | 41 (100.0%) | 8 (100.0%) | 4 (100.0%) | 1 (100.0%) | 1 (100.0%) | NS |
| Neurological disease | 10 (22.9%) | 1 (12.5%) | 0 (0.0%) | 0 (0.0%) | 1 (100.0%) | NS |
| Haematological disease | 15 (36.6%) | 4 (50.0%) | 1 (25.0%) | 0 (0.0%) | 0 (0.0%) | NS |
| Immunological disease (Anti-dsDNA, anti-Sm, anti-phospholipid Ab) | 24 (58.3%) | 5 (62.5%) | 3 (75.0%) | 1 (100.0%) | 1 (100.0%) | NS |
| ANA | 29 (70.7%) | 7 (87.5%) | 2 (50.0%) | 0 (0.0%) | 1 (100.0%) | NS |

*Not significant, anti-dsDNA: antibodies to the double stranded DNA, anti-SM: anti-Smith antibodies (specific markers for SLE), and ANA: antinuclear antibodies.

The first study to correlate this polymorphism with SLE susceptibility was done on Caucasians and the carriage of IL-1RN*2 allele was reported to be associated with severity rather than susceptibility to SLE [14]. The association strengthened with extensive disease and particularly with the presence of photosensitivity and discoid skin lesions. The association of the IL1-RN*2 allele with SLE was confirmed for Japanese patients and it was again increased with photosensitivity [15]. Similarly, increased frequencies of malar rash and photosensitivity were observed among patients with IL1-RN*2 compared to patients without the allele [16]. In our study we have not observed any association between that polymorphism and ACR criteria. However, we have observed a higher frequency of the IL-1RN*2 allele and 1/2 + 2/2 genotype in patients with SLE which is in line with the results of most of the previous studies [14–18]. Our results correlate well with the results of a recent meta-analysis [19].

In Malaysia, however, the risk allele associated with SLE susceptibility was IL-1RN*1 [20] while other authors could not find any association between that polymorphism and SLE [21–23]. Quite surprisingly Mohammadoo-Khorasani et al. [24] found an association between the IL-1RN*4 allele and the 1RN* 1/4 genotype and the development of SLE in Iranian cohort. Such discrepancies could be attributed to interethnic variations [25], low frequency of the IL-1RN*2 allele, small sample size which lacks statistical power, or influence of other polymorphisms. Furthermore, it was shown that IL-1RA 2/2 was not individually associated with SLE but the combination of the FcγRIIa R/R and IL-1RN 2/2 genotypes is associated with SLE in Caucasian patients [26]. The studies concerning the polymorphisms in the IL-1RN gene could have practical aspects since they might affect the response towards Anakinra, which is a recombinant form of human IL-1RA [27].

The frequency of the IL-1RN*2 allele was low among the DM patients and no statistically significant associations were found in allele and genotype distribution. Our results correlate with the results of other authors [8]. Interestingly Rider et al. [28] have found the IL-1RN*1 allele being associated with juvenile idiopathic inflammatory myopathies (JIIM) in Caucasians, while the IL-1RN*3 allele was associated with JIIM in African-Americans.

In summary, our results indicate that IL-1RN VNTR polymorphism might play a role in the susceptibility of SLE but not DM in Bulgarian patients.

## Conflict of Interests

The authors state no conflict of interests.

## Acknowledgments

The genetic analysis was performed at the Molecular Medicine Center, Medical University, Sofia, supported by an infrastructure Grant DUNK01-2/2009 by the National Science Fund, Ministry of Education, Youth and Science.

## References

[1] J. J. O'Shea, A. Ma, and P. Lipsky, "Cytokines and autoimmunity," *Nature Reviews Immunology*, vol. 2, no. 1, pp. 37–45, 2002.

[2] J. K. Tarlow, A. I. F. Blakemore, A. Lennard et al., "Polymorphism in human IL-1 receptor antagonist gene intron 2 is caused by variable numbers of an 86-bp tandem repeat," *Human Genetics*, vol. 91, no. 4, pp. 403–404, 1993.

[3] M. Dale and M. J. H. Nicklin, "Interleukin-1 receptor cluster: gene organization of IL1R2, IL1R1 IL1RL2 (IL-1Rrp2), IL1RL1 (T1/ST2), and IL18R1 (IL-1Rrp) on human chromosome 2q," *Genomics*, vol. 57, no. 1, pp. 177–179, 1999.

[4] D. M. Chang, "Interleukin-1 and interleukin-1 receptor antagonist in systemic lupus erythematosus," *Immunological Investigations*, vol. 26, no. 5-7, pp. 649–659, 1997.

[5] G. S. Baird and T. J. Montine, "Multiplex immunoassay analysis of cytokines in idiopathic inflammatory myopathy," *Archives of Pathology & Laboratory Medicine*, vol. 132, no. 2, pp. 232–238, 2008.

[6] C. Gabay, F. Gay-Croisier, P. Roux-Lombard et al., "Elevated serum levels of interleukin-1 receptor antagonist in polymyositis/dermatomyositis: a biologic marker of disease activity with a possible role in the lack of acute-phase protein response," *Arthritis and Rheumatism*, vol. 37, no. 12, pp. 1744–1751, 1994.

[7] B. Brugos, E. Kiss, C. Dul et al., "Measurement of interleukin-1 receptor antagonist in patients with systemic lupus erythematosus could predict renal manifestation of the disease," *Human Immunology*, vol. 71, no. 9, pp. 874–877, 2010.

[8] K. Son, Y. Tomita, T. Shimizu, S. Nishinarita, S. Sawada, and T. Horie, "Abnormal IL-1 receptor antagonist production in patients with polymyositis and dermatomyositis," *Internal Medicine*, vol. 39, no. 2, pp. 128–135, 2000.

[9] A. M. Prieur, A. Dayer, P. Roux-Lombard, and J. M. Dayer, "Levels of cytokine inhibitors: a possible marker of disease activity in childhood dermatomyositis and polymyositis," *Clinical and Experimental Rheumatology*, vol. 15, no. 2, pp. 211–214, 1997.

[10] A. Bohan and J. B. Peter, "Polymyositis and dermatomyositis," *The New England Journal of Medicine*, vol. 292, no. 7, pp. 344–347, 1975.

[11] A. Bohan and J. B. Peter, "Polymyositis and dermatomyositis II," *The New England Journal of Medicine*, vol. 292, no. 8, pp. 403–407, 1975.

[12] I. N. Targoff, F. W. Miller, T. A. Medsger Jr., and C. V. Oddis, "Classification criteria for the idiopathic inflammatory myopathies," *Current Opinion in Rheumatology*, vol. 9, no. 6, pp. 527–535, 1997.

[13] S. S. Witkin, S. Gerber, and W. J. Ledger, "Influence of interleukin-1 receptor antagonist gene polymorphism on disease," *Clinical Infectious Diseases*, vol. 34, no. 2, pp. 204–209, 2002.

[14] A. I. F. Blakemore, J. K. Tarlow, M. J. Cork, C. Gordon, P. Emery, and G. W. Duff, "Interleukin-1 receptor antagonist gene polymorphism as a disease severity factor in systemic lupus erythematosus," *Arthritis and Rheumatism*, vol. 37, no. 9, pp. 1380–1385, 1994.

[15] H. Suzuki, Y. Matsui, and H. Kashiwagi, "Interleukin-1 receptor antagonist gene polymorphism in Japanese patients with systemic lupus erythematosus," *Arthritis & Rheumatism*, vol. 40, no. 2, pp. 389–390, 1997.

[16] C.-M. Huang, M.-C. Wu, J.-Y. Wu, and F.-J. Tsai, "Interleukin-1 receptor antagonist gene polymorphism in Chinese patients with systemic lupus erythematosus," *Clinical Rheumatology*, vol. 21, no. 3, pp. 255–257, 2002.

[17] C. G. Parks, G. S. Cooper, M. A. Dooley et al., "Systemic lupus erythematosus and genetic variation in the interleukin 1 gene cluster: a population based study in the southeastern United States," *Annals of the Rheumatic Diseases*, vol. 63, no. 1, pp. 91–94, 2004.

[18] F. Tjernström, G. Hellmer, O. Nived, L. Truedsson, and G. Sturfelt, "Synergetic effect between interleukin-1 receptor antagonist allele (IL1RN*2) and MHC class II (DR17,DQ2) in determining susceptibility to systemic lupus erythematosus," *Lupus*, vol. 8, no. 2, pp. 103–108, 1999.

[19] G. G. Song, J. H. Kim, Y. H. Seo, S. J. Choi, J. D. Ji, and Y. H. Lee, "Associations between interleukin 1 polymorphisms and susceptibility to systemic lupus erythematosus: a meta-analysis," *Human Immunology*, vol. 75, no. 1, pp. 105–112, 2014.

[20] T. P. Lau, L. H. Lian, S. Y. Tan, and K. H. Chua, "VNTR polymorphisms of the IF-1RN gene: IL-1RN*1 allele and the susceptibility of SLE in the Malaysian population," *International Journal of Biomedical and Pharmaceutical Sciences*, vol. 2, no. 1, pp. 32–37, 2009.

[21] J. Heward, A. Allahabadia, C. Gordon et al., "The interleukin-1 receptor antagonist gene shows no allelic association with three autoimmune diseases," *Thyroid*, vol. 9, no. 6, pp. 627–628, 1999.

[22] S. D'Alfonso, M. Rampi, D. Bocchio, G. Colombo, R. Scorza-Smeraldi, and P. Momigliano-Richardi, "Systemic lupus erythematosus candidate genes in the Italian population: evidence for a significant association with interleukin-10," *Arthritis & Rheumatism*, vol. 43, no. 1, pp. 120–128, 2000.

[23] V. A. Danis, M. Millington, Q. Huang, V. Hyland, and D. Grennan, "Lack of association between an interleukin-1 receptor antagonist gene polymorphism and systemic lupus erythematosus," *Disease Markers*, vol. 12, no. 2, pp. 135–139, 1995.

[24] M. Mohammadoo-Khorasani, S. Salimi, E. Tabatabai, M. Sandoughi, and Z. Zakeri, "Association of interleukin-1 receptor antagonist gene 86bp VNTR polymorphism with systemic

lupus erythematosus in south east of Iran," *Zahedan Journal of Research in Medical Sciences*, vol. 16, no. 12, pp. 51–54, 2014.

[25] P. K. Manchanda, H. K. Bid, and R. D. Mittal, "Ethnicity greatly influences the interleukin-1 gene cluster(IL-1b promoter, exon-5 and IL-1Ra) polymorphisms: a pilot study of a north Indian population," *Asian Pacific Journal of Cancer Prevention*, vol. 6, no. 4, pp. 541–546, 2005.

[26] A. Jönsen, A. A. Bengtsson, G. Sturfelt, and L. Truedsson, "Analysis of HLA DR, HLA DQ, C4A, FcgammaRIIa, FcgammaRIIIa, MBL, and IL-1Ra allelic variants in Caucasian systemic lupus erythematosus patients suggests an effect of the combined FcgammaRIIa R/R and IL-1Ra 2/2 genotypes on disease susceptibility," *Arthritis research & therapy.*, vol. 6, no. 6, pp. R557–562, 2004.

[27] N. J. Camp, A. Cox, F. S. di Giovine, D. McCabe, W. Rich, and G. W. Duff, "Evidence of a pharmacogenomic response to interleukin-1 receptor antagonist in rheumatoid arthritis," *Genes and Immunity*, vol. 6, no. 6, pp. 467–471, 2005.

[28] L. G. Rider, C. M. Artlett, C. B. Foster et al., "Polymorphisms in the IL-1 receptor antagonist gene VNTR are possible risk factors for juvenile idiopathic inflammatory myopathies," *Clinical & Experimental Immunology*, vol. 121, no. 1, pp. 47–52, 2000.

# 29

# Superpulsed $CO_2$ Laser with Intraoperative Pathologic Assessment for Treatment of Periorbital Basal Cell Carcinoma Involving Eyelash Line

**Ali Ebrahimi,**[1] **Mansour Rezaei,**[2] **Reza Kavoussi,**[1] **Mojtaba Eidizadeh,**[1] **Seyed Hamid Madani,**[1] **and Hossein Kavoussi**[1,3]

[1] *Kermanshah University of Medical Sciences (KUMS), Kermanshah, Iran*
[2] *Health School, Family Health Research Center of Kermanshah University of Medical Sciences (KUMS), Kermanshah, Iran*
[3] *Hajdaie Dermatology Clinic, Golestan Ave, Kermanshah 6714653113, Iran*

Correspondence should be addressed to Hossein Kavoussi; hkawosi@kums.ac.ir

Academic Editor: Elizabeth Helen Kemp

*Background.* Periorbital basal cell carcinoma (BCC) is considered a high risk case because it is associated with high rate of recurrence and complication. Superpulsed $CO_2$ laser with intraoperative pathologic assessment could be an alternative and appropriate treatment for periocular lesions where Mohs micrographic surgery is not available. *Objective.* To evaluate the efficacy of superpulsed $CO_2$ laser therapy with intraoperative pathologic assessment on periocular BCC involving eyelash line. *Method.* This follow-up study was performed on 20 patients with a total of 21 BCC lesions that were pathologically documented. Firstly, debulkation of tumoral mass was done by curettage. Then, irradiation and intraoperative pathologic evaluation were done by concurrent $CO_2$ laser. The patients were followed up for a period of 36 months. *Results.* Out of 21 lesions, the nodular type accounted for 15 (71.4%) lesions, and 12 (57.1%) lesions were seen in the lower lid as the most common clinical type and site involvement. Twenty BCC lesions (95.2%) were treated after one session. Damage to eyelash was seen in 2 (10%) patients, but ectropion and other complications were not seen in any patient. *Conclusion.* Treatment with superpulsed $CO_2$ laser and intraoperative pathologic evaluation for periorbital BCC lesions much close to conjunctiva could be an effective method with minimal complications without major danger of recurrence. This modality can be used with care in the inner canthus and high risk pathologic lesions.

## 1. Introduction

Although basal cell carcinoma (BCC) is the most common malignant tumor of periorbital area, it rarely results in death [1–3].

BCC is associated with disfiguration and very high cost especially in large lesion, recurrent forms, aggressive pathologic subtype, poorly defined tumor, immunosuppression, and high risk locations such as periorbital region [1, 4, 5].

The periorbital BCC is the most common cause of orbital exenteration, especially in recurrent BCCs, infiltrative pathologic subtype, and medial canthal lesions [6].

Several optional treatments have been suggested for periorbital BCC such as chemotherapy [7, 8], traditional surgical excision [9–11], photodynamic therapy [12, 13], Mohs micrographic surgery [14–16], and laser ablation [17–20].

The use of superpulsed mode of $CO_2$ laser compared with its traditional one results in precise destruction of lesion with minimum damage to the normal surrounding tissue due to minimal thermal diffusion; therefore, it is associated with low risk of hypertrophic or atrophic scar [21].

This study was carried out to evaluate the treatment outcome and complications of the superpulsed mode $CO_2$

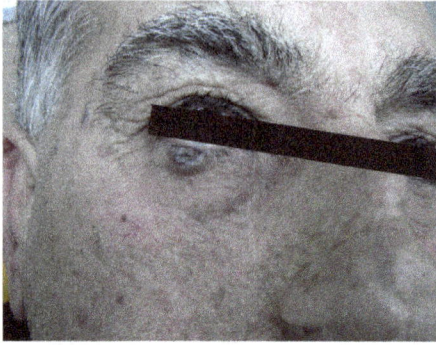

FIGURE 1: A man with 2 BCC lesions in lower lid.

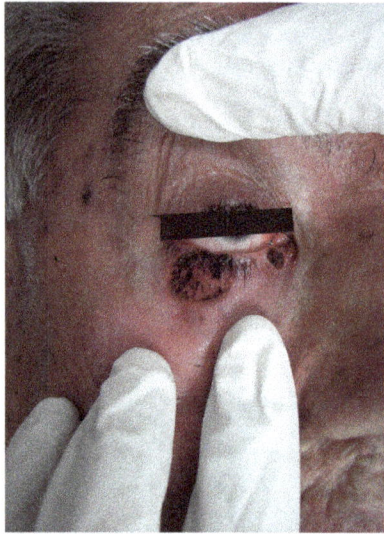

FIGURE 3: Shave sample of induced defect after $CO_2$ laser indicates presence of malignant cells (H&E stain ×100).

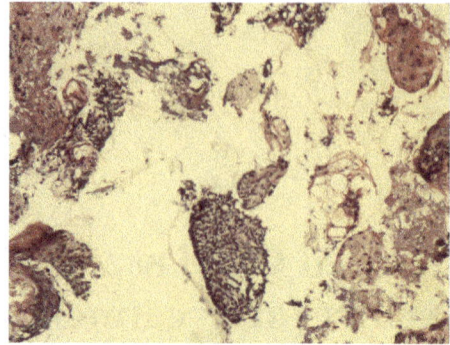

FIGURE 2: Induced defects after laser therapy.

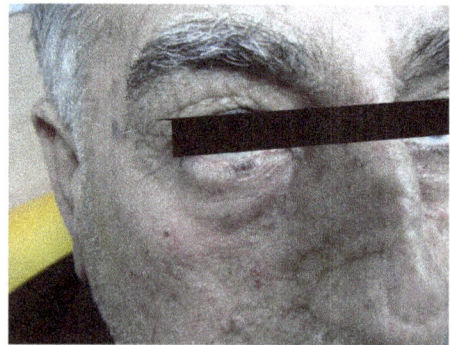

FIGURE 4: Six months after laser treatment.

laser with concomitant pathologic assessment of periorbital BCC treatment.

## 2. Methods

This clinical follow-up study was carried out on 20 patients at Hajdaie Dermatology Clinic of Kermanshah University of Medical Sciences in Iran over a period of 48 months from 2007 to 2012. Biopsy was done in the patients that were clinically suspected of periorbital BCC extended to eyelash line. The patients with histopathologically documented BCC were enrolled in our study. Patients were given information about this procedure and asked for their consent. We consulted with ophthalmologist about any ocular problems and existence of any contraindication in the patients. The exclusion criteria included lesions with a diameter larger than 2 cm, pregnancy, patients younger than 30 years old, recurrence after excision, wide extension to conjunctiva, morphoeic form, immunosuppression, keloid former, and any orbital contraindication for laser therapy.

We delineated 3 mm of normal appearing marginal skin around the BCC and this region was anesthetized with an injection of lidocaine 2% with or without epinephrine

1/100000, if there was no contraindication of epinephrine. The tumoral mass of BCC was removed by a very sharp curettage that resulted in an even defect. We treated the induced defect and marginal skin by 4 passes of superpulsed $CO_2$ laser with appropriate eye protection. We selected the following laser therapy parameters (12-watt power and 600–800-microsecond pulse duration), and between laser passes the char was wiped away with saline-soaked gauze (Figures 1 and 2).

In the end of procedure, the histopathological sample was obtained by a very sharp curettage from the base and margin of the treated site. In the presence of any malignant cells (Figure 3), retreatment was done by $CO_2$ laser. This cycle of laser therapy and histopathology evaluation was performed until no malignant cells were seen.

Postoperative care included washing with normal saline and dressing with tetracycline ophthalmic ointment for 7–10 days. The induced defect was repaired by secondary intention (Figure 4).

This study was approved by the Ethics Committee of Kermanshah University of Medical Sciences and registered in the IRCT database (IRCT201404036403N4).

Analysis of data was carried out using the SPSS software version 16. Analysis of qualitative data was done by Chi-square and Fisher's exact test, and KS test was used for analysis of quantitative data. Levene's and the independent sample $t$-test were also used for comparison of variance and the means.

TABLE 1: Characteristics of patients.

| Variables | Number |
|---|---|
| Number of patients | 20 |
| Sex of patients | |
| Female | 7 |
| Male | 13 |
| Number of lesions | 21 |
| Mean of age | 61.43 |
| Mean of size | 10.62 |

## 3. Results

Our study recruited 20 patients (7 females and 13 males) with 21 lesions. The age range of participants was between 42 and 80 with mean age of 61.43. The mean size of lesions was 10.62 mm (ranged between 5 and 20 mm) (Table 1).

The lesions were located in lower lid, inner canthus, upper lid, and outer canthus 12 (57.1%), 7 (33.3%), 1 (4.8%), and 1 (4.8%), respectively (Table 2).

The most common clinical and histopathological forms were nodular and solid.

The cure rate was observed in 20 (95.2%) lesions and recurrent rate was seen in 1 (4.8%) lesion in the follow-up period (Table 2).

Because there was 1 recurrence, it was not possible to run statistical test between recurrence and other variables.

Recurrence was seen in a 75-year-old male patient with nodular clinical lesion and infiltrative pathology with 20 mm diameter at inner canthus.

Damage to eyelash was seen in 2 (10%) cases, but other complications such as ectropion, trichiasis, atrophic and hypertrophic scar, and damage to eye structure were not seen in any patient (Table 2).

## 4. Discussion

Superpulsed $CO_2$ laser with intraoperative histopathological evaluation is a highly appropriate modality for the treatment of periorbital BCC with high cure rate (95.2%) and low complication rate during 36 months of follow-up period.

The aim of periorbital BCC treatment is eradication of the tumor to prevent local recurrence, good aesthetic outcome, and preservation of lid function without any injury to eye structure [9].

The best treatment for BCC is Mohs micrographic surgery, a method of tumor removal with histologic margin control for residual malignant cells, which is superior to other treatments. However, it is expensive and time consuming and requires skilled surgical and pathological team [14–16]; it is also not generally available in most areas of the world including Iran.

Determination of BCC pathologic subtype in order to appropriate treatment is very important [22].

High recurrence rate of BCC in eyelid area must be expected according to histopathological type [23].

Cystic and nodular histopathologic subtypes of BCC are relatively well defined margin, but morphoeic, micronodular,

TABLE 2: Characteristics of lesion, outcome, and complication of treatment.

| Variables | Frequency | Percent |
|---|---|---|
| Clinical type | | |
| Nodular | 15 | 71.4 |
| Pigmented | 5 | 23.8 |
| Superficial | 1 | 4.8 |
| Histopathologic subtype | | |
| Solid | 15 | 71.4% |
| Cystic | 2 | 9.5% |
| Superficial | 1 | 4.8% |
| Infiltrative | 1 | 4.8% |
| Micronodular | 1 | 4.8% |
| Basosquamous | 1 | 4.8% |
| Location of treatment | | |
| Lower lids | 12 | 57.1 |
| Medial canthal | 7 | 33.3 |
| Lateral canthal | 1 | 4.8 |
| Upper lids | 1 | 4.8 |
| Outcome | | |
| Cure | 20 | 95.2 |
| Recurrence | 1 | 4.8 |
| Complication | | |
| Damage to eyelash | 2 | 9.5 |
| Atrophic and hypertrophic scars | 0 | 0 |
| Ectropion | 0 | 0 |

infiltrative, and basosquamous BCCs have frequently ill-defined margin and are considered as high risk or aggressive histopathologic subtypes [5].

Traditional and new versions of $CO_2$ laser were used for treatment of BCC on the head and neck and other sites of body [17–21, 24–29], but Bandieramonte et al. [17] reported the use of $CO_2$ laser microsurgery in the treatment of 26 superficial BCC tumors combined with intraoperatory histopathological examination. They concluded that $CO_2$ laser microsurgery appears to be the most effective treatment method only for primary superficial BCC of the eyelid margins without any complication.

Humphreys et al. [26] used pulsed $CO_2$ laser for the treatment of primary superficial BCC and concluded that ultrapulse $CO_2$ laser is the most favorable treatment for superficial BCC.

Campolmi et al. [27] treated 140 patients with superficial and nodular BCC by superpulsed $CO_2$ laser. In the end of laser therapy, the bed of the treated site was excised for histopathological examination. This technique, in addition to clinical efficacy for superficial BCC, is associated with minimal thermal damage to the surrounding tissue and permits intraoperative histopathological evaluation.

Multiple passes of pulsed mode $CO_2$ laser combined with intraoperatory histopathological examination have been used for the treatment of 21 superficial, 28 nodular, and 2 infiltrative BCC tumors, but laser ablation is a reliable method for patients with multiple superficial BCCs [28].

Previous studies have treated special clinical and histopathological types of BCC mostly on the trunk by $CO_2$ laser, but we treated various clinical (nodular, superficial, and pigmented) and histopathological types of BCC on the periorbital area that involved eyelash line by superpulsed $CO_2$ laser.

We performed concurrent histopathological study for complete removal of malignant cells and prevention of local recurrence as well as preservation of marginal normal tissue and consequently prevention of complications such as ectropion.

The anatomic distortion and scar induced following incomplete excision and repair of primary BCC obscure the malignant cells, which leads to recurrence and identification of tumor margin becomes more difficult [30, 31].

One of the main advantages of this form of therapy in contrast to surgical excision is that it induces no anatomic distortion. Therefore, any remaining malignant cells during laser therapy do not result in irregular growth of malignant cells; it even results in easy and early detection and extent of tumor [20].

BCC on the periorbital area not only is considered a high risk tumor [1–5] but also is associated with a number of complications such as ectropion, trichiasis, and damage to eyelash after surgical excision [32, 33].

In our method, the recurrence rate was reported in 1 (4.8%) lesion, which occurred in a BCC on the medial canthal lesion, infiltrative histopathological subtype with 20 mm diameter.

Damage to eyelash was seen in 2 (10%) patients, one in the lower lid with infiltrative pathologic subtype and another in medial canthal BCC, both of which had a diameter more than 10 mm. Therefore, patients need to be informed about the probability of eyelash damage in periorbital BCC with high risk infiltrative pathologic subtype and diameter more than 10 mm.

## 5. Conclusion

Our study indicated recurrence occurring in one case of nodular clinical type with 20 mm diameter and infiltrative histopathological subtype in the medial canthal lesion. Therefore, this method is an appropriate modality for small, other than inner canthal region, and nonhigh risk histopathological subtype but should be used with caution for large and high risk histopathological subtype in the medial canthal region.

## Conflict of Interests

The authors declare that there is no conflict of interests regarding the publication of this paper.

## Acknowledgment

The authors thank the patient for agreeing to publish his photo in the paper.

## References

[1] A. G. Quinn and W. Perkins, "Non-melanoma skin cancers and other epithermal skin tumor," in *Rooks Textbook of Dermatology*, T. Burns, S. Breathnach, N. Cox, and C. Griffiths, Eds., vol. 3, pp. 1–3, Wiley-Blackwell, Oxford, UK, 8th edition, 2010.

[2] J. Salomon, A. Bieniek, E. Baran, and J. C. Szepietowski, "Basal cell carcinoma on the eyelids: own experience," *Dermatologic Surgery*, vol. 30, no. 2, part 2, pp. 257–263, 2004.

[3] B. E. Cook Jr. and G. B. Bartley, "Epidemiologic characteristics and clinical course of patients with malignant eyelid tumors in an incidence cohort in Olmsted County, Minnesota," *Ophthalmology*, vol. 106, no. 4, pp. 746–750, 1999.

[4] F. Urbach, "Incidence of nonmelanoma skin cancer," *Dermatologic Clinics*, vol. 9, no. 4, pp. 751–755, 1991.

[5] V. Smith and S. Walton, "Treatment of facial basal cell carcinoma: a review," *Journal of Skin Cancer*, vol. 2011, Article ID 380371, 7 pages, 2011.

[6] A. Iuliano, D. Strianese, G. Uccello, A. Diplomatico, S. Tebaldi, and G. Bonavolont, "Risk factors for orbital exenteration in periocular basal cell carcinoma," *The American Journal of Ophthalmology*, vol. 153, no. 2, pp. 238.e1–241.e1, 2012.

[7] M. N. Luxenberg and T. H. Guthrie Jr., "Chemotherapy of basal cell and squamous cell carcinoma of the eyelids and periorbital tissues," *Ophthalmology*, vol. 93, no. 4, pp. 504–510, 1986.

[8] M. N. Luxenberg and T. H. Guthrie Jr., "Chemotherapy of eyelid and periorbital tumors," *Transactions of the American Ophthalmological Society*, vol. 83, pp. 162–180, 1985.

[9] S. Hamada, T. Kersey, and V. T. Thaller, "Eyelid basal cell carcinoma: non-Mohs excision, repair, and outcome," *British Journal of Ophthalmology*, vol. 89, no. 8, pp. 992–994, 2005.

[10] D. B. David, M. L. Gimblett, M. J. Potts, and R. A. Harrad, "Small margin (2 mm) excision of peri-ocular basal cell carcinoma with delayed repair," *Orbit*, vol. 18, no. 1, pp. 11–15, 1999.

[11] N. Kakudo, Y. Ogawa, K. Suzuki, S. Kushida, and K. Kusumoto, "Clinical outcome of surgical treatment for periorbital basal cell carcinoma," *Annals of Plastic Surgery*, vol. 63, no. 5, pp. 531–535, 2009.

[12] C. Hintschich, J. Feyh, C. Beyer-Machule, K. Riedel, and K. Ludwig, "Photodynamic laser therapy of basal-cell carcinoma of the lid," *German Journal of Ophthalmology*, vol. 2, no. 4-5, pp. 212–217, 1993.

[13] B. D. Wilson, T. S. Mang, H. Stoll, C. Jones, M. Cooper, and T. J. Dougherty, "Photodynamic therapy for the treatment of basal cell carcinoma," *Archives of Dermatology*, vol. 128, no. 12, pp. 1597–1601, 1992.

[14] L. Kvannli, R. Benger, A. Gal, and B. Swamy, "The method of en face Frozen section in clearing periocular basal cell carcinoma and squamous cell carcinoma," *Orbit*, vol. 31, no. 4, pp. 233–237, 2012.

[15] R. Malhotra, S. C. Huilgol, N. T. Huynh, and D. Selva, "The Australian Mohs database, part I: periocular basal cell carcinoma experience over 7 years," *Ophthalmology*, vol. 111, no. 4, pp. 624–630, 2004.

[16] G. Lindgren, B. Lindblom, and O. Larkö, "Moh's micrographic surgery for basal cell carcinomas on the eyelids and medial canthal area. II. Reconstruction and follow-up," *Acta Ophthalmologica Scandinavica*, vol. 78, no. 4, pp. 430–436, 2000.

[17] G. Bandieramonte, P. Lepera, D. Moglia, A. Bono, C. de Vecchi, and F. Milani, "Laser microsurgery for superficial T1-T2 basal cell carcinoma of the eyelid margins," *Ophthalmology*, vol. 104, no. 7, pp. 1179–1184, 1997.

[18] J. D. Hsuan, R. A. Harrad, M. J. Potts, and C. Collins, "Small margin excision of periocular basal cell carcinoma: 5 year results," *British Journal of Ophthalmology*, vol. 88, no. 3, pp. 358–360, 2004.

[19] A. P. Murchison, J. D. Walrath, and C. V. Washington, "Non-surgical treatments of primary, non-melanoma eyelid malignancies: a review," *Clinical and Experimental Ophthalmology*, vol. 39, no. 1, pp. 65–83, 2011.

[20] H. Kavoussi, A. Ebrahimi, and M. Rezaei, "Treatment and cosmetic outcome of superpulsed $CO_2$ laser for basal cell carcinoma," *Acta Dermatovenerologica Alpina, Pannonica et Adriatica*, vol. 22, no. 3, pp. 57–61, 2013.

[21] E. R. Hobbs, P. L. Bailin, R. G. Wheeland, and J. L. Ratz, "Super-pulsed lasers: minimizing thermal damage with short duration, high irradiance pulses," *Journal of Dermatologic Surgery and Oncology*, vol. 13, no. 9, pp. 955–964, 1987.

[22] M. P. Szewczyk, J. Pazdrowski, A. Dańczak-Pazdrowska et al., "Analysis of selected recurrence risk factors after treatment of head and neck basal cell carcinoma," *Postępy Dermatologii i Alergologii*, vol. 31, no. 3, pp. 146–151, 2014.

[23] C.-J. Wang, H.-N. Zhang, H. Wu et al., "Clinicopathologic features and prognostic factors of malignant eyelid tumors," *International Journal of Ophthalmology*, vol. 6, no. 4, pp. 442–447, 2013.

[24] R. G. Wheeland, P. L. Bailin, J. L. Ratz, and R. K. Roenigk, "Carbon dioxide laser vaporization and curettage in the treatment of large or multiple superficial basal cell carcinomas," *Journal of Dermatologic Surgery and Oncology*, vol. 13, no. 2, pp. 119–125, 1987.

[25] M. Landthaler, R. M. Szeimies, and U. Hohenleutner, "Laser therapy of skin tumors," *Recent Results in Cancer Research*, vol. 139, pp. 417–421, 1995.

[26] T. R. Humphreys, R. Malhotra, M. J. Scharf, S. M. Marcus, L. Starkus, and K. Calegari, "Treatment of superficial basal cell carcinoma and squamous cell carcinoma in situ with a high-energy pulsed carbon dioxide laser," *Archives of Dermatology*, vol. 134, no. 10, pp. 1247–1252, 1998.

[27] P. Campolmi, B. Brazzini, C. Urso et al., "Superpulsed $CO_2$ laser treatment of basal cell carcinoma with intraoperatory histopathologic and cytologic examination," *Dermatologic Surgery*, vol. 28, no. 10, pp. 909–912, 2002.

[28] N. Horlock, A. O. Grobbelaar, and D. T. Gault, "Can the carbon dioxide laser completely ablate basal cell carcinomas? A histological study," *The British Journal of Plastic Surgery*, vol. 53, no. 4, pp. 286–293, 2000.

[29] S. Iyer, L. Bowes, G. Kricorian, A. Friedli, and R. E. Fitzpatrick, "Treatment of basal cell carcinoma with the pulsed carbon dioxide laser: a retrospective analysis," *Dermatologic Surgery*, vol. 30, no. 9, pp. 1214–1218, 2004.

[30] K. Mosterd, M. R. T. M. Thissen, A. M. W. van Marion et al., "Correlation between histologic findings on punch biopsy specimens and subsequent excision specimens in recurrent basal cell carcinoma," *Journal of the American Academy of Dermatology*, vol. 64, no. 2, pp. 323–337, 2011.

[31] R. S. Batra and L. C. Kelley, "Predictors of extensive subclinical spread in nonmelanoma skin cancer treated with Mohs micrographic surgery," *Archives of Dermatology*, vol. 138, no. 8, pp. 1043–1051, 2002.

[32] S. N. Stafanous, "The switch flap in eyelid reconstruction," *Orbit*, vol. 26, no. 4, pp. 255–262, 2007.

[33] G. Santos and J. Goulão, "One-stage reconstruction of full-thickness lower eyelid using a Tripier flap lining by a septal mucochondral graft," *Journal of Dermatological Treatment*, vol. 25, no. 5, pp. 446–447, 2014.

# 30

# Different Trichoscopic Features of Tinea Capitis and Alopecia Areata in Pediatric Patients

**Abd-Elaziz El-Taweel, Fatma El-Esawy, and Osama Abdel-Salam**

*Dermatology & Andrology Department, Faculty of Medicine, Benha University, Benha, Al Qalyubia 13512, Egypt*

Correspondence should be addressed to Osama Abdel-Salam; oselfady452003@yahoo.com

Academic Editor: Giuseppe Argenziano

*Background.* Diagnosis of patchy hair loss in pediatric patients is often a matter of considerable debate among dermatologists. Trichoscopy is a rapid and noninvasive tool to detect more details of patchy hair loss. Like clinical dermatology, trichoscopy works parallel to the skin surface and perpendicular to the histological plane; like the histopathology, it thus allows the viewing of structures not discovered by the naked eye. *Objective.* Aiming to compare the different trichoscopic features of tinea capitis and alopecia areata in pediatric patients. *Patients and Methods.* This study included 40 patients, 20 patients with tinea capitis and 20 patients with alopecia areata. They were exposed toclinical examination, laboratory investigations (10% KOH and fungal culture), and trichoscope examination. *Results.* Our obtained results reported that, in tinea capitis patients, comma shaped hairs, corkscrew hairs, and zigzag shaped hairs are the diagnostic trichoscopic features of tinea capitis. While in alopecia areata patients, the most trichoscopic specific features were yellow dots, exclamation mark, and short vellus hairs. *Conclusion.* Trichoscopy can be used as a noninvasive tool for rapid diagnosis of tinea capitis and alopecia areata in pediatric patients.

## 1. Introduction

Losing hair is not usually health threatening; it can scar a young child's vulnerable self-esteem by causing immense psychological and emotional stress, not only to the patient, but also to the concerned parents and siblings [1]; so the cause of hair loss should be diagnosed and treated early to overcome the resulting problems [2]. The most frequent causes of hair loss in pediatric patients include tinea capitis, alopecia areata, traction alopecia, and trichotillomania. The clinician must be able to separate the types and causes of hair loss into those that reflect primary dermatologic conditions and those that represent reaction to systemic disease [3].

Tinea capitis is a superficial fungal infection of the scalp. The disease is primarily caused by dermatophytes in the *Trichophyton* and *Microsporum* genera that invade the hair shaft. The clinical presentation is typically a single or multiple patches of hair loss, sometimes with a "black dot" pattern, that may be accompanied by inflammation, scaling, pustules, and itching [4]. Alopecia areata (AA) is a medical condition in which hair is lost from some or all areas of the body, usually from the scalp [5]. Typical first symptoms of alopecia areata

are small bald patches; the underlying skin looks superficially normal. These patches can take many shapes but are most usually round or oval [6].

The cause of focal hair loss may be diagnosed by the appearance of the patch and examination for fungal agents. A scalp biopsy may be necessary if the cause of hair loss is unclear [7].

Trichoscopy is a noninvasive diagnostic tool that allows the recognition of morphologic structures not visible by the naked eye. The trichoscope, despite its ease of handling, is not a mere magnifying glass but a more complex instrument, allowing the superimposition of the skin layers. This is entirely different from the image obtained in histopathology, where the visualization is total, with the possibility to observe any surface or deep skin layer [8]. Trichoscopy is useful for the diagnosis and follow-up of hair and scalp disorders. However, it is not widely used in the management of hair disorders. This will enable dermatologists to make fast diagnoses of tinea capitis and alopecia areata, distinguish early androgenetic alopecia from telogen effluvium, and differentiate scarring from nonscarring alopecia [9].

*Aim of Work.* The aim of this work is to detect different trichoscopic features of tinea capitis and alopecia areata in pediatric patients with localized patches of hair loss.

## 2. Patients and Methods

This observational analytical study included forty patients, twenty patients with tinea capitis and twenty patients with alopecia areata, without sex predilection, their age (≤12 years) presented with solitary or multiple lesions of patchy hair loss of the scalp. This study was conducted at Cairo Hospital of Dermatology and Andrology (Al-Haud Al-Marsoud), during the period from October 2012 to March 2013. The *exclusion criteria* were (1) patients with any concomitant dermatological diseases and (2) history of using any topical (1 month) or systemic treatment (3 month) for tinea capitis or alopecia areata prior to the study. *Consent* was taken from a parent of each patient before participation in the study which was approved by Ethics Committee Human Research of Benha University.

All patients were subjected to the following: (1) history taking, clinical examination, and digital photography of any lesion of patchy hair loss by using Panasonic LUMIX S5 16 mega pixel, (2) microscopic examination of skin scraping and plucked hairs using KOH 10% and fungal culture and (3) trichoscopic examination.

*2.1. Laboratory Examination.* The specimen was collected in a sufficient amount from the edge of the area of hair loss (scales or plucked hairs). Hair roots and skin scraping were mounted in 10% potassium hydroxide solution. The slide was gently heated and microscopically examined for spores. The culture was done on Sabouraud's agar media; the cultures were incubated at 30°C and examined frequently for 4 weeks.

*2.2. Trichoscope Examination.* In this study, a hand-held trichoscope (DermLite DL3, Gen, USA) which can block light reflection from the skin surface without immersion gels was used. Characteristics and specifications of the DermLite DL3 trichoscope used in the study were 20x and 40x magnification with focusing optics. It consisted from light emitting diodes (LEDs) bulbs, piece handle and head, and replaceable batteries (rechargeable lithium).

The trichoscope is switched on and placed away from the lesion by about 1 cm or gently over the lesion after covering the lesion with gel, so that it is in the center of the contact plate. The examiner's eyes should be as close as possible to the eyepieces, with the free hand adjusting the focusing ring until a clearly focused image is obtained (in most cases it is only necessary to set up the focus once). Disinfection of the lens with alcohol swab to avoid transmission of infection. Digital photography of the lesion(s) were taken through the DermLite DL3 Gen Trichoscope. Findings obtained were evaluated by the same two dermatologists.

*2.3. Statistical Analysis.* All collected data were revised for completeness and accuracy. Precoded data was entered on the computer using the statistical package of social science software program, version 15 (SPSS), to be statistically analyzed.

## 3. Results

*3.1. Clinical Data.* In alopecia areata patients, the study was carried on 13 female 65% and 7 males 35%. Their age ranged from 1.5–11 years with median ± inter quartile range (IQR) 5.25 (3.3, 8.0). The duration of lesions ranged from 2 to 12 weeks with median ± IQR 4.00 (2.3, 11.0). The number of lesion(s) ranged from 1 to 2 with median ± IQR 1.0 (1.0, 2.0). The size of the lesion(s) ranged from 0.5 to 3 cm with median ± IQR (2.0 ± 0.6 × 1.5 ± 0.7). In tinea capitis patients, the study was carried on 15 male 75.0% and 5 females 15.0%. Their age ranged from 2–11 years with median ± IQR 5.0 (3.5, 7.1), the duration of the lesion(s) ranged from 2 to 12 weeks with median ± IQR 4.00 (2.3, 11.0). The number of lesion(s) ranged from 1 to 2 with median ± IQR 1.0 (1.0, 1.0). The size of the lesion(s) ranged from 1 to 3 cm with median ± IQR (2.1 ± 0.8 × 1.6 ± 0.8).

*3.2. Laboratory Results.* Direct microscopic examination of the collected specimens from the lesion(s) after being mounted by KOH 10% was done for all patients and revealed that 13 patients, 32.5%, of tinea capitis gave positive result, 7 patients, 17.5%, gave false negative results, and all cases of alopecia areata gave negative results. The dermatophytes isolated are as follows: *T. violaceum* in 6 patients, 15.0%, *M. canis* in 6 patients, 15.0%, *T. rubrum* in 3 patients, 7.0%, and *T. verrucosum* in 5 patients, 13.0%.

*3.3. Trichoscopic Results.* In patients with tinea capitis, the most common trichoscopic feature (Figure 1) was short broken hairs seen in 18 patients, 90.0%, followed by black dots in 13 patients, 65.0%, comma shaped hairs in 11 patients, 55.0%, or corkscrew hairs in 9 patients, 45.0%, and zigzag shaped hair in 5 patients, 25.0% (Table 1).

In patients with alopecia areata the most common trichoscopic feature (Figure 2) was black dots in 12 patients, 60.0%, followed by yellow dots seen in 11 patients, 55.0%, exclamation mark in 11 patients, 55.0%, white hairs in 9 patients, 45.0%, short vellus hairs in 8 patients, 40.0%, short broken hairs in 8 patients, 40.0%, and pig tail growing hairs in 3 patients, 15.0% (Table 2).

## 4. Discussion

Tinea capitis and alopecia areata are considered to be the most common causes of hairless patches of the scalp in pediatrics [10]. Tinea capitis especially nonscaly type may have the same clinical appearance of alopecia areata, so trichoscopy has recently become a useful diagnostic tool for alopecia areata and tinea capitis, especially in doubtful cases as lab investigations like fungal culture or biopsy may take several weeks [11, 12].

The studies regarding trichoscopic finding of patients with tinea capitis were few and included few patients [13]. In the present study we found in tinea capitis patients by trichoscope examination, comma shaped hairs, zigzag shaped hairs, corkscrew hairs, black dots, and shortbroken hairs are considered characteristic trichoscopic features of tinea capitis as conducted by Ekiz et al. [14].

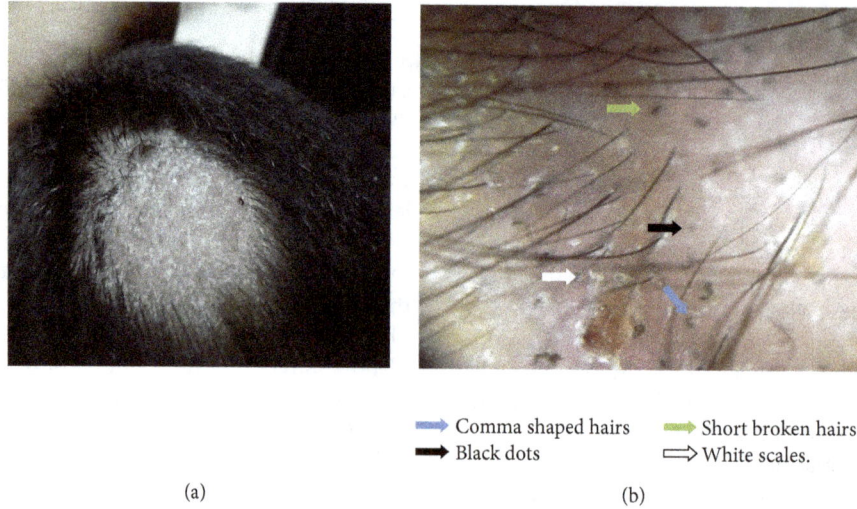

Comma shaped hairs ➡ Short broken hairs
Black dots ➡ White scales.

(a)                                                    (b)

FIGURE 1: Tinea capitis (a) macroscopic view, (b) trichoscopic view at 20x magnification, dermoscopy shows comma shaped hairs (blue arrow), black dot (black arrow), short broken hairs (green arrow), and white scales (white arrow).

TABLE 1: Different trichoscopic features of tinea capitis.

|                      | Frequency ($N = 20$) | Percent (%) |
| -------------------- | -------------------- | ----------- |
| Comma shaped hairs   |                      |             |
| Present              | 11                   | 55.0        |
| Absent               | 9                    | 45.0        |
| Zigzag shaped hairs  |                      |             |
| Present              | 5                    | 25.0        |
| Absent               | 15                   | 75.0        |
| Black dots           |                      |             |
| Present              | 13                   | 65.0        |
| Absent               | 7                    | 35.0        |
| Short broken hairs   |                      |             |
| Present              | 18                   | 90.0        |
| Absent               | 2                    | 10.0        |
| Corkscrew hairs      |                      |             |
| Present              | 9                    | 45.0        |
| Absent               | 11                   | 55.0        |

The most common trichoscopic feature was short broken hairs followed by black dots, but both of them are nonspecific as they were detected in other conditions of hair loss. Comma shaped hairs, corkscrew hairs, and zigzag shaped hairs are the diagnostic trichoscopic features of tinea capitis.

In the present study, comma shaped hairs were seen in 55% (11 out of 20 patients); this finding was detected in other studies that included few number of patients [14–16]. Comma hairs, which are slightly curved and fractured hair shafts, are associated with ectothrix and endothrix type fungal invasion. The authors believe that comma hair is probably shaped as a result of subsequent cracking and bending of a hair shaft filled with hyphae [15].

In the current study, zigzag shaped hairs were seen in 25.0% (5 out of 20 patients) and corkscrew hairs in 45.0% (9 out of 20 patients); these findings were detected in other studies with different number of patients [14, 16]. The zigzag shaped hairs or corkscrew hair seems to be a variation of the comma hair, manifesting in black patients [16].

Short broken hairs were observed in the present study in 90.0% (18 out of 20 patients) of tinea capitis cases; this finding was conducted with other studies [13, 14]. Short broken hairs may be nonspecific trichoscopic finding of tinea capitis but may be a sign of severity of the disease.

Black dots were reported in our study in 65.0% (13 out of 20 patients) of tinea capitis cases, as conducted by Sandoval et al. [17]. Black dots are remnants of broken hairs or dystrophic hairs [18].

Hughes et al. [16] stated that comma shaped hairs, corkscrew hairs were detected in zoophilic infection. In the present study T. violaceum, M. canis, and T. verrucosum were isolated; this result may be due to farming and low socioeconomic status of our patients.

To conclude the most common trichoscopic features are short broken hairs, followed by black dots, comma shaped hairs, or corkscrew hairs. However, comma shaped hairs, zigzag shaped hairs, or corkscrew hairs are characteristic trichoscopic features of tinea capitis. Black dots and short broken or dystrophic hairs are not specific to tinea capitis, as they can be observed also in alopecic areata and trichotillomania but could be used as a sign of severity of tinea capitis.

There are large scale studies in patients with alopecia areata. Yellow dots, black dots, broken hairs, exclamation mark, and short vellus hairs are considered as characteristic trichoscopic features in AA [14, 19].

In the present study yellow dots are detected in 55% (11 out of 20 patients) of alopecia areata patients; this finding was detected in other studies [20, 21]; these are marked by distinctive array of yellow to yellow-pink, round or polycyclic dots that vary in size and are uniform in color. They are more easily observed using video trichoscopy than with handheld trichoscopy [18]. The combination of large numbers of yellow dots and short growing hairs is a feature of AA incognita [22]. For the diagnosis of alopecia areata, other signs of alopecia areata should be taken into account, because isolated yellow dots may be seen in trichotillomania, hypotrichosis simplex, and even tinea capitis, as stated by Inui [23].

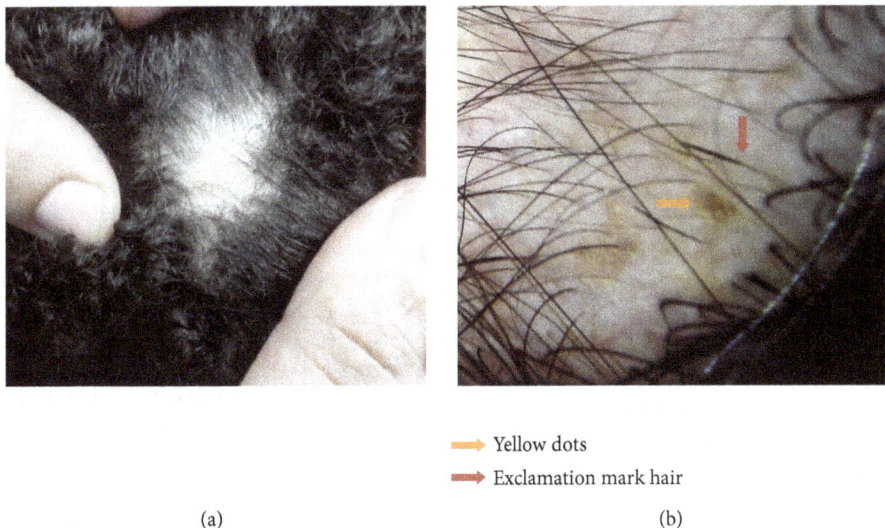

⟹ Yellow dots
⟹ Exclamation mark hair

(a)                                    (b)

FIGURE 2: Alopecia areata (a) macroscopic view, (b) trichoscopic view at 40x magnification, shows yellow dots (orange arrow) and exclamation mark hair (pink arrow).

TABLE 2: Different trichoscopic features of alopecia areata.

|                        | Frequency ($N = 20$) | Percent (%) |
|------------------------|:--------------------:|:-----------:|
| Black dots             |                      |             |
| Present                | 12                   | 60.0        |
| Absent                 | 8                    | 40.0        |
| Yellow dots            |                      |             |
| Present                | 11                   | 55.0        |
| Absent                 | 9                    | 45.0        |
| Microexclamation mark  |                      |             |
| Present                | 11                   | 55.0        |
| Absent                 | 9                    | 45.0        |
| Short vellus hairs     |                      |             |
| Present                | 8                    | 40.0        |
| Absent                 | 12                   | 60.0        |
| Pig tail regrowing hair |                     |             |
| Present                | 3                    | 15.0        |
| Absent                 | 17                   | 85.0        |
| Short broken hairs     |                      |             |
| Present                | 8                    | 40.0        |
| Absent                 | 12                   | 60.0        |
| White hairs            |                      |             |
| Present                | 9                    | 45.0        |
| Absent                 | 11                   | 55.0        |

In alopecia areata patients, the most common trichoscopic feature was black dots but it is nonspecific for alopecia areata, as it is found in other conditions as trichotillomania and tinea capitis. But the specific features were yellow dots, exclamation mark, and short vellus hairs.

In the current study under trichoscopic examination exclamation mark hair was detected in 55.0% (11 out of 20 patients) of alopecia areata cases; this finding was detected in other studies [14, 18, 20]. This term, tapering hair, is preferred over "exclamation mark hair" because the affected hair is not typical exclamatory mark in shape. It occurs due to the narrowing of hair shafts toward the follicles which is more readily perceived using trichoscopy than by naked eye [18]. In the present study we believe that tapering hairs are diagnostic feature of alopecia areata as reported by authors [12, 14, 19]. We discovered that it was more sensitive and diagnostic when associated with yellow dots, short vellus hairs, or pig tail growing hairs. We detected that it was sign of active alopecia areata, as it was seen in the active cases of alopecia areata at the periphery of the lesion(s).

In our study under trichoscopic examination black dots were detected in 60.0% (12 out of 20 patients) of tinea capitis patients; this finding was detected in other studies [19, 20]. Black dots as remnants of exclamation mark hairs or broken hairs occur when hair shaft, fractured before emerging from the scalp, provides a sensitive marker for disease activity as well as severity of AA [18]. The present study showed that black dots are the most common trichoscopic finding and can be used as a sensitive feature of alopecia areata only if associated with other specific trichoscopic features of alopecia areata as yellow dots, tapering hairs, or short vellus hairs. As in the present study, black dots were detected also in cases of trichotillomania and tinea capitis, and black dots were not detected by Ekiz et al. [14].

In the present study under trichoscopic examination short vellus hair was detected in 40.0% (8 patients out of 20 patients) of alopecia areata cases; this finding was detected in other studies [14, 19, 20]. Short vellus hairs were seen as new, thin, and nonpigmented hairs within the patch, which may or may not be clinically detectable [24]. Our obtained data showed that short vellus hair is also a diagnostic feature of AA, which can provide useful prognostic information (indicating the nondestructive nature of AA) as stated by Inui et al. [18]. They also mentioned that the appearance of clusters of short vellus hairs is a possible sign of spontaneous remission or adequate treatment, but in the present study it was a sign of spontaneous remission as the cases were not treated before the study.

In the current study pig tail regrowing hair was reported in 15.0% (3 out of 20 patients) of alopecia areata patients; this finding was detected in other studies [19]. We observed that pig tail growing hair is not common, but if present it is a diagnostic trichoscopic finding and is a possible sign of spontaneous remission of alopecia areata.

In the present study short broken hairs were detected in 40.0% (8 out of 20 patients) of alopecia areata cases conducted with other authors [18–20]. Inui et al. [18] mentioned that broken hairs were considered as being clinical markers of the disease activity and severity of AA. They are nondiagnostic as in our study we detected broken hairs in tinea capitis cases as mentioned by Köse and Güleç [19] and Ekiz et al. [14].

In the present study white hairs were detected in 45.0% (9 out of 20 patients) of alopecia areata cases; we suggested that it is a diagnostic trichoscopic finding and a sign of spontaneous remission of alopecia areata.

Some of the trichoscopic features can be used to predict the activity and severity of AA. Tapering hair is considered as a marker of disease activity and known to reflect exacerbation of disease. These trichoscopic findings will be helpful for management of patients with hair disorders. Yellow dots and short vellus hairs enable AA to be screened from other hair loss disorders. Abundant numbers of the yellow dots seen in AA can differentiate it from trichotillomania which can have limited number of yellow dots. In addition, black dots, tapering hairs, and broken hairs are specific for AA, except for trichotillomaniasingle trichoscopic feature which may not reliably diagnose AA [20]. Inui et al. [18] found that a combination of cadaverized hairs, exclamation mark hairs, broken hairs, and yellow dots could sensitively detect difficult-to-clinically diagnose types of AA like alopecia areata incognita, and broken hairs may be found in tinea capitis and trichotillomania.

To conclude the most common trichoscopic feature was black dots, followed by yellow dots, exclamation mark, white hairs, short vellus hairs, short broken hairs, and pig tail growing hairs. However, yellow dots, exclamation mark hair, and short vellus hair are specific to alopecia areata; if not detected under trichoscopy, further clinical and histopathological examination will be required.

## 5. Conclusion

Trichoscopy has been shown to improve the clinical diagnostic performance in the daily practice; it can be used to differentiate between tinea capitis by its characteristic findings as comma shaped hairs and zigzag shaped hairs or corkscrew hairs which are not present in alopecia areata. Alopecia areata also has characteristic findings as yellow dots or exclamation mark which are not present in tinea capitis. Trichoscopy can nowadays be seen as the dermatologists' stethoscope.

## Conflict of Interests

The authors declare that there is no conflict of interests regarding the publication of this paper.

## References

[1] V. Mendiratta and M. Jabeen, "Hair loss and its management in children," *Expert Review of Dermatology*, vol. 6, no. 6, pp. 581–590, 2011.

[2] E. Sarifakioglu, A. E. Yilmaz, C. Gorpelioglu, and E. Orun, "Prevalence of scalp disorders and hair loss in children," *Cutis*, vol. 90, no. 5, pp. 225–229, 2012.

[3] J. H. Phillips, S. L. Smith, and J. S. Storer, "Hair loss, common-congenital and acquiredcauses," *Postgraduate Medicine*, vol. 79, no. 5, pp. 207–215, 1986.

[4] G. F. Kao, "Tinea capitis," in *Fungal Infection: Diagnosis and Management*, M. Richardson, Ed., Medical Mycology, WB Saunders, Philadelphia, Pa, USA, 3rd edition, 1993.

[5] J. Shapiro and S. Madani, "Alopecia areata: diagnosis and management," *International Journal of Dermatology*, vol. 38, no. 1, pp. 19–24, 1999.

[6] R. Paus, E. A. Oslen, and A. G. Messenger, "Hair growth disorders," in *Fitzpatrick's Dermatology in Generalmedicine*, K. Wolff, L. A. Goldsmith, and S. I. Katz, Eds., p. 763, McGraw-Hill, New York, NY, USA, 7th edition, 2008.

[7] A. L. Mounsey and S. W. Reed, "Diagnosing and treating hair loss," *American Family Physician*, vol. 80, no. 4, pp. 356–374, 2009.

[8] G. Campos-do-Carmo and M. Ramos-e-Silva, "Dermoscopy: basic concepts," *International Journal of Dermatology*, vol. 47, no. 7, pp. 712–719, 2008.

[9] M. Miteva and A. Tosti, "Hair and scalp dermatoscopy," *Journal of the American Academy of Dermatology*, vol. 67, no. 5, pp. 1040–1048, 2012.

[10] K. Hillmann and U. Blume-Peytavi, "Diagnosis of hair disorders," *Seminars in Cutaneous Medicine and Surgery*, vol. 28, no. 1, pp. 33–38, 2009.

[11] E. C. Haliasos, M. Kerner, N. Jaimes-Lopez et al., "Dermoscopy for the pediatric dermatologist part I: dermoscopy of pediatric infectious and inflammatory skin lesions and hair disorders," *Pediatric Dermatology*, vol. 30, no. 2, pp. 163–171, 2013.

[12] A. Lencastre and A. Tosti, "Role of trichoscopy in children's scalp and hair disorders," *Pediatric Dermatology*, vol. 30, no. 6, pp. 674–682, 2013.

[13] E. T. M. Mapelli, L. Gualandri, A. Cerri, and S. Menni, "Comma hairs in tinea capitis: a useful dermatoscopic sign for diagnosis of tinea capitis," *Pediatric Dermatology*, vol. 29, no. 2, pp. 223–224, 2012.

[14] O. Ekiz, B. B. Sen, E. N. Rifaioglu, and I. Balta, "Trichoscopy in paediatric patients with tinea capitis: a useful method to differentiate from alopecia areata," *Journal of the European Academy of Dermatology and Venereology*, 2013.

[15] M. Slowinska, L. Rudnicka, R. A. Schwartz et al., "Comma hairs: a dermatoscopic marker for tinea capitis. A rapid diagnostic method," *Journal of the American Academy of Dermatology*, vol. 59, supplement 5, pp. S77–S79, 2008.

[16] R. Hughes, C. Chiaverini, P. Bahadoran, and J.-P. Lacour, "Corkscrew hair: a new dermoscopic sign for diagnosis of tinea capitis in black children," *Archives of Dermatology*, vol. 147, no. 3, pp. 355–356, 2011.

[17] A. B. Sandoval, J. A. Ortiz, J. M. Rodriguez et al., "Dermoscopic pattern in tinea capitis," *Revista Iberoamericana de Micología*, vol. 27, no. 3, pp. 151–152, 2010.

[18] S. Inui, T. Nakajima, F. Shono, and S. Itami, "Dermoscopic findings in frontal fibrosing alopecia: report of four cases," *International Journal of Dermatology*, vol. 47, no. 8, pp. 796–799, 2008.

[19] Ö. K. Köse and A. T. Güleç, "Clinical evaluation of alopecias using a handheld dermatoscope," *Journal of the American Academy of Dermatology*, vol. 67, no. 2, pp. 206–214, 2012.

[20] M. Mane, A. K. Nath, and D. M. Thappa, "Utility of dermoscopy in alopecia areata," *Indian Journal of Dermatology*, vol. 56, no. 4, pp. 407–411, 2011.

[21] E. K. Ross, C. Vincenzi, and A. Tosti, "Videodermoscopy in the evaluation of hair and scalp disorders," *Journal of the American Academy of Dermatology*, vol. 55, no. 5, pp. 799–806, 2006.

[22] A. Tosti, F. Torres, C. Misciali et al., "Follicular red dots: a novel dermoscopic pattern observed in scalp discoid lupus erythematosus," *Archives of Dermatology*, vol. 145, no. 12, pp. 1406–1409, 2009.

[23] S. Inui, "Trichoscopy for common hair loss diseases: algorithmic method for diagnosis," *Journal of Dermatology*, vol. 38, no. 1, pp. 71–75, 2011.

[24] F. Lacarrubba, V. D'Amico, M. R. Nasca, F. Dinotta, and G. Micali, "Use of dermatoscopy and videodermatoscopy in therapeutic follow-up: a review," *International Journal of Dermatology*, vol. 49, no. 8, pp. 866–873, 2010.

# 31

# A Critical Review of Personal Statements Submitted by Dermatology Residency Applicants

**Jeannette Olazagasti,**[1,2] **Farzam Gorouhi,**[2] **and Nasim Fazel**[2,3]

[1] *School of Medicine, University of Puerto Rico, San Juan, PR 00936, USA*

[2] *University of California, Davis, Sacramento, CA 95816, USA*

[3] *Department of Dermatology, University of California, Davis School of Medicine, 3301 C Street, Suite 1400, Sacramento, CA 95816, USA*

Correspondence should be addressed to Nasim Fazel; nasim.fazel@ucdmc.ucdavis.edu

Academic Editor: Jane M. Grant-Kels

*Background.* A strong personal statement is deemed favorable in the overall application review process. However, research on the role of personal statements in the application process is lacking. *Objective.* To determine if personal statements from matched applicants differ from unmatched applicants. *Methods.* All dermatology residency applications ($n = 332$) submitted to UC Davis Dermatology in the year of 2012 were evaluated. Two investigators identified the characteristics and recurring themes of content present in the personal statements. Then, both investigators individually evaluated the content of these personal statements in order to determine if any of the defined themes was present. Chi-square, Fisher's exact, and reliability tests were used. *Results.* The following themes were emphasized more often by the matched applicants than the unmatched applicants as their reasons for going into dermatology are to study the cutaneous manifestations of systemic disease (33.8% versus 22.8%), to contribute to the literature gap (8.3% versus 1.1%), and to study the pathophysiology of skin diseases (8.3% versus 2.2%; $P \leq 0.05$ for all). *Conclusion.* The prevalence of certain themes in personal statements of dermatology applicants differs according to match status; nevertheless, whether certain themes impact match outcome needs to be further elucidated.

## 1. Introduction

Medical students applying for dermatology residency programs submit a less than 2-page personal statement in which they elaborate on themselves and their interest in dermatology.

While the Electronic Residency Application Service (ERAS) facilitates the residency application process as a centralized service that distributes all necessary documents to prospective residency programs including medical school transcripts, USMLE test scores, and letters of recommendation, it has a few shortcomings. First, the applications have become very standardized; therefore the personal statement is the only place the applicants can express their personality and interests. Second, ERAS provides limited instructions for composing the personal statements including allowed size limits and characters [1]. Nevertheless, the American

Medical Association (AMA) advises applicants to address three questions: (1) what got you interested in a particular residency? (2) what are you looking for in a residency program? and (3) what are your goals as that specialist? Furthermore, there are numerous residency guides appearing in Google web searches which often include variations of these three questions [1].

Successful matching into a dermatology residency program has become a competitive process [2]. Every year, approximately 500 medical students apply for approximately 370 dermatology residency positions [3]. While prospective candidates believe that a strong personal statement will increase their chances of matching, there is a lack of research on the impact it has on the overall application review and selection process [1]. Nonetheless, according to the "Results of the 2012 National Resident Matching Program (NRMP) Director Survey," 74% of dermatology program directors responded that the personal statement is more important than USMLE scores or clerkship grades in the residency candidate selection process [4].

We decided to evaluate the personal statements submitted by applicants to a dermatology residency program at a major academic teaching hospital with the objective of determining which themes of content were more frequently emphasized. Furthermore, we sought to investigate if the themes were different between the matched and unmatched groups and whether certain themes had a higher correlation with successful matching.

## 2. Materials and Methods

This study was approved by the University of California, Davis Institutional Review Board as an exemption. All applications ($n = 332$) to the UC Davis Dermatology Residency Program in the year 2012 were analyzed. Essays were deidentified by removing the applicant's name and other identifiable variables and a randomly generated identification number was used to link the essay to other ERAS application data. Reviewers were blinded to the candidate's other application data.

Two investigators (JO and FG) who were blinded to the match outcome initially evaluated 50 randomly selected personal statements in order to identify the characteristics and recurring themes of content. Then, both investigators individually evaluated the content of each of these 50 personal statements in order to determine if any of the defined themes was present. For this initial analysis, the interrater reliability was deemed to be satisfactory (93%) and any disagreements were resolved by consensus. The content of the remaining personal statements was subsequently evaluated by JO. Therefore, all personal statements ($n = 332$) submitted to UC Davis Dermatology Program in the year 2012 were evaluated. Match outcomes of the respective candidates were retrieved from the NRMP website.

Differences in the prevalence of the themes between the matched and unmatched groups were subsequently calculated along with their corresponding 95% confidence intervals (CIs). Chi-square and Fisher's exact tests were used when appropriate in order to assess whether these differences in the prevalence were statistically significant. $P$ values equal to or less than 0.05 were considered significant. STATA 12 statistical software (StataCorp LP) was used for this analysis.

## 3. Results

The content of all personal statements ($n = 332$) from the dermatology applicants was evaluated. The initial screening of the 50 randomly selected personal statements resulted in the description of 10 main themes of content, each with its own subdivisions, giving a total of 47 characteristic themes (Table 1). Each theme was defined in a measurable term to minimize interrater variability. Interrater reliability during the initial analysis of 50 randomly was satisfactory (93%), indicating that both investigators agreed with a high level of consistency on whether any of the defined

characteristic themes of content was present in a particular personal statement. The prevalence of the 47 characteristic themes reported in the personal statements of matched and unmatched dermatology applicants is shown in Table 1.

The most commonly stated themes in both the matched and unmatched groups were "discussion of a cutaneous disease," "why dermatology," and "story telling." Other specialties have found an increasing number of personal statements sharing common features. Max et al. conducted a study where they evaluated the content of personal statements submitted by anesthesiology residency applicants at a major academic teaching hospital [5]. They found that the personal statement in a typical anesthesiology residency application revolves around one of thirteen common themes [5]. Similarly, in a study examining the personal statements submitted by radiology residency applicants, the statements seemed to consistently mention at least one of eleven defined themes [6]. Therefore, a residency selection committee member recently suggested that statements should be more original and personal since the commonality noted across personal statements limits their utility in distinguishing between candidates who have similar academic records [7].

The prevalence of certain themes found in the statements varied according to whether the applicant successfully matched into dermatology residency or not. For example, personal statements sharing a personal story were less prevalent in the matched group (119/240 (49.6%)) as compared to the unmatched group (55/92 (59.8%)). However, this difference in prevalence did not reach statistical significance ($P = 0.09$). Also discussed less frequently in the matched group versus the unmatched group was the theme of having a family member within the field of medicine (9/240 (3.8%) versus 9/92 (9.8%), $P = 0.03$).

Candidates for dermatology residency positions believe explaining why they chose dermatology is the most important aspect of the personal statement, as this theme was present in about 70% of the submitted statements. Interestingly, a similar observation was also made by Smith et al. They showed that candidates applying to radiology also feel that providing reasons for choosing the field is the most important aspect of the personal statement, since this theme was present in 29 of 30 (96.7%) of the statements [6]. While they did not analyze if these applicants matched or not into radiology residency, they do demonstrate that this theme is of importance for the members of the selection committee since they ranked it the highest out of all the categories of content they defined [6]. While discussing reasons for choosing dermatology was one of the most commonly mentioned themes by residency applicants, these reasons differed significantly between the matched and unmatched applicants. Matched candidates more frequently emphasized their desire to study the cutaneous manifestations of systemic diseases, to contribute to the literature gap, and to understand better the pathophysiology of skin diseases, as their reasons for wanting to go into dermatology. A possible explanation for this finding could be that applicants who successfully match into dermatology often have more extensive research experience and scholar publications. In fact, according to the last "Charting Outcomes in the Match," matched applicants in

TABLE 1: Characteristic themes of content that appeared in the personal statements.

| Characteristic | Prevalence, % | | | Difference | | |
|---|---|---|---|---|---|---|
| | Matched | Not matched | % | 95% CI | P value |
| (1) Story telling | 64.58 | 72.83 | −8.24 | (−19.16, 2.68) | 0.1533 |
|   Personal story | 49.58 | 59.78 | −10.20 | (−22.05, 1.65) | 0.0958 |
|   Case presentation | 39.58 | 32.61 | 6.97 | (−4.43, 18.38) | 0.2404 |
|   Personal illness | 15.83 | 16.30 | −0.471 | (−9.32, 8.34) | 0.9165 |
|   Family illness | 15.00 | 14.13 | 0.869 | (−7.56, 9.30) | 0.8415 |
|   Family relevance to dermatology | 5.83 | 5.43 | 0.399 | (−5.10, 5.90) | 0.8887 |
|   Family relevance to medicine | 3.75 | 9.78 | −6.03 | (−12.56, 0.496) | 0.0298 |
| (2) Why medicine? | 17.50 | 19.57 | −2.07 | (−11.49, 7.36) | 0.6616 |
| (3) Why dermatology? | 75.42 | 69.57 | 5.85 | (−5.01, 16.72) | 0.2779 |
|   Multidisciplinary | 34.17 | 32.61 | 1.56 | (−9.75, 12.86) | 0.7881 |
|   Visual | 24.58 | 19.57 | 5.02 | (−4.75, 14.78) | 0.3322 |
|   Cutaneous manifestations of systemic disease | 33.75 | 22.83 | 10.92 | (0.467, 21.38) | 0.0535 |
|   Social/psychosocial issues | 39.17 | 35.87 | 3.30 | (−8.29, 14.88) | 0.5801 |
|   Chronicity of disease | 7.50 | 8.70 | −1.20 | (−7.85, 5.46) | 0.7167 |
|   Literature gap | 8.33 | 1.09 | 7.25 | (3.16, 11.33) | 0.0152 |
|   Complexity of the field | 19.17 | 19.57 | −0.398 | (−9.91, 9.12) | 0.9343 |
|   Technology | 5.00 | 4.35 | 0.652 | (−4.34, 5.65) | 0.8039 |
|   Patients of all ages | 10.00 | 8.70 | 1.30 | (−5.59, 8.20) | 0.7185 |
|   Better understanding of the pathophysiology of skin disease | 8.33 | 2.17 | 6.16 | (1.57, 10.75) | 0.0434 |
|   Lifestyle | 0.417 | 1.09 | −0.670 | (−2.94, 1.60) | 0.4799 |
| (4) Accomplishment | 61.25 | 56.52 | 4.73 | (−7.13, 16.59) | 0.4313 |
|   Fellowship/research | 62.08 | 58.70 | 3.39 | (−8.40, 15.17) | 0.5709 |
|   Publications | 25.00 | 23.91 | 1.09 | (−9.21, 11.38) | 0.8371 |
|   Volunteer service | 32.50 | 25.00 | 7.50 | (−3.15, 18.15) | 0.1837 |
|   Skin cancer screenings | 7.92 | 6.52 | 1.39 | (−4.70, 7.49) | 0.6664 |
|   Leadership | 10.00 | 10.87 | −0.870 | (−8.28, 6.54) | 0.8151 |
| (5) Quotation | 23.75 | 25.00 | −1.25 | (−11.61, 9.11) | 0.8116 |
|   By famous figures | 4.17 | 7.61 | −3.44 | (−9.42, 2.54) | 0.2028 |
|   Other or self-quotation | 12.92 | 14.13 | −1.21 | (−9.50, 7.07) | 0.7703 |
| (6) Career goal | 51.25 | 47.83 | 3.42 | (−8.58, 15.43) | 0.5765 |
|   Purely clinician | 4.17 | 5.43 | −1.27 | (−6.55, 4.01) | 0.6185 |
|   Physician scientist | 36.67 | 32.61 | 4.06 | (−7.30, 15.41) | 0.4893 |
|   Physician educator | 22.50 | 21.74 | 0.761 | (−9.19, 10.71) | 0.8815 |
| (7) Subspecialty within dermatology | 12.92 | 16.30 | −3.39 | (−12.05, 5.27) | 0.4239 |
|   Procedural dermatology/MOHs micrographic surgery | 2.92 | 3.26 | −0.344 | (−4.55, 3.86) | 0.8695 |
|   Pediatric dermatology | 5.42 | 6.52 | −1.11 | (−6.90, 4.70) | 0.6980 |
|   Dermatopathology | 2.08 | 3.26 | −1.18 | (−5.23, 2.88) | 0.5312 |
|   Immunodermatology | 2.50 | 3.26 | −0.761 | (−4.89, 3.37) | 0.7024 |
| (8) Name a cutaneous disease | 76.25 | 71.74 | 7.79 | (−0.798, 16.38) | 0.1031 |
|   Mentions > 5 | 20.83 | 13.04 | 4.51 | (−6.15, 15.17) | 0.3956 |
| (9) Significant other | 2.50 | 3.26 | −7.61 | (−4.89, 3.37) | 0.7024 |
| (10) Personalized application | 13.75 | 8.70 | 5.05 | (−2.17, 14.45) | 0.2103 |
|   Interest in California | 5.00 | 3.26 | 1.74 | (−2.82, 6.30) | 0.4947 |
|   Interest in UC Davis | 8.75 | 6.52 | 2.23 | (−3.96, 8.41) | 0.5062 |
|   Mentions UC Davis Faculty | 1.25 | 2.17 | −0.924 | (−4.22, 2.37) | 0.5362 |
|   Interest in other institutions | 25.00 | 30.43 | −5.43 | (−16.32, 5.45) | 0.3153 |
|   Mentions the faculty of other institutions | 29.17 | 29.35 | −0.181 | (−11.12, 10.76) | 0.9741 |

dermatology have a mean number of 3.7 research experiences and 7.5 publications, higher than the unmatched applicants who have a mean number of 2.9 and 4.2, respectively [3].

The aforementioned reasons for choosing dermatology of the matched applicants revolved essentially around characteristics specific to the study of dermatology. Interestingly, Max et al. also noticed that personal statements written by anesthesiology applicants tend to be focused about 60% of the time on themes that are specific to the study of anesthesiology, such as interest in physiology and pharmacology [5]. While they did not see if this frequency was different between the matched and unmatched applicants, they did report that stating an interest in the relevant physiology and pharmacology was associated with an invitation to interview at their institution. Their results were unanticipated as they had hypothesized that statements including recurrent, common themes would be viewed less favorably by the selection committee. They thought that reading repeatedly similar subject matter would cause reviewers to view those statements with common themes as less appealing. However, this was not the case since their study showed a strong correlation between the number of common themes in personal statements and an invitation to interview [5].

The idea that personal statements should be more original and personal is supported in different specialties [7–9]. Interestingly, in our study, applicants that successfully matched into dermatology seemed to place less emphasis on a unique storytelling theme or even an applicant-related storyline (Table 1). This was somewhat unexpected considering that the personal statement provides applicants the opportunity to express their personal attributes rather than the explicit details of their CVs and therefore to distinguish themselves from other applicants. According to Smith et al., it is possible that some candidates might have hesitation in sharing their personal qualities for fear of being perceived as conceited [6]. Nonetheless, they believe that this should not be so since their study shows that radiology residency committee members rated the theme of personal attributes highly [6]. It is not feasible to determine, with our current results, if dermatology applicants should in fact try to reveal more of their personalities.

Also less of importance for the matched applicants was to mention if they had a physician relative. This theme was observed significantly less frequently in the statements from the matched group when compared to those from the unmatched group. This falls into accord with the thoughts of residency selection committee members that have an aversion to applicants who sound as if they are going into a specialty just because their parents or family members are in the field. Furthermore, very few applicants (2/332 (0.6%)) admitted that they wanted to go into dermatology for the easy lifestyle. In the past years, residency selection committee members have been trying to differentiate these candidates from the ones that are going into the field because of a genuine desire and passion for the field. Hence, prospective applicants are generally advised not to mention dermatology's lifestyle as their main reason for applying to it. Nevertheless, one of the two applicants who mentioned this theme in our study successfully matched.

A significant limitation of our study was that the personal statements of applicants applying to a single program (UC Davis) were analyzed. Therefore, further research is needed to determine whether or not these results are generalizable to all dermatology residency applicants. While it is possible that our results remain specific only to those applying for a dermatology residency at our institution, it is rather unlikely since the 332 applications reviewed represent 65.4% of the total national pool of applicants to PGY-2 dermatology residencies in 2012 [10]. Another limitation is that the analysis of each personal statement is inevitably subjective; however, the initial analysis of 50 randomly selected personal statements showed that both reviewers showed strong interrater reliability in their assessments. We believe that the personal statement has an important role in the initial residency application screening process. However, its ultimate impact on successful matching into dermatology residency was not investigated, which is a significant limitation of our study. In addition, the role of other factors such as volunteerism and community service in the residency screening process was not explored in this study and would be worthy of further investigation.

The available literature on the topic suggests that the value placed on personal statements might vary depending on the specialty. Crane and Ferraro found that personal statements were the least important factor for selecting emergency medicine residents [11]. Similarly, a study by Taylor et al. showed that obstetrics and gynecology directors ranked personal statements last in importance for interview invitation [12]. The latter study also presented that family practice program directors consider them the second most important factor, implying that different specialties have differing views on the overall significance of personal statements [12]. Nevertheless, the fact that a personal statement's content correlates with clinical aspects of training, as shown by Ferguson et al., suggests that these could potentially be of value for all specialties [13]. Ferguson et al. compared the impact of grades, personal statements, and letters of recommendation to predict performance over the five years of a medical degree and found that personal statements with greater number of common themes were reliable predictors of positive clinical performance [13].

In spite of the research done so far in the field, there is sparse evidence to help medical students and more often than not they still agonize on what they should write in their statements. We understand that our study is the first attempt to analyze the contents of personal statements submitted by dermatology applicants in order to instigate if there are characteristics in them that increase the chance of matching. We impart our results not only to inform students and faculty involved in the match process of what are the trends seen in the personal statements of dermatology applicants, but also to stimulate continued research on this important subject.

## 4. Conclusion

Personal statements of dermatology applicants discuss a number of common, repeated themes. The prevalence of certain themes differs according to whether the applicant successfully matched into residency or not. For example, describing why they chose dermatology was more commonly recognized in the statements of the matched group. On the other hand, stating a personal story was more frequently observed in those of the unmatched group. However, the possibility that describing certain themes in personal statements impacts match outcome is currently under investigation and needs to be further elucidated.

## Conflict of Interests

The authors declare that there is no conflict of interests regarding the publication of this paper.

## Authors' Contribution

Jeannette Olazagasti, Farzam Gorouhi, and Nasim Fazel had full access to all of the data in the study and take responsibility for the integrity of the data and the accuracy of the data analysis. Study concept and design were carried out by Jeannette Olazagasti, Farzam Gorouhi, and Nasim Fazel. Acquisition of data was carried out by Jeannette Olazagasti, Farzam Gorouhi, and Nasim Fazel. Analysis and interpretation of data were carried out by Jeannette Olazagasti, Farzam Gorouhi, and Nasim Fazel. Drafting of the paper was carried out by Jeannette Olazagasti. Critical revision of the paper for important intellectual content was carried out by Jeannette Olazagasti, Farzam Gorouhi, and Nasim Fazel. Statistical analysis was carried out by Jeannette Olazagasti, Farzam Gorouhi, and Nasim Fazel. Administrative, technical, or material support was held by Jeannette Olazagasti, Farzam Gorouhi, and Nasim Fazel. Study supervision was carried out by Jeannette Olazagasti, Farzam Gorouhi, and Nasim Fazel.

## References

[1] B. A. A. White, M. Sadoski, S. Thomas, and M. Shabahang, "Is the evaluation of the personal statement a reliable component of the general surgery residency application?" *Journal of Surgical Education*, vol. 69, no. 3, pp. 340–343, 2012.

[2] E. J. Stratman and R. M. Ness, "Factors associated with successful matching to dermatology residency programs by reapplicants and other applicants who previously graduated from Medical School," *Archives of Dermatology*, vol. 147, no. 2, pp. 196–202, 2011.

[3] National Resident Matching Program, *Charting Outcomes in the Match. Characteristics of Applicants Who Matched to Their Preferred Specialty in the 2011 Main Residency Match*, National Resident Matching Program, Washington, DC, USA, 4th edition, 2011.

[4] National Resident Matching Program, *Results of the 2012 NRMP Program Director Survey*, National Resident Matching Program, Washington, DC, USA, 2012.

[5] B. A. Max, B. Gelfand, M. R. Brooks, R. Beckerly, and S. Segal, "Have personal statements become impersonal? An evaluation of personal statements in anesthesiology residency applications," *Journal of Clinical Anesthesia*, vol. 22, no. 5, pp. 346–351, 2010.

[6] E. A. Smith, B. Weyhing, Y. Mody, and W. L. Smith, "A critical analysis of personal statements submitted by radiology residency applicants," *Academic Radiology*, vol. 12, no. 8, pp. 1024–1028, 2005.

[7] J. W. Heitz, "Making the personal statement more personal," *Journal of Clinical Anesthesia*, vol. 24, no. 1, p. 75, 2012.

[8] J. Miller, O. F. Miller III, and I. Freedberg, "Dear dermatology applicant," *Archives of Dermatology*, vol. 140, no. 7, article 884, 2004.

[9] R. E. Johnstone, "Describing oneself: what anesthesiology residency applicants write in their personal statements," *Anesthesia and Analgesia*, vol. 113, no. 2, pp. 421–424, 2011.

[10] National Resident Matching Program, *Results and Data: 2012 Main Residency Match*, National Resident Matching Program, Washington, DC, USA, 2012.

[11] J. T. Crane and C. M. Ferraro, "Selection criteria for emergency medicine residency applicants," *Academic Emergency Medicine*, vol. 7, no. 1, pp. 54–60, 2000.

[12] C. A. Taylor, L. Weinstein, and H. E. Mayhew, "The process of resident selection: a view from the residency director's desk," *Obstetrics and Gynecology*, vol. 85, no. 2, pp. 299–303, 1995.

[13] E. Ferguson, D. James, F. O'Hehir, and A. Sanders, "Pilot study of the roles of personality, references, and personal statements in relation to performance over the five years of a medical degree," *British Medical Journal*, vol. 326, no. 7386, pp. 429–432, 2003.

# 32

# Quantitative Fraction Evaluation of Dermal Collagen and Elastic Fibres in the Skin Samples Obtained in Two Orientations from the Trunk Region

**Naveen Kumar,[1] Pramod Kumar,[2] Satheesha Nayak Badagabettu,[1] Keerthana Prasad,[3] Ranjini Kudva,[4] and Coimbatore Vasudevarao Raghuveer[5]**

[1] *Department of Anatomy, Melaka Manipal Medical College, Manipal University, Manipal Campus, Manipal, India*
[2] *Consultant Plastic Surgeon, King Abdulaziz Hospital, Al Jouf, Saudi Arabia*
[3] *Department of Information Science, Manipal School of Information Science, Manipal University, Manipal, India*
[4] *Department of Pathology, Kasturba Medical College, Manipal University, Manipal, India*
[5] *Department of Pathology, Yenepoya University, Deralakatte, Mangalore, India*

Correspondence should be addressed to Pramod Kumar; pkumar86@hotmail.com

Academic Editor: Markus Stucker

*Background.* Histomorphic evaluation of dermal collagen and elastic fibres was analysed by image analysis technique. The quantification of dermal elements was performed in skin tissues, collected in horizontal and vertical directions from trunk region and discussed under the perspective of consequences of scar related complications. *Materials and Method.* Total number of 200 skin samples collected from 5 areas of trunk region were processed histologically and subjected to tissue-quant image analysis. Statistical analysis involving mean with SEM and paired $t$ test by SPSS were employed to the percentage values obtained from image analysis. *Result.* Among the chosen 5 areas of trunk region, abdomen showed the statistically significant difference for both collagen and elastic content between horizontal and vertical orientations ($P < 0.05$), whereas upper back, presternal, and lateral chest areas showed significant difference ($P < 0.05$) only for collagen and groin only for elastic content. *Conclusion.* The differences in the distribution of dermal collagen and elastic fibres in 2 directions of the samples from the same areas might be attributed to final outcome of wound healing process by influencing the appearance and behaviour of scar related complications in the region of trunk.

## 1. Introduction

The mechanical qualities of skin provide a unique arrangement of strength and elasticity. These functional qualities are achieved due to the predominate content of collagen network and to a lesser extent elastin and extracellular matrix substances in the underlying dermis [1]. Functionally, it is believed that these fibres support and nourish the skin to maintain its moisture and elasticity. However, the existence of these proteins in the dermis plays a vital role that determines the appearance and behaviour of scar related problems resulting from the natural process of wound healing. Changes in the morphology of dermis vary among anatomic location,

sex, and age of the individual. Children have relatively thin skin, which progressively thickens until the fourth or fifth decade of life when it begins to thin. This thinning is also primarily a dermal change, with loss of elastic fibres, epithelial appendages, and ground substance [2]. Collagen is the most ubiquitous and most durable proteins in nature among the proteins in the body. On other hand, elastin of the skin provides elasticity and this property is made for maximum stretch. Excessive lay down of collagen associated with stretching of scar is more in the skin with abundant elastic content as in children or young adults [3].

The arrangement of dermal collagen, mostly in random form, is designed for its major role in strength and function of the human integument. It appears less parallel in deep dermis when compared to superficial dermis of the normal skin [4] and its bundles show a basket weave-like pattern with random organisation [5].

Dermal elastic network is a strong determinant of skin resilience, texture, and quality but is not sufficiently regenerated following burn injury. In addition to its structural and mechanical roles, elastin has natural cell signalling properties that uphold a varied range of cellular responses including chemotaxis, cell attachment, proliferation, and differentiation. Elastic fibres undergo extensive changes during life. This change may be representing aging or elastotic degeneration due to chronic sun exposure. In very old persons, the fragmentation and disintegration of elastic fibres may be observed [6].

Dermal substitutes are intended to replace damaged dermal tissue in severe burn injuries. This varied nature of dermal connective tissue fibres along with their unequal distributions in the body suggested being probable role in wound healing properties [7]. Quantifying these elements in the skin samples oriented in different directions at the same region also exhibited remarkable asymmetrical distribution. This research study emphasizes similar context in trunk region of the human body. Hence, to find the anatomical cause difference in keloid appearance or scar related complications, the distribution of collagen and elastic tissue between the skin sections taken in 2 orientations perpendicular to each other from trunk region was carried out.

## 2. Materials and Method

*2.1. Sample Collection.* From each area chosen, elliptical (1 × 0.5 cm) skin sections were collected in two directions.

Quantitative fraction of dermal collagen and elastic fibres was evaluated in 200 skin samples of 2 directions obtained from 5 areas of the trunk region from 20 cadavers. Full thickness skin samples were collected from formalin embalmed adult human cadavers of either sex with the age ranging approximately around 55 ± 5 years. From each selected area, elliptical skin sections measuring 1 × 0.5 cm were collected in two directions which were perpendicular to each other. While the first sample was almost "horizontal" to the plane of the region, the second sample was across it and hence termed as "vertical" sample. The topographic site of sample collection was randomly selected and the uniformity was maintained in all the subjects as the following criteria (Figure 1).

*(1) Upper Back Area.* Skin overlying the upper border of trapezius muscle that is between the root of the neck and shoulder joint: sample along the border was "vertical" and across it was "horizontal."

*(2) Presternal Area.* Samples were collected at the midline over the sternum at the level of the 3rd rib. "Vertical" sample was parallel to plane of sternum and "horizontal" one was across it.

*(3) Lateral Chest Area.* Samples were obtained at the level of the 8th rib in the anterior axillary line. "Horizontal" samples

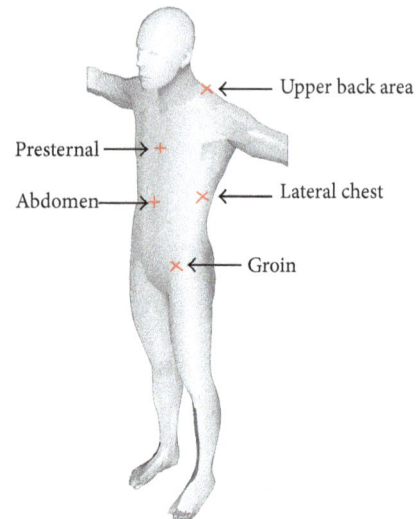

FIGURE 1: Topographic area on the trunk region where the skin samples were obtained in horizontal and vertical directions (adapted from http://www.3dcadbrowser.com/).

were taken along the direction of the rib; "vertical" samples were perpendicular to it.

*(4) Abdomen.* At the midline of abdomen, 1 cm below the umbilicus: parallel orientation to the linea alba represented as "vertical" and section across it as "horizontal."

*(5) Groin.* Over the midpoint of inguinal ligament: Sample taken along the direction of inguinal ligament served as "horizontal" direction, while perpendicular to it as "vertical".

*2.2. Histological Processing.* Skin samples were processed under histological techniques to obtain paraffin sections. These sections were treated through series of solutions till hydration. A special stain Verhoeff-van Gieson (VVG) was employed to selective demonstration of collagen and elastic fibres [8]. These slides were observed under light microscope to ascertain normal histological pattern of dermis. From each section stained, 3 photomicrographs were collected under 20x magnification using inverted phase contrast microscope attached with ProgRes CapturePro 2.1, Jenoptik, microscopic camera. Each image was captured with the resolution of 694 × 516 VGA for the image analysis by "tissue-quant" method [7]. Images were collected just beneath the epidermis including both papillary and reticular layers of the dermis in a random fashion.

*2.3. Image Analysis.* Image analysis of the VVG sections based on their property of colours acquired by the stain employed was done by the software "tissue-quant" version 1.0. The tissue-quant software work on the principle of scoring the number of pixels assigned to the shades of the colour to be analysed. The software has the option of obtaining strength of staining in terms of a colour score. Selection of positively stained area in the image is measured by means

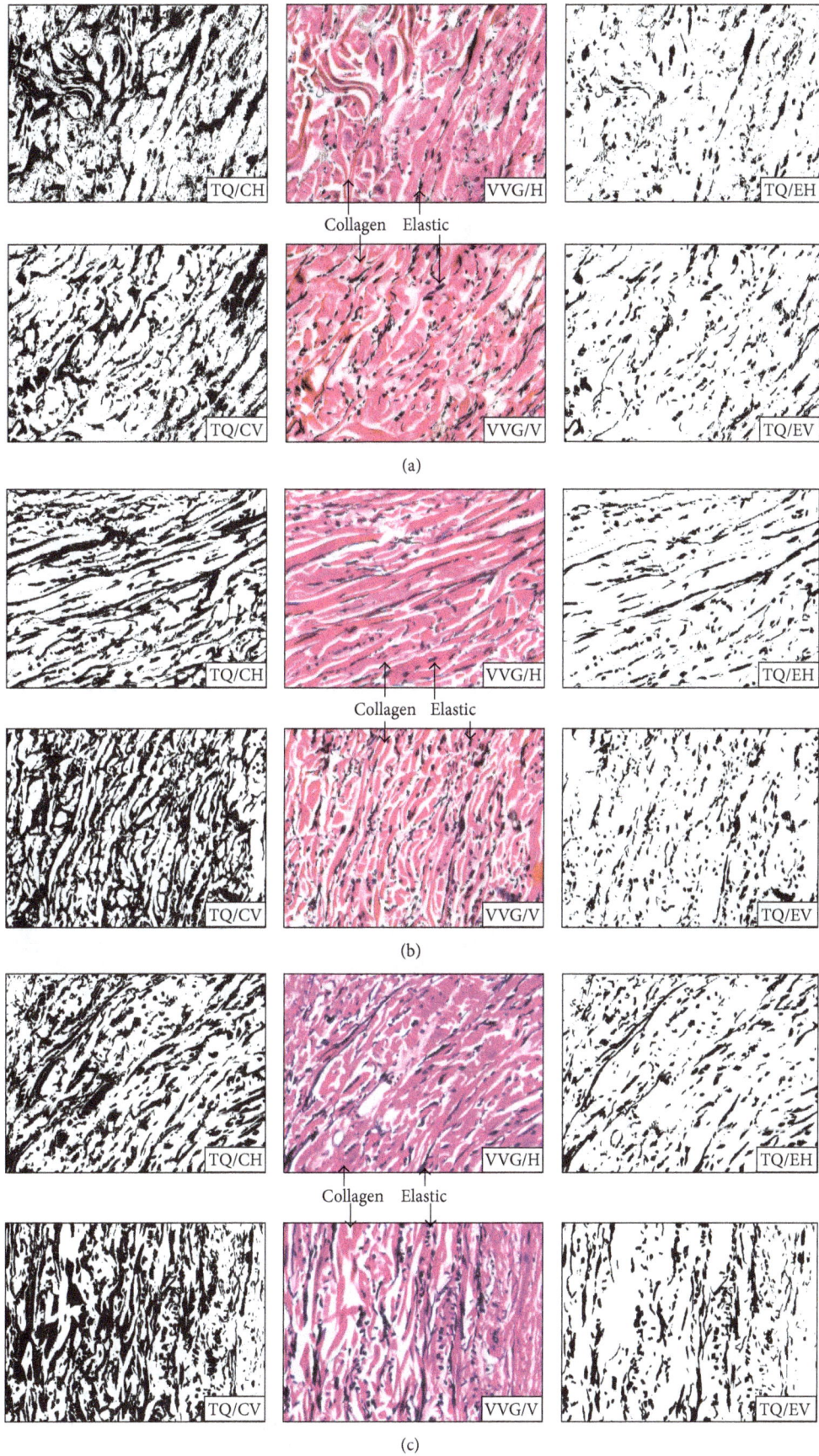

Collagen    Elastic

(a)

Collagen    Elastic

(b)

Collagen    Elastic

(c)

FIGURE 2: Continued.

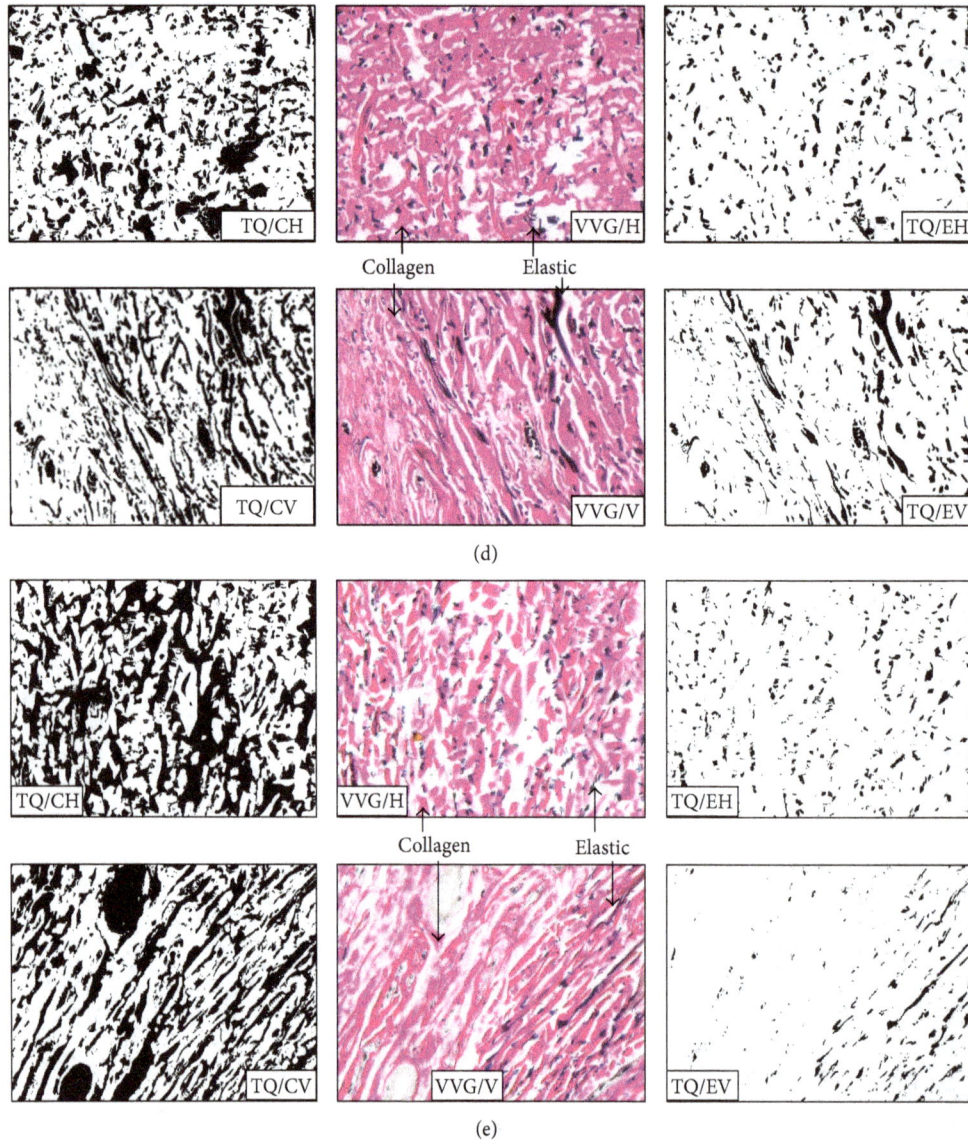

FIGURE 2: Photograph showing the pattern of collagen (stained pink) and elastic (black stain) fibres as in Verhoeff-van Gienson (VVG) stain (×20) in horizontal (VVG/H) and vertical (VVG/V) samples of upper back (a), presternal (b), lateral chest (c), abdomen (d), and groin (e) areas of trunk region. Segmentation of collagen and elastic fibres by tissue-quant (TQ) image analysis is shown in adjacent photographs. TQ/CH and TQ/EH: for collagen and elastic fibres in horizontal section, respectively, and TQ/CV and TQ/EV: as in vertical sections, respectively.

of number of pixels assigned by it. This corresponds to the quantitative fraction of the structure to be measured. This process is prerequisite by the segmentation of colour and its shades of interest from the rest of the colours (Figure 2). Total number of pixels corresponding to the colour of interest is then converted to percentage value by proper calculation [9]. The results obtained from all 3 images of each section were aggregated for further statistical evaluation.

*2.4. Statistical Analysis.* Mean value with standard error of mean was calculated from the percentage values of quantitative fraction; in addition, paired sample *t* test with 95% confidence level was employed to compare all the variables between two different directions separately for collagen and

elastic fibres. The $P < 0.05$ is considered to be statistically significant.

## 3. Results

Results of quantitative fraction of dermal collagen and elastic fibres measured based on percentage area occupied by them in the samples obtained in horizontal and vertical direction with their level of significance are tabulated in Table 1.

Upon analysis of content of dermal elements in the trunk region by image analysis method, it has been observed that the consistency of collagen remained more dominant in horizontally oriented sections than its vertical counterpart in all the areas tested. The difference in collagen distribution

TABLE 1: Mean quantitative fraction (%) with SEM and the result of paired sample $t$ test between 2 directions for collagen and elastic fibre quantity measured by tissue-quant image analysis.

| Topographic area | Collagen | | | Elastic | | |
|---|---|---|---|---|---|---|
| | Horizontal section Mean (%) with SEM | Vertical section Mean (%) with SEM | $P$ value | Horizontal section Mean (%) with SEM | Vertical section Mean (%) with SEM | $P$ value |
| Upper back | 51.9 ± 1.6 | 49.2 ± 1.8 | 0.03* | 9.7 ± 0.6 | 10.5 ± 1 | 0.25 |
| Presternal | 52.3 ± 2.1 | 47.5 ± 1.8 | 0.01* | 13.6 ± 1 | 12.4 ± 0.9 | 0.18 |
| Lateral chest | 54.1 ± 1.8 | 49.7 ± 2.2 | 0.02* | 10.3 ± 0.8 | 11.6 ± 0.8 | 0.16 |
| Abdomen | 52.1 ± 1.9 | 47.1 ± 1.9 | 0.009* | 14.7 ± 1.2 | 12.8 ± 1.1 | 0.04* |
| Groin | 51.5 ± 2.2 | 49.8 ± 2.2 | 0.25 | 11.5 ± 0.8 | 13.4 ± 1 | 0.02* |

*Indicates statically significant ($P < 0.05$) difference between "horizontal" and "vertical" directions of samples taken.

between 2 directions was also found to be statistically significant ($P < 0.05$) in all areas tested except in the groin area. Contrary to this, the elastic fibre content exhibited an asymmetric pattern of predominance as far as orientations of the section were concerned. It was observed to be great in the vertically oriented than in horizontal sections of upper back, lateral chest, and groin area with the significant difference in groin region ($P < 0.05$) only. On the other hand, in presternal and abdomen areas, the elastic dominance was found to be more in horizontally directed samples with the significant difference at the abdomen area ($P < 0.05$).

## 4. Discussion

Tissue injury resulting in irreversible cell death and connective tissue disruption initiates the repair process. Wounds heal by scarring where a new cell population resides in a newly deposited connective tissue matrix. In certain regions of the body, surgical wounds heal with a better and less noticeable scar if they are lying in a particular direction. This is because of number of factors including skin tension and naturally formed wrinkle lines. Skin tension is due to protrusion of underlying structures and direction of underlying muscle and joint movements. Though the anatomists and surgeons have attempted to produce a body map to indicate the best direction for elective incision to obtain the most aesthetic scar, these maps frequently differ in regions, specifically on face [10].

Histomorphic assessment of collagen and elastic fibres of abdominal skin after abdominoplasty procedure performed on obese females for weight loss revealed the deficiency of collagen fibre network mainly in epigastrium region without damaging elastic fibres [11]. This is possibly because of opposed action of elastic fibres by stretching the skin, which in turn exerts the stretching force on the scar [7].

Hypertrophic scarring is mostly developed in wounds at anatomic locations with high tension, such as shoulders, neck, presternum, knees, and ankles [12, 13], whereas risk of keloid formation is higher at anterior chest, shoulders, earlobes, upper arms, and cheeks [14]. Scar stretching occurs most frequently in the lower third of the scar overlying the xiphisternum and extending onto the abdomen [15].

Although the importance of dermal connective tissue fibres is widely approved, no uniform evaluation method was available for the reliable quantification in terms of their amount of area of occupancy. For research that focuses on wound healing and scar formation, polarised light is the established method for the evaluation of these structures. However, an image analysis technique reported to be more accurate than observer ratings [15]. Thus, we employed a simple and reliable-method of quantification based on their area of occupancy in the field of image measured by tissue-quant software.

Concepts of skin lines in aesthetic approach gained much importance, though there was no clear explanation for individuals view. However, universal agreement as widely accepted is that if a scar follows a certain direction, a better scar will be produced than if it is at right angles to that direction. Lack of evidence for this fact made each researcher attempt the explanation based on 3 factors of skin tensions: physical, anatomic, and functional or experimental (empirical) methods [16].

This actuality is being supported by plastic surgeons, as in the living individuals gaping of the wound may be produced by anatomical (due to dermal elastic content) or functional (at joints) or physical (closure under tension) reasons. The later factor is dependent on surgeons, as, whenever skin is closed under tension, the scar is often unacceptable due to physical reason. Similarly, over the joints, a horizontal scar heals better due to less physical tension on the healing wounds, irrespective of anatomical differences in elastic fibers in different orientation.

On the other hand, the concept of Langer's line has been established by the observation of gaping (elliptical shaped opening) on the skin by the puncture wound made at particular direction. The direction which produced less gaping was considereda Langer's line of that particular area, without any explanation for this [16]. And also, one can explain the difference in collagen content in 2 different directions. The collagen content is meant for the strength of the structure or scar. Therefore, collagen content will be often more on one or both directions (horizontal/vertical) depending on the repeated stress due to associated elastic fiber content, physical stretching, or functional reason. Accordingly, present findings can be justified as follows:

*In the Upper Back Area.* Anatomical cause is subsided, as there was no significant difference in the elastic content between

2 directions. Hence, it is expected that anatomical factors will not be important in determination of quality of scars at the upper back area. It is in accordance with general experience of surgeons that, at this area, scar in any direction is usually unaesthetic. But, due to functional reason, repeated stretching over the back, in particular, direction as a result of flexion of spines in daily activities, might produce more stress in horizontal direction. Therefore, collagen content along the horizontal direction is supplementary to augment the strength of dermis as evident from our findings.

*Presternal Area.* Here, too, anatomical factor is not playing significant role in the formation of unacceptable scar, as there was no significant difference in the elastic content between 2 directions. Thus, Langer's line concept for aesthetic scar will not be acceptable in presternal area as is the general experience of surgeons. However, due to functional reason, repeated stretching in upward and oblique direction by the shoulder movements, the collagen content is expected to be more in horizontal direction (H > V) than in vertical one.

*Lateral Chest Area.* Anatomical factor at lateral chest area is also not playing major role in the formation of unacceptable scar, due to elastic content. The functional cause, during each respiration leading to chest expansion, produces maximum stretch in vertical direction and therefore the collagen content is significantly higher in vertical direction than in its horizontal counterpart.

*Abdomen.* At abdomen region, both the collagen and elastic content are significantly higher in horizontal direction, indicating that more collagen in horizontal direction cannot be explained due to anatomical reason. Continuous abdominal movement due to pushing down of abdominal content by the diaphragmatic movement may be appropriate functional reason. Increased collagen in horizontal plane explains more stress along the horizontal direction which is not due to anatomical reason as explained by elastic fiber content. Hence, increased elastic content in horizontal direction in abdomen area is responsible for an unacceptable scar in vertical direction. Thus, Langer's line concept holds well over the abdomen.

*Groin.* Elastic fiber content is extremely higher on vertical direction with the statistical significant difference between 2 directions. Thus, scar along the crease is expected to be under stress, giving rise to unaesthetic result, which is contrary to routine observation by the surgeons. This may be explained by nullified action of elastic fibre by flexed posture of hip joint during most of the activities (functional). The collagen content difference is insignificant.

*Conclusion.* Often, collagen content will be more in a particular direction depending on the repeated stress due to associated elastic fibre content, physical stretching or functional reason. These facts are confirmed with the results of present research study by the asymmetric distribution of dermal collagen and elastic fibre content along horizontal and vertical orientations of the skin samples obtained.

## Conflict of Interests

The authors declare that there is no conflict of interests.

## Authors' Contribution

Naveen Kumar contributed to the integrity and accuracy of the data analysis; Pramod Kumar and Satheesha Nayak Badagabettu contributed to the study concept and design; Keerthana Prasad contributed to the data analysis; Coimbatore Vasudevarao Raghuveer and Ranjini Kudva contributed to the critical revision of the paper; Pramod Kumar contributed to the study supervision.

## References

[1] E. E. Peacock, *Structure Synthesis and Interaction of Fibrous Protein and Matrix in Wound Repair*, WB Saunders Company, Philadelphia, Pa, USA, 3rd edition, 1984.

[2] D. A. Burns, S. M. Breathnach, N. Cox, and C. E. Griffiths, *Rook's Textbook of Dermatology*, Blackwell Science, Malden, Mass, USA, 7th edition, 2004.

[3] B. Berman, M. H. Viera, S. Amini, R. Huo, and I. S. Jones, "Prevention and management of hypertrophic scars and keloids after burns in children," *Journal of Craniofacial Surgery*, vol. 19, no. 4, pp. 989–1006, 2008.

[4] P. P. M. van Zuijlen, J. J. B. Ruurda, H. A. van Veen et al., "Collagen morphology in human skin and scar tissue: no adaptations in response to mechanical loading at joints," *Burns*, vol. 29, no. 5, pp. 423–431, 2003.

[5] H. A. Linares, "Pathophysiology of the burn scar," in *Total Burn Care*, D. N. Herdon, Ed., pp. 383–397, WB Saunders, London, UK, 1st edition, 1996.

[6] D. E. Elder, *Lever's Histopathology of the Skin*, Lippincott Williams & Wilkins, Philadelphia, Pa, USA, 10th edition, 2009.

[7] K. Naveen, K. Pramod, P. Keerthana, and N. B. Satheesha, "A histological study on the distribution of dermal collagen and elastic fibres in different regions of the body," *International Journal of Medicine and Medical Sciences*, vol. 4, no. 8, pp. 171–176, 2012.

[8] D. B. John, " Theory and practice of histological techniques (5th edition)," in *Marilyn Gamble*, pp. 127–156, Churchill Livingstone, Philadelphia, Pa, USA, 2002.

[9] K. Prasad, P. B. Kumar, M. Chakravarthy, and G. Prabhu, "Applications of "TissueQuant"—a color intensity quantification tool for medical research," *Computer Methods and Programs in Biomedicine*, vol. 106, no. 1, pp. 27–36, 2012.

[10] S. Standring, *Gray's Anatomy: The Anatomical Basis of Clinical Practice*, Elsevier Churchill Livingstone, 39th edition, 2005.

[11] L. From and D. Assad, "Neoplasms, pseudo-neoplasms and hyperplasia of supporting tissue origin," in *Dermatology in General Medicine*, J. D. Jeffers and M. R. Englis, Eds., pp. 1198–1199, McGraw-Hill, New York, NY, USA, 1993.

[12] H. K. Hawkins, "Pathophysiology of the burn scar," in *Total Burn Care*, D. N. Herndon, Ed., pp. 608–619, Saunders Elsevier, Philadelphia, Pa, USA, 2007.

[13] F. B. Niessen, P. H. M. Spauwen, J. Schalkwijk, and M. Kon, "On the nature of hypertrophic scars and keloids: a review," *Plastic and Reconstructive Surgery*, vol. 104, no. 5, pp. 1435–1458, 1999.

[14] D. Elliot, R. Cory-Pearce, and G. M. Rees, "The behaviour of presternal scars in a fair-skinned population," *Annals of the*

*Royal College of Surgeons of England*, vol. 67, no. 4, pp. 238–240, 1985.

[15] P. P. M. van Zuijlen, H. J. C. de Vries, E. N. Lamme et al., "Morphometry of dermal collagen orientation by Fourier analysis is superior to multi-observer assessment," *The Journal of Pathology*, vol. 198, no. 3, pp. 284–291, 2002.

[16] A. F. Borges, "Relaxed skin tension lines (RSTL) versus other skin lines," *Plastic and Reconstructive Surgery*, vol. 73, no. 1, pp. 144–150, 1984.

# 33

# Effect of Oral PUVAsol on the Quality of Life in Indian Patients Having Chronic Plaque Psoriasis

**Pratik Gahalaut, Nitin Mishra, Puneet S. Soodan, and Madhur K. Rastogi**

*Department of Dermatology, Shri Ram Murti Smarak Institute of Medical Sciences, Bareilly 243202, India*

Correspondence should be addressed to Pratik Gahalaut; drpratikg@rediffmail.com

Academic Editor: Lajos Kemény

*Background.* Psoriasis is associated with a high impact on health-related QoL (quality of life). PUVAsol has been successfully used for treating psoriasis instead of standard PUVA therapy in developing countries. However, data for PUVAsol therapy and its effect on QoL in psoriatic patients is meagre. *Objective.* To investigate the effect of PUVAsol on the quality of life in patients having chronic plaque psoriasis. *Materials and Methods.* An observational prospective study done in patients having chronic plaque psoriasis. PASI and DLQI were calculated before initiating treatment with oral PUVAsol. These were compared with the respective scores after 12 weeks of regular treatment with PUVAsol. Statistical analysis was done using SPSS version 20.0. *Results.* Both PASI and DLQI showed statistically significant reduction after 12 weeks of regular treatment. 90% of patients responded favourably to PUVAsol therapy in the study and all the domains of DLQI showed significant reduction except domain of "work and school." *Conclusion.* Our results show that regular PUVAsol treatment improves the physical appearance of disease as evident by decrease in PASI scores. It also improves the QoL of the patients. This study will add upon the growing evidence of efficacy of PUVAsol.

## 1. Introduction

Psoriasis is a common, chronic, inflammatory, and proliferative condition of the skin [1]. In India, the prevalence of psoriasis varies from 0.44 to 2.8% [2]. There is evidence that psoriasis is associated with a high impact on health-related QoL (quality of life) [2]. For a psoriatic patient, measures of morbidity have a far greater relevance compared to mortality. It is currently accepted that the evaluation of disease severity should include clinical, psychological, and social factors [3]. QoL assessment has become an important endpoint in clinical trials in addition to the traditional clinical outcomes [4]. In developing countries QoL issues have not yet gained popularity due to lack of awareness among workers in health sector [4]. Any treatment of psoriasis should be considered ineffective until it improves QoL in patients. Patients with moderate to severe psoriasis generally require phototherapy (e.g., narrowband ultraviolet B radiation), photochemotherapy (oral psoralen plus ultraviolet A radiation), or systemic agents (e.g., cyclosporine, methotrexate, oral retinoids, and fumaric acid esters) to control their disease adequately [5]. Photochemotherapy (PUVA) is the combined use of the drug

psoralen and UVA (ultra violet A) radiation to achieve an effect not achieved with the individual components alone [6]. PUVAsol is the intake of psoralen followed by sun exposure as a source of UVA [6, 7]. PUVAsol has been used successfully for treating psoriasis [7–10]. Though a wealth of international data is available regarding QoL in psoriasis, data for PUVAsol therapy and its effect on QoL in psoriatic patients is meagre [4, 11]. There is no data in the literature regarding changes in the quality of life in terms of dermatology life quality index (DLQI) for patients of psoriasis after PUVAsol therapy. Hence this study was designed primarily to measure the effect of PUVAsol therapy on QoL in patients having psoriasis.

## 2. Objective

Primary objective of the study was to investigate the effect of PUVAsol on the quality of life in patients having chronic plaque psoriasis.

## 3. Materials and Methods

This study was done in the Department of Dermatology at Shri Ram Murti Smarak Institute of Medical Sciences,

Bareilly (India), from January 2012 to June 2013. All the patients presenting in psoriasis clinic were screened and enrolled in the study based on below mentioned inclusion and exclusion criteria. Inclusion criteria were patients of chronic plaque psoriasis; aged ≥18 years; having >10% body surface area involvement; literate; diagnosed with psoriasis for ≥3 months; willing for treatment, inclusion in study, and regular follow-up. Patients with hepatic or renal impairments, photodermatoses, past or present history of any malignancy or immunobullous disorder, any chronic systemic disorder, and pustular or erythrodermic psoriasis, patients having psoriatic arthropathy and concurrent administration of any phototoxic drugs, and patients who took treatment irregularly, chronic alcoholics and/or smokers and pregnant or lactating females were excluded from the study. A washout period of 2 and 4 weeks was given for topical and systemic therapies, respectively, before including the patients in study.

Written informed consent from all the subjects was taken before recruitment in study. Ethical review committee of our institution approved the study. History, examination, baseline PASI (psoriasis area severity index) score, and relevant investigations were recorded in a specially designed proforma. Patients were also asked to fill a validated Hindi version of DLQI (Dermatology Life Quality Index) questionnaire [12]. PASI and DLQI scores were assessed by a single investigator in the present study. The PASI and the DLQI are the most cited and most often used tools for experimental and descriptive studies due to their high degree of reliability, applicability, and reproducibility [13].

PASI is a physician assessed score. It is recognized by the USA Food and Drug Administration to assess the efficacy of psoriasis therapies in clinical trials. It takes into account the extent of involved skin surface area and severity of erythema, desquamation, and plaque induration [14]. DLQI is a self-administered, easy and user-friendly, dermatology-specific quality of life instrument/questionnaire with an average completion time of 126 s [4]. The total DLQI ranges between 0 (no impairment) and 30 (maximum impairment). The 10 questions in the DLQI can be subdivided into six domains that relate to different aspects of a person's health-related QoL as follows: symptoms and feelings (questions 1, 2), daily activities [3, 4], leisure [5, 6], work/school [7], personal relationships [8, 9], and treatment [10]. Higher scores mean greater impairment of the patient's QoL and vice versa [4].

The patients were counselled about the duration of treatment, the need for regular followup, and probable side effects that could be encountered during treatment. Patients were then started on oral PUVAsol therapy. In the absence of a standard protocol for PUVAsol, the most frequently followed protocol was selected which is described below [15]. For oral PUVAsol, 8-methoxypsoralen (8-MOP) was administered orally in morning with breakfast followed by sunlight exposure, after an interval of 2 hours on 3 alternate days in a week. The 8-methoxypsoralen (8-MOP) was administered at a fixed dose of 0.6 mg/kg. The sunlight exposure was for 5 minutes initially, preferably between 11 a.m. and 3 p.m., and then exposure time was increased by 5 minutes to a maximum of 30 minutes at every alternate subsequent exposure depending on side effects. We could not

calculate the minimal phototoxicity dose (MPD) of patients due to financial constraints. Hence it was pertinent to start PUVAsol for the minimal acceptable time period to avoid side effects. Though there is no standard protocol for treating patients with PUVAsol, authors selected the most frequently followed schedule which recommends initial exposure time limit of 5 minutes [16]. PUVAsol exposure daytime limit was chosen based on the above mentioned protocol because solar ultraviolet irradiation is maximum in midnoon. In the past Balasaraswathy et al. measured UVA and UVB irradiance in India and recommended that ideal time for PUVAsol should be between 9:30 a.m. and 3:30 p.m. [17]. Eye protection with UVA blocking glasses was requested from the time of ingestion of psoralen until sunset on the day of exposure. The standard topical therapy was emollients in the form of light liquid paraffin only. End point of treatment was completion of 12 weeks of regular treatment. DLQI and PASI were again assessed at the end of 12 weeks of regular treatment and compared with the respective baseline scores. Hepatic and renal function tests were done at baseline and then repeated at an interval of 4 weeks till the end of study time period.

Statistical analysis was done using SPSS version 20.0. Paired and unpaired $t$-tests were used for comparing the DLQI and PASI scores and results are expressed as mean ± SD. $P$ value of <.05 at a CI of 95% was taken as statistically significant.

## 4. Results

Altogether, 187 patients were screened and only 88 patients were deemed fit to be enrolled in the study due to various inclusion/exclusion criteria. However, only 65 patients gave consent for enrolment in the study. Out of these 65, only 40 patients completed the study. 15 patients took the treatment irregularly and hence were excluded from the study. Another 10 patients withdrew voluntarily due to privacy issues as they had difficulty in exposing their bodies to sunlight. Hence final analysis was done on 40 patients (Figure 1).

Table 1 describes the demographic and clinical characteristics of study patients. All our patients had Fitzpatrick skin phototype IV. To assess the efficacy of PUVAsol, patients in the study groups were classified depending on the site of lesions on their body into different subgroups, namely, exposed (lesions only on exposed parts), unexposed (patients having lesions on unexposed parts only), and mixed (lesions present on both exposed and unexposed parts of the body). However, none of the patients had lesions in only exposed parts. Subsequently the patients were divided into 2 subgroups: those having lesions at the unexposed sites only and others having lesions at mixed sites. PASI scores in different subgroups of study patients have been described in Table 2. Table 3 describes the DLQI scores in study patients.

90% (36/40) of patients responded to the treatment and achieved reduction in PASI scores after 12 weeks of regular PUVASOL. While 20% of patients (8/40) achieved ≥75% reduction from baseline PASI scores, 40% (16/40) of patients had 50–74% reduction, 10% (4/40) of patients showed 40–49% reduction in PASI scores, and 20% (8/40) of patients achieved 30–39% reduction in baseline PASI scores after 12

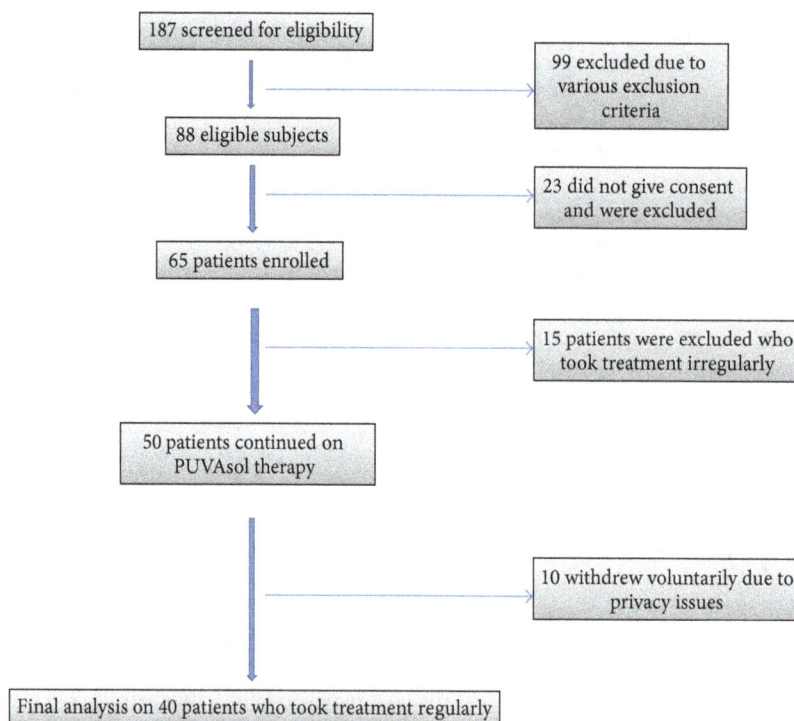

FIGURE 1: Schematic flowchart of study subjects.

TABLE 1: Demographic and baseline clinical characteristics.

| Variables | Study group ($n = 40$) |
|---|---|
| Age in years (mean) (range) | 40.55 (21–70) |
| Sex ratio (M : F) | 4 : 1 |
| Duration in years (mean) (range) | 3.98 (1–10) |
| Family history of psoriasis (%) | 16 (40%) |
| Body site of affliction | |
|   Exposed only | 0 |
|   Nonexposed only | 32 (80%) |
|   Mixed | 8 (20%) |
| Previous treatment taken | |
|   Topical only | 4 (10%) |
|   Systemic only | 4 (10%) |
|   Both topical and systemic | 32 (80%) |
| Occupation | |
|   Housewife | 6 (15%) |
|   Farmer | 14 (35%) |
|   Labourer | 10 (25%) |
|   Student | 4 (10%) |
|   Business | 6 (15%) |
| Household background | |
|   Urban | 12 (30%) |
|   Rural | 28 (70%) |

weeks of regular treatment. Rest 10% (4/40) of the patients reported worsening of the condition, that is, increase in PASI, even after regular treatment.

As per Table 4, after regular treatment with PUVASOL for 12 weeks, all the domains of DLQI scores showed statistically significant reduction except the domain of "work and school." It is noteworthy that the domain of DLQI (symptom and feeling) having highest score at baseline showed highly significant reduction after regular treatment.

During haematological investigations no hepatic or renal impairment was detected in the study patients. 28 patients (70%) experienced side effects. These were nausea in 26/40 (65%), hyperpigmentation in 12/40 (30%), headache in 8/40 (20%), pruritus in 4/40 (10%), and phototoxicity in 4/40 (10%) of study patients. However, none of the patients withdrew from the study due to these side effects.

## 5. Discussion

PUVA has a beneficial effect in psoriasis and other skin diseases [6]. While artificial UV radiation, which allows precise dosing, has been available for last few decades, the recognition of the therapeutic effect of sunlight, of which UV light comprises a proportion, goes back to ancient times [6]. Though, the controlled irradiance of an artificial light source is preferable, 8-methoxypsoralen in conjunction with sunlight exposure is also effective [18]. In a tropical country like India, sun is an inexpensive and inexhaustible source of UVA almost throughout the year. PUVAsol is the most commonly used mode of phototherapy for treating psoriasis in India as artificial chambers for photochemotherapy are not readily available [6]. PUVASOL does not require a costly set-up, can be administered at home, and has better compliance as compared with PUVA [6, 7]. Moreover, clinical efficacy

TABLE 2: PASI scores in study group at baseline and after 12 weeks of regular treatment.

| Study subjects | Pretreatment (baseline) | Posttreatment (after 12 weeks) | P value |
|---|---|---|---|
| Total cases ($n = 40$) | 22.94 ± 9.03 | 14.16 ± 10.99 | 0.0002 |
| Patients having lesions at mixed sites ($n = 8$) | 29.38 ± 7.30 | 24.20 ± 16.09 | 0.0780 |
| Patients having lesions at unexposed sites ($n = 32$) | 19.79 ± 7.03 | 10.81 ± 5.64 | 0.0001 |

TABLE 3: DLQI scores in study group at baseline and after 12 weeks of regular treatment.

| Type of study subjects | Pretreatment (baseline) | Posttreatment (after 12 weeks) | P value |
|---|---|---|---|
| Total cases ($n = 40$) | 14.45 ± 3.19 | 9.40 ± 6.52 | 0.0004 |
| Patients having lesions at mixed sites ($n = 8$) | 14.27 ± 2.66 | 8.33 ± 4.87 | 0.0001 |
| Patients with lesions at unexposed sites ($n = 32$) | 14.20 ± 5.01 | 11.20 ± 7.73 | 0.0587 |
| Patients who achieved ≥75% PASI improvement ($n = 8$) | 12.25 ± 3.06 | 4.00 ± 2.73 | 0.0001 |
| Patients who achieved 50–75% PASI improvement ($n = 16$) | 13.38 ± 2.83 | 5.75 ± 1.24 | 0.0001 |
| Patients with <50% PASI improvement ($n = 12$) | 16.5 ± 2.39 | 14.67 ± 4.41 | 0.1737 |
| Patients reporting worsening of disease ($n = 4$) | 16.00 ± 2.31 | 19.75 ± 2.63 | 0.0006 |

of PUVAsol is comparable to PUVA and PUVAsol has a favourable cost effectiveness ratio [7].

In the present study, males constituted the majority of patients. This is in concurrence with most of the Indian studies which have reported a higher prevalence of psoriasis in males [9, 10, 19–23]. It can be attributed to the fact that the male patients come forward for examination and treatment. On the other hand, there is hesitancy on the part of females to come forward for treatment, which may be due to fear of social stigma and/or rejection.

Mean baseline PASI score of 22.94 in the present study is much more than an earlier Indian study describing the clinical efficacy of PUVAsol [7]. The difference may be due to the varied severity of patients included in these studies. Besides PASI is a semiquantitative and subjective score with limited interrater reliability [24].

90% of the patients responded to PUVAsol therapy in the present study. This is more than the response seen in past studies [7, 9, 10]. Recently Aggarwal et al. reported positive response in 75% of psoriatics after 12 weeks of PUVAsol therapy [7]. Kar et al. and Talwarkar et al. reported marked improvement in 44% of patients and >50% improvement in 63% of patients, respectively, with PUVAsol [9, 10]. The difference in response rate may be attributable to the different study period in past studies or the difference in the baseline severity of psoriasis among patients included in the above mentioned studies. Further, quantification of ultraviolet light in PUVAsol depends on the season, time of the day, latitude, conditions of the atmosphere, and time of exposure [18].

In the present study, the decrease in PASI scores was not statistically significant among patients having lesions on mixed sites. This may be due to the small sample size and higher baseline PASI score in these patients compared to patients having lesions on only unexposed sites.

In our study, 24/40 (60%) of study subjects achieved at least ≥50% of improvement in PASI scores after 12 weeks of regular treatment. Marquis and Rangwala reported marked improvement in 79.2% of patients in 8–12 weeks with PUVAsol [8]. In a recent study 65% of patients of chronic plaque psoriasis achieved PASI 90 within 8 weeks [7].

Although sunlight is largely beneficial, in a small minority of patients psoriasis may be provoked by strong sunlight and cause summer exacerbations in exposed skin [25]. This may be a possible explanation for the worsening of disease in 10% of patients after PUVAsol therapy.

The baseline psoriasis severity of patients included in the present study, in terms of mean DLQI, was 14.45. This is comparable to mean DLQI scores of 10.6 to 18.83 reported among psoriatic patients in various past studies done worldwide [11, 26]. Finlay et al. have proposed a banding system to felicitate the clinical interpretation of DLQI scores [4, 27]. The baseline DLQI scores indicate that the patients who presented for treatment in the present study had "very large effect" on overall health-related quality of life (HRQoL) [4].

Many clinical trials have demonstrated the ability of DLQI to detect changes in patients' QoL before and after treatment [4]. In the present study, after 12 weeks of regular treatment, the mean DLQI score reduced to 9.40. In other

TABLE 4: Comparison of different domains of DLQI at baseline and after 12 weeks of treatment.

| Domain | DLQI (mean ± SD) before treatment | DLQI (mean ± SD) after treatment | $P$ value |
|---|---|---|---|
| Symptoms and feelings | 4.20 ± 1.20 | 2.75 ± 1.62 | 0.0003 |
| Daily activities | 3.10 ± 0.91 | 2.30 ± 1.81 | 0.04 |
| Leisure | 2.25 ± 0.72 | 1.45 ± 0.89 | 0.003 |
| Work and school | 1.45 ± 0.69 | 1.00 ± 1.21 | 0.07 |
| Personal relationships | 2.10 ± 1.55 | 1.45 ± 1.50 | 0.0004 |
| Treatment | 1.25 ± 0.55 | 0.45 ± 0.51 | 0.0004 |

words, after 12 weeks of treatment, there was statistically significant improvement and a favourable band shift in the DLQI scores from "very large effect" to "moderate effect" [4]. The difference in the mean values of DLQI before and after treatment is clinically meaningful according to the proposed minimal clinical important difference (MCID) of 3.2 for DLQI in psoriasis [28]. Patient reported outcomes, based on DLQI scores, are more sensitive to treatment and precede clinical outcomes in psoriasis [14]. Recent studies have stated that improvement in DLQI paralleled the changes in PASI scores [14].

Interestingly present study also demonstrates that a reduction in PASI of as low as 50% may also translate into significant improvement of QoL in patients treated with PUVAsol. This is in sharp contrast to various earlier studies for psoriasis where endpoint of PASI 75 translated into significant QoL improvement [28]. However, Carlin et al. reported earlier that 50% to <75% improvement in PASI score is associated with improvement in QoL scores and therefore it is a clinically meaningful degree of improvement [29]. This implies that PUVAsol is indeed an effective treatment for psoriasis.

DLQI scores in both the subgroups of patients were comparable at baseline ($P = 0.9571$) and after treatment ($P = 0.1747$). In a past study from developing nation, there was no significant difference in quality of life among patients having either localized or disseminated lesions [30]. After treatment, DLQI scores decreased significantly only in patients belonging to mixed group. Hence patients having lesions on both exposed and unexposed parts of the body had a greater and significant improvement in QoL after 12 weeks of regular PUVAsol therapy. Facial involvement and widespread disease in psoriasis is associated with greater impact of disease on QoL [31]. In the present study also, a relatively lesser improvement in widespread psoriatic lesions and in psoriatic lesions on the exposed parts of the body transcended into a much greater improvement in QoL.

DLQI and PASI scores were compared in the 2 subgroups of patients, depending on the site of lesion. Though the patients having lesions on the unexposed parts had significant reduction in PASI during study period, statistically significant decrease in DLQI score was observed in the other subgroup of patients, which had lesions on mixed sites. DLQI provides a multidimensional view of the effect of disease and treatment. It thereby enables assessment of treatment benefit beyond that demonstrated by clinical measures alone [14]. To identify the areas that were most influenced by the treatment, the DLQI scores were divided into six domains as explained above. The greatest pre/posttreatment difference in DLQI was seen in "symptoms and feelings," followed by "personal relationships," "treatment," "leisure," and "daily activities." There are a couple of past studies which have reported similar strong impairments in the domain of "symptoms and feelings" [11, 32]. The variation in total DLQI scores in the present and earlier studies may be a reflection of the differences in geography and cultural practices.

The domain of "work and school" failed to show any statistically significant fall in DLQI scores in the present study. Since our medical college is located in a suburban locality, majority of patients presenting in our department are from lower socioeconomic status and hail from a rural background (Table 1). Occupation of such patients may not be affected by the presence or absence of psoriasis. On the other hand, perceptions of relatives and coworkers towards psoriasis may have a much greater impact on such patients. This perception may be reflected as high scores for the domain of "symptoms and feelings" on QoL index in our study. A recent Brazilian study stated that psoriatic patients having occupation, which involved interaction with familiar or restricted groups of people (retired and rural workers and housekeepers), failed to show any correlation between PASI and DLQ-Bra (Brazilian version of DLQI) both before and after treatment [13].

## 6. Limitations

In our study design, we had no control group and therefore we cannot draw any conclusions about the efficacy of PUVAsol treatment compared to other modalities of treatment for psoriasis. Further a small sample size is another limitation of the present study. It is possible that the patients who were excluded from the study, due to irregular treatment, may have showed lesser or no response. Besides only one disease-specific instrument, that is, DLQI, was used to measure HRQoL. Doubts have been raised in the past regarding the inadequate measurement properties of DLQI [33]. Still, these shortcomings cannot negate the results of the present study.

## 7. Conclusion

The present study shows that PUVAsol has a definitive role in improving QoL in patients having chronic plaque psoriasis. This study will add upon the growing evidence for utility of PUVAsol as well as DLQI in daily practice. This should help dermatologists in a developing country or resource poor settings to make a better and informed decision to promote PUVAsol as a fruitful, convenient, and effective therapy for managing psoriasis. However, large randomized trials are needed to substantiate the results of the present study as the quest for an ideal treatment of psoriasis seems everlasting.

## Conflict of Interests

The authors declare that there is no conflict of interests regarding the publication of this paper.

## Authors' Contribution

Pratik Gahalaut conceptualised the study and prepared the initial draft. Puneet S. Soodan collected the data and analysed it. Nitin Mishra and Madhur K. Rastogi designed the study and revised the paper. All the authors approved the final version of the paper. Pratik Gahalaut was the principal investigator and shall act as the guarantor.

## Acknowledgments

The authors would like to thank Albatross Pharmaceuticals and Palsons Pharmaceuticals (India) for providing methoxsalen tablets free of cost for conducting the study.

## References

[1] J. E. Gudjonsson and J. T. Elder, "Psoriasis," in *Fitzpatrick's Dermatology in General Medicine*, L. A. Goldsmith, S. I. Katz, B. A. Gilchrest, A. S. Paller, D. J. Leffell, and K. Wolff, Eds., p. 197, McGrawHill Medical, New Delhi, India, 8th edition, 2012.

[2] S. Dogra and S. Yadav, "Psoriasis in India: prevalence and pattern," *Indian Journal of Dermatology, Venereology and Leprology*, vol. 76, no. 6, pp. 595–601, 2010.

[3] A. Y. Finlay, G. K. Khan, D. K. Luscombe, and M. S. Salek, "Validation of sickness impact profile and psoriasis disability index in psoriasis," *British Journal of Dermatology*, vol. 123, no. 6, pp. 751–756, 1990.

[4] M. K. A. Basra, R. Fenech, R. M. Gatt, M. S. Salek, and A. Y. Finlay, "The dermatology life quality index 1994–2007: a comprehensive review of validation data and clinical results," *British Journal of Dermatology*, vol. 159, no. 5, pp. 997–1035, 2008.

[5] L. Naldi and C. E. M. Griffiths, "Traditional therapies in the management of moderate to severe chronic plaque psoriasis: an assessment of the benefits and risks," *British Journal of Dermatology*, vol. 152, no. 4, pp. 597–615, 2005.

[6] R. Rai and C. R. Srinivas, "Photohterapy : an Indian perspective," *Indian Journal of Dermatology*, vol. 52, pp. 169–175, 2007.

[7] K. Aggarwal, S. Khandpur, N. Khanna, V. K. Sharma, and C. S. Pandav, "Comparison of clinical and cost-effectiveness of psoralen+ultraviolet A versus psoralen+sunlight in the treatment of chronic plaque psoriasis in a developing economy," *International Journal of Dermatology*, vol. 52, no. 4, pp. 478–485, 2013.

[8] L. Marquis and M. G. Rangwala, "Photochemotherapy of psoriasis with oral methoxsalen (8-MOP) and solar irradiation

[9] P. K. Kar, P. K. Jha, and P. S. Snehi, "Evaluation of psoralen with solar ultraviolet light (puvasol) and adjunctive topical tar therapy in psoriasis," *Journal of the Indian Medical Association*, vol. 92, no. 4, pp. 120–121, 1994.

[10] P. G. Talwalkar, R. B. Gadgil, C. Oberai, and V. D. Parekh, "Evaluation of 8-methoxypsoralen and solar ultraviolet light (puvasol) in psoriasis," *Indian Journal of Dermatology, Venereology and Leprology*, vol. 47, no. 1, pp. 17–20, 1981.

[11] N. Meyer, C. Paul, D. Feneron et al., "Psoriasis: an epidemiological evaluation of disease burden in 590 patients," *Journal of the European Academy of Dermatology and Venereology*, vol. 24, no. 9, pp. 1075–1082, 2010.

[12] Dermatology Life Quality Index (DLQI), "Different Language Versions," Department of Dermatology and Wound Healing, School of Medicine, Cardiff University, Cardiff, UK, 2014, http://www.dermatology.org.uk/quality/dlqi/quality-dlqi-languages.html.

[13] M. F. P. Silva, M. R. Parise-Fortes, L. D. B. Miot, and S. A. Marques, "Psoriasis: correlation between clinical severity (PASI) and quality of life index (DLQI) in patients assessed before and after systemic treatment," *Anais Brasileiros de Dermatologia*, vol. 88, pp. 760–763, 2013.

[14] M. Lebwohl, K. Papp, C. Han et al., "Ustekinumab improves health-related quality of life in patients with moderate-to-severe psoriasis: results from the PHOENIX 1 trial," *British Journal of Dermatology*, vol. 162, no. 1, pp. 137–146, 2010.

[15] P. Gahalaut, P. S. Soodan, N. Mishra, M. K. Rastogi, H. S. Soodan, and S. Chauhan, "Clinical efficacy of psoralen + sunlight vs. combination of isotretinoin and psoralen + sunlight for the treatment of chronic plaque-type psoriasis vulgaris: a randomized hospital-based study," *Photodermatology Photoimmunology and Photomedicine*, 2014.

[16] N. Khanna and T. R. Tejasvi, *Step by Step Psoriasis Management*, Jaypee Brothers Medical Publishers, New Delhi, India, 1st edition, 2012.

[17] P. Balasaraswathy, U. Kumar, C. R. Srinivas, and S. Nair, "UVA and UVB in sunlight, optimal utilization of UV rays in sunlight for phototherapy," *Indian Journal of Dermatology, Venereology and Leprology*, vol. 68, no. 4, pp. 198–201, 2002.

[18] C. R. Srinivas and S. Pai, "Psoralens," *Indian Journal of Dermatology Venereology and Leprology*, vol. 63, pp. 276–287, 1997.

[19] T. Sharma and G. C. Sepha, "Psoriasis—clinical study," *Indian Journal of Dermatology Venereology and Leprology*, vol. 30, pp. 191–197, 1964.

[20] K. C. Verma and N. C. Bhargava, "Psoriasis—a clinical and some biochemical investigative study," *Indian Journal of Dermatology, Venereology and Leprology*, vol. 45, pp. 32–38, 1979.

[21] S. Lal, "Clinical pattern of psoriasis in Punjab," *Indian Journal of Dermatology, Venereology*, vol. 35, pp. 5–12, 1966.

[22] K. Inderjeet, K. Bhushan, and K. S. Vinod, "Epidemiology of psoriasis in a clinic from North India," *Indian Journal of Dermatology Venereology and Leprology*, vol. 52, pp. 208–212, 1986.

[23] P. S. Chauhan, I. Kaur, S. Dogra, D. de, and A. J. Kanwar, "Narrowband ultraviolet B versus psoralen plus ultraviolet A therapy for severe plaque psoriasis: an Indian perspective," *Clinical and Experimental Dermatology*, vol. 36, no. 2, pp. 169–173, 2011.

[24] L. Naldi, "Scoring and monitoring the severity of psoriasis. What is the preferred method? What is the ideal method? Is PASI passé? facts and controversies," *Clinics in Dermatology*, vol. 28, no. 1, pp. 67–72, 2010.

[25] C. E. M. Griffiths and J. N. W. N. Barker, "Psoriasis," in *Rook's Textbook of Dermatology*, T. Burns, S. Breathnach, N. Cox, and C. Griffiths, Eds., p. 20.3, Wiley-Blackwell, Sussex, NJ, USA, 8th edition, 2010.

[26] A. K. Wahl, C. Mørk, B. Mørk Lillehol et al., "Changes in quality of life in persons with eczema and psoriasis after treatment in Departments of Dermatology," *Acta Dermato-Venereologica*, vol. 86, no. 3, pp. 198–201, 2006.

[27] Y. Hongbo, C. L. Thomas, M. A. Harrison, M. S. Salek, and A. Y. Finlay, "Translating the science of quality of life into practice: what do dermatology life quality index scores mean?" *Journal of Investigative Dermatology*, vol. 125, no. 4, pp. 659–664, 2005.

[28] P. L. Mattei, K. C. Corey, and A. B. Kimball, "Psoriasis Area Severity Index (PASI) and the Dermatology Life Quality Index (DLQI): the correlation between disease severity and psychological burden in patients treated with biological therapies," *Journal of the European Academy of Dermatology and Venereology*, vol. 28, pp. 333–337, 2014.

[29] C. S. Carlin, S. R. Feldman, J. G. Krueger, A. Menter, and G. G. Krueger, "A 50% reduction in the Psoriasis Area and Severity Index (PASI 50) is a clinically significant endpoint in the assessment of psoriasis," *Journal of the American Academy of Dermatology*, vol. 50, no. 6, pp. 859–866, 2004.

[30] M. W. Ludwig, M. Oliviera, M. C. Muller, and J. F. Moraes, "Quality of life and site of the lesion in dermatological patients," *Anais Brasileiros de Dermatologia*, vol. 84, pp. 143–150, 2009.

[31] F. Valenzuela, P. Silva, M. P. Valdés, and K. Papp, "Epidemiology and quality of life of patients with psoriasis in Chile," *Actas Dermo-Sifiliograficas*, vol. 102, no. 10, pp. 810–816, 2011.

[32] J. Prinz, K. Rauner, E. Schubert, S. Sohn, and K. Reich, "Costs and quality of life in patients with moderate to severe plaque-type psoriasis in Germany: a multi center study," *Journal der Deutschen Dermatologischen Gesellschaft*, vol. 5, pp. 209–218, 2007.

[33] J. Twiss, D. M. Meads, E. P. Preston, S. R. Crawford, and S. P. McKenna, "Can we rely on the dermatology life quality index as a measure of the impact of psoriasis or atopic dermatitis," *Journal of Investigative Dermatology*, vol. 132, no. 1, pp. 76–84, 2012.

# 34

# Cosmetic Contact Sensitivity in Patients with Melasma: Results of a Pilot Study

**Neel Prabha, Vikram K. Mahajan, Karaninder S. Mehta, Pushpinder S. Chauhan, and Mrinal Gupta**

*Department of Dermatology, Venereology & Leprosy, Dr. R. P. Govt. Medical College, Kangra, Tanda, Himachal Pradesh 176001, India*

Correspondence should be addressed to Vikram K. Mahajan; vkmahajan1@gmail.com

Academic Editor: Craig G. Burkhart

*Background*. Some of the patients with melasma perhaps have pigmented cosmetic dermatitis. However, cosmetic contact sensitivity in melasma remains poorly studied particularly in the Indian context. *Objectives*. To study cosmetic contact sensitivity in patients with melasma. *Materials and Methods*. 67 (F : M = 55 : 12) consecutive patients with melasma between 19 and 49 years of age were patch tested sequentially during January–December, 2012, with Indian Cosmetic and Fragrance Series, Indian Sunscreen Series, *p*-phenylenediamine, and patient's own cosmetic products. *Results*. 52 (78%) patients were in the age group of 20–40 years. The duration of melasma varied from 1 month to 20 years. Centrofacial, malar, and mandibular patterns were observed in 48 (72%), 18 (27%), and 1 (1%) patients, respectively. Indian Cosmetics and Fragrance Series elicited positive reactions in 29 (43.3%) patients. Cetrimide was the most common contact sensitizers eliciting positivity in 15 (52%) patients, followed by gallate mix in 9 (31%) patients and thiomersal in 7 (24%) patients. Only 2 of the 42 patients showed positive reaction from their own cosmetics while the other 5 patients had irritant reaction. Indian Sunscreen Series did not elicit any positive reaction. *Conclusion*. Cosmetics contact sensitivity appears as an important cause of melasma not associated with pregnancy, lactation, or hormone therapy.

## 1. Introduction

The use of cosmetics and skin care products for grooming of both men and women has seen tremendous rise the world over in the last few years. Fairness creams/lotions and sunscreen are perhaps the most sought after cosmetics for daily use particularly in India and other Asian countries. The cosmetics are different from drugs, they lack diagnostic and therapeutic properties, and they are used topically to cleanse, beautify, perfume, protect from body odors, or promote attractiveness. Additionally, the cosmetic allergens may come in contact with skin from a product used by the partner/other persons, airborne vapors/droplets, or accidental transfer by hands to more sensitive areas like eyelids and after contact with an allergen-contaminated surface. Occasionally, patients may experience numerous allergic reactions to cosmetics or photosensitivity from photo-allergens in a cosmetic product and exposure to sunlight especially ultraviolet (UV)-A. The reported prevalence of cosmetic allergy varied between 29 and 36% during 1999 to 2008 while fragrances and preservatives were the most common allergens [1–4]. Similarly, sunscreen chemicals, used as such or as ingredients in other cosmetics, are a common cause of irritant or allergic contact dermatitis. They often interact with *Myroxylon pereirae* (balsam of Peru) and/or fragrance additives (cinnamic acid, cinnamic aldehyde, and cinnamon oils) and elicit contact reactions [5, 6]. Moreover, benzophenones are well-known cause of photoallergic reactions [6]. However, cosmetics have been rarely implicated to cause melasma [7]. Pigmented cosmetic dermatitis, as proposed by Nakayama et al. [8], is a variant of pigmented contact dermatitis where cosmetic ingredients are the primary allergens and the face is involved predominantly. Clinically, diffuse or patchy brown hyperpigmentation occurs over cheeks and/or forehead or the entire face making its differentiation difficult from melasma. However, this aspect of cosmetic contact sensitivity in melasma remains poorly studied. In this pilot study, we present our observations on cosmetic contact sensitivity in patients with melasma.

## 2. Material and Methods

67 (F : M = 55 : 12) patients aged ≥18 years with melasma were enrolled for the study during January–December 2012 after a written/informed consent. The study was approved by the Institutional Protocol Review Board and Institutional Ethics Committee (Registration no. ECR/490/Inst/HP/2013). Pregnant or lactating women and patients taking oral contraceptives/other medications or having other pigmentary disorders, endocrinopathies, or family history of melasma were excluded. Details about age, sex, occupation, onset, duration, and progress of melasma, clinical patterns of melasma, aggravating factor, use of cosmetics, and medications were recorded. All patients were patch tested sequentially by Finn chamber method using Indian Cosmetic and Fragrance Series (Table 1) and IndianSunscreen Series (Table 2).

Additionally, personal cosmetic products brought by the patients were also patch tested (as is) along with $p$-phenylenediamine (PPD, 1.0% pet), a constituent of commonly used hair coloring agents. The patch tests were applied on upper back and the patients returned for reading of results after 48 hrs (D2) and 72 hrs (D3). The results were graded according to the International Contact Dermatitis Research Group criteria [9]. Reactions persisting on D3 were considered positive for final analysis. Other 10 volunteers were also patch tested similarly as controls. They were using similar cosmetics and did not have melasma. Relevance of positive patch test results was determined clinically. Side effects (adhesive tape reaction, discomfort and itching, flare up of dermatitis, angry back phenomenon, active sensitization, and pigment alteration at test site), if any, were noted.

## 3. Results and Observations

The study comprised 55 (82%) females aged between 19 and 49 years and 12 (17.9%) males in the age group of 20 to 32 years. 52 (77.6%) patients were in the age group of 20–40 years and constituted the majority. The duration of melasma varied from 1 month to 20 (mean 3.3 years) years. The majority, 38 (56.7%) patients, had melasma for 1 to 5 years and 19 (28.3%) patients had melasma for <1 year while its duration was more than 5 years in 10 (14.9%) patients, respectively. All patients had well delineated clinical patterns of melasma; 48 (71.6%) patients had centrofacial pattern, 18 (26.8%) patients had malar pattern, and one (1.4%) patient had mandibular pattern (Table 3).

Common cosmetics/skin care products used were cold creams and skin moisturizers (50 patients), medicated soaps (58 patients), fairness creams (39 patients), hair colors (17 patients), facial bleach (13 patients), and sunscreens (7 patients), respectively (Figure 1).

All 67 patients were patch tested with Indian Cosmetics and Fragrance Series but only 46 patients turned up for sequential patch testing with Indian Sunscreen Series. Patch test results with Indian Cosmetics and Fragrance Series were positive in 29 (43.3%, $n = 67$) patients and none showed positive result from Indian Sunscreen Series. Cetrimide was the most common contact sensitizers in 15 (52%, $n = 29$)

TABLE 1: Indian Cosmetic and Fragrance Series*.

| Sr. number | Allergen |
|---|---|
| 1 | Abitol (10%) |
| 2 | Amerchol L 101 (50%) |
| 3 | Benzyl alcohol (10%) |
| 4 | Benzyl salicylate (10%) |
| 5 | Bronopol (0.25%) |
| 6 | Butylated hydroxyanisole (BHA) (2.0%) |
| 7 | Butylated hydroxytoluene (2.0%) |
| 8 | Cetyl alcohol (5.0%) |
| 9 | Chloroacetamide (0.2%) |
| 10 | Chloroxylenol (0.5%) |
| 11 | Gallate mix (1.5%) |
| 12 | Geranium oil (2%) |
| 13 | Benzophenone (10%) |
| 14 | Drometrizole (1.0%) |
| 15 | Imidazolidinyl urea (2.0%) |
| 16 | Isopropyl myristate (2.0%) |
| 17 | Jasmine absolute Egyptian (2.0%) |
| 18 | Lavender absolute (2.0%) |
| 19 | Musk mix (3.0%) |
| 20 | Phenyl salicylate (1.0%) |
| 21 | Polyoxyethylene sorbitan (5.0%) |
| 22 | Rose oil (2.0%) |
| 23 | Sorbic acid (2.0%) |
| 24 | Sorbitan monooleate (Span 80) (5.0%) |
| 25 | Sorbitan sesquioleate (arlacel 83) (20.0%) |
| 26 | Stearyl alcohol (30.0%) |
| 27 | Tert-butyl hydroquinone (1.0%) |
| 28 | Thiomersal (0.1%) |
| 29 | Triclosan (2.0%) |
| 30 | Triethanolamine (2.0%) |
| 31 | Vanillin (2.0%) |
| 32 | Oleamidopropyl dimethylamine (0.4%) |
| 33 | Cetrimide (0.5%) |
| 34 | Jasmine synthetic (2.0%) |
| 35 | Hexamine (2.0%) |
| 36 | Control (100%) |
| 37 | Chlorhexidine digluconate (0.5%) |
| 38 | Phenyl mercuric acetate (0.01%) |
| 39 | Cocamidopropyl betaine (1.0%) |
| 40 | Diazolidinyl urea (germall II) (2.0%) |
| 41 | Ethylene diamine dihydrochloride (1.0%) |
| 42 | Quaternium 15 (Dowiell 200) (1.0%) |
| 43 | Propylene glycol (5.0%) |
| 44 | Kathon CG (1.3%) |

patients followed by gallate mix in 9 (31%) patients, respectively. Thiomersal elicited positive results in 7 (24%) patients

TABLE 2: Indian Sunscreen Series*.

| Sr. number | Allergen |
|---|---|
| 1 | 4-Tert-butyl-4-methoxy-dibenzoyl-methane (10%) |
| 2 | Homosalate (5%) |
| 3 | PABA (10%) |
| 4 | 3-(4-Methylbenzylidene) camphor (10%) |
| 5 | 2-Ethylhexyl-4-dimethyl-aminobenzoate (10%) |
| 6 | Benzophenone-3 (10%) |
| 7 | 2-Ethyl hexyl-4-methoxycinnamate (10%) |
| 8 | 2-Hydroxy-4-methoxy-4-methyl-benzophenone (10%) |
| 9 | Phenyl benzimidazole sulfonic acid (10%) |
| 10 | Octyl triazone (10%) |
| 11 | Octyl triazone (10%) |
| 12 | Drometrizole trisiloxane (10%) |
| 13 | Octocrylene (10%) |
| 14 | Octyl Salicylate (5%) |
| 15 | Ethylhexyl triazone (10%) |
| 16 | Isoamyl-p-methoxy cinnamate (10%) |
| 17 | Bis-ethylhexyloxyphenol methoxyphenyl triazine (10%) |
| 18 | Methylene bis-benzotriazolyl tetramethyl butyl phenol (10%) |
| 19 | 2-(4-Diethylamino-2 hydroxybenzoyl) benzoic acid hexylester (10%) |
| 20 | Diethyl hexyl butamido triazone (10%) |

*Note: both Indian Cosmetic and Fragrance Series and Indian Sunscreen Series are recommended by Contact Dermatitis and Occupational Dermatoses Forum of India and were purchased from Systopic India Limited, New Delhi (India).

among 39 patients using fairness creams (Fair & Lovely, Fair & Handsome, Garnier Lite, Olay). Isopropyl myristate, jasmine synthetic, sorbic acid, bronopol, chloroacetamide, vanillin, 2-(2-hydroxy-5-methyl-phenyl) benzotriazole, germall 115, quaternium 15, triethanolamine, geranium oil, butylated hydroxyanisole, and hexamine elicited positive reactions in one patient each. Polysenstivity, that is, positive patch test reactions to ≥2 allergens, was observed in 11 (38%, $n = 29$) patients; 5 patients had sensitivity to 2 allergens, 5 patients to 3 allergens, and 1 patient to 5 allergens, respectively. One patient showed sensitivity to gallate mix, thiomersal, and jasmine synthetic simultaneously. One patient showed sensitivity to gallate mix, thiomersal, and cetrimide simultaneously. One patient showed sensitivity to chloroacetamide, phenyl salicylate, and cetrimide simultaneously. One patient showed sensitivity to bronopol, cetrimide, and foundation lotion. One patient showed sensitivity to PPD and gallate mix. Two patients each were positive to gallate mix and cetrimide simultaneously.

42 patients were patch tested with their own cosmetics/skin care products "as is." One male patient showed positive reaction to fairness creams ("Fair & Handsome" and "Fair & Lovely" cream). One female patient showed positive reaction to her foundation lotion. Five patients showed irritant reaction to "Lifebuoy" soap and one each to a soap containing sandalwood oil (Santoor soap) and fairness creams (as above), face wash (Fair & Lovely and Soundarya face wash), and after shave lotion (Gillete), respectively.

Ten (M : F 5 : 5) controls aged between 26 and 48 years were healthy volunteers or attendants accompanying the patients. One controls subject had positive reactions from gallate mix, polyoxyethylene sorbitan, sorbitan sesquioleate, and stearyl alcohol. PPD elicited positive reaction in another female who never had contact dermatitis clinically despite using hair colors.

## 4. Discussion

Melasma is a common acquired hypermelanosis involving the face, and being of long-standing nature has significant effect on psychology and quality of life. Although the exact prevalence of melasma is unknown, it accounts for 0.25 to 4% of the patients seen in dermatology clinics in South East Asia and is also a common pigment disorder among Indians [10, 11]. The disease affects all races but Hispanics and Asians predominate [12]. Genetic predisposition, pregnancy, oral contraceptives, endocrine dysfunction, hormone treatments, or exposure to UV light is the most implicated etiologic factors in melasma [7]. Drugs containing phototoxic agents, phenothiazines, and anticonvulsants have been particularly linked to melasma. However, cosmetics have been rarely considered in the list of causes of melasma [7, 10]. There is a predilection for the involvement of cheeks, forehead, upper lip, nose, chin, and sometimes neck as well. However, three distinctly recognized clinical patterns include centrofacial, malar, and mandibular. The most common centrofacial pattern was seen in 55% and 75% while malar pattern and the mandibular pattern occurred in 43% and 24% and 2% and 1.5% patients in two separate studies, respectively [12, 13]. Melasma affects predominantly women, men comprising only 10% of all cases or perhaps men consult less often for aesthetic motives, but it rarely manifests before puberty [12, 14]. The majority 52 (77.6%) patients in our study were in the age group of 20–40 years and predominately comprised females (82%) in the age group of 19–49 years corroborating above clinicoepidemiological findings. Similarly, they also did not differ in duration and age of onset from what has been reported previously [12]. Men comprised only 18% in our study as compared to 10% of all cases in a previous study [14]. Similarly, our patients also had centrofacial pattern in 48 (71.6%), malar pattern in 18 (26.8%), and mandibular pattern in 1 (1.4%) patients in order of frequency corroborating with earlier studies [12, 13].

Cosmetics are complex mixtures of perfumes, preservatives, emulsifiers and stabilizers, various lipids, and higher alcohols. Various chemicals in cosmetics (colophony, PPD, balsam peru, cetostearyl alcohol, lanolin, bees wax, formaldehyde, fragrances, musk mix, vanillin, rose oil, triclosan, or other antiseptics) have been implicated to cause primary irritant reactions, allergic contact dermatitis, photoallergic contact dermatitis, contact urticaria, pigment alteration, photosensitivity, brittle hair and nails, and so on (Figure 2). Hyperpigmentation, as in Berloque dermatitis,

TABLE 3: Clinical patterns of Melasma as observed in this study.

| Clinical patterns of Melasma | Definition | Number of Patients |
| --- | --- | --- |
| (1) Centrofacial | Pigmentation on cheeks, forehead, upper lip, nose, and chin | 48 (71.6%) |
| (2) Malar | Pigmentation present only on cheeks and nose | 18 (26.8%) |
| (3) Mandibular | Pigmentation on ramus of the mandible | 1 (1.4%) |

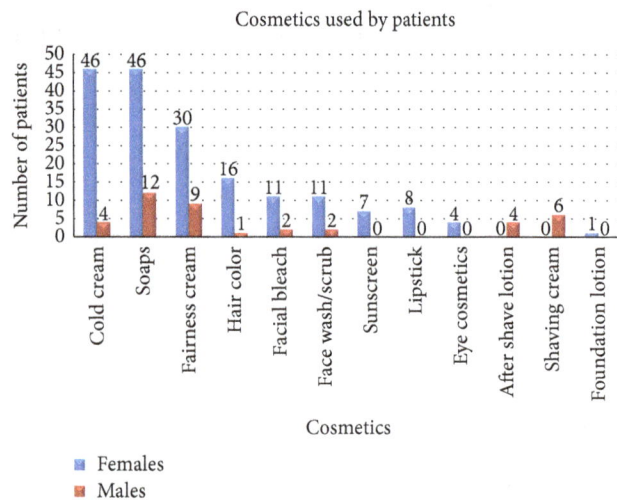

FIGURE 1: Common cosmetics used by the patients.

Riehl's melanosis, poikiloderma of Civatte, and erythrosis pigmentata faciei of Brocq, has been attributed to bergamot oil in eau-de-Cologne or from tars in cosmetics. Our 29 (43.2%) patients with melasma showed positive patch test results from cosmetic chemicals. Cetrimide was the most frequent allergen accounting for 52% of the positive results (Figure 3). Cetrimide is an antiseptic and major formulation excipient chemical in cosmetics and reported to elicit positive reactions in 12% of 50 patients with cosmetic dermatitis [15]. The formulation excipients are inert substances that serve to solubilize, emulsify, sequester, thicken, foam, lubricate, or color the active component in a product. However, they can be responsible for allergic contact dermatitis or can act as irritants when used in higher concentrations particularly in locations of direct contact with the allergen-containing products. Our patients who were patch test positive with cetrimide were using various facial cosmetics (cold creams, fairness creams, antiseptic soaps, face wash/scrubs, shaving creams, and aftershave lotions). One male patient with cetrimide positivity had also reported irritant reaction to aftershave lotion. However, we tend to agree with Beltrani et al. [16] that predicting the precise allergen in suspected cosmetics is difficult in view of ubiquity of these chemicals in cosmetic products. Dodecyl gallate, octyl gallate, and propyl gallate (gallate mix) are antioxidant substances used as preservatives in cosmetics (lipstick, liposome containing creams, body lotions, facial moisturizers, facial cleanser, body wash and cleansers, hair conditioners, and foundation lotions), foods, and the topical pharmaceutical preparations. The use of liposome containing creams has been implicated for rise in

propyl gallate allergy observed in patients patch tested from 1988 to 2005 over the previous decade [17, 18]. Gallate mix was the second most frequent allergen eliciting positive results in 31% of our patients who have been using various facial cosmetics/skin care products (Figure 4).

Skin lightening soaps and fairness creams usually contain inorganic mercury (ammoniated mercury) while organic mercury compounds (ethyl mercury or thiomersal, phenyl mercuric salts) are used as preservatives in cosmetics, eye drops, contact lens solutions, vaccines, and antiseptics. Thiomersal is considered uncommon allergen and the reported thiomersal contact sensitivity in patients of cosmetic dermatoses or pigmented cosmetic dermatitis varies from 8% to 77% [19–21]. However, discretion is recommended in interpretation of positive patch test reaction to thiomersal as primary sensitization may be from childhood vaccination. Nevertheless, chronic use of topical mercury may itself cause increased pigmentation due to accumulation of mercury granules in the dermis via absorption through hair follicles and sebaceous glands. Boonchai et al. [1] also observed that ammoniated mercury showed a significantly increased tendency to cause cosmetic allergies over a 10-year period. Interestingly, mercury is rarely listed as a component of commercially available cosmetics. Al-Saleh and Al-Doush [22] after analyzing 38 commercially available skin lightening creams in 1997 noted that 45% of the tested samples contained mercury at levels far surpassing 1 ppm (the maximum permitted limit by FDA). More recently in 2005, they also analyzed "Fair & Lovely" fairness cream and found traces of mercury that was otherwise not its listed component [23]. Thiomersal was third common allergen in order of frequency eliciting positive reactions in our 7 (24%) patients who were using various fairness creams (Figure 5).

Another patient who had positive patch test from phenyl salicylate, chloroacetamide, and cetrimide was using 5 different varieties of face creams. Phenyl salicylate is a preservative, denaturant for alcohol and fragrance ingredient in cosmetics, face and hand creams, mouthwashes, and sunscreen preparations. It has a pleasant odor somewhat similar to that of oil of wintergreen. There are reports of cheilitis from lip salve containing phenyl salicylate wherein both lip salve and phenyl salicylate elicited positive patch test reactions [24, 25]. Similarly, Fimiani et al. [26] reported a 17-year-old woman of hand dermatitis from galenic cream and showed positive reactions to both phenyl salicylate and her galenic cream but not to the petrolatum. However, our patient had no positivity from her cosmetic creams. PPD is a strong sensitizer and sensitization may occur from PPD in textile or fur dyes, black rubber, temporary tattoos, photocopying, and printing inks. In addition to PPD induced acute allergic dermatitis, uncommon presentations such as pigmentary

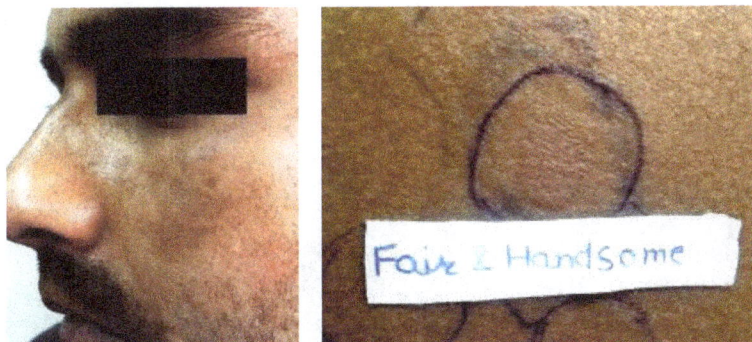

FIGURE 2: Irritant patch test (Janus type) reaction from Fair & Handsome cream in a male with malar pattern.

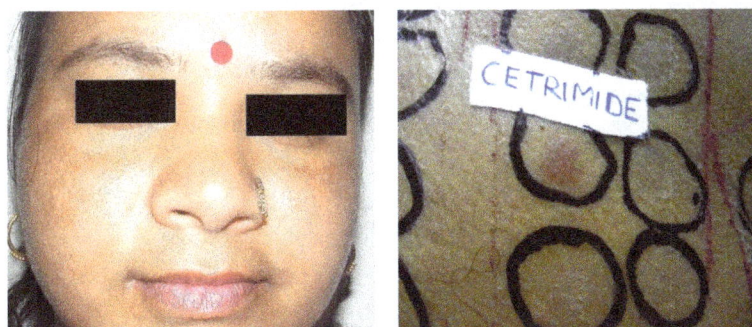

FIGURE 3: A patient with malar pattern of melasma and positive patch test from cetrimide.

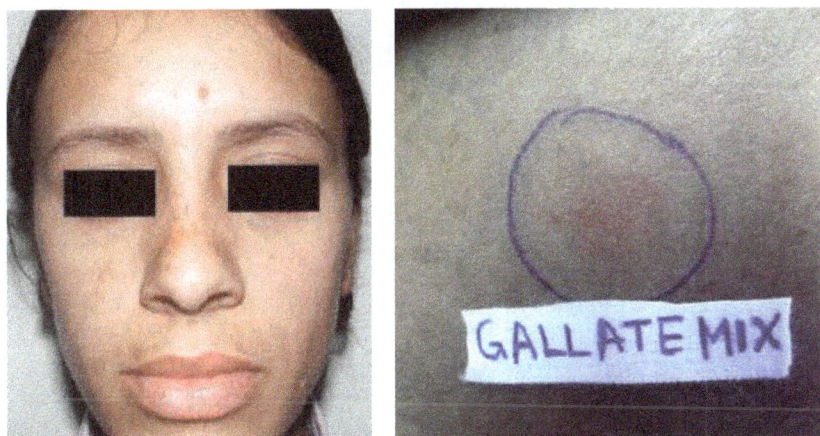

FIGURE 4: A patient with malar pattern of melasma and positive reaction from gallate mix.

changes too have been ascribed to its use. Dandale et al. [21] documented positive reactions from PPD in 8.6% patients of facial melanosis. Mehta et al. [27] also described a case of pigmented contact cheilitis from PPD. Our 2 patients and one control had positive reaction to PPD but never had clinical contact dermatitis despite using hair colors in the past or perhaps being subtle clinically it remained unnoticed. Jasmine synthetic, chloroacetamide, isopropyl myristate, vanillin, bronopol, sorbic acid, 2-(2-hydroxy-5-methyl-phenyl) benzotriazole, germall 115, hexamine, quaternium 15, geranium oil, butylated hydroxyanisole, and triethanolamine, the common additives to cosmetics/skin care

products, appear to be uncommon sensitizers. One female patient who had positive patch test from jasmine synthetic, a common fragrance in cosmetics, also showed positive reaction to gallate mix and thiomersal. She was using "Ayur" body lotion and "Fair & Lovely" fairness cream but had no positive reaction from them. Positive reactions from gallate mix and thiomersal in her could be from reasons vide supra. Chloroacetamide, a common preservative, is a well known cause of cosmetic allergy from baby lotion, cleansing lotion, eye cream, massage cream, facial cream, hand lotion, and antiwrinkle serum in Europe [28]. Although in our study none of the patient's own cosmetics elicited positive reaction,

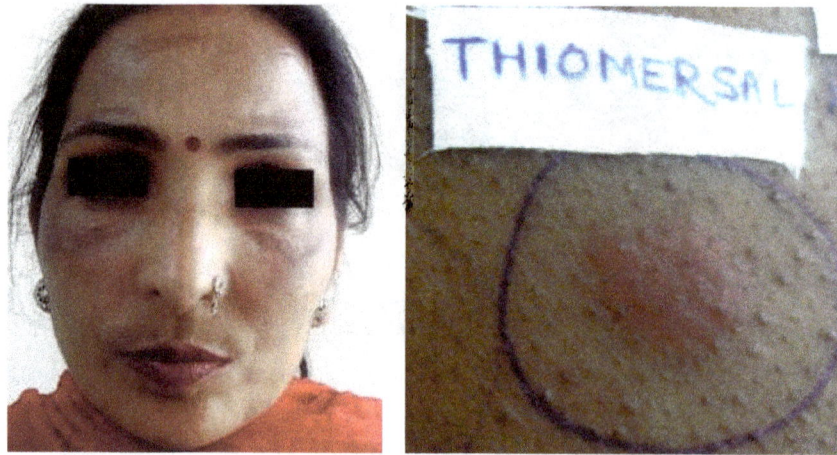

FIGURE 5: A patient with centrofacial melasma and positive reaction from thiomersal.

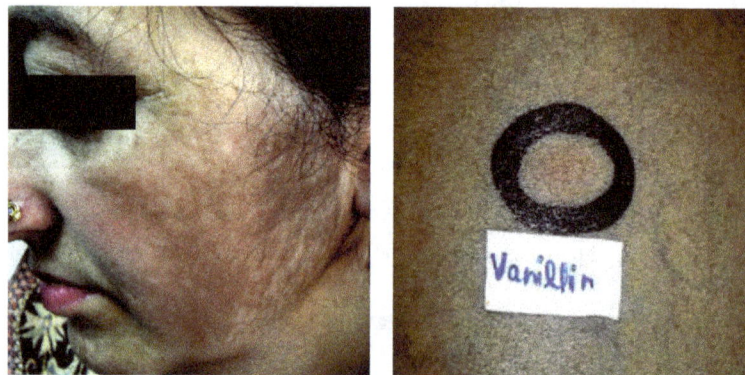

FIGURE 6: Positive patch test from vanillin in a patient with diffuse-to-reticulated mandibular pattern of melasma.

it is possible that our patient was sensitized from other cosmetics or pharmaceuticals used in the past. The reported sensitivity from isopropyl myristate, an emollient, fragrance, and skin-conditioning agent, was 1.2% in 244 patients with cosmetic contact dermatitis in a study from Israel [29]. Although our patient showed positive patch test reaction from isopropyl myristate, cosmetic cream itself did not elicit positive reaction in her despite isopropyl myristate being one of the listed ingredients in "Fair & Lovely" cream that she had been using for over 6 years. Perhaps this ingredient is present in much lower concentration in finished cosmetics product than used for patch testing. Although vanillin, a substituted aromatic aldehyde and a fragrance, is known to induce skin sensitization in humans [30], it is often considered secondary allergen in patients sensitized to *Myroxylon pereirae* and positive reactions to vanillin (pure or 10%) were reported in 8/142 and 21/164 of such patients [31]. Vanillin elicited positive reaction in a female (Figure 6) who had been using various cosmetics (cold creams, soap).

Bronopol, a formaldehyde-releasing preservative in topical medications and cosmetics specially the foundation lotion, had elicited 10 (0.12%) irritant and 38 (0.47%) allergic reactions in a series of 8149 patients who were patch tested in seven European contact dermatitis clinics; only 17 (0.21%)

were considered to be of current or past clinical relevance [32]. Bronopol caused contact sensitization in one of 202 patients with cosmetic dermatitis in another series [33]. The only patients who had positive reaction to bronopol in our series also had positive reaction from her foundation lotion. Sorbic acid, a common preservative in antiaging cream, cleansers, shampoos, exfoliant/scrub, shaving creams, and aftershave lotion, elicited positive reaction in one male patient who showed positive reaction to sorbic acid (Figure 7) and was using face wash (Johnson's), walnut scrub (Everyouth), after shave, and shaving cream (Gillette). Silva et al. [34] patch tested 147 patients with suspected cosmetic dermatitis and sorbic acid produced positive reactions in 9 patients.

Another female patient who was using fairness (Fair & Lovely) cream, various soaps, and shampoo had positive reaction from cetrimide, 2-(2-hydroxy-5-methyl-phenyl) benzotriazole, germall 115, hexamine, and quaternium 15. She also showed irritant reaction to "Fair & Lovely" fairness cream and "Lifebouy soap." 2-(2-Hydroxy-5-methyl-phenyl) benzotriazole is used as a UV absorber in cosmetics and dental materials and has caused contact sensitivity in 1 patient in an earlier study of 50 patients with cosmetic dermatitis [15]. Germall 115 (imidazolidinyl urea) is a formaldehyde-releasing preservative in creams/lotions, hair conditioner/shampoos,

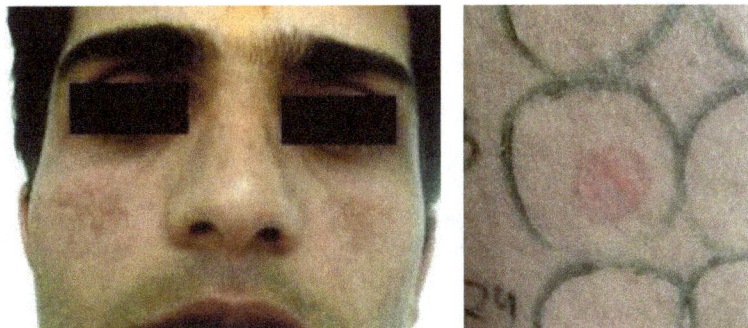

FIGURE 7: Positive patch test from sorbic acid in a patient with malar pattern of melasma.

and deodorants while hexamine is used as a solvent in cosmetics. Quaternium 15, a preservative in creams/lotions, shampoos, and soaps, elicited positive reaction in 1 (2.8%) of 35 patients of cosmetic dermatoses [20]. Geranium oil, another fragrance ingredient, caused positive reaction in our one male patient along with positive reactions from gallate mix and phenyl salicylate and he was using face wash, shaving cream, after shave lotion, soaps and hair color. Geranium oil contact sensitivity has also been reported previously in 10% of 50 patients with cosmetic dermatitis [15]. One male patient who had positive patch test from butylated hydroxyanisole (antioxidant in cosmetics), triethanolamine (surface-active agent in soaps, shampoos), and gallate mix was using fairness creams, antiacne (herbal) cream, and soaps but elicited no positive reaction from these products. The reported positivity from these cosmetic ingredients is 8.7% in patients with cosmetic contact dermatitis [35].

Sunscreens are common causes of photoallergic contact dermatitis and are frequently present in cosmetics such as moisturizers, lip and hair preparations, and foundations. They are capable of causing allergic contact dermatitis even in the absence of photo activation [16]. None of our 46 patients, however, showed positive results from sunscreen series. As photo patch testing was not performed, whether melasma among them is from photo allergic contact dermatitis remains unknown.

Overall, it was observed that there was dissociation between the patch test results from individual cosmetics ingredients and the cosmetic product when patch tested as such in our 42 patients. Dogra et al. [36] also made similar observations that ingredients of cosmetics showed more frequent sensitivity as compared to the cosmetics applied as such perhaps because of exposure to similar ingredients present in other products/medicaments and presence of ingredients in much lower concentration in finished products/cosmetics. Moreover, manufacturers usually do not list most of the ingredients on the package. This is quite evident in a study of allergic contact dermatitis from gallates and a skin repair cream was one of products suspected of causing allergic reactions [37]. The list of ingredients of current packaging did not specify presence of gallates whereas previous older packaging stated that it contained propyl gallate. The researchers could not ascertain whether the formulation had changed or

the product contained such miniscule quantities that its name was deleted from the ingredient list. Interestingly, none of our patients experienced symptoms of contact sensitivity from their cosmetics or attributed melasma to use of cosmetics. It has been suggested that there are perhaps subtle signs of preceding dermatitis in few patients and others may not observe any skin changes or itching attributable to the cosmetic use prior to or during the development of the pigmentation [38].

## 5. Conclusion

Pigmented cosmetic dermatitis and cosmetics contact sensitivity should be considered in the etiologic factors when melasma is not associated with pregnancy, lactation, or hormone therapy. However, some of these cases having diffuse-to-reticulated pattern of hyperpigmentation (brown, slate-gray, gray-brown, red-brown, or blue-brown depending upon the causal agent) and diagnosed clinically as melasma are perhaps due to pigmented cosmetic dermatitis. It is also possible that positive patch test results to various cosmetic or their ingredients, listed or unlisted, are coincidental or false positive but the hyperpigmentation is primarily postinflammatory as has been suggested by Nakayama et al. [8]. Sun exposure only deepens the pigmentation further. Accordingly, the cosmetics perhaps cause low-grade inflammation and hyperpigmentation by way of cytolysis and melanin incontinence at basal layer level following irritant reaction or after absorption of allergen from daily application in concentrations enough to elicit contact hypersensitivity. This is also evident in our 2 patients and one control having positive reaction to PPD without apparent clinical contact dermatitis despite using hair colors previously. As manufacturers do not list most of the ingredients in a cosmetic product, the relevance of positive reactions may not possibly be ascertained in all. Furthermore, dissociation between the patch test results from individual cosmetics ingredients and the cosmetic product when patch tested as such could be due to presence of ingredients in much lower concentration in finished products of cosmetics [37]. Avoidance of cosmetic contact hypersensitivity is perhaps a first step in preventing/treating melasma.

## Conflict of Interests

The authors declare that there is no conflict of interests regarding the publication of this paper.

## References

[1] W. Boonchai, R. Desomchoke, and P. Iamtharachai, "Trend of contact allergy to cosmetic ingredients in Thais over a period of 10 years," *Contact Dermatitis*, vol. 65, no. 6, pp. 311–316, 2011.

[2] K. A. Biebl and E. M. Warshaw, "Allergic Contact Dermatitis to Cosmetics," *Dermatologic Clinics*, vol. 24, no. 2, pp. 215–232, 2006.

[3] E. M. Warshaw, H. J. Buchholz, D. V. Belsito et al., "Allergic patch test reactions associated with cosmetics: retrospective analysis of cross-sectional data from the North American Contact Dermatitis Group, 2001-2004," *Journal of the American Academy of Dermatology*, vol. 60, no. 1, pp. 23–38, 2009.

[4] L. Kohl, A. Blondeel, and M. Song, "Allergic contact dermatitis from cosmetics: retrospective analysis of 819 patch-tested patients," *Dermatology*, vol. 204, no. 4, pp. 334–337, 2002.

[5] R. L. Rietschel and J. F. Fowler Jr., "Medications from plants," in *Fisher's Textbook of Contact Dermatitis*, R. L. Rietschel and J. F. Fowler Jr., Eds., p. 175, BC Decker Inc., Hamilton, New Zealand, 6th edition, 2008.

[6] R. L. Rietschel and J. F. Fowler Jr., "Photocontact dermatitis," in *Fisher's Textbook of Contact Dermatitis*, R. L. Rietschel and J. F. Fowler Jr., Eds., pp. 460–461, BC Decker Inc, Hamilton, Ontario, Canada, 6th edition, 2008.

[7] P. E. Grimes, "Melasma: etiologic and therapeutic considerations," *Archives of Dermatology*, vol. 131, no. 12, pp. 1453–1457, 1995.

[8] H. Nakayama, S. Matsuo, K. Hayakawa, K. Takhashi, T. Shigematsu, and S. Ota, "Pigmented cosmetic dermatitis," *International Journal of Dermatology*, vol. 23, no. 5, pp. 299–305, 1984.

[9] R. L. Rietschel and J. F. Fowler Jr., "Practical aspects of patch testing," in *Fisher's Textbook of Contact Dermatitis*, R. L. Rietschel and J. F. Fowler Jr., Eds., pp. 11–29, BC Decker, Hamilton, Canada, 6th edition, 2008.

[10] A. Sivayathorn, "Melasma in orientals," *Clinical Drug Investigation*, vol. 10, pp. 24–40, 1995.

[11] J. S. Pasricha, B. K. Khaitan, and S. Dash, "Pigmentary disorders in India," *Dermatologic Clinics*, vol. 25, no. 3, pp. 343–352, 2007.

[12] A. Achar and S. K. Rathi, "Melasma: a clinico-epidemiological study of 312 cases," *Indian Journal of Dermatology*, vol. 56, no. 4, pp. 380–382, 2011.

[13] C. Guinot, S. Cheffai, J. Latreille et al., "Aggravating factors for melasma: a prospective study in 197 Tunisian patients," *Journal of the European Academy of Dermatology and Venereology*, vol. 24, no. 9, pp. 1060–1069, 2010.

[14] M. Vazquez, H. Maldonado, C. Benmaman, and J. L. Sanchez, "Melasma in men. a clinical and histologic study," *International Journal of Dermatology*, vol. 27, no. 1, pp. 25–27, 1988.

[15] J. Tomar, V. K. Jain, K. Aggarwal, S. Dayal, and S. Gupta, "Contact allergies to cosmetics: testing with 52 cosmetic ingredients and personal products," *Journal of Dermatology*, vol. 32, no. 12, pp. 951–955, 2005.

[16] V. S. Beltrani, I. L. Bernstein, D. E. Cohen, and L. Fonacier, "Contact dermatitis: a practice parameter," *Annals of Allergy, Asthma and Immunology*, vol. 97, no. 2, pp. S1–S38, 2006.

[17] R. L. Rietschel and J. F. Fowler Jr., "Preservatives and vehicles in cosmetics and toiletries," in *Fisher's Contact Dermatitis*, R. L. Rietschel and J. F. Fowler Jr., Eds., pp. 266–318, BC Decker, Ontario, Canada, 6th edition, 2008.

[18] A. Perez, D. A. Basketter, I. R. White, and J. McFadden, "Positive rates to propyl gallate on patch testing: a change in trend," *Contact Dermatitis*, vol. 58, no. 1, pp. 47–48, 2008.

[19] G. Smita, "Study of pigmented cosmetic dermatitis, poster presentation," in *Proceedings of the 21st International Pigment Cell Conference*, vol. 24 of *Pigment Cell & Melanoma Research*, pp. 742–863, 2011.

[20] A. K. Nath and D. M. Thappa, "Patch testing in cosmetic dermatoses: a report from South India," *The Internet Journal of Dermatology*, vol. 5, article 1, 2006.

[21] A. Dandale, S. Chavan, and R. Dhurat, "Patch test in facial melanosis. Poster presentation. P97 21st International pigment cell conference 20–24 September 2011," *Pigment Cell and Melanoma Research*, vol. 24, pp. 742–863, 2011.

[22] I. Al-Saleh and I. Al-Doush, "Mercury content in skin-lightening creams and potential hazards to the health of Saudi women," *Journal of Toxicology and Environmental Health*, vol. 51, no. 2, pp. 123–130, 1997.

[23] I. Al-Saleh, I. El-Doush, N. Shinwari, R. Al-Baradei, F. Khogali, and M. Al-Amodi, "Does low mercury containing skin-lightening cream (Fair & Lovely) affect the kidney, liver, and brain of female mice?" *Cutaneous and Ocular Toxicology*, vol. 24, no. 1, pp. 11–29, 2005.

[24] C. Hindson, "Phenyl salicylate (Salol) in a lip salve," *Contact Dermatitis*, vol. 6, no. 3, p. 216, 1980.

[25] C. D. Calnan, E. Cronin, and R. J. G. Rycroft, "Allergy to phenyl salicylate," *Contact Dermatitis*, vol. 7, no. 4, pp. 208–211, 1981.

[26] M. Fimiani, L. Casini, and S. Bocci, "Contact dermatitis from phenyl salicylate in a galenic cream," *Contact Dermatitis*, vol. 22, no. 4, p. 239, 1990.

[27] V. Mehta, S. Nayak, and C. Balachandran, "Pigmented contact cheilitis to paraphenylenediamine," *Indian Journal of Dermatology*, vol. 55, no. 1, pp. 119–120, 2010.

[28] A. C. de Groot and J. W. Weyland, "Contact allergy to chloroacetamide in an "anti-wrinkle serum,"" *Contact Dermatitis*, vol. 15, no. 2, pp. 97–98, 1986.

[29] A. Trattner, Y. Farchi, and M. David, "Cosmetics patch tests: first report from Israel," *Contact Dermatitis*, vol. 47, no. 3, pp. 180–181, 2002.

[30] Bibra working group, "CAS Registry Number: 121-33-5 Toxicity Effects: The British Industrial Biological Research Association 8," 1990, http://ntp.niehs.nih.gov/testing/status/chemid/hsdb-121-33-5.html.

[31] G. D. Clayton and F. E. Clayton, Eds., *Patty's Industrial Hygiene and Toxicology. Volumes 2A, 2B, 2C, 2D, 2E, 2F: Toxicology*, John Wiley & Sons, New York, NY, USA, 4th edition, 1993.

[32] P. J. Frosch, I. R. White, R. J. Rycroft et al., "Contact allergy to bronopol," *Contact Dermatitis*, vol. 22, pp. 24–26, 1990.

[33] C. Laguna, J. de la Cuadra, B. Martín-González, V. Zaragoza, L. Martínez-Casimiro, and V. Alegre, "Allergic contact dermatitis to cosmetics," *Actas Dermo-Sifiliográficas*, vol. 100, no. 1, pp. 53–60, 2009.

[34] E. A. Silva, M. R. M. Bosco, and É. Mozer, "Study of the frequency of allergens in cosmetics components in patients with suspected allergic contact dermatitis," *Anais Brasileiros de Dermatologia*, vol. 87, no. 2, pp. 263–268, 2012.

[35] A. Trattner, Y. Farchi, and M. David, "Cosmetics patch tests: First report from Israel," *Contact Dermatitis*, vol. 47, no. 3, pp. 180–181, 2002.

[36] A. Dogra, Y. C. Minocha, V. K. Sood, and S. P. Dewan, "Contact dermatitis due to cosmetics and their ingredients," *Indian Journal of Dermatology, Venereology and Leprology*, vol. 60, no. 2, pp. 72–75, 1994.

[37] S. E. Gamboni, A. M. Palmer, and R. L. Nixon, "Allergic contact stomatitis to dodecyl gallate? A review of the relevance of positive patch test results to gallates," *Australasian Journal of Dermatology*, vol. 54, no. 3, pp. 213–217, 2013.

[38] P. E. Osmundsen, "Pigmented contact dermatitis," *British Journal of Dermatology*, vol. 83, no. 2, pp. 296–301, 1970.

# 35

# Chronic Urticaria: Indian Context—Challenges and Treatment Options

**Sujoy Khan,[1] Anirban Maitra,[2] Pravin Hissaria,[3] Sitesh Roy,[4] Mahesh Padukudru Anand,[5] Nalin Nag,[6] and Harpal Singh[7]**

[1] Consultant Allergist & Immunologist, Department of Allergy & Immunology, Apollo Gleneagles Hospital, 58 Canal Circular Road, Kolkata, West Bengal 700 054, India

[2] Department of Paediatric Pulmonology, Vision Care Hospital, Mukundapur, Kolkata West Bengal 700099, India

[3] Department of Allergy, Immunology and Arthritis, Apollo Hospitals International Ltd., Bhat GIDC, Gandhinagar, Ahmedabad, Gujarat 382428, India

[4] Dr. Niphadkar's Asthma and Allergy Health Clinic, Hindu Colony Lane No. 1, Dadar (East), Mumbai 400 014, India

[5] Department of Pulmonary Medicine, JSS Medical College, JSS University, Mysore, Karnataka 570 004, India

[6] Department of Medicine, Indraprastha Apollo Hospital, Mathura Road, Jasola Vihar, New Delhi 110076, India

[7] Clinical Marketing Manager, Phadia/IDD, Thermo Fisher Scientific, Units No. 7, 10 & 11, Splendor Forum, Plot No. 3, Disttrict Centre, Jasola, New Delhi 110025, India

Correspondence should be addressed to Sujoy Khan; sujoykhan@gmail.com

Academic Editor: Tadamichi Shimizu

Urticaria is a common condition that occurs in both children and adults. Most cases have no specific allergic trigger and the aetiology of urticaria remains idiopathic and occasionally spontaneous in nature. Inappropriate advice such as avoidance of foods (milk, egg, prawn, and brinjal) is common place in certain sections of India mostly by nonspecialists that should not be routinely recommended. It is important to look for physical urticarias such as pressure urticaria in chronic cases, which may be present either alone or in combination with other causes. Autoimmune causes for chronic urticaria have been found to play an important role in a significant proportion of patients. Long-acting nonsedating antihistamines at higher than the standard doses is safe and effective. Quality of life is affected adversely in patients with chronic symptomatic urticaria and some may require multidisciplinary management.

## 1. Background

Urticaria is a common condition and the chronic form usually has no allergic trigger. Longacting non-sedating antihistamines at higher than the standard doses is safe and effective.

Urticaria is characterized by itchy, red, raised (wheal), and flared skin reactions that last usually for a few hours (typically <24 hours). It is classified as chronic urticaria (CU) if it lasts for more than 6 weeks. The chronic spontaneous form of urticaria does not need any stimulus and sometimes it is also referred to as chronic idiopathic urticaria (CIU) [1–6]. It is now well recognized that CIU consists of a myriad group of diseases and development of skin lesions and/or angioedema is seen in all different types and subtypes [4–6]. The terms CIU and CU have been used interchangeably in the article, although strictly CIU would refer to patients without a proven autoimmune component to the urticaria [5–9].

The wheal has a central swelling surrounded by a reflex erythema that is itchy while the angioedema is associated with pronounced swelling of the lower dermis and subcutaneous tissue with the occasional involvement of mucous membranes (lips, tongue) in some patients. Acute urticaria appears more commonly in children and young adults of which common causes are infections, food, drugs (intravenous more than oral forms), and insect stings. It is important to take a detailed clinical history to identify whether the urticaria is chronic (or acute or chronic), as occasionally a patient may be wrongly labeled as drug allergic when it may be that the urticaria was present *before* the drug was started [1–3]. There are some drugs, however, that are notorious in causing urticaria due to a nonspecific mast cell stimulation such as opiates, high-osmolar radiocontrast media, and vancomycin. A physical examination (combined with history taking) is important as the diagnosis of urticaria remains a clinical one, apart from a few supportive investigations that could only label the cause as autoimmune.

This paper aims to discuss existing guidelines of urticaria in the Indian context, with an attempt to demystify some of the myths surrounding this condition based on our collective experience and extensive publications in this field. This paper is, therefore, applicable or relevant to physicians working in India or South East Asia where nonspecialists deal with the majority of cases of urticaria, and higher specialist training in the field of Allergology is yet to begin. This article does not aim to review the urticarias but to discuss the current level of understanding of the patients and treatment options (feasible and otherwise) to the physicians.

## 2. Consensus Guidelines on Urticaria

The EAACI/GA$^2$LEN/EDF/WAO consensus guideline for the diagnosis and management of urticaria was published in 2009. These were based on expert recommendations from the Third International Consensus Meeting on Urticaria (Urticaria 2008), joint initiative of the EAACI Dermatology Section, Global Allergy and Asthma European Network (GA$^2$LEN), European Dermatology Forum (EDF), and World Allergy Organization [1, 2]. Since then, several other societies have also published guidelines but have essentially maintained the messages of the 2009 guidelines. The important messages for clinicians and researchers in this field were (1) the absence of reliable assessment tools including specific laboratory markers and (2) the absence of effective long-term treatments for this common condition. A subsequent update from the GA$^2$LEN task force also identified several unmet clinical needs in patients with chronic spontaneous urticaria [3].

The worldwide incidence is 0.1%–3% of the population with women affected twice more likely than men. It is estimated that about 1 in 5 people will have urticaria once in their lifetime and this seems to be the case across all age groups. Up to 1% of the population suffers from chronic urticaria (CU) and all age groups appear to be affected, although the peak incidence is between 20 and 40 years of age. In most cases, the disease lasts between 1 or 5 years, but the duration can be longer for those with severe urticaria, those with concurrent angioedema, those with the physical component, and those with a positive autologous serum skin test.

Although up to half of the patients with CIU have an IgG autoantibody directed against the alpha subunit of the high-affinity IgE receptor (FcεRlα) which is believed to be the pathophysiological basis of autoimmune urticaria, the role of antithyroid antibodies on persistent cutaneous mast cell and basophil activation remains unproven [5–9].

The role of the coagulation cascade (particularly the extrinsic pathway) is interesting as patients with severe disease have an increased thrombin generation; higher fragment F(1+2), D-dimer, and activated factor VII plasma levels, while increasing tissue factor reactivity in the skin. Takeda and colleagues showed that levels of fibrinogen, D-dimer, fibrin and fibrinogen degradation products were significantly raised in CU patients with a hypercoagulable state on APTT waveform analyses [10]. It is, therefore, not surprising that acute phase reactants like C-Reactive Protein (CRP) and procalcitonin levels are raised in patients with severe CU as compared to healthy controls or mild CU patients, including several other cytokines [11–24] and the soluble serum factor that leads to the release of histamine from basophils [25, 26]. Although histamine plays a significant role in diseases like CU and eczema, prostaglandins, leukotrienes (LTs), and cytokines such as IL-31 seem to prolong the inflammatory process.

## 3. Myths about Urticaria and Reality

*Myth 1.* Patients with urticaria have multiple allergies.

*Reality.* Most patients with urticaria do not have allergies, and patients who have positive specific IgE to allergens usually do not find any objective improvement on the avoidance of such allergens [27]. It is well accepted that a very high total IgE (usually a feature of atopy but also seen in some patients with urticaria) leads to low-level "false-positive" specific IgE results. Clinicians need to consider this before interpreting the results and advising patients to avoid multiple "triggers" for the urticaria. It is, therefore, not useful to do IgE levels in patients with only CU as it does not affect the management plan.

*Myth 2.* Patients with urticaria should be given an extensive list of foods that must be avoided.

*Reality.* Our collective experience has shown that patients are often asked by nonspecialists to avoid egg, milk, brinjal, spinach, prawn, and fish as these are the "triggers" for urticaria. Strict avoidance has little or no effect on the frequency of urticarial eruptions. There are some foods that do, however, have or can release more histamine and clinical advice often entails educating patients to avoid eating most of the foods that are high in histamine during acute urticarial eruptions until the "episode" settles down. Skin prick testing to these foods in patients with chronic urticaria does not show any wheal or flare response suggesting the absence of a specific IgE or the supposed "trigger" factor(s).

A small cohort of paediatric patients with CU underwent skin testing to foods that were being avoided based on ELISA allergy results at one centre (further details with Dr. Sujoy Khan, Apollo GleneaglesHospital, Kolkata). None of the 30 children with CU (mean (±SD) age was 10.9 (±4.2) years, 13 males and 17 females) demonstrated skin test reactivity to milk, egg white, egg yolk, prawn, brinjal, and spinach which were the foods on the exclusion list. All patients were able to resume a normal diet on high dose antihistamines that controlled the urticaria.

In selected patients with supportive histories, presence of IgE to specific foods or sensitivity (non-IgE mediated reactions) to certain dyes or coloring agents in food (pseudo allergies) could have a relevance to their chronic urticaria symptoms, but careful elimination and reintroduction are needed to establish the same [28].

*Myth 3.* Patients with urticaria should undergo testing to exclude specific allergies.

*Reality.* Whilst the concurrent presence of house dust mite (*D. pteronyssinus, D. farinae,* and *Blomia sp.*) allergy or other aeroallergen sensitivities can be found in some patients [27, 29–31], these tests should be reserved for patients who complain of allergic rhinitis symptoms that occur without urticaria.

In view of this perception that allergy testing is mandatory, another observational study at one centre on 43 consecutive patients with chronic urticaria (dermographism, autoimmune thyroiditis excluded) with skin prick testing to aeroallergens was carried out (further details with Dr. Sujoy Khan, Apollo Gleneagles Hospital, Kolkata). Skin prick tests (SPT) were done after a 7-day antihistamine free period to house dust mites (*Dermatophagoides pteronyssinus, Dermatophagoides farinae,* and *Blomia tropicalis*), cockroach, pollens, moulds, and animal dander in all patients. Positive control was histamine (10 mg/mL) and positive SPT was defined as >3 mm than the negative control (saline).

Nonparametric statistical data were calculated using the GraphPad Prism software Version 5.04 (GraphPad Software, Inc., La Jolla, CA, USA). Fisher's exact test was used to see the relationship between CIU, mite reactivity status, and with/without respiratory symptoms (allergic rhinitis, asthma).

The mean (±SD) age was 33.28 (±14.97) years that included 23 males and 20 females. Range of duration of the symptoms of CIU was 6 months to 13 years. SPT demonstrated immediate reactivity to dust mite in 24 patients (55.8%), cockroach 6 (14%), pollens 8 (18.5%), moulds 5 (11.6%), and dander 0 (0%). Five patients were polysensitized (dust mites, cockroach, pollens, or moulds). The mean (±SD) age of patients with CIU and mite allergy was 31.1 (±14.7) years compared to 36.1 (±15.2) years in CIU patients without mite allergy (nonsignificant, 2-tailed $t$-test 0.2849). Among mite positive patients with CIU, there was a slight female predominance (13 females, 11 males) that was statistically nonsignificant ($P = 0.3586$). However, 16 CIU patients with respiratory symptoms had dust mite reactivity as compared to 3 CIU patients with respiratory symptoms but without mite reactivity (highly significant, $P = 0.0016$).

We conclude from this study that house dust mite reactivity in CIU is linked with respiratory allergy. Avoidance of these allergens will, therefore, have little effect on urticaria, except in a few cases where there is a strong consistent history of contact urticaria on exposure to dust, but antihistamine and nasal spray treatment will have an effect on the rhinitis and will encourage the patient to continue on antihistamines

that will control the urticaria. Routine skin prick testing or specific IgE allergy tests when no trigger is identified on history taking cannot be recommended. Again, in some highly atopic individuals, allergens such as grass pollens, molds, animal dander, house dust mites, and latex might aggravate chronic urticaria but this is usually not the primary cause for the urticaria.

*Myth 4.* Patients should not receive high doses of antihistamine medications and definitely not in pregnancy.

*Reality.* Almost all physicians dealing with CIU patients recognize that standard or recommended doses of antihistamines are ineffective in treating this condition. Consensus guidelines do take this seriously and specifically comment that higher doses, even up to four fold higher, are safe and have been verified in studies [1–6]. This is true for all classes of antihistamines such as desloratidine, levocetirizine, fexofenadine, and even antiplatelet activating factor blocker rupatadine. First generation antihistamines should preferably be avoided in infants and children as well as adults especially those dealing with heavy machinery or engaged in skilled tasks such as driving. At least two long-term studies on healthy volunteers have shown that fexofenadine at 240 mg once daily for a year is safe, well tolerated, and does not lead to sedation at these supratherapeutic doses [32, 33]. Cetirizine and levocetirizine have sedative effects in therapeutic and supratherapeutic doses, and it is, therefore, best to check with the patient whether sedation has been a problem in the past.

The EAACI/GA$^2$LEN/EDF/WAO consensus guidelines mention that loratidine and possibly desloratidine are safe in pregnancy but supratherapeutic doses should be carefully considered. The product literature of fexofenadine HCl (Sanofi, Aventis Pharma Ltd., CDS version 5 dated Nov 2006) does not mention pregnancy as a contraindication to its use, other than to use it if the benefit outweighs the potential risks. Cetirizine, loratidine, and hydroxyzine have been shown to be safe in pregnancy with no difference in spontaneous or therapeutic abortions, birth weight, mode of delivery, gestational age, and rate of live births, neonatal distress, and major fetal congenital malformations [34, 35].

## 4. Quality of Life

It is now well recognized that patients with CU have a poor quality of life (QoL) (see Table 1, [36–42]). Although not specifically addressed in some studies, the "uncertainty" factor of appearance of skin lesions, especially in social gatherings or workplace, plays an important role in affecting the QoL. Several other issues related to poor QoL would include cost of therapy, fatigue associated with use of antihistamines, and inability to explain the skin lesions that may add to social isolation including frustration in dealing with the chronic condition.

Several tools are available for assessment of impairment of QoL in patients affected by chronic diseases. QoL studies on patients with psoriasis enabled healthcare providers to understand that there were several areas that required attention apart from simply controlling the disease with multiple

TABLE 1: Quality of life (QoL) studies in patients with chronic urticarial.

| Study design, place | Methods used | Outcome | Reference |
|---|---|---|---|
| Questionnaire based study on 170 consecutive patients, London (UK) | Dermatology life quality index (DLQI) assessment in different urticarial groups | Moderate impairment in QoL in CU with physical urticaria; significantly higher impairment in patients with DPU and cholinergic urticaria (QoL affected areas: work/study, symptoms/feelings, leisure) | [37] |
| Interview/questionnaire-based study on 100 in-patients (96 age- and sex-matched controls), University of Mainz (Germany) | Assessed using Skindex-29 on overall QoL and three defined QoL aspects | CU patients had a markedly reduced QoL compared to controls, all 3 areas affected, psychiatric comorbidity was made worse | [39] |
| Questionnaire based study on 157 CU patients, Berlin (Germany) | CU-QoL, DLQI, and Skindex-29 questionnaires were completed | 70% data variance in CU-QoL in functioning, sleep, itching/embarrassment, mental status, swelling/eating, and appearance; sleep and mental health significant areas are affected and women are more affected by pruritis | [41] |
| Mental disorder assessment on 100 patients, University Medical Center Mainz (Germany) | Specialised diagnostic interviews and psychometric instruments and SCL-90R GSI | 48% of patients had one or more psychosomatic disorders; high emotional stress impairing quality of life | [42] |
| Cross-sectional observational study ($n = 249$), Suwon (Korea) | CU-QoL and UAS; multiple linear regression for CU-QoL predictors | DPU, sunlight exposure, and emotional stress significantly influenced the overall CU-QoL scores (univariate analysis); multivariate regression models indicated that dermatographism and emotional stress were significant predictors of impairment of all four QoL domains | [40] |

Abbreviations: QoL: quality of life, CU-QoL: chronic urticaria-quality of life, DLQI: dermatology life quality index, DPU: delayed pressure urticarial, and SCL-90R GSI.

medications. Staubach and colleagues in an interdisciplinary interview/questionnaire-based study on 100 CU patients found that significantly low quality of life (functioning and emotions) and psychiatric comorbidity (depression, anxiety, somatoform disorders) made this worse even in those without a formal psychiatric diagnosis [39]. In another study by the same group and of 100 patients with CU who were formally assessed for psychiatric illnesses, nearly half (48%) of the patients had one or more psychosomatic disorders, of which anxiety disorders were predominant followed by depressive and somatoform disorders [42]. As the authors rightly concluded, patients with CSU frequently experience anxiety, depression, and somatoform disorders, that with time become inextricably linked to an increased emotional distress.

Studies on fexofenadine-treated patients (180 mg) have shown significantly greater improvements in mean dermatology life quality index (DLQI) total score than those treated with placebo. These were not only seen in areas such as symptoms and feelings, activities of daily living including less impairment while working, leisure, and personal relationships but also greater improvement in Urticaria Activity Score (wheals and pruritis) when compared with placebo.

Indeed it is interesting that while this disease itself causes distress, chronic urticaria is also recognized as a stress-vulnerable disease in which psychological stressors can trigger or increase itching. It is suggested that effective management processes should take into account the psychological factors in some of the patients and the treatment

regimen should be tailored to the individual patient's needs and circumstances [36, 38, 39, 42].

## 5. Treatment Options

The consensus guidelines have adopted the management of urticaria into (1) avoidance measures and (2) pharmacotherapy nonspecific and specific. The avoidance approach outlines elimination or treatment of eliciting stimulus or cause (such as nonsteroidal anti-inflammatory drug-induced urticaria/angioedema, physical causes, treatment of an infectious trigger, etc.) that is not possible in all cases (i.e., those with CIU) [1–6]. In line with this "infectious trigger," the approach that is gaining relevance is the consideration of *Helicobacter pylori* induced gastritis and urticaria, and several reports of long-lasting remission of urticaria can be seen in patients after eradication therapy [43–47].

The second approach is lowering or inhibiting mast cell mediator release and the most commonly used drugs (nonspecific approach) that inhibit mast cell release are corticosteroids. Continuous or prolonged use with corticosteroids to treat urticaria is not recommended as the risks and long-term side effects outweigh the benefits. Specific treatment approaches involve the use of nonsedating long-acting antihistamine (anti-H1) drugs such as cetirizine, levocetirizine, loratadine, desloratadine, and fexofenadine that provide both antiallergic and anti-inflammatory effects, such as inhibition of cytokines release from basophiles and

TABLE 2: Overview of medications available in India for urticaria and angioedema.

| Type | Generic name | Availability | Price CIMS India[*] |
|---|---|---|---|
| Antihistamine H1 | Cetirizine | Widely available (41 brands) | Re[$] 1/tablet to Rs 4.75/tab |
| Antihistamine H1 | Chlorphenamine | Widely available (17 brands) | 4 mg (500 tablets) from Rs 25.79 to Rs 29.12; Syrup (0.5 mg/5 mL) 60 mL at Rs 23.80 |
| Antihistamine H1 | Desloratadine | Widely available (11 brands) | Rs 1.99/tablet to Rs 5.50/tablet |
| Antihistamine H1 | Fexofenadine | Widely available (11 brands) | 30 mg 10 tablets for Rs 31.00 120 mg 10 tabs from Rs 40 to Rs 99.15 180 mg 10 tabs from Rs 60 to Rs 111.80 |
| Antihistamine H1 | Hydroxyzine | Widely available (4 brands) | 10 mg 10 tablets for Rs 9.00 25 mg 10 tablets from Rs 16.00 to Rs 23.00 Syrup (10 mg/5 mL) 100 mL at Rs 40.18 |
| Antihistamine H1 | Levocetirizine | Widely available (60 brands) | 5 mg 10 tablets from Rs 8.90 to 55.32 Syrup (2.5 mg/5 mL) 30 mL from Rs 18.90 to Rs 29.00 |
| Antihistamine H1 | Loratidine | Widely available (6 brands) | 10 mg 10 tablets from Rs 19.50 to Rs 150.00 Syrup (5 mg/5 mL) 30 mL for Rs 46.00 Suspension 1 mg 30 mL for Rs 17.85 |
| Leukotriene receptor antagonist (LTRA) | Montelukast Zafirlukast | Montelukast is widely available (14 brands) Zafirlukast is not available | 4 mg 10 tablets from Rs 62.50 to 89.00 5 mg 10 tablets from Rs 70 to 98.00 10 mg 10 tablets from Rs 83.20 to 149 Sachet 4 mg 1 sachet costs Rs 5.85 |
| Combinations anti-H1 + LTRA | Levocetirizine 5 mg + Montelukast 4/5/10 mg | Widely available (16 brands) | Rs 5.90 to Rs 16/tablet (adult) Rs 3.80 to Rs 6.30/tablet (kid) |
| Combinations anti-H1 + LTRA | Fexofenadine 120 mg + Montelukast 4/10 mg | Limited to no availability in smaller cities | 10 tablets for Rs 125.00 |
| Anti-PAF | Rupatadine 10 mg | Limited availability (3 brands) | 10 mg tablets Rs 5-6/tablet |
| Combinations anti-PAF + LTRA | Rupatadine 10 mg + Montelukast 10 mg | Limited availability | 10 tablets for Rs 84.60 (Rs 8.46/tablet) |
| Immunosuppressant | Hydroxychloroquine | Widely available | 200 mg tablets 10 from Rs 59 to Rs 80 |
| Immunosuppressant | Methotrexate | Widely available | 2.5 mg tablets 10 from Rs 15.00 to 57.85 |
| Immunosuppressant | Cyclosporin | Widely available | 25 mg tablets from Rs 21.60–32.60/tab 50 mg tablets from Rs 43.20–65.20/tab 100 mg tablets from Rs 82.60–130.40/tab |
| Anti-IgE | Omalizumab (Xolair, Novartis) | Very limited availability, expensive, and available through select Central Govtenment Health Schemes at reduced costs in India | 150 mg injection, frequency, and dose calculated on body weight and IgE level is £256.15 + VAT per vial (NHS, UK) or US$10,000/year (1-2 injections/month) |

[*]Ref: CIMS 115 Oct 2011 (Update-4); costs of the last 4 of 5 drugs were obtained from Medline India.
[$]Indian currency in Rupees (Rs), exchange rate Rs 56.83 = 1 US$ (as on 6 June, 2013).
Abbreviations: PAF: platelet activating factor, LTRA: leukotriene receptor antagonist, IgE: immunoglobulin E, and NHS: national health service.

mast cells as well as reduction of chemotactic activity of eosinophils. Doxepin, a tricyclic antidepressant, is the only agent that blocks both H1- and H2-receptors, and can be useful in the selected patients who experience significant psychosomatic symptoms of depression and anxiety due to the urticaria.

Table 2 provides a list (not comprehensive) of antihistamine medications available in India, including combination formulations that may not be suitable in all patients although they may prove to be cost-effective.

Montelukast is an orally active leukotriene receptor antagonist (LTRA) licensed the maintenance treatment of asthma and to relieve symptoms of seasonal allergies. Montelukast binds to and blocks the action of leukotriene D4 (LTD4) on the cysteinyl-leukotriene receptor CysLT1 in the lungs, with almost no interaction with other antiallergy drugs. This reduces the bronchoconstrictive and inflammatory effects of LTD4 in the airways. Other LTs such as LTC4, LTD4, and LTE4 have important roles in the pathophysiologic mechanisms of allergic inflammation after binding to activating receptors, cystenyl-LT1 (CysLT1) receptor and Cys-LT2 receptor. Hence, LTRAs such as montelukast 10 mg once daily or zafirleukast 20 mg twice daily has been employed either as monotherapy or in combination with H1-receptor and/or H2-receptor antagonists, to treat different forms of CU, including cold urticaria, urticaria related to food additives, chronic autoimmune urticaria, steroid-dependent urticaria, and delayed-pressure urticaria, and CIU and dermographism with varying results [48–54]. Our report on montelukast as an added therapy to anti-H1 and anti-H2 blockers showed that it was effective in controlling the urticaria in about 50% of the patients (UK based study). However, we were unable to delineate any specific clinical features (such as age, gender, duration, or severity of urticaria) or laboratory features (such as thyroid autoimmunity, antinuclear antibody positivity, or basophil histamine release potential) that could predict a response to montelukast [54].

Other treatment options that have significant activity on mediator release on basophils include the calcineurin inhibitor cyclosporin A [55–60], and occasionally ultraviolet therapy [59–62]. As for immunosuppressive therapy with cyclosporin, a recent study suggests that history of hives, shorter duration of urticaria (mean of 55.2 weeks versus 259.6 weeks, $P = 0.03$), and CU index >10 ($P = 0.05$) predict a favorable response to cyclosporin [60].

The most specific and promising therapy for the future appears to be anti-IgE therapy, Omalizumab (Xolair, Novartis) [63–66]. A typical dose of 150 mg every 2nd/4th week or 300 mg/month for 4–6 doses can have lasting efficacy of up to 15 months with significant improvement in QoL [65–67]. The significant downside is the high cost associated with the treatment (1-2 subcutaneous injections/month at US $10,000/year) and its yet unknown side effects with regard to parasitic infectious disease burden with its use in India or Asia [68–70].

## 6. Conclusions

1. Chronic urticaria is a relatively common condition in India and most cases have no specific allergic trigger and remain idiopathic.

2. Autoimmune causes have been found to be associated with up to 30-40% cases.

3. It is important to look for physical urticarias such as pressure urticaria in chronic cases.

4. Avoidance of foods without appropriate testing for food allergy should not be routinely recommended.

5. Long-acting nonsedating antihistamines at even higher than standard doses if necessary are safe and effective.

6. Quality of life is affected adversely in many patients with chronic urticaria.

7. Psychological stressors can play an important role in this disease and require special attention.

## Conflict of Interests

Sujoy Khan, Anirban Maitra, Pravin Hissaria, Sitesh Roy, Mahesh PA, Nalin Nag have declared that they have no relevant conflict of interests. Harpal Singh is the Medical Advisor and Clinical Marketing Manager for Phadia India/IDD Thermo Fisher Scientific, the company that pioneered the ImmunoCAP technology for in-vitro allergy diagnostics.

## Acknowledgments

All authors in this paper are part of GGAPI (Group for Guidelines for Allergy Practice in India) and we are grateful to other Consultants of GGAPI for their help with the paper. GGAPI is in the final stages of being registered under Indian Societies Registration Act, XXI of 1860.

## References

[1] T. Zuberbier, R. Asero, C. Bindslev-Jensen et al., "EAACI/GA$^2$LEN/EDF/WAO guideline: definition, classification and diagnosis of urticaria," *Allergy*, vol. 64, no. 10, pp. 1417–1426, 2009.

[2] T. Zuberbier, R. Asero, C. Bindslev-Jensen et al., "EAACI/GA$^2$LEN/EDF/WAO guideline: management of urticaria," *Allergy*, vol. 64, pp. 1427–1443, 2009.

[3] M. Maurer, K. Weller, C. Bindslev-Jensen et al., "Unmet clinical needs in chronic spontaneous urticaria. A GA$^2$LEN task force report," *Allergy*, vol. 66, no. 3, pp. 317–330, 2011.

[4] L. Fromer, "Treatment options for the relief of chronic idiopathic urticaria symptoms," *Southern Medical Journal*, vol. 101, no. 2, pp. 186–192, 2008.

[5] K. Godse, V. Zawar, D. Krupashankar et al., "Consensus statement on the management of urticaria," *Indian Journal of Dermatology*, vol. 56, no. 5, pp. 485–489, 2011.

[6] G. N. Konstantinou, R. Asero, M. Ferrer et al., "EAACI task-force position paper: evidence for autoimmune urticaria and proposal for defining diagnostic criteria," *Allergy*, vol. 68, pp. 27–36, 2013.

[7] S. Pastore, I. Berti, and G. Longo, "Autoimmune chronic urticaria: transferability of autologous serum skin test," *European Journal of Pediatrics*, vol. 172, p. 569, 2013.

[8] L. Brunetti, R. Francavilla, V. L. Miniello et al., "High prevalence of autoimmune urticaria in children with chronic urticaria," *Journal of Allergy and Clinical Immunology*, vol. 114, no. 4, pp. 922–927, 2004.

[9] K. S. Wan and C. S. Wu, "The essential role of anti-thyroid antibodies in chronic idiopathic urticaria," *Endocrine Research*, vol. 38, pp. 85–88, 2013.

[10] T. Takeda, Y. Sakurai, S. Takahagi et al., "Increase of coagulation potential in chronic spontaneous urticaria," *Allergy*, vol. 66, no. 3, pp. 428–433, 2011.

[11] Z. Huilan, L. Runxiang, L. Bihua, and G. Qing, "Role of the subgroups of T, B, natural killer lymphocyte and serum levels of interleukin-15, interleukin-21 and immunoglobulin e in the pathogenesis of urticaria," *Journal of Dermatology*, vol. 37, no. 5, pp. 441–447, 2010.

[12] U. Raap, D. Wieczorek, M. Gehring et al., "Increased levels of serum IL-31 in chronic spontaneous urticaria," *Experimental Dermatology*, vol. 19, no. 5, pp. 464–466, 2010.

[13] A. Lopes, D. Machado, S. Pedreiro et al., "Different frequencies of tc17/tc1 and th17/th1 cells in chronic spontaneous urticaria," *International Archives of Allergy and Immunology*, vol. 161, pp. 155–162, 2013.

[14] J. C. dos Santos, M. H. Azor, V. Y. Nojima et al., "Increased circulating pro-inflammatory cytokines and imbalanced regulatory T-cell cytokines production in chronic idiopathic urticaria," *International Immunopharmacology*, vol. 8, no. 10, pp. 1433–1440, 2008.

[15] W.-C. Chen, B.-L. Chiang, H. E. Liu, S.-J. Leu, and Y.-L. Lee, "Defective functions of circulating CD4$^+$CD25$^+$ and CD4$^+$CD25$^-$ T cells in patients with chronic ordinary urticaria," *Journal of Dermatological Science*, vol. 51, no. 2, pp. 121–130, 2008.

[16] F. D. Lourenço, M. H. Azor, J. C. Santos et al., "Activated status of basophils in chronic urticaria leads to interleukin-3 hyper-responsiveness and enhancement of histamine release induced by anti-IgE stimulus," *British Journal of Dermatology*, vol. 158, no. 5, pp. 979–986, 2008.

[17] M. Caproni, B. Giomi, L. Melani et al., "Cellular infiltrate and related cytokines, chemokines, chemokine receptors and adhesion molecules in chronic autoimmune urticaria: comparison between spontaneous and autologous serum skin test induced wheal," *International Journal of Immunopathology and Pharmacology*, vol. 19, no. 3, pp. 507–515, 2006.

[18] A. Puccetti, C. Bason, S. Simeoni et al., "In chronic idiopathic urticaria autoantibodies against FcεRII/CD23 induce histamine release via eosinophil activation," *Clinical and Experimental Allergy*, vol. 35, no. 12, pp. 1599–1607, 2005.

[19] A. Kasperska-Zajac, Z. Brzoza, and B. Rogala, "Increased concentration of platelet-derived chemokinesin serum of patients with delayed pressure urticaria," *European Cytokine Network*, vol. 19, no. 2, pp. 89–91, 2008.

[20] M. Caproni, B. Giomi, W. Volpi et al., "Chronic idiopathic urticaria: infiltrating cells and related cytokines in autologous serum-induced wheals," *Clinical Immunology*, vol. 114, no. 3, pp. 284–292, 2005.

[21] M. Caproni, C. Cardinali, B. Giomi et al., "Serological detection of eotaxin, IL-4, IL-13, IFN-γ, MIP-1α, TARC and IP-10 in chronic autoimmune urticaria and chronic idiopathic urticaria," *Journal of Dermatological Science*, vol. 36, no. 1, pp. 57–59, 2004.

[22] J. C. Santos, C. A. de Brito, E. A. Futata et al., "Up-regulation of chemokine C-C ligand 2 (CCL2) and C-X-C chemokine 8 (CXCL8) expression by monocytes in chronic idiopathic urticaria," *Clinical and Experimental Immunology*, vol. 167, no. 1, pp. 129–136, 2012.

[23] F. Bossi, B. Frossi, O. Radillo et al., "Mast cells are critically involved in serum-mediated vascular leakage in chronic urticaria beyond high-affinity IgE receptor stimulation," *Allergy*, vol. 66, no. 12, pp. 1538–1545, 2011.

[24] M. Ferrer, J. M. Nuñez-Córdoba, E. Luquin et al., "Serum total tryptase levels are increased in patients with active chronic urticaria," *Clinical and Experimental Allergy*, vol. 40, no. 12, pp. 1760–1766, 2010.

[25] J.-I. Kashiwakura, T. Ando, K. Matsumoto et al., "Histamine-releasing factor has a proinflammatory role in mouse models of asthma and allergy," *Journal of Clinical Investigation*, vol. 122, no. 1, pp. 218–228, 2012.

[26] R. Asero, M. Lorini, S. U. Chong, T. Zuberbier, and A. Tedeschi, "Assessment of histamine-releasing activity of sera from patients with chronic urticaria showing positive autologous skin test on human basophils and mast cells," *Clinical & Experimental Allergy*, vol. 34, pp. 1111–1114, 2004.

[27] K.-L. Chang, Y.-H. Yang, H.-H. Yu, J.-H. Lee, L.-C. Wang, and B.-L. Chiang, "Analysis of serum total IgE, specific IgE and eosinophils in children with acute and chronic urticaria," *Journal of Microbiology, Immunology and Infection*, vol. 46, no. 1, pp. 53–58, 2013.

[28] T. Zuberbier, "The role of allergens and pseudoallergens in urticaria," *Journal of Investigative Dermatology Symposium Proceedings*, vol. 6, no. 2, pp. 132–134, 2001.

[29] K. Kulthanan and C. Wachirakahan, "Prevalence and clinical characteristics of chronic urticaria and positive skin prick testing to mites," *Acta Dermato-Venereologica*, vol. 88, no. 6, pp. 584–588, 2008.

[30] P. A. Mahesh, P. A. Kushalappa, A. D. Holla, and P. K. Vedanthan, "House dust mite sensitivity is a factor in chronic urticaria," *Indian Journal of Dermatology, Venereology and Leprology*, vol. 71, no. 2, pp. 99–101, 2005.

[31] Z. Caliskaner, S. Ozturk, M. Turan, and M. Karaayvaz, "Skin test positivity to aeroallergens in the patients with chronic urticaria without allergic respiratory disease," *Journal of Investigational Allergology and Clinical Immunology*, vol. 14, no. 1, pp. 50–54, 2004.

[32] A. F. Finn Jr., A. P. Kaplan, R. Fretwell, R. Qu, and J. Long, "A double-blind, placebo-controlled trial of fexofenadine HCl in the treatment of chronic idiopathic urticaria," *Journal of Allergy and Clinical Immunology*, vol. 104, no. 5, pp. 1071–1078, 1999.

[33] H. S. Nelson, R. Reynolds, and J. Mason, "Fexofenadine HCl is safe and effective for treatment of chronic idiopathic urticaria," *Annals of Allergy, Asthma and Immunology*, vol. 84, no. 5, pp. 517–522, 2000.

[34] C. Weber-Schoendorfer and C. Schaefer, "The safety of cetirizine during pregnancy. A prospective observational cohort study," *Reproductive Toxicology*, vol. 26, no. 1, pp. 19–23, 2008.

[35] M. S. Blaiss and ACAAI-ACOG(American College of Allergy, Asthma, and Immunology and American College of Obstetricians and Gynecologists), "Management of rhinitis and asthma in pregnancy," *Annals of Allergy, Asthma and Immunology*, vol. 90, pp. 16–22, 2003.

[36] D. R. Weldon, "Quality of life in patients with urticaria," *Allergy and Asthma Proceedings*, vol. 27, no. 2, pp. 96–99, 2006.

[37] E. Poon, P. T. Seed, M. W. Greaves, and A. Kobza-Black, "The extent and nature of disability in different urticarial conditions," *British Journal of Dermatology*, vol. 140, no. 4, pp. 667–671, 1999.

[38] J.-J. Grob and C. Gaudy-Marqueste, "Urticaria and quality of life," *Clinical Reviews in Allergy and Immunology*, vol. 30, no. 1, pp. 47–51, 2006.

[39] P. Staubach, A. Eckhardt-Henn, M. Dechene et al., "Quality of life in patients with chronic urticaria is differentially impaired and determined by psychiatric comorbidity," *British Journal of Dermatology*, vol. 154, no. 2, pp. 294–298, 2006.

[40] Y. M. Ye, J. W. Park, S. H. Kim et al., "Clinical evaluation of the computerized chronic urticaria-specific quality of life questionnaire in Korean patients with chronic urticaria," *Clinical and Experimental Dermatology*, vol. 37, pp. 722–728, 2012.

[41] A. Młynek, M. Magerl, M. Hanna et al., "The German version of the chronic urticaria quality-of-life questionnaire: factor analysis, validation, and initial clinical findings," *Allergy*, vol. 64, no. 6, pp. 927–936, 2009.

[42] P. Staubach, M. Dechene, M. Metz et al., "High prevalence of mental disorders and emotional distress in patients with chronic spontaneous urticaria," *Acta Dermato-Venereologica*, vol. 91, no. 5, pp. 557–561, 2011.

[43] S. Fukuda, T. Shimoyama, N. Umegaki, T. Mikami, H. Nakano, and A. Munakata, "Effect of Helicobacter pylori eradication in the treatment of Japanese patients with chronic idiopathic urticaria," *Journal of Gastroenterology*, vol. 39, no. 9, pp. 827–830, 2004.

[44] M. K. Yadav, J. P. Rishi, and S. Nijawan, "Chronic urticaria and *Helicobacter pylori*," *Indian Journal of Medical Sciences*, vol. 62, no. 4, pp. 157–162, 2008.

[45] E. Magen, J. Mishal, M. Schlesinger, and S. Scharf, "Eradication of *Helicobacter pylori* infection equally improves chronic urticaria with positive and negative autologous serum skin test," *Helicobacter*, vol. 12, no. 5, pp. 567–571, 2007.

[46] A. Campanati, R. Gesuita, M. Giannoni et al., "Role of small intestinal bacterial overgrowth and *Helicobacter pylori* infection in chronic spontaneous urticaria: a prospective analysis," *Acta Dermato-Venereologica*, vol. 93, pp. 161–164, 2013.

[47] G. W. Scadding and G. K. Scadding, "Recent advances in antileukotriene therapy," *Current Opinion in Allergy and Clinical Immunology*, vol. 10, no. 4, pp. 370–376, 2010.

[48] B. J. Lipworth, "Leukotriene-receptor antagonists," *The Lancet*, vol. 353, no. 9146, pp. 57–62, 1999.

[49] G. E. Rovati and V. Capra, "Cysteinyl-leukotriene receptors and cellular signals," *The Scientific World Journal*, vol. 7, pp. 1375–1392, 2007.

[50] Z. Erbagci, "The leukotriene receptor antagonist montelukast in the treatment of chronic idiopathic urticaria: a single-blind, placebo-controlled, crossover clinical study," *Journal of Allergy and Clinical Immunology*, vol. 110, no. 3, pp. 484–488, 2002.

[51] M. Kosnik and T. Subic, "Add-on montelukast in antihistamine-resistant chronic idiopathic urticaria," *Respiratory Medicine*, vol. 105, no. 1, pp. S84–S88, 2011.

[52] K.-S. Wan, "Efficacy of leukotriene receptor antagonist with an anti-H1 receptor antagonist for treatment of chronic idiopathic urticaria," *Journal of Dermatological Treatment*, vol. 20, no. 4, pp. 194–197, 2009.

[53] G. di Lorenzo, A. D'Alcamo, M. Rizzo et al., "Leukotriene receptor antagonists in monotherapy or in combination with antihistamines in the treatment of chronic urticaria: a systematic review," *Journal of Asthma and Allergy*, no. 2, pp. 9–16, 2009.

[54] S. Khan and N. Lynch, "Efficacy of montelukast as added therapy in patients with chronic idiopathic urticaria," *Inflammation and Allergy*, vol. 11, no. 3, pp. 235–243, 2012.

[55] E. di Leo, E. Nettis, A. M. Aloia et al., "Cyclosporin-A efficacy in chronic idiopathic urticaria," *International Journal of Immunopathology and Pharmacology*, vol. 24, no. 1, pp. 195–200, 2011.

[56] C. Boubouka, C. Charissi, D. Kouimintzis, D. Kalogeromitros, P. Stavropoulos, and A. Katsarou, "Treatment of autoimmune urticaria with low-dose cyclosporin a: a one-year follow-up," *Acta Dermato-Venereologica*, vol. 91, no. 1, pp. 50–54, 2011.

[57] A. Kessel and E. Toubi, "Cyclosporine-A in severe chronic urticaria: the option for long-term therapy," *Allergy*, vol. 65, no. 11, pp. 1478–1482, 2010.

[58] H. Serhat Inaloz, S. Ozturk, C. Akcali, N. Kirtak, and M. Tarakcioglu, "Low-dose and short-term cyclosporine treatment in patients with chronic idiopathic urticaria: a clinical and immunological evaluation," *Journal of Dermatology*, vol. 35, no. 5, pp. 276–282, 2008.

[59] K. V. Godse, "Cyclosporine in chronic idiopathic urticaria with positive autologous serum skin test," *Indian Journal of Dermatology*, vol. 53, no. 2, pp. 101–102, 2008.

[60] S. M. Hollander, S. S. Joo, and H. J. Wedner, "Factors that predict the success of cyclosporine treatment for chronic urticaria," *Annals of Allergy, Asthma and Immunology*, vol. 107, no. 6, pp. 523–528, 2011.

[61] S. Darras, M. Ségard, L. Mortier, A. Bonnevalle, and P. Thomas, "Treatment of solar urticaria by intravenous immunoglobulins and PUVAtherapy," *Annales de Dermatologie et de Venereologie*, vol. 131, no. 1, pp. 65–69, 2004.

[62] K. Aydogan, S. K. Karadogan, S. Tunali, and H. Saricaoglu, "Narrowband ultraviolet B (311nm, TL01) phototherapy in chronic ordinary urticaria," *International Journal of Dermatology*, vol. 51, no. 1, pp. 98–103, 2012.

[63] B. Engin, M. Özdemir, A. Balevi, and I. Mevlitoğlu, "Treatment of chronic urticaria with narrowband ultraviolet B phototherapy: a randomized controlled trial," *Acta Dermato-Venereologica*, vol. 88, no. 3, pp. 247–251, 2008.

[64] G. Monfrecola, A. de Paulis, E. Prizio et al., "In vitro effects of ultraviolet A on histamine release from human basophils," *Journal of the European Academy of Dermatology and Venereology*, vol. 17, no. 6, pp. 646–651, 2003.

[65] A. C. Lefévre, M. Deleuran, and C. A. Vestergaard, "A long term case series study of the effect of omalizumab on chronic spontaneous urticaria," *Annals of Dermatology*, vol. 25, pp. 242–245, 2013.

[66] M. Maurer, K. Rosén, H. J. Hsieh et al., "Omalizumab for the treatment of chronic idiopathic or spontaneous urticaria." *The New England Journal of Medicine*, vol. 368, pp. 924–935, 2013.

[67] C. H. Song, S. Stern, M. Giruparajah, N. Berlin, and G. L. Sussman, "Long-term efficacy of fixed-dose omalizumab for patients with severe chronic spontaneous urticaria," *Annals of Allergy, Asthma & Immunology*, vol. 110, pp. 113–117, 2013.

[68] L. S. Cox, "How safe are the biologicals in treating asthma and rhinitis?" *Allergy, Asthma and Clinical Immunology*, vol. 5, no. 4, article 4, 2009.

[69] P. J. Cooper, G. Ayre, C. Martin, J. A. Rizzo, E. V. Ponte, and A. A. Cruz, "Geohelminth infections: a review of the role of IgE and assessment of potential risks of anti-IgE treatment," *Allergy*, vol. 63, no. 4, pp. 409–417, 2008.

[70] S. K. Chow, "Management of chronic urticaria in Asia: 2010 AADV consensus guidelines," *Asia Pacific Allergy*, vol. 2, pp. 149–160, 2012.

# 36

# Health-Care Delay in Malignant Melanoma: Various Pathways to Diagnosis and Treatment

**Senada Hajdarevic,[1] Åsa Hörnsten,[1] Elisabet Sundbom,[2] Ulf Isaksson,[1] and Marcus Schmitt-Egenolf[3]**

[1] Department of Nursing, Umeå University, Umeå, Sweden
[2] Department of Clinical Sciences, Division of Psychiatry and Medical Psychology, Umeå University, Umeå, Sweden
[3] Department of Public Health and Clinical Medicine, Dermatology and Venereology, Umeå University, Umeå, Sweden

Correspondence should be addressed to Senada Hajdarevic; senada.hajdarevic@nurs.umu.se

Academic Editor: Giuseppe Argenziano

We aimed to describe and compare patients diagnosed with malignant melanoma (MM), depending on their initial contact with care and with regard to age, sex, and MM type and thickness, and to explore pathways and time intervals (lead times) between clinics from the initial contact to diagnosis and treatment. The sample from northern Sweden was identified via the Swedish melanoma register. Data regarding pathways in health care were retrieved from patient records. In our unselected population of 71 people diagnosed with skin melanoma of SSM and NM types, 75% of patients were primarily treated by primary health-care centres (PHCs). The time interval (delay) from primary excision until registration of the histopathological assessment in the medical records was significantly longer in PHCs than in hospital-based and dermatological clinics (Derm). Thicker tumors were more common in the PHC group. Older patients waited longer times for wide excision. Most MM are excised rapidly at PHCs, but some patients may not be diagnosed and treated in time. Delay of registration of results from histopathological assessments within PHCs seems to be an important issue for future improvement. Exploring shortcomings in MM patients' clinical pathways is important to improve the quality of care and patient safety.

## 1. Introduction

Malignant melanoma (MM) incidence is increasing globally, and Sweden is among the top 10 countries in the world with regard to incidence [1]. During the last decade, MM has become the sixth most common form of cancer in Sweden [2]. MM is a skin cancer with fatal outcome, if not diagnosed and treated in time [3]. A critical point in the development of MM is the penetration of the dermal-epidermal basement membrane, which highly increases the risk for metastases [4]. The optimal way to cure MM is therefore early detection and excision. The reduction of both patient and doctor's delay is of key importance for early diagnosis and clinical outcome of MM.

One reason for delayed diagnosis relates to patients' care-seeking patterns for suspected MM [5]. A review of the literature concerning patient delay highlights health beliefs, low sense of severity, and susceptibility related to melanoma as reasons for delayed care seeking. Other reasons are related to gender, age, and living conditions [5–7].

In the health-care organization, reasons for late diagnosis of cancer in general have been related to accessibility, difficulties and complexity in procedures of diagnosis and incorrect referrals [8–12]. Despite its importance, reasons for health-care and doctor's delay in MM have been only sparsely investigated. Earlier studies emphasized difficulties in diagnostics [5, 13], as well as low access to general practitioners (GPs) [14], and gatekeeping [11]. Baade et al. [13] have described the diagnostic process and highlighted the important role of GPs and the emerging role of primary care skin clinics. They also reported that older people from rural areas needed special attention and intervention since both patient delay and health-care delay are prolonged.

TABLE 1: Characteristics of included participants: gender related to age, tumor type, tumor thickness, and initial contact clinic.

| Total | All ($n$ = 71) | Women ($n$ = 38) | Men ($n$ = 33) | $P$-value |
|---|---|---|---|---|
| Age (yrs) | | | | |
|   Median | 60.0 | 56.5 | 63.0 | 0.059[1] |
|   Range | 30–80 | 30–79 | 32–80 | |
|   ≤60 ($n$ (%)) | 38 (53.5%) | 24 (63.2%) | 14 (42.4%) | 0.081[2] |
|   >60 ($n$ (%)) | 33 (46.5%) | 14 (36.8%) | 19 (57.6%) | |
| Tumor type ($n$ (%)) | | | | |
|   In situ | 22 (31.0%) | 18 (47.0%) | 4 (12.0%) | 0.006[2] |
|   SSM | 38 (53.5%) | 15 (40.0%) | 23 (70.0%) | |
|   NM | 11 (15.5%) | 5 (13.0%) | 6 (18.0%) | |
| Tumor thickness (mm) | | | | |
|   Mean (SD) | 1.01 (1.19) | 0.84 (1.26) | 1.21 (1.09) | |
|   Median (range) | 0.75 (0.00–5.90) | 0.25 (0.00–5.90) | 0.90 (0.00–4.10) | 0.023[1] |
|   ≤0.70 ($n$ (%)) | 35 (49.3%) | 23 (60.5%) | 12 (36.4%) | 0.042[2] |
|   >0.70 ($n$ (%)) | 36 (50.7%) | 15 (39.5%) | 21 (63.6%) | |
| Initial contact clinic ($n$ (%)) | | | | |
|   PHCs | 53 (74.6%) | 30 (78.9%) | 23 (69.7%) | 0.372[2] |
|   Derm | 18 (25.4%) | 8 (21.1%) | 10 (30.3%) | |

[1]Mann-Whitney $U$ test. [2]Chi-square test. SSM: superficial spreading melanoma, NM: nodular melanoma, PHCs: primary health-care centres, Derm: dermatological and other specialist clinics.

The need for quality assurance in the health-care system has become generally appreciated. Analysis of clinical pathways and lead times can detect opportunities for improvement. Murchie et al. [14] compared melanoma health-care delay during the diagnostic pathways in the United Kingdom, Sweden, and the Netherlands and found differences in time delay in secondary care between countries, in which Scotland had the highest delay.

Guidelines for treatment of MM [3, 15] are important for patients' clinical pathways to know how to act and, if needed, where to refer patients with suspected MM. Since prognosis is strongly related to tumor thickness [16], timely treatment is essential for optimal outcomes. In some guidelines, time limits for referrals or excision of suspected melanomas are pronounced, where the primary excision of a suspected lesion should be done within two weeks [3, 17]. European consensus declares that the definitive surgical excision should be performed with wide safety margins, preferably within 4–6 weeks after initial diagnosis [3]. Swedish guidelines omit such recommendations [15, 18].

Only a few studies have described pathways and lead times between clinics from initial care seeking to diagnosis and treatment for MM [13, 14, 19]. The aim of this study was to describe and compare patients diagnosed with MM, depending on their initial contact with care, with regard to age, sex, and MM type and thickness, and to explore pathways and lead times between clinics from the initial contact to diagnosis and treatment.

## 2. Materials and Methods

*2.1. Participants.* The melanoma register identified 134 people meeting the inclusion criteria: aged 18–80 years and diagnosed with skin melanoma—superficial spreading melanoma

(SSM), nodular melanoma (NM), or melanoma *in situ*—between January 2008 and December 2010. Less frequent subtypes such as ALM (acral lentiginous melanoma) and LMM (lentigo maligna melanoma) were excluded, since they have a differing biological behaviour.

Completing data about the clinical pathways were collected from the computerized patient records. Deceased people ($n$ = 5), those who had moved to other counties ($n$ = 2), people with documented severe mental illness ($n$ = 1), and those diagnosed with melanoma more than once ($n$ = 3) were excluded. In all, 123 people were asked to participate. Among those, 35 declined, 17 did not respond after two reminders, and 71 (58%) participants gave informed consent and were included in the study. Characteristics of the participants are given in Table 1.

The participants were divided into two groups, depending on where they initially sought care. The first group were patients who were recruited from the public primary health-care centers (PHCs) and the second group from dermatological clinics at hospitals, other hospital specialist clinics, or private skin clinics (Derm). Data were analyzed following the clinical pathways and lead times for each patient as documented in their medical records. The elapsed time between the milestones in the pathway was analyzed and compared between groups of patients, based on age, sex, and MM characteristics.

*2.2. Data Collection.* During the spring of 2011, we collected data from the National Quality Register for Melanoma of the Skin of the northern Swedish region and patients' medical records from the County of Västerbotten in northern Sweden. The data collection consisted of dates for important events (milestones) between clinics and examinations in accordance with the regional guidelines for MM [18]

TABLE 2: (a) Definition of milestones. (b) Mean, median, and range (in days) between milestones in the clinical pathway of melanoma patients seeking care at either PHCs or Derm clinics.

(a)

| Milestones | Event marked by milestone |
|---|---|
| 0 = initial contact | Patient booked the first appointment |
| A = assessment by physician | The first assessment by a physician |
| B = preexcision referral | Referral for primary excision |
| C = primary excision | Primary excision |
| D = histopathological diagnosis I | Result from first histopathological diagnosis |
| E = referral for wide excision | Referral for wide excision |
| F = wide excision | Wide excision surgery |
| G = histopathological diagnosis II | Result from second histopathological diagnosis |
| H = follow-up referral | Referral for follow-up |
| I = follow-up | Follow-up visit |

(b)

| Milestone transition | PHCs (days) | | | Derm (days) | | | $P^*$ | Participants (n) |
|---|---|---|---|---|---|---|---|---|
| | Mean | Median | Range | Mean | Median | Range | | |
| A → B | 11.8 | 0 | 0–98 | 3.0 | 0 | 0–13 | ns | 24 |
| B → C | 41.6 | 35.0 | 13–131 | 19.0 | 20.0 | 5–34 | 0.024 | 24 |
| A → C | 19.9 | 0 | 0–131 | 14.1 | 4.5 | 0–67 | ns | 71 |
| C → D | 16.0 | 13.0 | 1–134 | 7.2 | 6.5 | 1–17 | 0.001 | 71 |
| D → E | 7.2 | 5.0 | 0–28 | 22.1 | 4.0 | 0–121 | ns | 53 |
| E → F | 74.4 | 50.0 | 20–374 | 121.5 | 57.5 | 15–528 | ns | 52 |
| F → G | 13.2 | 12.0 | 0–64 | 9.3 | 8.0 | 1–25 | ns | 65 |
| G → H | 10.6 | 7.0 | 0–60 | 11.9 | 2.0 | 0–63 | ns | 44** |
| H → I | 63.4 | 42.5 | 1–353 | 54.3 | 43.0 | 4–148 | ns | 43** |

*Mann-Whitney U test.
**Seven patients excluded, as referral was sent before registration of histopathology diagnosis II.

(Tables 2(a) and 2(b)). Data regarding tumor thickness, histogenetic subtype of melanoma, registered result from first histopathological diagnosis, and the reporting clinics were collected from the register.

*2.3. Statistical Analysis.* Descriptive statistics were used to describe the background data. In order to explore differences in lead times between patients seeking care at either a PHC or Derm, the pathway was divided into important milestones (Tables 2(a) and 2(b)). The Chi-square test was used for dichotomous data and Mann-Whitney U test for continuous data to compare differences between the groups due to skewness in distribution of data. A P value <0.05 was chosen as the level for significance in all tests. For all analyses, SPSS, ver. 18.0 was used.

*2.4. Ethics.* The study obtained approval from the Regional Ethics Review Board in Umeå (Dnr 2011-88-32). Before sending invitations and reminders to patients, we updated information about deceased persons from the Swedish Population Register, with the intention of sparing the relatives unnecessary distress.

## 3. Results

The results showed that 53 (75%) patients had initially sought care and were primarily treated for suspected MM at PHCs (Table 1). The remaining 18 (25%) patients sought care at other clinics (Derm), that is, the public dermatological hospital clinic, 11 (15.4%); other hospital clinics, 4 (5.6%); and private skin clinics, 3 (4%).

From the physician's assessment to primary excision, 38 (72%) patients were managed within their own clinics in the PHC group compared to 12 (67%) in the Derm group (P = ns). Patients whose lesions had not been excised within their own clinics were referred to surgery clinics for primary excision. In total, 24 patients were referred once, and 7 patients were referred twice before primary excision. Ten percent (n = 7) of all patients underwent a biopsy before the primary excision. After receiving results from the histopathological diagnosis, 36 (95%) patients from the PHC group were referred to surgical clinics for wide excision compared to eight (40%) patients from the Derm group who were referred to another clinic for wide excision. A wide excision, that is, a margin of 5–20 mm, depending on the initial Breslow thickness, was performed on 67 (94%) patients, 87% at surgical clinics (n = 58) and 13% at

TABLE 3: Comparison between primary health-care centers (PHC) and dermatological and other clinic groups (Derm) as related to age, sex, tumor thickness, and type.

| | Total | PHCs | Derm | P-value |
|---|---|---|---|---|
| Age (yrs) | | | | |
|   Median | 60 | 58 | 60.5 | 0.726[1] |
|   ≤60 (n (%)) | 38 (53.5) | 29 (54.7) | 9 (50.0) | 0.729[2] |
| Sex | | | | |
|   Women (n (%)) | 53 (74.6) | 30 (56.6) | 8 (44.4) | 0.372[2] |
|   Men (n (%)) | 18 (25.4) | 23 (43.4) | 10 (56.6) | |
| Tumor thickness (mm) | | | | |
|   Mean/median | 1.01/0.75 | 1.12/0.80 | 0.70/0.37 | 0.140[1] |
|   >0.70 (n (%)) | 36 (50.7) | 29 (54.7) | 7 (38.9) | 0.246[2] |
| Tumor type (n (%)) | | | | |
|   SSM | 38 (53.5) | 28 (52.8) | 10 (55.6) | 0.360[2] |
|   NM | 11 (15.5) | 10 (18.9) | 1 (5.6) | |
|   In situ | 22 (31.0) | 15 (28.3) | 7 (38.9) | |

[1]Mann-Whitney $U$ test. [2]Chi-square test. SSM: superficial spreading melanoma, NM: nodular melanoma, PHCs: primary health-care centers, Derm: dermatological and other clinics.

dermatological clinics ($n = 9$). The remaining patients (6%) were diagnosed within dermatological clinics as having *in situ* MM and were followed up there. Sixty-four patients (91%) were followed up after treatment. Four percent were assessed as not in need of any follow-up. Among those, two participants had *in situ* melanoma, and one had SSM 0.60 mm. For the remaining 5%, information was lacking in the patient records.

The results showed that PHCs primarily treated patients with more severe types of MM (Table 1). Furthermore (not presented in tables), in the PHC group, *in situ* MM was more common among women than among men (86.7% versus 13.3%, $P = 0.020$). There were no significant differences in age or sex between patients of the PHC and Derm groups (Table 3).

The time from first physician's assessment to the preexcision referral was significantly higher and almost doubled in the PHC group compared to the Derm group (35 versus 20 days, $P = 0.024$) (Tables 2(a) and 2(b)).

The range from the physician's assessment to primary excision was wide in both groups (0–131 and 0–67 days, resp.); however, no significant differences between groups were found.

Significant differences in time interval (delay) were found between the PHC and Derm groups from primary excision until registration of the histopathological diagnosis in the medical records. The delay was significantly longer at PHCs (13 versus 6.5 days, $P = 0.001$) (Tables 2(a) and 2(b)).

One result (not presented in tables) showed that people with thicker melanomas (>0.70 mm) waited significantly longer to be referred for follow-up than those with thinner MM (10 versus 0 days, $P = 0.001$). People older than 60 years waited significantly longer from first histopathological diagnosis to wide excision than younger patients (38 versus 28 days, $P = 0.005$) and also from referral for wide excision to wide excision (35 versus 21.5 days, $P = 0.029$).

We found that women waited a shorter time from the first physician's assessment to the primary excision compared to men (0 versus 18 days, $P = 0.052$) and also waited a shorter time from referral for wide excision to wide excision (21 versus 35.5 days, $P = 0.031$). In addition, women had a tendency towards a shorter waiting time from first physician's assessment to follow-up, compared to men (108.5 versus 150 days, $P = 0.059$).

## 4. Discussion

We found differences in health-care pathways and lead times between groups, depending on where people started to seek care. The time from primary excision until the result of the histopathological diagnosis recorded in the medical records was nearly twice as long for those who were seeking care at PHCs as for those who were seeking care at hospital or dermatological clinics. More precisely, it differed by 6.5 days just for registration, which is not optimal among patients with an aggressive cancer such as MM, since the histopathological diagnosis is a crucial moment for a physician to decide upon further treatment [3]. This delay, documented in medical patient records, is consistent with a national report [20] that revealed long waiting times from primary excision until patients received information about the diagnosis. The report presented differences of 4.3 times (in days) between the lowest and the highest median waiting time.

It is difficult to analyze the reasons for this difference, due to the complexity of the administrative health-care system. Our investigation is based on registration dates in patient records. One explanation might be that PHCs professionals are overloaded [21], which could account for a delayed document registration in the medical patient record. The number of patient visits at PHCs has increased 10% during 2005–2009, while specialist care visits only increased by 2%. We also found that the median of time from the first physician's assessment to primary excision was short, independent of initial contact clinic, which is encouraging. However, the ranges within both groups were unfortunately wide (Table 2(b)). Although such results are difficult to interpret, it is important to present them, in order to identify obstacles in the clinical pathways for patients with malignant melanoma, and thereby improve patient safety. Organizational problems during vacation periods, or incorrect referrals or misconceptions between clinics could also contribute to such delay [20].

We also found that patients who sought care at PHCs had more severe and thicker melanoma than patients treated at hospital and dermatological clinics (Table 3). Melanoma, in general and particularly NM, is more common among older people [22], who traditionally more often seek care at PHCs. This may explain why thicker melanoma is more common there. Older patients in our study waited a longer time for wide excision. The National Board of Health and Welfare [20] has recently reported that older people with cancer in general wait longer for appointments with physicians and for care, which we also found. Accessibility, lack of information, and long wait times to diagnosis are common problems within health care, particularly within cancer care [23]. Nurses could preferably act as coordinators to speed up the process of diagnosis and treatment.

Furthermore, we observed that about 10% of all participants underwent biopsies before primary excision, which is not in line with guidelines [3, 15]. This implies that physicians do not suspect some of those lesions as MM, and thereby contribute to a delayed diagnosis [24].

Women's shorter health-care delay regarding primary excision and referral for wide excision to wide excision can be related to their thinner tumors and better prognosis. Since women's care-seeking delay is shorter and they more often detect MM by themselves than men do [5, 7], they may request quicker further treatment. The highest delay in both PHC and Derm groups concerned the time from the referral for wide excision to the wide excision, which in median was 50.0 versus 57.5 days and thereby something that certainly could be improved (Table 2(b)).

## 5. Methodological Discussion

The total local population of all people 18–80 years diagnosed with SSM, NM, and in situ MM during the past 3 years was identified by the melanoma register and invited to participate. The Swedish law requires informed consent for this kind of study. Unfortunately, we were only able to achieve a 58% rate of acceptance. However, the sample concurs with the distribution of melanoma in the area of the study, which indicates a representative sample. Furthermore, a missing-case analysis showed no significant differences between participants and nonparticipants concerning gender (male gender 46.5% versus 42.3%, $P = 0.646$), mean age (57.92 years versus 58.00 years, $P = 0.973$), mean tumor thickness (1.02 mm versus 1.16 mm, $P = 0.602$), or type of melanoma (in situ 31% versus 25%; SSM 53.5% versus 57.3%; NM 15.5% versus 17.3%, $P = 0.766$). However, we cannot totally exclude the possibility that the missing data may affect the results.

The reliability of the documentation of the first contact with the health-care service is a limitation of using data from patients' records. Records show that most patients had their melanomas excised at day one. However, we estimate that many patients had contacted a nurse or physician by telephone to get an appointment time at least 1–7 days before the first visit, sometimes longer. Nevertheless, if not registered in the record, we cannot verify if and/or when such a precontact was made.

## 6. Conclusions

PHCs were, during the period of data collection, the primary contact clinic for MM patients in this region of Northern Sweden. Most MMs are excised rapidly, but for some patients the time for diagnosis and treatment may have been prolonged. Delay from primary excision until registration of the results from histopathological diagnosis within PHCs seems to be an important issue for future improvement. Exploring delay in MM patients' clinical pathways is important for improving the quality of care and patient safety. To reduce total delay of treatment in MM, future studies should focus on the time interval between first discovery of a suspect lesion through final treatment, since patient delay far exceeds health-care delay.

## Conflict of Interests

The authors declare that they have no conflict of interests.

## Authors' Contribution

Senada Hajdarevic, Åsa Hörnsten, Elisabet Sundbom, and Marcus Schmitt-Egenolf carried out study design. Senada Hajdarevic and Åsa Hörnsten collected data. All authors contributed to the paper preparation. Senada Hajdarevic and Ulf Isaksson performed the statistical analysis. All authors read and approved the final paper.

## Acknowledgments

The authors acknowledge with thanks funding provided by the County Council of Västerbotten, the Edvard Welanders and Finsen Foundation, the Cancer Research Foundation in Northern Sweden, the Department of Nursing at Umeå University, and Faculty of Medicine, Umeå University. The authors would also like to thank the Strategic Research Programme in Care Sciences, Umeå University. The authors would especially like to thank the participants for their contribution to the study and Katarina Örnkloo from Regionalt Cancercentrum Norr for help with data collection.

## References

[1] J. Ferlay, H. R. Shin, F. Bray, D. Forman, C. Mathers, and D. M. Parkin, GLOBOCAN 2008 v1.2, Cancer Incidence and Mortality Worldwide: IARC CancerBase No. 10, 2010, http://globocan.iarc.fr/.

[2] Socialstyrelsen [The National Board of Health and Welfare], Cancer Incidence in Sweden 2010, Socialstyrelsen, Stockholm, 2011.

[3] C. Garbe, K. Peris, A. Hauschild et al., "Diagnosis and treatment of melanoma: European consensus-based interdisciplinary guideline," *European Journal of Cancer*, vol. 46, no. 2, pp. 270–283, 2010.

[4] M. S. Ko and M. P. Marinkovich, "Role of dermal-epidermal basement membrane zone in skin, cancer, and developmental disorders," *Dermatologic Clinics*, vol. 28, no. 1, pp. 1–16, 2010.

[5] A. Blum, C. Ingvar, M. Avramidis et al., "Time to diagnosis of melanoma: same trend in different continents," *Journal of Cutaneous Medicine and Surgery*, vol. 11, no. 4, pp. 137–144, 2007.

[6] P. D. Baade, D. R. English, P. H. Youl, M. McPherson, J. M. Elwood, and J. F. Aitken, "The relationship between melanoma thickness and time to diagnosis in a large population-based study," *Archives of Dermatology*, vol. 142, no. 11, pp. 1422–1427, 2006.

[7] J. Baumert, G. Plewig, M. Volkenandt, and M.-H. Schmid-Wendtner, "Factors associated with a high tumour thickness in patients with melanoma," *British Journal of Dermatology*, vol. 156, no. 5, pp. 938–944, 2007.

[8] S. K. Byrne, "Healthcare avoidance: a critical review," *Holistic Nursing Practice*, vol. 22, no. 5, pp. 280–292, 2008.

[9] M. Lövgren, H. Leveälahti, C. Tishelman, S. Runesdotter, K. Hamberg, and H. Koyi, "Time spans from first symptom to treatment in patients with lung cancer - The influence of symptoms and demographic characteristics," *Acta Oncologica*, vol. 47, no. 3, pp. 397–405, 2008.

[10] A. Molassiotis, B. Wilson, L. Brunton, and C. Chandler, "Mapping patients' experiences from initial change in health to cancer diagnosis: a qualitative exploration of patient and system factors mediating this process," *European Journal of Cancer Care*, vol. 19, no. 1, pp. 98–109, 2010.

[11] R. S. Andersen, P. Vedsted, F. Olesen, F. Bro, and J. Søndergaard, "Does the organizational structure of health care systems influence care-seeking decisions? A qualitative analysis of Danish cancer patients' reflections on care-seeking," *Scandinavian Journal of Primary Health Care*, vol. 29, no. 3, pp. 144–149, 2011.

[12] E. Mitchell, S. Macdonald, N. C. Campbell, D. Weller, and U. Macleod, "Influences on pre-hospital delay in the diagnosis of colorectal cancer: a systematic review," *British Journal of Cancer*, vol. 98, no. 1, pp. 60–70, 2008.

[13] P. D. Baade, P. H. Youl, D. R. English, J. M. Elwood, and J. F. Aitken, "Clinical pathways to diagnose melanoma: a population-based study," *Melanoma Research*, vol. 17, no. 4, pp. 243–249, 2007.

[14] P. Murchie, N. C. Campbell, E. K. Delaney et al., "Comparing diagnostic delay in cancer: a cross-sectional study in three european countries with primary care-led health care systems," *Family Practice*, vol. 29, no. 1, Article ID cmr044, pp. 69–78, 2012.

[15] Regionala Cancercentrum i samverkan [Regional Cancer Centres], Malignt melanom-Natioenellt vårdprogram [Malignant melanoma—Swedish national Melanoma Guidelines], 2013, http://www.cancercentrum.se/Global/RCC%20Samverkan/Dokument/V%C3%A5rdprogram/NatVP_Malignt_melanom_130-520_final%5Bl%C3%A5ng%5D.pdf.

[16] A.-V. Giblin and J. M. Thomas, "Incidence, mortality and survival in cutaneous melanoma," *Journal of Plastic, Reconstructive and Aesthetic Surgery*, vol. 60, no. 1, pp. 32–40, 2007.

[17] J. R. Marsden, J. A. Newton-Bishop, L. Burrows et al., "Revised UK guidelines for the management of cutaneous melanoma 2010," *Journal of Plastic, Reconstructive and Aesthetic Surgery*, vol. 63, no. 9, pp. 1401–1419, 2010.

[18] Regionalt Cancercentrum Norr[Regional Cancer Centre North], Malignt melanom—Vårdprogram Norra regionen [Malignant melanoma—treatment guidelines, Northren region], 2011, http://www.vinkcancer.se/Global/OCNorra/RCC%20dokument/v%c3%a5rdprogram/melanom_regionalt%20vp_2011.pdf.

[19] P. Murchie, "Treatment delay in cutaneous malignant melanoma: from first contact to definitive treatment," *Quality in Primary Care*, vol. 15, no. 6, pp. 345–351, 2007.

[20] Socialstyrelsen [The National Board of Health and Welfare], Väntetider inom cancervården—från remiss till behandlingsstart [Waiting times for cancer—from referral to start of treatment], Socialstyrelsen, Stockholm, Sweden, pp 1-81, 2011.

[21] Socialstyrelsen [The National Board of Health and Welfare], Lägesrapport 2011, hälso- och sjukvård och socialtjänst [Progress report 2011, health-care and social services], Socialstyrelsen, Stockholm. pp. 1-183, 2011.

[22] A. C. Geller, M. Elwood, S. M. Swetter et al., "Factors related to the presentation of thin and thick nodular melanoma from a population-based cancer registry in queensland australia," *Cancer*, vol. 115, no. 6, pp. 1318–1327, 2009.

[23] E. H. Wagner, E. J. A. Bowles, S. M. Greene et al., "The quality of cancer patient experience: perspectives of patients, family members, providers and experts," *Quality and Safety in Health Care*, vol. 19, no. 6, pp. 484–489, 2010.

[24] T. J. Matzke, A. K. Bean, and T. Ackerman, "Avoiding delayed diagnosis of malignant melanoma," *Journal for Nurse Practitioners*, vol. 5, no. 1, pp. 42–46, 2009.

# Permissions

The contributors of this book come from diverse backgrounds, making this book a truly international effort. This book will bring forth new frontiers with its revolutionizing research information and detailed analysis of the nascent developments around the world.

We would like to thank all the contributing authors for lending their expertise to make the book truly unique. They have played a crucial role in the development of this book. Without their invaluable contributions this book wouldn't have been possible. They have made vital efforts to compile up to date information on the varied aspects of this subject to make this book a valuable addition to the collection of many professionals and students.

This book was conceptualized with the vision of imparting up-to-date information and advanced data in this field. To ensure the same, a matchless editorial board was set up. Every individual on the board went through rigorous rounds of assessment to prove their worth. After which they invested a large part of their time researching and compiling the most relevant data for our readers.

The editorial board has been involved in producing this book since its inception. They have spent rigorous hours researching and exploring the diverse topics which have resulted in the successful publishing of this book. They have passed on their knowledge of decades through this book. To expedite this challenging task, the publisher supported the team at every step. A small team of assistant editors was also appointed to further simplify the editing procedure and attain best results for the readers.

Apart from the editorial board, the designing team has also invested a significant amount of their time in understanding the subject and creating the most relevant covers. They scrutinized every image to scout for the most suitable representation of the subject and create an appropriate cover for the book.

The publishing team has been an ardent support to the editorial, designing and production team. Their endless efforts to recruit the best for this project, has resulted in the accomplishment of this book. They are a veteran in the field of academics and their pool of knowledge is as vast as their experience in printing. Their expertise and guidance has proved useful at every step. Their uncompromising quality standards have made this book an exceptional effort. Their encouragement from time to time has been an inspiration for everyone.

The publisher and the editorial board hope that this book will prove to be a valuable piece of knowledge for researchers, students, practitioners and scholars across the globe.

# List of Contributors

**Megan J. Schlichte and Rajani Katta**
Baylor College of Medicine, Houston, TX 77030, USA

**Wanjarus Roongpisuthipong**
Division of Dermatology, Department of Medicine Vajira Hospital, Navamindradhiraj University, Bangkok 10300, Thailand

**Sirikarn Prompongsa**
Research Center, Navamindradhiraj University, Bangkok 10300, Thailand

**Theerawut Klangjareonchai**
Department of Medicine, Faculty of Medicine, Ramathibodi Hospital, Mahidol University, Bangkok 10400, Thailand

**S. Kaur**
Clinic of Dermatology, University of Tartu, 31 Raja Street, 50417 Tartu, Estonia

**K. Zilmer and M. Zilmer**
Institute of Biomedicine and Translational Medicine, Department of Biochemistry, the Centre of Excellence for Translational Medicine, University of Tartu, 19 Ravila Street, 50411 Tartu, Estonia

**V. Leping**
Institute of Computer Science, University of Tartu, 2 J. Liivi Street, 50409 Tartu, Estonia

**Yasemin Oram and A. Deniz Akkaya**
Department of Dermatology, V.K. Foundation American Hospital of Istanbul, Turkey

**Pramod Kumar**
Dermatology Department, KMC Hospital, Manipal University, Attavar, Mangalore 575 001, India

**Rekha Paulose**
Ahalia Hospital, P.O. Box 2419, Abu Dhabi, UAE

**Sanjiv Jain**
Skin Care Clinic, 108 Darya Ganj, New Delhi 110002, India

**Mingwei Joel Ye**
Department of Dermatology, Western Hospital, Footscray, VIC 3011, Australia
Department of Medicine, Dentistry and Health Sciences, University of Melbourne, Parkville, VIC 3010, Australia

**Joshua Mingsheng Ye**
Department of Medicine, Dentistry and Health Sciences, University of Melbourne, Parkville, VIC 3010, Australia

**José Maria Pereira de Godoy**
Cardiology and Cardiovascular Surgery Department, Medicine School in São José do Rio Preto (FAMERP), Avenida Constituição 1306, 15025-120 São José do Rio Preto, SP, Brazil

**Renata Lopes Pinto**
Research Group Godoy Clinic, São José do Rio Preto, Brazil

**Ana Carolina Pereira de Godoy**
Research Group Godoy Clinic, São José do Rio Preto, Brazil
Medicine School of ABC, São Paulo, Brazil

**Maria de Fátima Guerreiro Godoy**
Research Group Godoy Clinic, São José do Rio Preto, Brazil
Medicine School in São José do Rio Preto (FAMERP), São José do Rio Preto, Brazil
Post-Graduate Specialization Course on Lymphovenous Rehabilitation (FAMERP), São José do Rio Preto, Brazil

**Narges Alizadeh, Hamed Monadi Nori, Javad Golchi, Shahriar S. Eshkevari and Abbas Darjani**
Department of Dermatology, Razi Hospital, Guilan University of Medical Sciences, Rasht 41448, Iran

**Ehsan Kazemnejad**
Department of Preventive and Community Medicine, Guilan University of Medical Sciences, Rasht, Iran

**Farzam Gorouhi and Nasim Fazel**
Department of Dermatology, University of California, Davis, 3301 C Street, Sacramento, CA 95816, USA

**Ali Alikhan**
Department of Dermatology, Mayo Clinic, Rochester, MN, USA

**Arash Rezaei**
Department of Civil & Environmental Engineering, University of California, Davis, USA

**Christopher D. Roche and Joelle S. Dobson**
St George's, University of London, Cranmer Terrace, London SW17 0RE, UK

**Sion K. Williams**
The National Hospital for Neurology, 23 Queen Square, LondonWC1N 3BG, UK

**Mara Quante**
Department of Histopathology, Royal Sussex County Hospital, Eastern Road, Brighton BN2 5BE, UK

**Joyce Popoola**
Department of Renal Medicine and Transplantation, St George's Healthcare NHS Trust, Blackshaw Road, London SW17 0QT, UK

**Jade W. M. Chow**
St George's, University of London, Cranmer Terrace, London SW17 0RE, UK
International Medical University, Jalan Jalil Perkasa 19, 57000 Kuala Lumpur, Malaysia

**Aimen Ismail**
School of Medicine, University of Alabama at Birmingham, Birmingham, AL 35294, USA

**Nabiha Yusuf**
Department of Dermatology, University of Alabama at Birmingham, VH 566A, 1670 University Boulevard, Birmingham, AL 35294, USA

**Ladan Dastgheib, Ahmad Adnan Abdorazagh and Maryam Sadat Sadati**
Molecular Dermatology Research Center, Dermatology Department, Shiraz University of Medical Sciences, Shiraz, Iran

**Zohreh Mostafavi-pour**
Maternal-Fetal Medicine Research Center, Hafez Hospital, Shiraz University of Medical Sciences, Shiraz, Iran

**Zahra Khoshdel**
Recombinant Protein Laboratory, Department of Biochemistry, Shiraz University of Medical Sciences, Shiraz, Iran

**Iman Ahrari**
Student Research Committee, Shiraz University of Medical Sciences, Shiraz, Iran

**Sajjad Ahrari**
Department of Biology, Shiraz University, Shiraz, Iran

**Mahsa Ghavipisheh**
Student Research Committee, Fasa University of Medical Sciences, Fasa, Iran

**Dan Yi, Ji Bihl, Mackenzie S. Newman and Yanfang Chen**
Department of Pharmacology and Toxicology, Boonshoft School of Medicine, Wright State University, 3640 Colonel Glenn Hwy, Dayton, OH 45435, USA

**Richard Simman**
Department of Pharmacology and Toxicology, Boonshoft School of Medicine, Wright State University, 3640 Colonel Glenn Hwy, Dayton, OH 45435, USA
Department of Plastic and Reconstructive Surgery, Boonshoft School of Medicine, Wright State University, 3640 Colonel Glenn Hwy, Dayton, OH 45435, USA

**Olaide Olutoyin Oke**
Dermatology Unit, Department of Internal Medicine, Federal Medical Centre, Abeokuta 110222, Nigeria

**Olaniyi Onayemi, Olayinka Abimbola Olasode and Olumayowa Abimbola Oninla**
Department of Dermatology & Venereology, Obafemi Awolowo University, Ile-Ife, Nigeria

**Akinlolu Gabriel Omisore**
Department of Community Medicine, Osun State University, Osogbo, Nigeria

**Haydar Ucak and Mustafa Arica**
Department of Dermatology, Faculty of Medicine, Dicle University, 21070 Diyarbakir, Turkey

**Betul Demir, Demet Cicek and Selma Bakar Dertlioglu**
Department of Dermatology, Faculty of Medicine, Firat University, Elazig, Turkey

**Ilker Erden**
Department of Dermatology, Elazig Training and Research Hospital, Elazig, Turkey

**Suleyman Aydin**
Department of Biochemistry, Faculty of Medicine, Firat University, Elazig, Turkey

**Amir Hossein Siadat, Naser Zeinali, Fariba Iraji, Kioumars Jamshidi and Parastoo Khosravani**
Department of Dermatology, Skin Diseases and Leishmaniasis Research Center, Isfahan University of Medical Sciences, Isfahan, Iran

**Bahareh Abtahi-Naeini**
Department of Dermatology, Skin Diseases and Leishmaniasis Research Center, Students' Research Committee, Isfahan University of Medical Sciences, Isfahan, Iran

**Mohammad Ali Nilforoushzadeh**
Skin and Stem Cell Research Center, Tehran University of Medical Sciences, Tehran, Iran

**Jill Henley**
College of Osteopathic Medicine Glendale, Midwestern University, 13989 N59th Avenue, Glendale, AZ 85308, USA

**Jerry D. Brewer**
Division of Dermatologic Surgery, Department of Dermatology Mayo Clinic, Mayo Clinic College of Medicine Rochester, 200 First Street SW, Rochester, MN 55905, USA

**Sumeet Reddy, Falah El-Haddawi, Michael Fancourt, Glenn Farrant, William Gilkison, Nigel Henderson, Stephen Kyle and Damien Mosquera**
Department of General Surgery, Taranaki Base Hospital, Private Bag 2016, New Plymouth 4342, New Zealand

**Vikram K. Mahajan**
Department of Dermatology, Venereology & Leprosy, Dr. R. P. Govt. Medical College, Kangra, Tanda, Himachal Pradesh 176001, India

**K. Chanprapaph, V. Vachiramon and P. Rattanakaemakorn**
Division of Dermatology, Faculty of Medicine Ramathibodi Hospital, Mahidol University, 270 Rama VI Road, Rajthevi, Bangkok 10400, Thailand

**Mrinal Gupta, Vikram K. Mahajan, Karaninder S.Mehta and Pushpinder S. Chauhan**
Department of Dermatology, Venereology & Leprosy, Dr. R. P. Govt. Medical College, Kangra (Tanda), Himachal Pradesh 176001, India

**Sangaré Abdoulaye, Kourouma Sarah Hamdan, Kouassi Yao Isidore, Ecra Elidjé Joseph, Kaloga Mamadou and Gbery Ildevert Patrice**
Department of Dermatology of the University Teaching Hospital of Treichville, Riviera, BP 408 Cidex 03 Abidjan, Cote d'Ivoire

**Mansooreh Bagheri, Mandana Bagheri and Mohammadreza Talebnejad**
Poostchi Ophthalmology Research Center, Shiraz University of Medical Sciences, Shiraz, Iran

**Masoomeh Eghtedari**
Ophthalmology Department, Shiraz University of Medical Sciences, Shiraz, Iran

**Bita Geramizadeh**
Pathology Department, Liver Transplant Research Center, Shiraz University of Medical Sciences, Shiraz, Iran

**Chrysovalantis Korfitis**
Department of Dermatology, Veterans Administration Hospital, 10-12 Monis Petraki Street, 11521 Athens, Greece

**Stamatis Gregoriou and Dimitris Rigopoulos**
Department of Dermatology, Attikon Hospital, 1 Rimini Street, Haidari, 12462 Athens, Greece

**Christina Antoniou and Andreas D. Katsambas**
Department of Dermatology, Andreas Sygros Hospital, 5 I. Dragoumi Street, 16121 Athens, Greece

**Federica Dassoni**
Ayder Referral Hospital, Mekelle, Ethiopia
INMP Istituto Nazionale per la Promozione della Salute delle Popolazioni Migranti ed il Contrasto delle Malattie della Povertà, Via di San Gallicano 25, 00153 Roma, Italy
Unità Operativa di Dermatologia, Università di Milano, I.R.C.C.S. Fondazione Ca' Granda Ospedale Maggiore Policlinico, 20122 Milano, Italy

**Zerihun Abebe**
Ayder Referral Hospital, Mekelle, Ethiopia

**Federica Ricceri**
Dipartimento di Chirurgia e Medicina Traslazionale, Sezione di Dermatologia, Università degli Studi di Firenze, Viale Michelangelo 41, 50125 Firenze, Italy

**Aldo Morrone**
Ospedale S. Camillo Forlanini, Piazza Carlo Forlanini 1, 00151 Rome, Italy

**Cristiana Albertin**
Dipartimento di Dermatologia, Università di Padova, Via Mocenigo 8, 35127 Padova, Italy

**Bernard Naafs**
Stichting Tropen Dermatologie, Gracht 15, 8485KN15 Munnekeburen Friesland, The Netherlands

**Basheir A. Hassan**
Pediatrics Department, Faculty of Medicine, Zagazig University, Zagazig 44519, Egypt

**Khalid S. Shreef**
Surgery Department, Faculty of Medicine, Zagazig University, Zagazig 44519, Egypt

**Zornitsa Kamenarska, Gyulnas Dzhebir, Radka Kaneva and Vanio Mitev**
Molecular Medicine Center and Department of Medical Chemistry and Biochemistry, Medical University-Sofia, 2 Zdrave Street, 1431 Sofia, Bulgaria

**Maria Hristova**
Department of Clinical Laboratory and Clinical Immunology and Department of Nephrology, Medical University-Sofia, 1 Georgi Sofijski Street, 1431 Sofia, Bulgaria

**Alexey Savov**
National Genetic Laboratory, Maichin Dom Hospital, 2 Zdrave Street, 1431 Sofia, Bulgaria

**Anton Vinkov**
28 Diagnostic and Consultative Center-Sofia, 1 Iliya Beshkov Street, 1592 Sofia, Bulgaria

**Lyubomir Dourmishev**
Department of Dermatology and Venereology, Medical University-Sofia, 1 Georgi Sofijski Street, 1431 Sofia, Bulgaria

**Ali Ebrahimi, Reza Kavoussi, Mojtaba Eidizadeh and Seyed Hamid Madani**
Kermanshah University of Medical Sciences (KUMS), Kermanshah, Iran

**Mansour Rezaei**
Health School, Family Health Research Center of Kermanshah University of Medical Sciences (KUMS), Kermanshah, Iran

**Hossein Kavoussi**
Kermanshah University of Medical Sciences (KUMS), Kermanshah, Iran
Hajdaie Dermatology Clinic, Golestan Ave, Kermanshah 6714653113, Iran

**Abd-Elaziz El-Taweel, Fatma El-Esawy and Osama Abdel-Salam**
Dermatology & Andrology Department, Faculty of Medicine, Benha University, Benha, Al Qalyubia 13512, Egypt

**Jeannette Olazagasti**
School of Medicine, University of Puerto Rico, San Juan, PR 00936, USA
University of California, Davis, Sacramento, CA 95816, USA

**Farzam Gorouhi**
University of California, Davis, Sacramento, CA 95816, USA

**Nasim Fazel**
University of California, Davis, Sacramento, CA 95816, USA
Department of Dermatology, University of California, Davis School of Medicine, 3301 C Street, Suite 1400, Sacramento, CA 95816, USA

**Naveen Kumar and Satheesha Nayak Badagabettu**
Department of Anatomy, Melaka Manipal Medical College, Manipal University, Manipal Campus, Manipal, India

**Pramod Kumar**
Consultant Plastic Surgeon, King Abdulaziz Hospital, Al Jouf, Saudi Arabia

**Keerthana Prasad**
Department of Information Science, Manipal School of Information Science, Manipal University, Manipal, India

**Ranjini Kudva**
Department of Pathology, Kasturba Medical College, Manipal University, Manipal, India

**Coimbatore Vasudevarao Raghuveer**
Department of Pathology, Yenepoya University, Deralakatte, Mangalore, India

**Pratik Gahalaut, Nitin Mishra, Puneet S. Soodan and Madhur K. Rastogi**
Department of Dermatology, Shri Ram Murti Smarak Institute of Medical Sciences, Bareilly 243202, India

**Neel Prabha, Vikram K. Mahajan, Karaninder S. Mehta, Pushpinder S. Chauhan and Mrinal Gupta**
Department of Dermatology, Venereology & Leprosy, Dr. R. P. Govt. Medical College, Kangra, Tanda, Himachal Pradesh 176001, India

**Sujoy Khan**
Consultant Allergist & Immunologist, Department of Allergy & Immunology, Apollo Gleneagles Hospital, 58 Canal Circular Road, Kolkata, West Bengal 700 054, India

**Anirban Maitra**
Department of Paediatric Pulmonology, Vision Care Hospital, Mukundapur, Kolkata West Bengal 700099, India

**Pravin Hissaria**
Department of Allergy, Immunology and Arthritis, Apollo Hospitals International Ltd., Bhat GIDC, Gandhinagar, Ahmedabad, Gujarat 382428, India

**Sitesh Roy**
Dr. Niphadkar's Asthma and Allergy Health Clinic, Hindu Colony Lane No. 1, Dadar (East), Mumbai 400 014, India

**Mahesh Padukudru Anand**
Department of Pulmonary Medicine, JSS Medical College, JSS University, Mysore, Karnataka 570 004, India

**Nalin Nag**
Department of Medicine, Indraprastha Apollo Hospital, Mathura Road, Jasola Vihar, New Delhi 110076, India

**Harpal Singh**
Clinical Marketing Manager, Phadia/IDD, Thermo Fisher Scientific, Units No. 7, 10 & 11, Splendor Forum, Plot No. 3, Disttrict Centre, Jasola, New Delhi 110025, India

**Senada Hajdarevic, Åsa Hörnsten and Ulf Isaksson**
Department of Nursing, Umeå University, Umeå, Sweden

**Elisabet Sundbom**
Department of Clinical Sciences, Division of Psychiatry and Medical Psychology, Umeå University, Umeå, Sweden

**Marcus Schmitt-Egenolf**
Department of Public Health and Clinical Medicine, Dermatology and Venereology, Umeå University, Umeå, Sweden

www.ingramcontent.com/pod-product-compliance
Lightning Source LLC
Chambersburg PA
CBHW080503200326
41458CB00012B/4070